PRINCIPLES OF HEALTH

Obesity

PRINCIPLES OF HEALTH

Obesity

Editor
Dawn Rutherford, MS, RDN

SALEM PRESS
A Division of EBSCO Information Services, Inc.
Ipswich, Massachusetts

GREY HOUSE PUBLISHING

Publisher's Cataloging-In-Publication Data
(Prepared by The Donohue Group, Inc.)

Names: Rutherford, Dawn, editor.
Title: Principles of health. Obesity / editor, Dawn Rutherford, MS, RDN.
Other Titles: Obesity
Description: [First edition]. | Ipswich, Massachusetts : Salem Press, a division of EBSCO Information Services, Inc. ; Amenia, NY : Grey House Publishing, [2020] | Includes bibliographical references and index.
Identifiers: ISBN 9781642653854
Subjects: LCSH: Obesity.
Classification: LCC RC628 .P756 2020 | DDC 616.398—dc23

First Printing
PRINTED IN THE UNITED STATES OF AMERICA

Table of Contents

Publisher's Note

Principles of Health: Obesity is the second title in the new *Principles of Health* series by Salem Press. This series is joining the current *Principles of* line that includes *Principles of Science, Principles of Business,* and *Principles of Sociology. Pain Management,* the first *Principles of Health* volume, was published last year.

Covering important topics in the fields of obesity, nutrition and weight management using easy-to-understand language, *Principles of Health: Obesity* is designed to provide a solid background and understanding of obesity, its causes, and treatment options.

Following a detailed Editor's Introduction by Dawn Rutherford, MS, RDN, the 140 entries in this work are arranged in the following seven broad categories:

Causes and Risk Factors include genetic, environmental, and pathological factors that may contribute to obesity and being overweight.

Related Conditions, Diseases, and Comorbidities describe conditions that often co-exist with being overweight, or that may develop as a result of obesity. It also deals with the types of cancer that are associated with obesity, including esophageal, pancreatic, and liver cancers.

Treatment and Weight Management discusses different avenues through which obesity can be managed, including general nutritional guidelines, targeted weight-lose diets, and healthy lifestyle practices.

Conditions In Depth details several conditions and diseases that are often associated with obesity, including sleep apnea, type 2 diabetes, and coronary artery disease.

All entries include Category and References, and most include Key Terms. Many images and photographs throughout the volume illustrate concepts and treatments.

This work includes helpful appendixes, including:
- Bibliography;
- Organizations;
- Category Index;
- Subject Index.

Salem Press extends appreciation to all involved in the development and production of this work. Names and affiliations of contributors follow the Editor's Introduction.

Principles of Health: Obesity, as well as all Salem Press reference books, is available in print and as an e-book. Please visit www.salempress.com for more information.

Editor's Introduction

According to the Centers for Disease Control (CDC), approximately 42.4% of American adults were obese in 2018. This number increased by 10% from the previous decade. If this trend continues, over half of Americans will be obese by 2030. Obesity is defined by a body mass index (BMI) over 30 kg/m2, calculated by height and weight. Although obesity itself is physical, its cause is almost always a combination of genetic, biological, environmental and psychological factors. Physiological conditions that predispose people to obesity are hormonal imbalances, genetics, inflammation and slowed metabolic processes. Psychological factors, including depression, eating disorders, sleep deprivation, anxiety and stress may increase one's risk for obesity. Obese individuals often feel hopeless to reverse the condition. Awareness of the multifaceted issues resulting in obesity is crucial in preventing and treating this epidemic facing our country.

Genetics and Obesity

Obesity usually develops over time from a combination of biological risk factors that can be identified at a young age. Some people are predisposed to gaining weight based on epigenetics (gene expression) which plays a role in the size, number and regional distribution of fat cells in the body. Genes also determine an individual's resting metabolic rate. There is a theory (set point theory) that says the body's metabolism will slow down or speed up to maintain a certain predisposed weight.

Hormonal Causes of Obesity

In addition to genetics, hormones also play a major role in obesity. The hormone insulin is secreted by the pancreas when blood sugar levels rise after eating, which stimulates glucose which lowers blood sugar levels and tells the brain that the body is full. If a person becomes resistant to insulin, blood sugar levels remain high, no glucose is produced and the brain doesn't get the signal to stop eating. A lack of the hormone adiponectin may also contribute to obesity; it's made by fat cells to help improve insulin function. Leptin is a hormone produced by fat cells which senses energy stores and signals to the brain to decrease food intake, and low leptin levels may result in weight gain. The "hunger hormone" ghrelin increases appetite. Its levels typically decrease after eating but if this doesn't happen, weight gain can result.

Obesity and Low Income Individuals

Low income individuals are often forced to buy less expensive foods that are high in fat, sugar and sodium and low in healthy nutrients. Fast food restaurants often offer unhealthy menu items that are cheap and convenient. Since low-income neighborhoods are often where you'll find a large number of fast food chains and convenience stores, many folks who want to eat healthy do not have the physical access or financial means to healthier food choices. Therefore, millions of Americans are considered to be food insecure, which means they lack reliable access to a sufficient quantity of affordable, nutritious food. An obese individual may be suffering from malnutrition even though they appear to be well-nourished!

Psychosocial Causes of Obesity

Emotional Eating

People suffering from psychological issues, such as depression and anxiety, have a greater tendency to lose control of their eating patterns, and often lack the motivation to exercise regularly. Emotional eating – using food as a coping mechanism when they feel sad, lonely, angry or anxious – often results in people not understanding why they are gaining weight since they feel disconnected and distracted during the eating process. Eating under distress results in a vicious cycle – feeling guilty for overeating, but continuing for the short term pleasure. A genetic predisposition for weight gain and slowed metabolism, along with an environment lacking healthy food choices may create the perfect storm for obesity.

Eating Disorders

Eating disorders can be defined as food deprivation diseases such as anorexia nervosa and bulimia, as well as eating excessive amounts of food. Binge

Eating Disorder (BED), or 'mindless eating' occurs when people overeat at meals, engage in frequent snacking on high calorie foods or secretly eat at night. BED is characterized by episodes of over-eating at least 2 days a week over a 6 month period; eating quantities of food larger than typical portions; lack of control during these eating episodes; and guilt or distress following overeating. One major difference between BED and other eating disorders is that BED is not associated with any behavior that compensates for overeating. Anorexia and bulimia, for example, are often accompanied by fasting, purging or excessive exercise. Therefore, people suffering from BED become overweight and obese.

Psychosocial Impact of Obesity

American society is obsessed with the perfect body. Cultural messaging such as "thin is in" is not only extremely disheartening for an overweight individual, but dangerous to their health. Obese individuals are extremely aware of societal attitudes which result in feelings of shame and humiliation. A viscous cycle occurs – people are overweight because they overeat and then overeat because they are overweight. Obese individuals may refrain from social gatherings for fear of being judged, resulting in psychosocial isolation. A lack of nurturing from friends and family increase an individual's risk for depression, anxiety and loneliness.

Treatment for Obesity

One way to combat obesity is balancing energy intake with physical activity. Diet pills are not an easy solution. A lifestyle adjustment is mandatory to losing weight and maintaining that weight loss. Obesity prevention occurs when people listen to hunger and satiety cues within their own bodies. A registered dietitian nutritionist can be incredibly helpful in developing an appropriate, customized meal plan that is well-balanced and nutritious. An exercise physiologist can help customize an attainable exercise regime that fits specific needs and tastes. And a psychologist may help an individual overcome feelings of depression and hopelessness. Healthy mental health is important for healthy physical health.

Finally, it is my honor to have developed a work dedicated to understanding obesity. As a practicing clinical registered dietitian nutritionist, I treat and educate patients on managing conditions that often involve obesity. Dietary choices play a significant role in the challenges faced by individuals combating obesity. My goal is that this work will help alleviate misconceptions and increase understanding of the complex issues surrounding this disease. If you or a loved one is suffering from obesity related problems, please contact a registered dietitian nutritionist as a reliable counselor for how to receive adequate nutrition based on individual needs. I hope you find the following information interesting and valuable. Remember, you are what you eat, so practice moderation, eat well and enjoy!

Dawn Rutherford, MS, RDN

Sources for Further Study

Carr D, Friedman MA. (2005). Is obesity stigmatizing? Body weight, perceived discrimination, and psychological well-being in the United States. *Journal of Health and Social Behavior*, 46(3), 244-259. A comparative article, demonstrating the difference in interpersonal treatment of obese versus normal weight individuals.

Greenberg I., Perna F., Kaplan M., & Sullivan M. (2005). Behavioral and psychological factors in the assessment and treatment of obesity surgery patients. *Obesity Research*, 13(2), 244-249. Evidence-based guidelines influencing the screening for weight loss surgery candidates and the psychological impact post-surgery.

Swencionis C., & Rendell S. (2012). The psychology of obesity. Abdominal Imaging, 37(5), 733-737. DOI: 10.1007/s00261-012-9863-9. This article discusses obesity as a public health issue and suggests the importance of an interdisciplinary team to effectively change obesity related dysfunctional behaviors. It is implied that a collaborative approach with the additional use of mobile health technology can help combat the obesity epidemic.

Stunkard A., Grace W., & Wolff H. (1955). The night-eating syndrome: A pattern of food intake among certain obese patients. *American Journal of Medicine*, 19, 78-86. This handbook suggests that there are many physiological, as well as psychological factors which result in night-eating syndrome. It is a complex issues with many etiologies and side effects.

List of Contributors

Richard Adler, PhD
University of Michigan-Dearborn

Saeed Akhter, MD
Texas Technological University

Ananya Anand, MSc
Brown University

John J. B. Anderson, PhD
University of North Carolina, Chapel Hill

Bryan C. Auday, PhD
Gordon College

Veronica N. Baptista, MD
Stanford Medical Group

John A. Bavaro, EdD, RN
Slippery Rock University

Paul F. Bell, PhD
Heritage Valley Health System

Alvin K. Benson, PhD
Utah Valley State College

Matthew Berria, PhD
Weber State University

Silvia M. Berry, MSc, RVT,
Englewood Hospital and Medical Center, New Jersey

Tyler Biscontini
Independent Scholar

Robert W. Block, MD
University of Oklahoma

Paul R. Boehlke, PhD
Wisconsin Lutheran College

Michael A. Buratovich, PhD
Spring Arbor University

Gilberto Cabrera, MD
Independent Scholar

Lauren M. Cagen, PhD
University of Tennessee, Memphis

Byron D. Cannon, PhD
University of Utah

Carita Caple, RN, BSN, MSHS
Cinahl Information Systems

Richard P. Capriccioso, MD
University of Phoenix

Kim Carmichael, MD
EBSCO Information Services

Rosalyn Carson-DeWitt, MD
Independent Scholar

Donatella M. Casirola, PhD
New Jersey Medical School

Anne Lynn S. Chang, MD
Stanford University

Karen Chapman-Novakofski, RD, LDN, PhD
University of Illinois

Paul J. Chara Jr., PhD
Northwestern College

Kerry L. Cheesman, PhD
Capital University

Francis P. Chinard, MD
New Jersey Medical School

Leland J. Chinn, PhD
Biola University

James P. Cornell, MD
EBSCO Information Services

Arlene R. Courtney, PhD
Western Oregon State College

Tish Davidson, MA
Independent Scholar

LeAnna DeAngelo, PhD
Arizona State University

Patricia Stanfill Edens, PhD, RN, LFACHE
Independent Scholar

C. Richard Falcon
Roberts and Raymond Associates, Philadelphia

L. Fleming Fallon Jr., MD, PhD, MPH
Bowling Green State University

Elizabeth Farrington, AGPCNP-BC
Yale University

Marisela Fermin-Schon, RN
Yale University

K. Thomas Finley, PhD
State University of New York, Brockport

Michael J. Fucci, DO, FACC
EBSCO Information Services

Lenela Glass-Godwin, MWS
Texas A&M University

Angela Harmon
Independent Scholar

Dianne Haskins, RN, BSN
Independent Scholar

David Wason Hollar Jr., PhD
Rockingham Community College

Shih-Wen Huang, MD
University of Florida

Mary Hurd
East Tennessee State University

Albert C. Jensen, MS
Central Florida Community College

Roushig Grace Kalebjian, MA, RN
Yale University

Karen E. Kalumuck, PhD
The Exploratorium, San Francisco

Hillar Klandorf, PhD
West Virginia University

Jeffrey A. Knight, PhD
Mount Holyoke College

Marylane Wade Koch, MSN, RN
Independent Scholar

Bill Kte'pi, MA
Independent Scholar

Victor R. Lavis, MD
University of Texas, Houston

Nancy E. Macdonald, PhD
University of South Carolina, Sumter

Laura Gray Malloy, PhD
Bates College

Cherie Marcel, BS
Cinahl Information Systems

Bonita L. Marks
University of North Carolina at Chapel Hill

Geraldine Marrocco, EdD, APRN, CNS, ANP-BC
Yale University

Charles C. Marsh, PharmD
University of Arkansas for Medical Sciences

Jeffrey A. McGowan
West Virginia University

Trudy Mercadal, MA, PhD
EBSCO Information Services

Christen Miller, RD, LDE
Cinahl Information Systems

Roman J. Miller, PhD
Eastern Mennonite College

Paul Moglia, PhD
Mount Sinai South Nassau

Rodney C. Mowbray, PhD
University of Wisconsin, LaCrosse

Kathleen O'Boyle
Wayne State University

Cherie Oertel
University of Kansas

Kristin S. Ondrak, PhD
University of North Carolina at Chapel Hill

Daniel A. Ostrovsky, MD
EBSCO Information Services

Oliver Oyama, PhD
Duke/Fayetteville Area Health Education Center

Robert J. Paradowski
Rochester Institute of Technology

Cheryl Pawlowski, PhD
University of Northern Colorado

Nancy A. Piotrowski, PhD
Capella University

Lori Porter, RD, MBA
Ball State University

Victoria Price, PhD
Lamar University

Douglas Reinhart, MD
University of Utah

Andrew Ren, MD
Kaiser Permanente Los Angeles Medical Center

Sara Richards, MSN, RN
Cinahl Information Systems

Alice C. Richer, RD, MBA, LD
Independent Scholar

John L. Rittenhouse
Eastern Mennonite College

Connie Rizzo, MD, PhD
Columbia University

Michael Ruth
Independent Scholar

Lauren Ruvo
Harvard Graduate School of Education

Tulsi B. Saral, PhD
University of Houston, Clear Lake

Zachary Sax, DPM
Mount Sinai South Nassau

Tanja Schub, BS
EBSCO Information Services

R. Baird Shuman, PhD
University of Illinois, Urbana-Champaign

Marcie L. Sidman, MD
EBSCO Information Services

Sanford S. Singer, PhD
University of Dayton

Caroline M. Small
Independent Scholar

Nathalie Smith, RN, MSN, CNP
Aspen Medical Communications

Claire L. Standen, PhD
University of Massachusetts Medical School

Sharon W. Stark, RN, APRN, DNSc
Monmouth University

Sue Tarjan
Independent Scholar

Alyssa Tedder-King
University of Kansas

Bethany Thivierge
Technicality Resources

Janine Ungvarsky
Independent Scholar

Eugenia M. Valentine, PhD
Independent Scholar

Charles Vigue, PhD
University of New Haven

Bradley R.A. Wilson, PhD
University of Cincinnati

Michael Woods, MD, FAAP
EBSCO Information Services

Rachel Zahn, MD
Independent Scholar

Causes and Risk Factors

■ Adipose tissue

CATEGORY: Biology

Adipose tissue is the anatomical name for body fat found in humans and other mammals. Adipose tissue is composed of a loose collection of adipocytes, or cells specially designed to provide storage for lipids and triglycerides. Lipids and triglycerides are naturally occurring, non-water soluble molecules that store energy for the body's future use. These fat reserves help insulate and protect the body. They provide a source of energy when food is unavailable. When more energy is consumed than the body needs, the quantity of adipose tissue grows, leading to obesity.

For many years, scientists believed that adipose tissue functioned simply as a storage container, holding energy in fat for future use. Twenty-first-century research has shown that it takes an active role in a number of key body functions, including regulating appetite, body weight, immunity, reproduction, and the way the body uses insulin and ingested fats. Although too much body fat can be a bad thing, adipose tissue plays an essential role in overall health.

Background

The two main forms of adipose tissue are white and brown. The center of most white adipocytes is a vacuole, or a sack surrounded by a membrane, filled with lipids. The remainder of the cell components surround the vacuole, giving the adipocyte a ring-like appearance. In brown adipocytes, lipids are dispersed in smaller drops throughout the cell. Brown adipocyte cells have a larger blood supply to help promote the provision of heat to the body. Adipocytes may be as small as 30 microns or larger than 230 microns. Brown cells are generally smaller than white cells. They are loosely held together by collagen fibers to form the third layer of the body under the skin.

White and brown adipose tissue are similar in composition but have some key differences. White adipose tissue stores energy and helps regulate other functions of the body. In addition, white adipose tissue is a poor conductor of heat, making it a very effective form of insulation for the body. This type is far more common and is the type people usually are referring to when they speak of body fat.

Brown adipose tissue is found more commonly in small mammals, such as mice and rats, and in

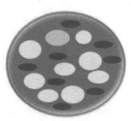

Lipid Droplet
Mitochondria
Nucleus

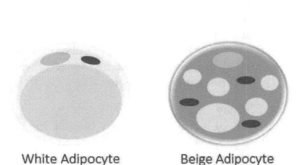

White Adipocyte   Beige Adipocyte   Brown Adipocyte

Morphology of three different classes of adipocytes. (Ktroike)

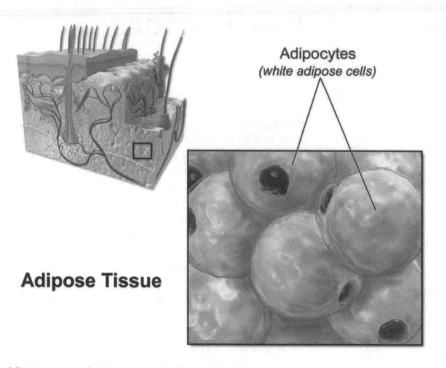

Adipocytes
(white adipose cells)

Adipose Tissue

Micro-anatomy of subcutaneous fat. (BruceBlaus)

human infants. The main function of brown adipose is to maintain body heat. Therefore, it is more common in small mammals, which are more vulnerable to cold because of their size. Human infants are generally unable to generate body heat by shivering, so the presence of a larger percentage of brown adipose tissue functions as an additional heat source.

As babies grow, brown adipose tissue disappears, and it is rarely present in adults. However, some individuals can develop so-called "beige" fat cells. This type of adipose tissue has been found in mice and in some people who exercise heavily. Exercise prompts skeletal muscles to release a protein called irisin, which in turn acts on white adipose cells to make them function like brown cells. An athlete's lean body can then compensate for the lack of insulating body fat by generating heat from the transformed white adipose tissue as if it were brown adipose tissue.

The number and type of adipose fat cells changes over an individual's lifetime. Each adipocyte has a life span of about ten years, after which it is replaced by a new cell. In humans, brown cells diminish, and white cells become more predominant. People have a tendency to gain weight with age, which is known to be the result of individual adipocytes growing in size. It is unclear, however, whether the body continues to increase the number of adipocytes it produces once an individual reaches adulthood or simply replaces worn out cells.

In addition to helping to regulate the body's temperature through insulation or heat generation, adipose tissue functions as an unofficial part of the endocrine system. The endocrine system regulates most of the body's important functions through the release of hormones from the thyroid, pancreas, pituitary gland, adrenal glands, and other glandular organs. Adipose tissue releases more than fifty adipokines, or substances that act like hormones, even though it is not technically part of the endocrine system.

Two of the more important adipokines produced by adipose tissue are adiponectin and leptin. Adiponectin affects how the body metabolizes fats and sugar; with more adiponectin, fats and sugars are more efficiently processed through the bloodstream. Among the more important results of this are increased glucose tolerance and decreased insulin resistance, leading to lower risk of diabetes. Leptin helps the hypothalamus regulate appetite; when leptin levels are low, individuals are more likely to overeat and become obese. In addition, a relationship exists between the amount of adipose tissue and the effectiveness of the adipokines, and researchers continue to study this relationship as a potential means to reduce the incidence of weight-related illnesses such as diabetes.

Topic Today

The role of adipose tissue in overall health is thought to be related to inflammation. Inflammation is the body's response to something harmful. Researchers have determined that high levels of adipose tissue—obesity—create a low level of persistent inflammation in a body, which affects the immune system and makes the body more susceptible to attack in the form of illnesses, including cancer. Adipose tissue has also been found to affect the function of the reproductive system, including the levels of the hormones necessary for fertility. The presence of either too much or too little adipose tissue can negatively affect fertility and reproduction.

Scientists continue to work to understand the complex interactions between adipose tissue and other body systems in the hopes of reducing or eliminating diseases such as type 2 diabetes and other weight-related conditions. They also are considering the unique aspects of adipose tissue to help find treatments for other conditions. For example, among the materials that make up adipocytes are stem cells, which are generally more abundant in and more easily harvested from adipose tissue than stem cells from bone marrow and other sources. These cells may help to treat bones that resist healing after breaks and other conditions.

—*Janine Ungvarsky, Geraldine Marrocco*

References

Bartelt, Alexander, and Joerg Heeren. "Adipose Tissue Browning and Metabolic Health." *Nature Reviews Endocrinology*, vol. 10, 2014, pp. 24-36, www.nature.com/nrendo/journal/v10/n1/full/nrendo.2013.204.html.

Bohler, Henry Jr., et al. "Adipose Tissue and Reproduction in Women." *Fertility and Sterility*, vol. 94, no. 3, Aug. 2010.

Catalán, V., et al. "Adipose Tissue Immunity and Cancer." *Frontiers in Physiology*, Oct. 2013.

Coelho, Marisa, et al. "Biochemistry of Adipose Tissue: An Endocrine Organ." *Archives of Medical Science*, vol. 9, no. 2, 2013.

Corvera, Sylvia, and Olga Gealekman. "Adipose Tissue Angiogenesis: Impact on Obesity and Type-2 Diabetes." *Molecular Basis of Disease*, vol. 1842, no. 3, Mar. 2014, www.science direct.com/science/article/pii/S0925443913002111.

Greenberg, Andrew S., and Martin S. Obin. "Obesity and the Role of Adipose Tissue in Inflammation and Metabolism." *The American Journal of Clinical Nutrition*, vol. 83, no. 2, Feb. 2006.

Tawonsawatruk, T., et al. "Adipose Derived Pericytes Rescue Fractures from a Failure of Healing—Non-union." *Scientific Reports*, vol. 6, 21 Mar. 2016.

■ Body mass index (BMI)

CATEGORY: Biology

Body mass index (BMI), refers to the measurement of a person using weight in relation to height. Despite its limitations, many studies have found correlations of correct BMI assessments with body fat rate, making it a reliable method. It is also useful to help assess the health risks of people who suffer from eating disorders such as anorexia nervosa and bulimia. It is not, however, a diagnostic tool. Improvements have been done on the BMI calculations through the decades. There are several ways to calculate BMI, and the most common relies on the mathematical formula weight(kg)/height(m^2). In general, the higher the BMI number, the more fat the body has. A high BMI may put the person at risk for chronic diseases such as heart disease and diabetes.

Brief History

The BMI measurement is also known as the Quetelet Index after its French inventor, Adolphe Quetelet, who designed it in the mid-nineteenth century. It became known as BMI and popularized in the early 1970s, after a study published by Ancel Benjamin Keys, the American scientist and nutritionist who invented the K-rations for US soldiers during World War II. Keys also identified the Mediterranean diet as a healthful alternative to the typical American diet. Based on the traditional diets of southern Europe, the Mediterranean diet has been linked to the health and longevity of the populations who consume it.

Since its invention in the 1800s and its revival in the 1970s, several organizations, such as the World Health Organization (WHO) and the US Centers for Disease Control (CDC), among others, have worked to consistently improve and modify the BMI measurement system. In general, BMI is an index to measure fatness or fat levels, which applies to adults preferably over 20 years of age. It can be also be used to measure weight levels in children and adolescents, but weight levels fluctuate so often through age and sex among children, that the CDC created weight charts for underage people based on percentiles according to sex and age.

The CDC has also added modifications to the BMI, in order to better assess the fat levels of some

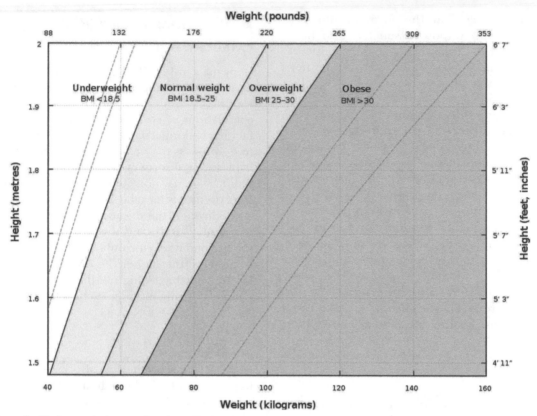

A graph of body mass index as a function of body mass and body height. The dashed lines represent subdivisions within a major class. (amfucla via Wikimedia Commons)

populations, such as the elderly and athletes. The basic BMI categories are as follows

- Underweight = 18.5 and below
- Normal weight = 18.5 to 24.9
- Overweight = 25 to 29.9
- Obesity = 30-39.9.
- Severe Obesity= >40

BMI is considered important because of the health risks associated with being overweight. According to some medical studies, excessive body weight—especially after middle age—is associated with myriad chronic diseases, health problems, and even death. For most of the adult population, BMI measurements are a good tool to estimate the healthy weight range of individuals. Therefore, medical personnel often use BMI to determine if a patient is overweight and often try to make some adjustments related to age and sex; the elderly, for example, may report a lower BMI due to muscle loss yet be overweight in reality.

Overview

Even though it is considered a reliable fat rate measurement and health risk predictor, experts warn against considering BMI estimates as a diagnosis. An in-depth examination aimed at determining a person's level of overweight and health risks needs to include other elements, such as measuring body fat by way of skinfold thickness using calipers, waist measurements, family medical history, ethnicity, occupation, and myriad other factors that should be taken into account when determining an individual's ideal weight and health risks. These should be performed by medical personnel or those highly trained in performing health screenings.

Despite its challenges and limitations, according to the CDC, paying attention to BMI is important because people who are extremely overweight or obese are at increased risk for many diseases and harmful health conditions, including hypertension, or high blood pressure, high low-density lipoprotein (LDL) cholesterol, type 2 diabetes, strokes, osteoarthritis, some cancers, some chronic conditions, and

Obesity and Body Mass Index (BMI)

$$BMI = \frac{weight\ (kg)}{height^2\ (m^2)}$$

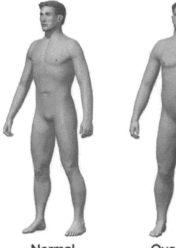
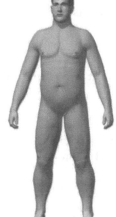
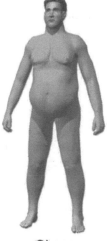

Normal	Overweight	Obese
<25 kg/m²	25 – 29 kg/m²	≥ 30 kg/m²

Source: BruceBlaus

even mental illness, such as anxiety and depression, among others. The CDC also recommends combining BMI calculations with other measurements when available, such as underwater weighing, bio-electrical impedance, dual energy x-ray absorptiometry, and isotope dilution. However, since these require trained personnel and are not always available, BMI remains a simple and inexpensive way of calculating healthy weight levels in individuals.

Although BMI is a common measure, it is also the subject of several criticisms. Among the most common critiques is that BMI is too general and even inaccurate; it does not, for instance, take into account that different populations have different degrees of fatness due to genetics or natural body shapes or proportions. It also cannot distinguish between healthy and unhealthy types of body mass. Fat gets distributed differently among different groups; for example, differences exist between Asian and some Pacific Asian groups. Moreover, some athletes may be perfectly healthy and not overweight, yet report a higher BMI due to increased muscle mass.

Therefore, BMI interpretations should take into account several biological and societal factors.

Some experts have proposed that the definitions for overweight in the WHO classification be amended to include these variants. In response, the WHO added cut-off points for observed health risks among different populations, which allows for better international comparisons.

The importance of using BMI has become clearer in the last decades, as the number of health studies grows which link body weight, health risks, and longevity. For example, close to 80 percent of individuals diagnosed with type 2 diabetes are also overweight or obese. Other chronic diseases that correlate with being overweight are hypertension, high cholesterol, heart disease and as a consequence of these, kidney damage, stroke, liver and gallbladder disease, as well as several types of cancer, among others. In some of these cases, scientists have not yet found the reason for these correlations. However, it is believed that excess weight serves as a catalyst for changes in cell structures and functions, and in other important bodily functions such as heart pumping and blood circulation, due to the overwork the organism undergoes because of the increased body mass caused by obesity.

—*Trudy Mercadal*

References

Bacon, Linda, and Lucy Aphramor. *Body Respect: What Conventional Health Books Get Wrong, Leave Out, and Just Plain Fail to Understand about Weight.* Benbella, 2014.

"BMI Classification." *Global Database on Body Mass Index.* World Health Organization. 27 July 2015.

"Body Mass Index (BMI)." *Centers for Disease Control and Prevention.* 15 May 2015.

Brown, Harriet. *Body of Truth: How Science, History and Culture Drive Our Obsession with Weight—And What We Can Do about It.* De Capo, 2015.

Flegal, Katherine M., Brian K. Kit, Heather Orpana, and Barry I. Graubard. "Association of All-Cause Mortality with Overweight and Obesity Using Standard Body Mass Index Categories: A Systematic Review and Meta-analysis." *The Journal of the American Medical Association,* vol. 309, no. 1, 2013, pp: 71–82.

■ Cholesterol

Cholesterol is a molecule that is a vital constituent of cell membranes and an essential substrate in the synthesis of vitamin D and steroid hormones (e.g., estradiol, testosterone, aldosterone, and cortisol). Cholesterol is also a component of bile, which facilitates the absorption of fats and fat-soluble vitamins. Although the body may synthesize cholesterol, it also utilizes the cholesterol provided by the diet, which is partially absorbed in the intestinal tract and transported into the liver, the organ that controls the concentration of cholesterol in the blood. Excessive cholesterol is secreted into the bile; part of it is then excreted into the feces while the rest is reabsorbed and return to the liver. Two lipoproteins play a major role in cholesterol transport through the blood, the high density lipoproteins (HDL) and low density lipoproteins (LDL). Cholesterol binds LDL in the liver to be transported to the tissues, while HDL removes cholesterol from cell membranes and transports it into the liver.

Action of Cholesterol

Cholesterol is used in the synthesis of the steroid hormones estradiol and testosterone, which are the main sex hormones, and the corticosteroids aldosterone and cortisol, which regulate the glucose metabolism, and the electrolytes concentration and water balance, respectively.

It contributes to the production of vitamin D and bile acids and assists in the absorption of fat and fat-soluble vitamins A, D, E, and K.

Sources of Cholesterol

Cholesterol is present in all animal-based fats in varying degrees. The following are rich sources of cholesterol:

- Egg yolk
- Butter
- Cheese
- Fatty meats

Excessive consumption of dietary fat (i.e., saturated and unsaturated fat) may contribute more significantly to dyslipidemia (i.e., a disorder of lipid and lipoprotein metabolism), and increased risk of atherosclerosis and cardiovascular diseases than the intake of dietary cholesterol itself.

High consumption of saturated fat, which is rich in saturated fatty acids, raises LDL-cholesterol blood levels. The following are sources of saturated fat:

- Fatty meats
- Fatty dairy products (i.e., whole milk, cream, butter, and cheese)
- Egg yolk
- Coconut and palm oils

Unsaturated fats can be monounsaturated (i.e., containing one double bond in its carbon chain) or polyunsaturated (i.e., containing more than one double bond). The following are sources of monounsaturated fat:

- Olive, canola, corn, sesame-seed, cod liver, and high-oleic sunflower-seed or safflower oils
- Avocados
- Almonds, peanuts, hazelnuts, macadamia nuts, pecans, pistachios, and cashews
- Soybeans
- Halibut, sablefish, and mackerel
- Monterey jack and parmesan cheese

The following are sources of polyunsaturated fat:
- Sesame-seed, safflower, soybean, corn flax-seed, and sunflower-seed oils
- Soybeans
- Pumpkin, sesame, flax, and sunflower seeds
- Fatty fish (e.g., salmon, mackerel, herring, trout, fresh tuna, and sardines)
- Walnuts

Trans fats exist in many foods naturally in small amounts but most are found in processed foods such as margarine, fast foods, packaged cookies and potato chips, and fried foods.

Recommended Intake of Cholesterol

The expert panel of the National Cholesterol Education Program on detection, evaluation and treatment of high blood cholesterol in adults (Adult Treatment Panel III - ATP III), recommends to consume < 200 mg/day of cholesterol.

It is recommended that whole milk be provided to babies (as appropriate following weaning from

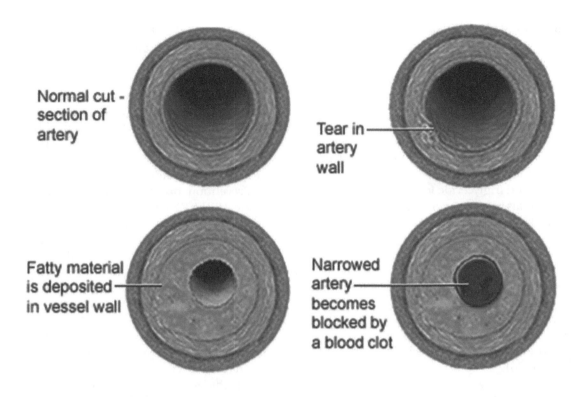

Normal cut - section of artery

Tear in artery wall

Fatty material is deposited in vessel wall

Narrowed artery becomes blocked by a blood clot

✳A.D.A.M.

High cholesterol levels can lead to hardening of the arteries, also called atherosclerosis. This occurs when fat, choles-terol, and other substances build up in the walls of arteries and form hard structures called plaques. Over time, these plaques can block the arteries and cause heart disease, stroke, and other symptoms or problems throughout the body. (MedlinePlus)

breast milk or formula feeding) up to 2 years of age as cholesterol is vital to achieve proper brain development during this time.

Dietary recommendations generally involve limiting intake of foods that increase LDL-cholesterol levels, particularly saturated and trans fats. It is currently recommended that dietary fat intake be limited as follows:

- Total dietary fat should comprise 25–35% of total caloric intake
- Saturated fat should comprise < 7 % of total caloric intake
- Trans fat should comprise < 1 % of total caloric intake

Cholesterol Deficiency

Conditions that disrupt the metabolism of cholesterol and lipoproteins and result in low levels of cholesterol (blood cholesterol level < 160 mg/dL) include:

- Tangier disease, a rare genetic disorder characterized by familial HDL deficiency
- Hypobetalipoproteinemia or abetalipoproteinemia, rare genetic disorders characterized by low total cholesterol, low or normal HDL, and low triglyceride levels
- Hyperthyroidism, liver disease, HIV infection/AIDS, or malnutrition, who are at risk of developing secondary hypocholesterolemia (i.e., low blood cholesterol levels).

Signs and symptoms of cholesterol deficiency are rare, and include:

- depression
- orange-yellow tonsils and enlarged liver and spleen in individuals with Tangier disease.

High Cholesterol (hypercholesterolemia)

Those at risk for high blood cholesterol level (recommended blood levels: total cholesterol < 200 mg/dL; LDL < 100 mg/dL; HDL > 60 mg/dL), include:

- persons with a genetic predisposition for hyperlipidemia (i.e., high blood lipid levels), hypercholesterolemia (i.e., high blood cholesterol levels), or hypertriglyceridemia (i.e., high blood triglyceride levels)
- individuals who are overweight or obese
- individuals with hypertension, diabetes mellitus (DM), hypothyroidism, polycystic ovary syndrome, or kidney disease
- individuals with alcoholism
- individuals with diets high in saturated fat, trans fat, and cholesterol
- persons with sedentary lifestyles
- individuals who smoke
- individuals with HDL-cholesterol levels < 40 mg/dL

Signs and symptoms of hypercholesterolemia include:

- Manifestations of atherosclerosis and coronary artery disease (CAD), such as
  - angina
  - shortness of breath
  - fatigue
  - weakness
  - a cardiac event, including sudden cardiac death

Risk of Interaction with Medications

The following substances can increase the risk for hypercholesterolemia:

- Birth control pills
- Estrogen
- Corticosteroids
- Some diuretics
- Beta blockers
- Some antidepressants

Research Findings

Investigators in a 2009 population study conducted in Australia estimated that a 10% reduction in LDL cholesterol could potentially save ~ 3,000 lives from CAD and stroke per year.

There is some criticism of the current public health recommendation in the U.S. for cholesterol consumption, as blood cholesterol is significantly impacted by other dietary factors. Researchers suggested that increasing intake of unsaturated fats and reducing intake of trans fat and saturated fat may have a more profound effect on LDL-cholesterol status and risk of cardiovascular diseases than simply limiting cholesterol intake alone.

Researchers conducted a prospective study in the Prevention of Renal and Vascular End-Stage Disease (PREVEND) cohort, in which they determined that higher blood HDL cholesterol is strongly related to lower risk for developing DM2.

Recent studies have revealed that individuals with cardiovascular diseases (e.g., atherosclerosis and hypercholesterolemia), DM2, and metabolic syndrome are at an increased risk for developing sporadic Alzheimer's disease (AD). Researchers studied mice fed an atherogenic diet to assess changes in metabolic and cognitive function. They observed that consuming an atherogenic diet caused changes in the hippocampus indicating defective insulin/IGF signaling resulting in an insulin resistant brain state, potentially contributing to the cognitive impairment seen in sporadic AD. While the mechanisms by which the atherogenic diet altered the brain insulin/IGF signaling are not fully understood, researchers believe that neuroinflammation is significant to the process, similar to the systemic/metabolic inflammation that results from diet-induced prediabietic and atherogenic conditions.

Red meats and saturated fats may increase the risk for CAD, but white meats, fish, and unsaturated fats (particularly monounsaturated fats) have shown potential for reducing the incidence of CAD and cancer risk by lowering LDL cholesterol in the blood.

While it is important to limit saturated fat and cholesterol intake, it is also important not to replace it with a diet high in simple carbohydrates. Diets high in simple carbohydrates are associated with dyslipidemia and DM. It is vital to emphasize that diet modification, for the prevention of CAD, should include unsaturated fats, lean proteins, complex carbohydrates, and fruits and vegetables.

Summary

Individuals should learn about the physiologic effects of cholesterol, including the contribution of high cholesterol to the development of atherosclerosis and CAD. Cholesterol intake, quantity and type of dietary fat intake may contribute to risk factors for obesity, hypertension, DM, CAD, and cancer. It is important to eat a balanced diet that includes low cholesterol and appropriate dietary fat options, balanced with protein and carbohydrate choices. There are potential interactions between cholesterol and any medications. Research suggests that increasing intake of unsaturated fats and reducing intake of trans fat and saturated fat is more beneficial than limiting cholesterol intake in general.

—*Cherie Marcel*

References

Blesso, Christopher N., and Maria Luz Fernandez. "Dietary Cholesterol, Serum Lipids, and Heart Disease: Are Eggs Working for or Against You?" Nutrients, vol. 10, no. 4, 2018, p. 426., doi:10.3390/nu10040426.

Dalvand, Sahar, et al. "Assessing Factors Related to Waist Circumference and Obesity: Application of a Latent Variable Model." Journal of Environmental and Public Health, vol. 2015, 2015, pp. 1–9., doi:10.1155/2015/893198.

Gjuladin-Hellon, Teuta, et al. "Effects of Carbohydrate-Restricted Diets on Low-Density Lipoprotein Cholesterol Levels in Overweight and Obese Adults: a Systematic Review and Meta-Analysis." Nutrition Reviews, vol. 77, no. 3, 2018, pp. 161–180., doi:10.1093/nutrit/nuy049.

Laclaustra, Martin, et al. "LDL Cholesterol Rises With BMI Only in Lean Individuals: Cross-Sectional U.S. and Spanish Representative Data." Diabetes Care, vol. 41, no. 10, 2018, pp. 2195–2201., doi:10.2337/dc18-0372.

Soliman, Ghada. "Dietary Cholesterol and the Lack of Evidence in Cardiovascular Disease." Nutrients, vol. 10, no. 6, 2018, p. 780., doi:10.3390/nu10060780.

■ Compulsive overeating

CATEGORY: Disorder

Signs

It is estimated that 4 million American adults are compulsive overeaters. The behavior is nearly twice as common in women as in men, and it typically begins before the age of twenty years. The primary sign of compulsive overeating is regularly eating large quantities of food uncontrollably without physical hunger. Other food related behaviors include eating rapidly, eating to the point of physical discomfort, eating alone and secretly, hiding food to eat later, hiding the evidence of eating, and eating food that has been discarded or is about to be discarded.

Compulsive overeaters have a preoccupation with food, spending an inordinate amount of time on meal planning, food shopping, and cooking and eating. They make furtive trips to convenience stores, fast food restaurants, and late night grocery stores. They recognize that their eating habits are not normal and feel powerless to stop eating voluntarily. They turn to food for comfort and yet use it as a reward. Their rapid weight gain brings them feelings of guilt, shame, disgust, and self-loathing. They cannot separate their identity from their weight; in weighing themselves, for example, how they feel about themselves is dictated by the number on the scale. They believe that they will be better persons once they are thin, so they try various diets with a sense of desperation. Although weight may be lost initially, it is often regained, plus more.

Underlying Causes

Researchers have not conclusively determined the underlying causes of compulsive overeating. Studies have investigated genetic predispositions to food addiction, in which a person's metabolism of foods, such as sugar, wheat, and fats, affects the same area of the brain affected by other addictive substances, such as cocaine. Other brain studies have examined compulsive overeating as a biochemically based impulse disorder somewhat similar to kleptomania, hypersexuality, compulsive shopping, and gambling addiction. A connection to dopamine in the brain has been shown, as well as hypersensitivity to the pleasurable properties of food.

Some medical professionals consider compulsive overeating to be a means of self-medicating for clinical depression. In some cases, the resulting rapid weight gain may be a protective mechanism to cope with physical or sexual abuse. The behavior also may serve to numb painful emotions of rejection, abandonment, and low self-esteem. One study showed that compulsive overeaters produce more cortisol in response to stress than do normal eaters;

cortisol is known to stimulate the drive to eat, leading to obesity. Chronic stress has an apparent connection to the preference for high-energy foods that contain large amounts of sugar and fat.

Negative Effects

The unbalanced diet of the compulsive overeater who typically chooses sweets and starches, has adverse health consequences, such as high serum cholesterol level, high blood pressure, and increased risks for heart attack, stroke, kidney failure, and diabetes. This diet may also result in lethargy, moodiness, irritability, and depression

In some cases, self-harming may be used to dissociate from emotional pain by substituting physical pain that releases endorphins. Compulsive overeaters who self-harm usually hold themselves to unreasonably high standards, have difficulty expressing their emotions, and are repulsed by their own bodies. The extreme and rapid weight gain contributes to varicose veins, blood clots in the legs, sciatica, arthritis, and bone deterioration. It may also cause shortness of breath and sleep apnea.

Treatment

Like alcohol use disorder, compulsive overeating is considered to be a disease in that it involves treatment and recovery and cannot be overcome by willpower alone. However, it is also a behavior that may be managed by behavior modification therapy. A typical initial exercise is to keep a food diary, a written record of the kind and quantity of food eaten, the time and place of eating, and the emotional context. This diary is then analyzed to identify habits, underlying emotions, and foods that trigger uncontrollable eating.

The next step usually is to consult a nutritionist to devise a healthy food plan with adequate calories for energy, necessary nutrients, and fiber for improved digestion. A third step is to identify and practice healthy activities—emotional coping mechanisms—that substitute for food; these activities may include exercise, meditation, and spending time with friends.

Persons can seek support from professional counseling or from a twelve-step program such as Overeaters Anonymous. In some cases, drug therapy with antidepressants may be appropriate.

—*Bethany Thivierge*

References

Boston University School of Medicine. "Evidence of Behavioral, Biological Similarities between Compulsive Overeating and Addiction." *ScienceDaily*, 17 Oct. 2019, www.sciencedaily.com/releases/2019/10/191017125240.htm.

Editorial Staff. "Compulsive Overeating." *American Addiction Centers*, 3 Feb. 2020, americanaddiction-centers.org/compulsive-overeating.

Kakoschke, Naomi, et al. "The Cognitive Drivers of Compulsive Eating Behavior." *Frontiers in Behavioral Neuroscience*, vol. 12, 2019, doi:10.3389/fnbeh.2018.00338.

Moore, Catherine F., et al. "Neuropharmacology of Compulsive Eating." *Philosophical Transactions of the Royal Society B: Biological Sciences*, vol. 373, no. 1742, 29 Jan. 2018, p. 20170024., doi:10.1098/rstb.2017.0024.

Moore, Catherine F., et al. "Neuroscience of Compulsive Eating Behavior." *Frontiers in Neuroscience*, vol. 11, 24 Aug. 2017, doi:10.3389/fnins.2017.00469.

■ Fast food

CATEGORY: Nutrition

Fast food typically refers to prepackaged, prepared foods that can be obtained quickly, easily, and usually inexpensively. Fast food restaurant chains (e.g., McDonald's, Taco Bell, Burger King) are a major source of fast food; other sources of fast foods include foods and drinks from vending machines and frozen dinners and premade packaged foods found in grocery stores. What is commonly referred to as the typical Western diet has become increasingly dependent on fast food options as a replacement for in-home food preparation and traditional family meals.

What's in Fast Food

Although fast foods are widely considered to be convenient, the harmful health implications cannot be ignored. Most fast foods are high in saturated and trans fats, cholesterol, sugar, high-fructose corn syrup (HFCS), and/or aspartame (i.e., a noncaloric sweetener). Consuming a diet that is high in these elements has been definitively linked to cardiovascular disease (CVD), coronary artery disease

(CAD), diabetes mellitus, type 2 (DM2), hypertension, hyperlipidemia, asthma, obesity, and cancer.

Because unsaturated fats are generally in liquid form at room temperature, food manufacturers hydrogenate them to form a solid in some cases. Hydrogenation also increases the shelf-life and stability of fatty acids. Most food sources of trans fats are processed and packaged foods (e.g., cookies, potato chips). Trans fats have been shown to increase the risk of heart disease by increasing blood levels of low-density lipoprotein (LDL) cholesterol, lowering high-density lipoprotein (HDL) cholesterol levels, and increasing platelet coagulation High intake of trans fats has been associated with a higher likelihood of developing DM2, dementia, gallstones, infertility, and certain cancers (e.g., colon and breast cancer).

For many persons, the beverage of choice with a meal of fast food is a soft drink. Global soft drink sales have increased by an estimated 300% in the past 20 years, making sugar-sweetened soft drinks the leading source of sugar in the Western diet, particularly in younger age groups (i.e., persons under 40 years of age). This increased consumption parallels the dramatic increase in rates of obesity over the past two decades.

A diet that is high in sugar is associated with CAD, dyslipidemia, and DM2. Most sugar-sweetened soft drinks use HFCS, which contains the monosaccharide (i.e., simple sugar) fructose as well as glucose and processed starches that accelerate the absorption of fructose. Unlike glucose, fructose cannot be stored as glycogen to be used as energy; if consumed in large amounts, fructose is likely to be converted to fat by the liver. Fat that is synthesized by the liver is released into the bloodstream as very low density lipoproteins (VLDL), which is a form of cholesterol known to contribute to CAD. Soft drinks that are sweetened with a non-caloric sweetener (typically aspartame) are referred to as diet soft drinks. However, substituting diet soft drinks for sugar-sweetened soft drinks does not appear to prevent obesity. Researchers report that compared with nondrinkers of diet soft drinks, consumers of diet soft drinks have a 70% larger waist circumference and intake of one or more diet soft drinks a day is linked to increased risk for stroke. The consumption of sugar-sweetened and diet soft drinks is associated with making poor dietary and lifestyle choices such as higher intake of fast foods, eating unhealthy snacks and sugary desserts, lower intake of fruits and vegetables, getting less night-time sleep, and engaging in exercise less regularly.

Research Findings

Evidence indicates that individuals tend to significantly underestimate the calorie content of the meals they eat at fast food restaurants. Researchers found that women were likely to choose lower calorie foods when provided with calorie information at the point of sale. Men's choices seemed unaffected by the provision of calorie information.

Results of recent studies show that adolescents who live near or attend school in close proximity to fast food restaurants eat fast food more often than adolescents who do not have the same access to sources of fast foods. Researchers report that Blacks who live in close proximity to fast food restaurants have a higher body mass index (BMI) than those who do not. This association is strongest among Blacks with lower economic status. Results of studies show that increasing the availability of fruits, vegetables, whole grains, and low-fat dairy products in the school setting can positively affect the food choices that students make. Many schools have vending machines that provide unhealthy food options to the students, which under mines the effectiveness of the school nutrition program.

Researchers report that preliminary results of a study indicate that fast food consumption is negatively associated with educational test scores. Along with the health risks (e.g., CAD, cancer, DM2) that are associated with consumption of trans fat, researchers report that there is a connection between trans fat intake and mental health. Results of a study involving older adults without dementia showed that high blood levels of trans fats were strongly linked with poor overall cognitive function. Results indicated that high consumption of trans fats has a detrimental effect on memory, language, attention, and speed of mental processing.

In a study including 5,038 men and 7,021 women with an average age of 37.5, researchers reported that individuals with the highest intake of trans fat were at a significantly elevated risk for developing depression.

Researchers report that individuals who consume diet soft drinks daily have a 36% higher risk of developing metabolic syndrome (i.e., a condition characterized by the combination of hyperglycemia, hypertension, abdominal obesity, and high

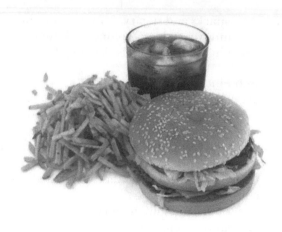

A basic and popular fast food meal, which includes a burger, french fries and a drink. (LukeB)

levels of triglycerides) and a 67% higher risk of developing DM2 compared with those who do not consume diet soft drinks regularly.

Summary

Individuals should learn about the health implications of fast food consumption. Health and diet history contribute to the risk factors for obesity, hypertension, DM2, CAD, and cancer. There are risks associated with regular fast food consumption and there are benefits of eating a balanced diet that includes appropriate dietary fat options, lean proteins, complex carbohydrates, and a variety of fruits and vegetables. Individuals should focus on healthier alternatives to high fat and sugar fast foods, including ordering smaller portions, adding salads or a serving of fruit or vegetables, and substituting water for soft drinks.

Counsel patients on the health benefits of preparing meals at home and packing meals to eat when away from home rather than relying on fast food. Provide examples of healthy meals and snacks that are quick and easy to prepare and are based around lean proteins, complex carbohydrates, fruits, vegetables and low fat dairy options.

—*Cherie Marcel*

References

Braithwaite, Irene, et al. "Fast-Food Consumption and Body Mass Index in Children and Adolescents: an International Cross-Sectional Study." BMJ Open, vol. 4, no. 12, 2014, doi:10.1136/bmjopen-2014-005813.

The Geisel School of Medicine at Dartmouth. "Fast Food Intake Leads to Weight Gain in Preschoolers." ScienceDaily, 14 Feb. 2020, www.sciencedaily.com/releases/2020/02/200214134723.htm.

NYU School of Medicine. "How Far Schoolkids Live from Junk Food Sources Tied to Obesity." ScienceDaily, 29 Oct. 2019, www.sciencedaily.com/releases/2019/10/191029080737.htm.

Poti, Jennifer M, et al. "The Association of Fast Food Consumption with Poor Dietary Outcomes and Obesity among Children: Is It the Fast Food or the Remainder of the Diet?" The American Journal of Clinical Nutrition, vol. 99, no. 1, 2013, pp. 162–171., doi:10.3945/ajcn.113.071928.

■ Food addiction

CATEGORY: Nutrition

What We Know

More than half of the adults in the United States are classified as overweight or obese, which increases risk for many chronic and/or life-threatening diseases. Each year, approximately 280,000 individuals die as a result of complications related to excess weight. The American Institute for Cancer Research (AICR) reports that more than 100,000 cases of cancer are associated with excess body fat in the U. S. each year. There are many risk factors for obesity, including sedentary lifestyle, family history of obesity, hormonal disturbances, eating disorders, and excessive caloric intake. Obesity is associated with negative social and psychological effects. For these reasons, weight loss and weight management is a major healthcare and societal concern. However, despite efforts to increase public awareness and millions of dollars spent on weight loss programs by consumers each year, reducing rates of obesity has proven to be especially difficult, with success rates for maintaining weight loss over 5 years hovering around 15%.

Similarities Between Food Addiction and Substance Addiction

- Food consumption can trigger the same reward-dysfunction mechanism (i.e., experiencing positive feedback from performing a negative, or unhealthy, action) experienced in substance addiction.

- Restriction of both foods (e.g., sugar) commonly considered addictive and substances of abuse can result in signs and symptoms of withdrawal.
- Behaviors associated with food addiction are similar to those associated with substance addiction, including:
  - insatiable cravings for hyperpalatable foods
  - lack of success to reduce caloric intake despite sincere attempts
  - continued over-eating regardless of negative consequences (e.g., obesity) and/or complications (e.g., developing diabetes mellitus and/or heart disease)

Differences Between Food Addiction and Substance Addiction

- Consumption of food is necessary for survival, unlike consumption of substances that are commonly abused.
- Hyperpalatable foods generally contain multiple ingredients, making it difficult to pinpoint the specifically addictive elements, whereas substances of abuse typically have one addictive component (e.g., ethanol, heroin).
- Foods are consumed early in life, resulting in repeated exposure during childhood, which can have long-lasting effects on dietary habits. Substances are typically introduced in adolescence or adulthood.

Medical Nutrition Therapy for Food Addiction

If food addiction parallels substance addiction, treatment protocols should theoretically be similar. For example, if hyperpalatable food intake is associated with decreased inhibition, then it would not be effective to rely on personal responsibility alone to stop overeating. Becoming involved with Overeaters Anonymous (OA) is one approach to treatment of food addiction.

Changing the food environment may be key to the success of weight loss and obesity prevention. Mandating labels of nutritional content and calories on food items and menus may help consumers to identify and avoid hyperpalatable foods.

Because food addiction involves neurologic system and psychological responses, it is important to resolve issues such as habitual, binge, stress-induced, and emotional eating with psychotherapy and, in some cases, pharmacotherapy when appropriate. Treatment of depression, anxiety, and post-traumatic stress disorder can be integral to the treatment of food addiction in many cases.

Research Findings

In recent years, research results show growing support for the theory that excessive food intake may be linked to addictive behaviors. Striking similarities have been found between the brain's response to consuming certain types of foods (e.g., foods high in fat and high in sugar) and its response to using substances (e.g., alcohol, drugs) that are commonly abused. The Yale Rudd Center for Food Policy and Obesity, a non-profit research and public policy organization, created the Yale Food Addiction Scale (YFAS) to identify signs of addiction associated with potentially addictive foods. The introduction of hyperpalatable foods (i.e., foods that are engineered to surpass the rewarding properties of natural foods [e.g., fruits, vegetables, nuts] by adding fat, sugar, salt, and food additives) has created a highly challenging public health dilemma in the fight against obesity and its complications.

Results of neuroimaging studies reveal that neurologic system responses to repeated exposure to foods that smell, look, and taste good are similar to neurologic system responses in substance addiction. Over time, the desire for appealing food becomes stronger and more difficult to satisfy. Researchers suggest that this phenomenon could cause an imbalance between hunger and reward centers in the brain and their regulation.

In the treatment of obesity, screening the obese individual for indicators of behavioral dependence and addiction is imperative to develop an individualized, successful weight loss and management regimen. Researchers suggest that more studies need to be conducted in order to understand the neurobiology of food addiction and to develop interventions that go beyond simple behavioral approaches, adding that the biochemical effects of such interventions should be closely examined.

Researchers suggest that it is possible that the addictive response to hyperpalatable foods may not be due to the sensory properties of the foods themselves, but rather a development resulting from a restriction-binge pattern of consumption. Such patterns are associated with higher risk for weight gain, obesity, depression, anxiety, substance abuse, and treatment difficulties/relapse.

Summary

Individuals experiencing food addition (and their family members) should understand the importance of resolving the behavioral and emotional issues associated with food consumption by accepting the help of trained professionals, including dietitians and psychotherapists, as recommended by the treating clinician. Family members should ensure individuals are receiving proper emotional support and education about food addiction, adhering to the prescribed treatment regimen, and continuing medical surveillance to monitor health status. Research suggests there are striking similarities between the brain's response to consuming certain types of foods and its response to using substances (e.g., alcohol, drugs) that are commonly abused.

—*Cherie Marcel*

References

Ayaz, Aylin, et al. "How Does Food Addiction Influence Dietary Intake Profile?" Plos One, vol. 13, no. 4, 2018, doi:10.1371/journal.pone.0195541.

Davis, Caroline. "From Passive Overeating to 'Food Addiction': A Spectrum of Compulsion and Severity." ISRN Obesity, 2013, pp. 1–20., doi:10.1155/2013/435027.

Ferrario, Carrie R. "Food Addiction and Obesity." Neuropsychopharmacology, vol. 42, no. 1, 2016, pp. 361–361., doi:10.1038/npp.2016.221.

Lerma-Cabrera, Jose Manuel, et al. "Food Addiction as a New Piece of the Obesity Framework." Nutrition Journal, vol. 15, no. 1, 2015, doi:10.1186/s12937-016-0124-6.

■ Freshman fifteen

CATEGORY: Nutrition; Physiology; Psychology

Introduction

Incoming college students hear about the dreaded freshman fifteen as often if not more than they hear about many of the other adjustments they will have to make during their first year living alone. Students are constantly told that the freshman fifteen is inevitable; however, recent research has shown that while college students are certainly likely to gain weight, they most likely won't gain the entire fifteen pounds and it is not guaranteed to happen over the course of one year. In fact, research shows that the freshman fifteen can happen over the course of several years. While the freshman fifteen does appear from the food choices students make, the many stressors that students are faced with are a big contributor to this weight gain. Studies have shown that college students often turn to food to feel they are in control and to cope with stress. Since the freshman fifteen is such a colloquial term, people often overlook the fact that this weight gain stems from many freshman not knowing how to control or manage their stress properly. Granted, gaining 10 or 15 pounds is not always a big deal; however, if this weight gain stems from the student not knowing how to properly cope, there can be detrimental consequences.

Freshman Fifteen

While the freshman fifteen can stem from the mere fact that college students are presented with many dining options and this is the first time that young adults have to make health conscious choices for themselves, there are two other underlying issues that commonly lead to the freshman fifteen weight gain. These are emotional eating and disordered eating. These two often go hand in hand as once people rapidly gain weight they want to see quick weight loss results. While there are plenty of healthy ways to go about losing the freshman fifteen, it is important to first understand emotional eating and disordered eating.

Emotional Eating

For the majority of college students, this is the first time that they have been away from home. Freshmen are faced with many stressors that often leave them feeling confused and vulnerable. Oftentimes, students try to numb these feelings by turning to drugs and alcohol, while others turn to and rely on food. Freshmen are facing the perils of making new friends and relationships, balancing their finances, academic rigor, and easily accessible alcohol. Many students underestimate how

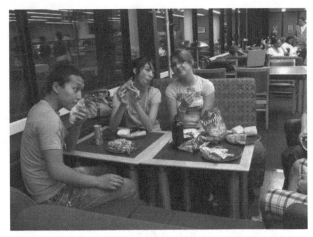

College freshman are often not presented with the healthiest options. (college.library via Wikimedia Commons)

difficult this transition will actually be, which is what leads to the overwhelming feeling of stress and anxiety. They feel like they do not have a support system like they did back in high school, so they turn to food.

Socialization is often seen as being easier when food is involved, which leads to many freshman relying on it as a way to make friends. Freshmen who use food as a way to help them make friends often end up gaining more weight when they are around people who do not make health conscious eating choices. Because of what researchers call a "shared environment," which is what all college students are in, there is an increased chance, about 57%, that if the freshman's roommate or best friend does not live a healthy lifestyle that the freshman will adopt the same unhealthy habits. Freshman often feel compelled to order the same or similar menu items as the person they are with, which can lead to weight gain.

Food is also used as a way to comfort themselves since it is something that they are used to. Every time someone feels stressed or sad and immediately reaches for their comfort food of choice, this is when it becomes emotional eating. Emotional eating oftentimes happens without people even realizing they are eating because they are stressed. In fact, most people do not realize they are eating when they are dealing with a difficult time until the difficult time has passed and they have put on a few pounds.

Along with the reliance on food to feel social, freshmen also drink to have "liquid courage."

Drinking helps people have the self-confidence they need to be social and oftentimes after having one or two drinks, people will end up eating and not making as healthy choices as they would have if they were sober. While getting food after a night out once in a while will not contribute to weight gain, this is an easy pattern to fall into, which leads to many people gaining the dreaded freshman fifteen.

Overcoming Emotional Eating

Now that the stress of going to college has been attributed to emotional eating as well as the freshman Fifteen, it is important to find ways that will allow students to keep their situational over-eating under control. According to *WebMD*, it is important to get into a regular pattern of eating. It is imperative to eat breakfast, lunch, and dinner and to not skip meals. It is also a good idea to keep healthy snacks on hand for when hunger strikes. By having healthy options in tow, it will be easier to ignore the unhealthy options the vending machine offers.

Another suggestion is to make sure that freshmen are only eating when they are truly hungry. Often the pressure from peers to go and get a snack or meal from the dining hall will leave the student feeling like he or she also has to get a snack, which is not the case. By only eating when actually hungry, students will be less likely to overeat.

Exercise is another way to combat emotional eating. Since freshman are likely to eat when they are stressed, it is suggested that instead of turning to food, freshman work out their emotions by going to the gym, trying a new exercise class, or going for a walk or run. Exercising is a great way to stay healthy and to maintain a good mindset. Exercise increases a person's endorphin levels, which leads to them feeling happier. Another benefit of exercise is that like eating, it does not have to be done alone. Students can join running clubs or other activities sponsored by their campus gym that will allow them to meet people and socialize, but in a healthy way.

Disordered Eating

Food becomes a way to exert control for many freshmen when they feel a loss of control in other areas of their lives. This desire for control often leads to people making poor and unhealthy lifestyle choices that can be detrimental to their overall health and ends up looking like the complete opposite of the freshman fifteen. According to WebMd, anorexia, bulimia, and excessive exercise are three of the most common forms of disordered eating amongst college students. The worry over gaining the freshman fifteen is a trigger for these students, which is what leads to them taking control of their bodies in such extreme ways. Similar to the idea that people gain weight when they are around other people who make unhealthy life choices, people who live amongst others who are concerned about gaining the freshman fifteen are more likely to develop disordered eating patterns than those who live with people who are not as concerned.

Overcoming Disordered Eating

People who exhibit disordered eating patterns display their symptoms in numerous ways, which makes it difficult for friends and family to know right away that a problem exists. While it is not the job of friends, family, or roommates to discover the disordered eating pattern, it is crucial to the person's recovery that he or she has support from his or her friends. Some people end up losing weight rapidly, but end up self-correcting the issue over the course of a year or two. However, there are others who are either hospitalized or need some form of outpatient therapy. It is important that when people are suffering from disordered eating that they receive the support they need. It is necessary that parents and friends focus on the root of the problem so that the student can overcome the disordered eating patterns and move forward.

Summary

While the freshman fifteen seems daunting, it does not have to be as detrimental to one's well-being as people assume. By making health conscious choices and sticking to a regular eating schedule, freshman will not have to combat the extra fifteen pounds. It is important that freshman have access to the appropriate resources so they feel capable of dealing with the many stressors placed on them without having to turn to emotional eating. It is also necessary that if the freshman student gain the dreaded extra weight, that friends and family

offer healthy advice on how to lose the weight and do not make the person feel badly about his or her weight gain so that disordered eating does not reoccur.

—*Lauren Ruvo*

References

Nguyen, Ngan. "Don't Fixate on Fifteen: Healthy Lifestyle Choices for College Freshmen." *University of Michigan School of Public Health*, 9 Sept. 2019, sph.umich.edu/pursuit/2019posts/freshman-fifteen.html.

Ordway, Denise-Marie. "The Freshman 15: Does College Cause Students to Gain Weight?" *Journalist's Resource*, 7 Feb. 2017, journalistsresource.org/studies/society/public-health/freshman-15-college-student-weight-gain/.

Prushinski, G., et al. "'The Freshman Fifteen:' Prevalence and Predictors of Weight Gain Among College Freshmen Students." *Journal of the Academy of Nutrition and Dietetics*, vol. 117, no. 9, 2017, doi:10.1016/j.jand.2017.06.336.

Smith-Jackson, Terisue, and Justine J. Reel. "Freshmen Women and the 'Freshman 15': Perspectives on Prevalence and Causes of College Weight Gain." *Journal of American College Health*, vol. 60, no. 1, 2012, pp. 14–20., doi:10.1080/07448481.2011.555931.

Vadeboncoeur, Claudia, et al. "A Meta-Analysis of Weight Gain in First Year University Students: Is Freshman 15 a Myth?" *BMC Obesity*, vol. 2, no. 1, 28 May 2015, doi:10.1186/s40608-015-0051-7.

■ Genetics

CATEGORY: Physiology

Risk Factors

Risk factors for obesity include advancing age, quitting smoking, working varied shifts, decreased activity, and a sedentary lifestyle. Other risk factors include an imbalance of excess calories versus decreased activity; a high level of fast-food intake; high alcohol consumption; eating foods with a high glycemic index, including carbohydrates, such as instant mashed potatoes, baked white potatoes, and instant rice; eating until full; and eating quickly

Etiology and Genetics

Genetic determinants play a significant part in the development of obesity. In October 2010 researchers from an international consortium, the Genetic Investigation of Anthropometric Traits (GIANT), published two papers in *Nature Genetics* regarding their identification of thirteen new DNA regions of genetic variation associated with body fat distribution and eighteen new regions associated with increased susceptibility of obesity, adding to the fourteen obesity-associated regions already known. Alternative alleles at most of these genes may marginally increase one's susceptibility to obesity, but environmental factors will still largely determine an individual's overall body size.

Although the gene function is not well understood, genetic variations at the *PTER* gene, are most strongly associated with childhood obesity and adult morbid obesity, according to a ten-year genome-wide association study of 1,380 Europeans with early-onset childhood obesity and adult morbid obesity, published in *Nature Genetics* in 2009. The same study found that these variations may contribute to as much as one-third of all childhood obesity and 20 percent of adult obesity.

Another major player mentioned in the study was the *NPC1* gene (at position 18q11.2), since its protein product seems to be involved in controlling appetite. The study estimated that allelic variations at this gene account for about 10 percent of childhood obesity and 14 percent of adult obesity. The *MAF* gene (at position 16q22–q23) encodes a protein that regulates the production of the hormones insulin and glucagon, key regulators of metabolism. The study estimated that variants at this locus account for about 6 percent of early-onset childhood obesity and 16 percent of adult morbid obesity. The *PRL* gene (at position 6p22.3) specifies the hormone prolactin, which not only stimulates lactation in women but also helps regulate the amount of food consumed.

An excellent animal model system to study obesity has been developed in mice, and these studies suggest that a protein known as leptin is particularly important for accelerating metabolism and reducing appetite. Leptin is specified by the *LEP* gene (at position 7q31), and four other genes have been identified whose protein products are necessary for proper functioning of leptin in the hypothalamus region of the brain: *PCSK1*, at position 5q15–q21; *LEPR*, at position 1q31; *POMC*, at position 2p23; and *MC4R*, at position 18q22. Mutations in any of these five genes can disrupt the normal leptin signaling pathway and result in obesity.

The 2010 GIANT Consortium report on obesity confirmed previous genome-wide association studies that found associations between body-mass index (BMI) and ten loci in or near the following genes: *FTO, MC4R, TMEM18, GNPDA2, BDNF, NEGR1, SH2B1, ETV5, MTCH2,* and *KCTD15.* The study also found eighteen new BMI-associated loci in or near the following genes: *RBJ, GPRC5B, MAP2K5, QPCTL, TNNI3K, SLC39A8, FLJ35779, LRRN6C, TMEM160, FANCL, CADM2, PRKD1, LRP1B, PTBP2, MTIF3, ZNF608, RPL27A,* and *NUDT3.*

Five years later, after an even larger study involving three hundred thousand individuals, GIANT announced that further progress had been made in the area through the discovery of more than 140 loci that contribute to different obesity traits. In addition to supporting the notion that obesity is linked to several genes rather than a single, this research revealed that the locations could be involved with neural processes connected to appetite control and energy use. The hope remained that scientists would be able to use the information obtained from the study to better understand how the genetic variations can increase the susceptibility to gain weight and subsequently come up with more targeted prevention and treatment methods.

Finally, a study of variations in the mitochondrial DNAs (deoxyribonucleic acids) of obese members of the Pima tribe of American Indians suggests that these mitochondrial DNA mutations affect enzymes in the mitochondrial respiratory chain and increase metabolic efficiency. The researchers suggest that an increased metabolic efficiency might have been advantageous at one time, since that perhaps would have allowed the Pimas to better survive the harsh dietary environment of the Sonoran Desert. In current times, with caloric overconsumption the norm, an increased efficiency may be unfavorable and contribute to the high incidence of obesity in these people.

Symptoms

Symptoms of obesity include increased weight, thickness around the midsection, and obvious areas of fat deposits. Complications of untreated obesity include decreased energy, heart disease, high blood pressure, high blood pressure during pregnancy, type 2 diabetes, gallstones, worsening arthritis symptoms, and an increased risk of certain cancers. Additional symptoms include gout, infertility, sleep apnea, poor self-image, depression, urinary incontinence, and the increased risk of death for individuals who have increased waist circumferences and waist-to-hip ratios.

Screening and Diagnosis

Obesity is diagnosed by visual exam and body measurements using height and weight tables, body mass index, a caliper to measure body folds, waist-to-hip ratio measurements, and water-displacement tests. The doctor may also order blood tests to rule out other medical conditions that may cause excess body weight.

Treatment and Therapy

Obesity is difficult to treat. Its treatment is affected by cultural factors, personal habits, lifestyle, and genetics. There are many different treatment approaches. Patients should talk to their doctors or ask for a referral to a specialist; the doctor and specialist can help develop the best treatment plan.

Plans for weight loss may include keeping a food diary, in which patients track everything they eat or drink. Patients should ask their doctors about an exercise program, which is another treatment option. Individuals can add bits of physical activity throughout their days, take stairs instead of elevators, and park a little farther away. Patients can also limit the amount of time they spend watching television and using the computer; this is important for children.

A dietitian can help patients with their total calorie intake goal, which is based on their current weights and weight loss goals. Portion size also plays an important role; using special portion control plates may help patients succeed.

The doctor may recommend that patients reduce saturated and trans fats, limit the amount of refined carbohydrates they eat, and keep fat intake under 35 percent of the total calories eaten daily. Behavior therapy may help patients understand when they tend to overeat, why they tend to overeat, and how to combat overeating habits.

Research on the effectiveness of weight-loss programs is limited. These programs do seem to work for some people. Some studies suggest that a partner or group may help a patient improve his or her diet and fitness.

Weight loss medications include sibutramine (Meridia), orlistat (Xenical), and metformin (Glucophage). Some medications have led to serious health complications. Patients should not use over-the-counter or herbal remedies without talking to their doctors.

Surgical procedures reduce the size of the stomach and rearrange the digestive tract. The smaller stomach can hold only a tiny portion of food at a time. Surgical operations include gastric bypass and laparoscopic gastric banding. These procedures can have serious complications, and they are an option only for people who are dangerously overweight.

Prevention and Outcomes

Preventing obesity can be difficult. There are many factors that influence an individual's weight. General recommendations include talking to a doctor or a dietician about an appropriate number of calories to eat per day and eating a diet with no more than 35 percent of daily calories from fat. Individuals can follow an appropriate exercise program; limit the amount of time they spend doing sedentary activities, including watching television or using the computer; and talk to their doctors or an exercise professional about working activity into their daily lives. Individuals can also ask a dietitian for help planning a diet that will help them maintain a healthy weight or lose weight if necessary. In addition, individuals can learn to eat smaller portions of food; most Americans eat portions that are too large.

—*Rosalyn Carson-DeWitt, Jeffrey A. Knight*

References

Carson-DeWitt, Rosalyn. "Overweight in Adults." *Health Library*. EBSCO, 27 May 2014.

Choquet, H., and Meyre, D. "Genetics of Obesity: What Have We Learned?" *Current Genomics*, vol. 12, no. 3, 2011, pp: 169–179.

DynaMed. "Morbid Obesity." *DynaMed*. EBSCO, 9 May 2014.

DynaMed. "Obesity in Children and Adolescents." *DynaMed*. EBSCO , 24 Mar. 2014.

Goldman, Lee, and Dennis Ausiello, eds. *Cecil Medicine*. 23d ed. Saunders, 2008.

Goroll, Allan H., and Albert G. Mulley, Jr., eds. *Primary Care Medicine: Office Evaluation and Management of the Adult Patient*. 7th ed. Wolters, 2014.

Heid, I. M., A. U. Jackson, J. C. Randall, et al. "Meta-Analysis Identifies 13 New Loci Associated with Waist-Hip Ratio and Reveals Sexual Dimorphism in the Genetic Basis of Fat Distribution." *Nature America*, 10 Oct. 2010.

"Largest Ever Genome-Wide Study Strengthens Genetic Link to Obesity." *Broad Institute*, 11 Feb. 2015.

■ High-fat diet

CATEGORY: Nutrition

Fat is an essential macronutrient that is formed by the combination of fatty acids and a glycerol molecule. Fatty acids are made of carbon atom chains, to which varying amounts of hydrogen and oxygen atoms are attached. One fat gram contains 9 calories, which is double that of carbohydrate or protein, making fat a significant source of energy. Fat stores excess calories, insulates the body, and helps to absorb and transport vitamins A, D, E, and K. The essential fatty acids (EFAs) linoleic and linolenic acid are vital for controlling inflammation, blood clotting, and brain development, particularly in the first 2 years of life.

Risks

High fat intake is associated with increased risk for coronary artery disease (CAD), diabetes mellitus, type 2 (DM2), obesity, and cancer. Overweight and obese individuals are at greater risk for cancer of the breast, colon, endometrium, gallbladder, esophagus, pancreas, and kidney. The contribution of fat intake to cancer risk or prevention varies according to the type of fat (e.g., saturated, unsaturated, or polyunsaturated), preparation of fat (e.g., by heating or hydrogenating), and the source of fat (e.g., animal or plant). Results of many studies show a correlation between intake of animal fat and increased cancer risk, although intake of fat from plant sources has not proven to be as significant a risk and monounsaturated fat (e.g., olive oil) is associated with a reduced incidence of breast cancer.

In general, it is recommended that fat intake is no more than 30% of the total daily calories consumed. The ketogenic diet (KD), which refers to a high-fat, low-carbohydrate, adequate protein diet implemented for the control of seizures, is an exception to this limitation. The KD is a structured and mathematically calculated diet that should only be implemented under close medical supervision.

Saturated and Unsaturated Fats

Fat is considered saturated or unsaturated based on the level of hydrogen in the fat compound. Fatty acid chains can be entirely filled with hydrogen atoms (i.e., saturated fatty acids) or can lack some hydrogen atoms (i.e., unsaturated fatty acids).

Saturated fats are responsible for raising levels of low-density lipoprotein (LDL) cholesterol (i.e., commonly called bad cholesterol). Diets that are high in saturated fat and cholesterol have been definitively linked to CAD, obesity, and cancer.

Unsaturated fats exist when one or more double bonds exist between carbons; the unsaturated fatty acid chain is called a monounsaturated or polyunsaturated fatty acid (PUFA), respectively. These fats are desirable in moderation because they can reduce the risk for heart disease by lowering LDL cholesterol and raising high-density lipoprotein (HDL) cholesterol(i.e., commonly called good cholesterol). HDL cholesterol appears to reduce the risk for CAD by transporting the cholesterol from areas of build-up in the arteries to the liver, where the cholesterol is eliminated.

Because unsaturated fats are generally in liquid form at room temperature, food manufacturers hydrogenate (i.e., add hydrogen to the double bond) them to achieve a solid form. This process of hydrogenation results in the creation of trans fats, which increase the risk for CAD and exhibit carcinogenic properties.

Most unsaturated fatty acids in food contain a mixture of mono- and polyunsaturated fatty acids. Foods that contain a higher amount of monounsaturated fatty acids are categorized as monounsaturated fatty acids, and foods that are higher in PUFAs are categorized as such

---

ACTION OF DIETARY FAT

Stores excess calories
Insulates the body
Assists in the absorption of vitamins A, D, E, and K
Controls inflammation
Contributes to blood clotting
Vital for brain development
Promotes satiety (i.e., feeling full after eating)

Essential Fatty Acids

EFAs are fatty acids that must be consumed because the body cannot synthesize them independently.

Linoleic acid is also called an omega-6 PUFA because it has a final double bond at the sixth carbon when one counts from the methyl end. Linoleic acid strengthens cell membranes, plays a role in the transport and metabolism of cholesterol, prolongs blood clotting time, enhances fibrinolytic activity (i.e., breaking down blood clots) and contributes to brain development.

Arachidonic acid is biosynthesized from linoleic acid in a multistep process. Arachidonic acid is vital for the synthesis of prostaglandins, which are hormone-like compounds that function as transmitters to regulate the contraction and relaxation of smooth muscle, dilation and constriction of blood vessels, aggregation of platelets in blood clotting, and inflammation.

Linolenic acid is also called an omega-3 PUFA because it has a final double bond at the third carbon when one counts from the methyl end. Linolenic acid exhibits anti-inflammatory activity, which promotes healthy lung function and prevents cardiovascular disease, arthritis, and other chronic diseases associated with inflammation. It also exhibits hypotensive properties (i.e., blood pressure lowering).

Oleic acid is a monounsaturated fatty acid that is biosynthesized from the triglycerides present in many natural oils. Oleic acid exhibits hypotensive properties and softens cell membranes, which enables linolenic acid to enter the cells.

Recommended Intake of Fat and Medication Interaction

It is currently recommended that dietary fat intake be limited as follows:

- Total dietary fat < 30% of total caloric intake but not < 20%
- Saturated fat < 10% of total caloric intake
- Trans fat < 1 % of total caloric intake

Diets that are high in fat and cholesterol are associated with CAD, obesity, and cancer. Signs and symptoms of CAD include angina, shortness of breath, fatigue, and/or weakness, and a cardiac event, including sudden cardiac death.

Individuals who are overweight and/or have been diagnosed with hypertension, DM2, heart disease, liver or kidney disease, or an intestinal disorder should be screened regularly for cancer.

Fat can enhance or decrease absorption of medications. It is important to follow the treating clinician's recommendation for correct intake of any medication (e.g., with or without food).

Research Findings

Results of many studies show a correlation between intake of animal fat and increased cancer risk, although intake of fat from plant sources has not proven to be as significant a risk. In fact, monounsaturated fatty acids (e.g., olive oil) are associated with a reduced incidence of breast cancer. Red meat and other sources of saturated fatty acids increase the risk for CAD, but white meat, fish, and unsaturated fatty acids (particularly monounsaturated fatty acids) have shown potential for reducing risk for CAD and cancer by lowering LDL cholesterol levels.

Results of a study that evaluated the impact of long-chain omega-3 fatty acids from diet and supplements on cause-specific and all-cause mortality revealed that consumption of omega-3 fatty acids is associated with a significantly reduced risk of all-cause mortality and mortality from cancer and a small reduction in risk of death from CVD.

The American Institute for Cancer Research (AICR) reports that in the U.S. each year more than 100,000 cases of cancer are associated with having excess body fat, including an estimated 49% of cases of endometrial cancer, 35% of cases of esophageal cancer, 28% of cases of pancreatic cancer, 24% of cases of kidney cancer, 21% of cases of gallbladder cancer, 17% of cases of breast cancer, and 9% of cases of colorectal cancer.

Although results of many studies link saturated fat to increased risk for certain types of cancer (e.g., breast, prostate, and pancreatic cancer), the hydrogenation of unsaturated fats to produce trans fats is

DIETARY SOURCES OF FAT	
Saturated Fat	Meat
	Fatty dairy products (e.g., whole milk, cream, butter, and cheese)
	Egg yolk
	Coconut and palm oils
Unsaturated Fat	
Monounsaturated fatty acids	Olive, canola, corn, sesame, cod liver, and high-oleic sunflower or safflower oils
	Avocados
	Almonds, peanuts, hazelnuts, macadamia nuts, pecans, pistachios, and cashews
	Soybeans
	Halibut, sablefish, and mackerel
	Monterey jack and parmesan cheese
Polyunsaturated fatty acids	Sesame, safflower, soybean, corn, flaxseed, and sunflower-seed oils
	Soybeans
	Pumpkin, sesame, flaxseed, and sunflower seeds
	Fatty fish, including salmon, mackerel, herring, trout, tuna, and sardines
	Walnuts
Trans Fat	Occurs naturally to a small degree in red meats
	Primarily found in processed foods such as cakes, cookies, chips, and margarines

considered to be as high or an even higher health risk. Trans fats are used in many processed foods, including cake, cookies, chips, and margarine. Currently more food manufacturers are producing foods that do not contain trans fats, but it remains important to check food labels for the presence of trans fats.

Although it is important to limit intake of saturated fat and cholesterol, it is also important to avoid replacing it with a diet that is high in simple carbohydrates. Diets that are high in simple carbohydrates are associated with dyslipidemia and DM2. Diet modification for the prevention of CAD should include regular intake of unsaturated fats, lean protein, complex carbohydrates, fruits, and vegetables.

Summary

Individuals should become knowledgeable about the physiologic effects of eating a high-fat diet. The quantity and type of dietary fat intake may affect risk factors for obesity, hypertension, DM2, CHD, and cancer. Eating a balanced diet that includes appropriate dietary fat options balanced with healthy choices of protein and carbohydrate is recommended. Individuals should be aware of potential interactions between dietary fat intake and any relevant medications they are receiving. Research suggests a high fat diet consisting of saturated and trans fats has numerous health risks, while a high fat diet consisting of essential fatty acids (MUFAs and PUFAs) may help reduce health risks for the same conditions.

—Cherie Marcel

References

Bell, Griffith A., et al. "Intake of Long-Chain Omega-3 Fatty Acids From Diet and Supplements in Relation to Mortality." *American Journal of Epidemiology*, vol. 179, no. 6, 3 Feb. 2014, pp. 710–720., doi:10.1093/aje/kwt326.

Chen, Michael A. "Coronary Heart Disease." *MedlinePlus*, U.S. National Library of Medicine, 13 Feb. 2018, medlineplus.gov/ency/article/007115.htm.

"HDL (Good), LDL (Bad) Cholesterol and Triglycerides." *American Heart Association*, 30 Apr. 2017, www.heart.org/en/health-topics/cholesterol/hdl-good-ldl-bad-cholesterol-and-triglycerides.

Kossoff, Eric. "Ketogenic Diet." *Epilepsy Foundation*, 25 Oct. 2017, www.epilepsy.com/learn/treating-seizures-and-epilepsy/dietary-therapies/ketogenic-diet.

Mazur, Erin E., et al., editors. "Diet and Cancer." *Lutz's Nutrition and Diet Therapy*, 7th ed., F.A. Davis, 2018, pp. 375–388.

Schlenker, Eleanor D. "Williams' Essentials of Nutrition and Diet Therapy." *Williams' Essentials of Nutrition and Diet Therapy*, edited by Eleanor D. Schlenker and Joyce Gilbert, 12th ed., Elsevier, 2018, pp. 55–67.

■ Hypothalamus

CATEGORY: Biology

Structure and Functions

The hypothalamus is a small, cone-shaped structure located near the center of the brain immediately below the thalamus. The hypothalamus has many nuclei and fiber tracts. It forms part of the walls and floor of the central chamber of the cerebral ventricles, which is known as the third ventricle. Neurons in the hypothalamus extend axons to the pituitary gland that is hanging on a stalk underneath the hypothalamus.

The hypothalamus controls many automatic functions of the body. Its overall function is to maintain normal, healthy conditions in the body by governing the autonomic nervous system and controlling pituitary output. Its specific functions are controlling the release of eight major hormones in the body, regulating body temperature, controlling food and water intake, controlling daily cycles in physiological state and behavior, mediating emotional responses, and regulating sexual behavior and reproduction.

Disorders and Diseases

If the hypothalamus is not functioning properly, the autonomic nervous system can send wrong neurosignals to the body that can make the victim feel stressed and emotionally empty. This can lead to disordered sleep, dysfunction of the immune system, altered body temperature, or multiple hormonal dysfunctions. These conditions often lead to depression, hyperactivity, malfunctioning of normal brain and limbic activities, or abnormal responses to stress. Disturbances in neural pathways that connect the hypothalamus and thalamus and control mood appear to be related to some of the symptoms of schizophrenia.

Obesity and related disorders are directly related to the critical role that the hypothalamus plays in the central regulation of appetite and metabolism. Insufficient production of antidiuretic hormone by the hypothalamus may cause diabetes insipidus. When the thirst center in the anterior hypothalamus is stimulated, polydipsia occurs, which can lead to polyuria.

Treatment of hypothalamic disorders depends on the cause of the dysfunction. If it is due to a tumor, the growth is either surgically removed or treated with radiation. If it is due to hormonal deficiencies, the missing hormones are replaced. Other specific treatments may be applied if the malfunction is due to infection, bleeding, or other causes.

—*Alvin K. Benson*

References

Jasmin, Luc. "Hypothalamus." *MedlinePlus*, 2 Nov. 2012.

Norwood, Diane Voyatzis. "Diabetes Insipidus." *Health Library*, 15 Mar. 2013.

Rennert, Nancy J. "Hypothalamus." *MedlinePlus*, 11 Dec. 2011.

Stoll, Walt, and Jan DeCourtney. *Recapture Your Health*. Sunrise Health Coach, 2006.

Swaab, Dick F. *Human Hypothalamus: Basic and Clinical Aspects, Part 2: Handbook of Clinical Neurology*. Elsevier, 2003.

■ Hypothyroidism

CATEGORY: Disorder

The thyroid gland is a butterfly-shaped organ located at the base of the neck which produces hormones that regulate heart rate, respiration, blood pressure, body weight (by controlling fat and carbohydrate metabolism), and temperature. Hypothyroidism refers to the inadequate production of the thyroid hormone, thyroxine (T4), by an underactive thyroid gland. As levels of T4 drop, metabolism begins to slow, and symptoms of hypothyroidism become apparent (for more information on hypothyroidism, see the related series of *Quick Lesson About* papers).

T4 Levels

T4 is excreted in response to the pituitary hormone thyroid stimulating hormone (TSH; also called thyrotropin); as T4 levels drop, the pituitary hormone is stimulated to produce more TSH, which in turn stimulates the thyroid to produce more T4.

Hypothyroidism is categorized as either subclinical (also called mild hypothyroidism) or overt, depending on the serum TSH level (normal level is 0.45–4.5mU/L). Subclinical hypothyroidism is characterized by TSH levels of 4.510mU/L. Overt hypothyroidism is characterized by TSH levels > 10mU/L.

Hypothyroidism in children can lead to poor physical and mental growth and development, short stature, delayed tooth development, and delayed puberty.

Causes

Causes of hypothyroidism are numerous, but 95% of cases are caused by thyroid gland dysfunction (primary hypothyroidism). Hypothyroidism can also be caused by pituitary gland dysfunction (secondary hypothyroidism) and disorders of the hypothalamus (tertiary hypothyroidism).

The most common cause of primary hypothyroidism in individuals > 8 years is Hashimoto's thyroiditis, an autoimmune disorder in which antibodies attack the cells of the thyroid gland. Hashimoto's thyroiditis is characterized by an enlarged thyroid, or goiter; indications of goiter include a visible swelling at the base of the neck, a sensation of choking, difficulty swallowing, and restricted breathing. Women are about 7 times more likely than men to develop Hashimoto's thyroiditis. Hashimoto's thyroiditis is also predisposed to developing other autoimmune disorders, including celiac disease (i.e., a chronic autoimmune disease characterized by intestinal hypersensitivity to gluten [i.e., a protein found in wheat, rye, and barley]). Cross-screening for these conditions is recommended in order to adequately treat each condition and prevent life-threatening complications.

Other causes of primary hypothyroidism include overtreatment of hyperthyroidism with radioactive iodine, antithyroid medications, or surgery (i.e., subtotal thyroidectomy), radiation therapy to the neck, medications (e.g., lithium), pregnancy, iodine deficiency, and congenital disease.

Overt hypothyroidism is treated with daily, lifelong, thyroid hormone replacement therapy (i.e., oral levothyroxine) to normalize TSH and T4 levels and prevent/reduce signs and symptoms; even with normalization of levels, some patients continue to experience symptoms of hypothyroidism. Subclinical hypothyroidism may be treated, or serum TSH levels evaluated every 6–12 months to monitor progress of the disease and treatment initiated if overt hypothyroidism develops.

Signs and Symptoms

Because T4 influences metabolism throughout the body, clinical signs/symptoms of hypothyroidism are numerous and varied, and can include nervousness, irritability, unexplained weight gain, elevated serum cholesterol, joint pain, bradycardia, coldness of the hands and feet, dry skin, chills, fatigue, constipation, difficulty concentrating, bradycardia, hoarseness, thickening of the tongue, hearing loss, memory impairment, brittle hair, and menstrual irregularities

Untreated hypothyroidism can lead to obesity, infertility, heart disease, goiter (i.e., enlarged thyroid), and myxedema (a rare, life-threatening severe form of hypothyroidism characterized by hypotension, bradypnea, hypothermia, and coma).

Medical Nutrition Therapy

Iodine is a trace mineral and essential nutrient that is primarily involved in the synthesis of the thyroid hormones T4 and triiodothyronine (T3). Eighty percent of the iodine in the body is stored within the thyroid gland. T3 and T4 are necessary for proper brain development (especially during the first three years of life), physical growth, sexual development, and metabolism and energy regulation.

Iodine must be consumed in the diet, as it is not produced within the body. Dietary sources of iodine include iodized table salt, seafood (e.g., cod, bass, haddock, and perch), kelp, dairy products, eggs, and produce from regions with iodine-rich soil.

Most environmental iodine is found in and around seawater; therefore, populations located in remote mountainous regions are at greater risk for

RECOMMENDED IODINE INTAKE

Infants 0–6 months of age	110 mcg/day
Infants 7–12 months of age	130 mcg/day
Children 1–8 years of age	90 mcg/day
Children 9–13 years of age	120 mcg/day
Males and females > 14 years of age	150 mcg/day
Pregnant females	220 mcg/day
Lactating females	290 g/day

iodine deficiency. In North America, supplementation programs (mostly in the form of iodized salt) are in place to prevent iodine deficiency in at-risk areas.

Iodine deficiency is endemic in much of the world and is responsible for the most common, preventable form of congenital mental retardation (due to maternal iodine deficiency during pregnancy). Endemic cretinism (i.e., congenital hypothyroidism resulting in stunted growth and cognition) affects up to 10% of the population in severely iodine-deficient regions (e.g., parts of India, Indonesia and China)

Mild iodine deficiency has been reported in Australia, New Zealand, and approximately 50% of continental Europe. It is suspected that many pregnant women in the Republic of Ireland and the United Kingdom are also deficient in iodine.

There is some speculation that eating goitrogenic foods (i.e., foods that can cause the thyroid gland to swell, such as sweet potato, soy, lima beans, and cruciferous vegetables including cabbage, Brussels sprouts, and broccoli) can interfere with thyroid hormone production; however, research has not shown that eating these foods can cause hypothyroidism in humans. Likewise, there is no significant evidence that diet can impact thyroid function in individuals that have hypothyroidism.

There is some concern that high-fiber meals or mineral-containing supplements (e.g., calcium, iron) can interfere with absorption of levothyroxine if consumed together; therefore, it is recommended that thyroid replacement hormones be taken several hours before or after meals or mineral-containing supplements.

Research Findings
Researchers have reported that subclinical hypothyroidism can develop in Chinese adults who consume about 800 mcg/day of iodine, suggesting that the current safe upper limit set for adults (i.e., 1100 mcg/daily iodine intake) is set too high for this population.

Similarly, an epidemiological survey of Chinese schoolchildren revealed a higher prevalence of goiter in areas in which the iodine content in drinking water is 150mcg/L, suggesting that the children are consuming excessive iodine.

Summary
Individuals should learn about hypothyroidism and diet to accurately assess health needs. Patients diagnosed with hypothyroidism should be educated on potential interactions between foods/supplements and any thyroid medications being taken. It is important to follow the prescribed treatment regime, report any health-related changes to the healthcare provider as soon as possible to prevent further damage and continue medical surveillance to monitor health status. Research suggests that excessive iodine intake may contribute to hypothyroidism.

—*Cherie Marcel*

References
Drake, Matthew T. "Hypothyroidism in Clinical Practice." *Mayo Clinic Proceedings*, vol. 93, no. 9, 2018, pp. 1169–1172., doi:10.1016/j.mayocp.2018.07.015.

Ferri, Fred F. "Hypothyroidism." *Ferri's Clinical Advisor 2020: 5 Books in 1*, edited by Fred F. Ferri, Elsevier, 2020, pp. 769–770.

Kearns, Ann. "Can Certain Foods Increase Thyroid Function in People with Hypothyroidism?" *Mayo Clinic*, Mayo Foundation for Medical Education and Research, 4 Sept. 2019, www.mayoclinic.org/diseases-conditions/hypothyroidism/expert-answers/hypothyroidism-diet/faq-20058554.

Leng, Owain, and Salman Razvi. "Hypothyroidism in the Older Population." *Thyroid Research*, vol. 12, no. 1, 8 Feb. 2019, doi:10.1186/s13044-019-0063-3.

Mcaninch, Elizabeth A., and Antonio C. Bianco. "The History and Future of Treatment of Hypothyroidism." *Annals of Internal Medicine*, vol. 164, no. 1, 5 Jan. 2016, p. 50., doi:10.7326/m15-1799.

Myers, Amy. *The Thyroid Connection: Why You Feel Tired, Brain-Fogged, and Overweight – and How to Get Your Life Back.* Little, Brown and Company, 2016.

■ Leptin

CATEGORY: Biology

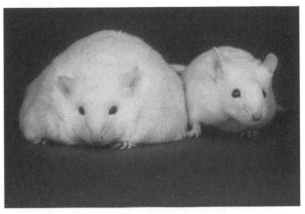

A comparison of a mouse unable to produce leptin, resulting in obesity, constant hunger, and lethargy (left), and an active normal weight mouse (right). (Oak Ridge National Laboratory)

Structure and Functions

Leptin (from the Greek *leptos*, meaning "thin") is a protein hormone with important effects in regulating body weight, metabolism, and reproductive function. It is the product of the obese (*ob*) gene occurring on chromosome 7 in the human. Leptin is produced primarily by adipocytes (white fat cells). It is also produced by cells of the epithelium of the stomach and in the placenta. It appears that as adipocytes increase in size because of accumulation of triglycerides (fat molecules), they synthesize more and more leptin. However, the mechanism by which leptin production is controlled is largely unknown. It is likely that a number of hormones modulate leptin output, including corticosteroids and insulin.

Disorders and Diseases

At first leptin was assumed to be simply a signaling molecule involved in limiting food intake and increasing energy expenditure. Studies published as early as 1994 showed a remarkable difference in weight gain in mice deficient in leptin (mice with a nonfunctional ob gene). Daily injections of leptin into these animals resulted in a reduction of food intake within a few days and a 50 percent decrease in body weight within a month.

More recent studies in the human have not been as promising. It appears that leptin's effects on body weight are mediated through effects on hypothalamic (brain) centers that control feeding behavior and hunger, body temperature, and energy expenditure. If leptin levels are low, appetite is stimulated and use of energy limited. If leptin levels are high, appetite is reduced and energy use stimulated. The most likely target of leptin in the hypothalamus is inhibition of neuropeptide Y, a potent stimulator of food intake. However, this inhibition alone could not account for the effects seen, and studies looking at other hormones are under way.

Leptin also affects reproductive function in humans. It has long been known that very low body fat in human females is associated with cessation of menstrual cycles, and the onset of puberty is known to correlate with body composition (fat levels) as well as age. Several studies have suggested that leptin stimulates hypothalamic output of gonadotropin-releasing hormone, which in turn causes increases of luteinizing and follicle-stimulating hormones from the anterior pituitary gland. These hormones stimulate the onset of puberty. Prepubertal mice treated with leptin become thin and reach reproductive maturity earlier than control mice. One report has also indicated that humans with mutations in the *ob* gene that prevent them from producing leptin not only become obese but also fail to achieve puberty.

Leptin has been identified in placental tissues; newborn babies show higher levels than those found in their mothers. Leptin has also been found in human breast milk. Together, these findings suggest that leptin aids in intrauterine and neonatal growth and development, as well as in regulation of neonatal food intake.

Finally, leptin appears to have a role in immune system function. Studies have suggested a role for leptin in production of white blood cells and in the control of macrophage function. Mice that lack leptin have depressed immune systems, but the mechanisms for this remain unclear.

Perspective and Prospects

Although early reports claimed that leptin could be useful in treating human obesity, clinical reports to date have not looked promising. It appears that deficiencies in leptin production are a rare cause of human obesity. However, since most obese individuals have plenty of leptin available, additional leptin will have no effect. In those individuals with a genetic deficiency of leptin, clinical use would require either daily injections of leptin or gene therapy. At this point neither of these options looks particularly promising.

—*Kerry L. Cheesman*

References

Friedman, Jeffrey M. "Leptin and the Endocrine Control of Energy Balance." *Nature Metabolism*, vol. 1, no. 8, 2019, pp. 754–764., doi:10.1038/s42255-019-0095-y.

Gruzdeva, Olga, et al. "Leptin Resistance: Underlying Mechanisms and Diagnosis." *Diabetes, Metabolic Syndrome and Obesity: Targets and Therapy*, vol. 12, 2019, pp. 191–198., doi:10.2147/dmso.s182406.

Hosoi, Toru, and Margherita Maffei. "Editorial: Leptin Resistance in Metabolic Disorders: Possible Mechanisms and Treatments." *Frontiers in Endocrinology*, vol. 8, 2 Nov. 2017, doi:10.3389/fendo.2017.00300.

"Leptin." *Hormone Health Network*, Endocrine Society, Nov. 2018, www.hormone.org/your-health-and-hormones/glands-and-hormones-a-to-z/hormones/leptin.

Quarta, Carmelo, et al. "Renaissance of Leptin for Obesity Therapy." *Diabetologia*, vol. 59, no. 5, 16 Mar. 2016, pp. 920–927., doi:10.1007/s00125-016-3906-7.

Yale University. "Biology of Leptin, the Hunger Hormone, Revealed." *ScienceDaily*, 18 June 2019, www.sciencedaily.com/releases/2019/06/190618113120.htm.

■ Lipids

CATEGORY: Biology

Structure and Functions

Lipids are a class of bio-organic compounds that are typically insoluble in water and relatively soluble in organic solvents such as alcohols, ethers, and hydrocarbons. Unlike the other classes of organic molecules found in biological systems (carbohydrates, proteins, and nucleic acids), lipids possess a unifying physical property-solubility behavior-rather than a unifying structural feature. Fats, oils,

some vitamins and hormones, and most of the non-protein components of cell membranes are lipids.

There are two categories of lipids-those that undergo saponification and those that are nonsaponifiable. The saponifiable lipids can be divided into simple and complex lipids. Simple lipids, which are composed of carbon, hydrogen, and oxygen, yield fatty acids and an alcohol upon saponification. Complex lipids contain one or more additional elements, such as phosphorus, nitrogen, and sulfur, yielding fatty acids, alcohol, and other compounds on saponification.

The fatty acid building blocks of saponifiable lipids may be either saturated, which means that as many hydrogen atoms as possible are attached to the carbon chain, or unsaturated, which means that at least two hydrogen atoms are missing. Saturated fatty acids are white solids at room temperature, while unsaturated ones are liquids at room temperature, because of a geometrical difference in the long carbon chains. The carbon atoms of a saturated fatty acid are arranged in a zigzag or accordion configuration. These chains are stacked on top of one another in a very orderly and efficient fashion, making it difficult to separate the chains from one another. When carbons in the chain are missing hydrogen atoms, the regular zigzag of the chain is disrupted, leading to less efficient packing, which allows the chains to be separated more easily. Saturated fatty acids have a higher melting temperature because they require more energy to separate their chains than do unsaturated fatty acids. Unsaturated fatty acids can be converted into saturated ones by adding hydrogen atoms through a process called hydrogenation.

Simple lipids can be divided into triglycerides and waxes. Waxes such as beeswax, lanolin (from lamb's wool), and carnauba wax (from a palm tree) are esters formed from an alcohol with a long carbon chain and a fatty acid. These compounds, which are solids at room temperature, serve as protective coatings. Most plant leaves are coated with a wax film to prevent attack by microorganisms and loss of water through evaporation. Animal fur and bird feathers have a wax coating. For example, the wax coating on their feathers is what allows ducks to stay afloat.

Edible fats and oils such as lard (pig fat), tallow (beef fat), corn oil, and butter are triglycerides. Triglyceride molecules are fatty acid esters in which three fatty acids (all saturated, all unsaturated, or mixed) combine with one molecule of the alcohol glycerol. Oils are triglycerides that are liquid at room temperature, while fats are solid at room temperature. The fluidity of a triglyceride is dependent on the nature of its fatty acid chains; the more unsaturated the triglyceride, the more fluid its structure. The triglycerides found in animals tend to have more saturated fatty acids than do those found in plants. Vegetable oils and fish oils are frequently polyunsaturated.

Complex lipids are classified as phospholipids or glycolipids. Structurally, phospholipids are composed of fatty acids and a phosphate group. Glycerol-based lipids called phosphoglycerides contain glycerol, two fatty acids, and a phosphate group. The phosphoglyceride structure contains a hydrophilic (polar) head, the phosphate unit, and two hydrophobic (nonpolar) fatty acid tails. The polar head can interact strongly with water, while the nonpolar tails interact strongly with organic solvents and avoid water. Egg yolks contain a large amount of the phosphoglyceride phosphatidylcholine (also called lecithin). This lipid is used to form the emulsion mayonnaise from oil and vinegar. Normally, oil and water do not mix. The hydrophobic oil forms a separate layer on top of the water. Since lecithin's structure contains both a hydrophobic and a hydrophilic region, it can attach to the water with its polar head and the oil with its nonpolar tail, preventing the two materials from separating. Lipids derived from the alcohol sphingosine are called sphingolipids. They contain one fatty acid, one long hydrocarbon chain and a phosphate group. Like the phosphoglycerides, sphingolipids have a head-and-two-tail structure. Sphingolipids are important components in the protective and insulating coating that surrounds nerves.

Glycolipids differ from phospholipids in that they possess a sugar group in place of the phosphate group. Their structure is again the polar head and dual tail arrangement in which the sugar is the hydrophilic unit. Cerebrosides, which are sphingosine-based glycolipids containing a simple sugar such as galactose or glucose, are found in large amounts in the white matter of the brain and in the myelin sheath. Gangliosides, which are found in the gray matter of the brain, in neural tissue, and in the receptor sites for neurotransmitters, contain a more complex sugar component.

Nonsaponifiable lipids do not contain esters of fatty acids as their basic structural feature. Steroids are an important class of nonsaponifiable lipids. All steroids possess an identical four-ring framework called the steroid nucleus, but they differ in the groups that are attached to their ring systems. Examples of steroids are sterols such as cholesterol, the bile acids secreted by the liver, the sex hormones, corticosteroids secreted by the adrenal cortex, and digitoxin from the digitalis plant, which is used to treat heart disease.

Lipids constitute about 50 percent of the mass of most animal cell membranes. Biological membranes control the chemical environment of the space they enclose. They are selective filters controlling what substances enter and exit the cell, since they constitute a relatively impermeable barrier against most water-soluble molecules. The three types of lipids involved are phospholipids (most abundant), glycolipids, and cholesterol. Phospholipids, when surrounded by an aqueous environment, tend to organize into a double layer of lipid molecules, a bilayer, allowing their hydrophobic tails to be buried internally and their hydrophilic heads to be exposed to the water. These phospholipids have one saturated and one unsaturated tail. Differences in tail length and saturation influence the packing efficiency of the molecules and affect the fluidity of the membrane. Short, unsaturated tails increase the fluidity of the membrane. Cholesterol is important in maintaining the mechanical stability of the lipid bilayer, thereby preventing a change from the fluid state to a rigid crystalline state. It also decreases the permeability of small water-soluble molecules.

The lipid bilayer provides the basic structure of the membrane and serves as a two-dimensional solvent for protein molecules. Protein molecules are responsible for most membrane functions; for example, they can provide receptor sites, catalyze reactions, or transport molecules across the membrane. These proteins may extend across the bilayer (transmembrane proteins) or be associated with only one face of the bilayer. Cell membranes also have carbohydrates attached to the outer face of the bilayer. These carbohydrates are bound to membrane proteins or part of a glycolipid. Typically, 2 to 10 percent of a membrane's total weight is carbohydrate. Evidence exists that cell-surface carbohydrates are used as recognition sites for chemical processes.

Lipids play an important role in health and well-being. The body acquires lipids directly from dietary lipids and indirectly by converting other nutrients into lipids. There are two fatty acids, linoleic and linolenic acids, which are called essential fatty acids. Since these fatty acids cannot be synthesized in the body in sufficient amounts, their supply must come directly from dietary sources. Fortunately, these acids are widely found in foodstuffs, so deficiency is rarely observed in adults.

About 95 percent of the lipids in foods are triglycerides, which provide 30 to 50 percent of the calories in an average diet. Triglycerides produce 4,000 calories of energy per pound, compared to the 1,800 calories per pound produced by carbohydrates or proteins. Since the triglyceride is such an efficient energy source, the body converts carbohydrates and proteins into adipose (reserve fatty) tissue for storage to be used when extra fuel is required.

While carbohydrates and proteins undergo major degradation in the stomach, triglycerides remain intact, forming large globules that float to the top of the mixture. Fats spend a longer time than other nutrients in the stomach, slowing molecular activity before continuing into the intestines. Thus, a fat-laden meal gives longer satiety than a low-fat one.

In the small intestine, bile salts split fat globules into smaller droplets, allowing enzymes called lipases to saponify the triglycerides. In some instances, the fatty acids at the two ends are removed, leaving one attached as a monoglyceride. About 97 percent of dietary triglycerides are absorbed into the bloodstream; the remainder are excreted. Although glycerol and fatty acids with short carbon chains are water-soluble enough to dissolve in the blood, the long-chain fatty acids and monoglycerides are not. These insoluble materials recombine to form new triglycerides. Since these hydrophobic triglycerides would form large globules if they were dumped directly into the blood, small triglyceride droplets are surrounded with a protective protein coat that can dissolve in water, taking the encapsulated triglyceride with it. This structure is an example of a lipoprotein.

Cholesterol is found in relatively small (milligram) quantities in foods, compared to triglycerides. Cholesterol supplies raw materials for the production of bile salts and to be used as a structural constituent of brain and nerve tissue. Since these functions are important to animals but serve no purpose in plants, cholesterol is found only in animals. Only about 50 percent of dietary cholesterol is absorbed into the blood; the rest is excreted. Much of the body's supply of cholesterol is produced in the liver. For most individuals, the amount of cholesterol synthesized in the body is larger than the amount absorbed directly from the diet.

Digested lipids released from the intestine and those synthesized in the liver compose the lipid content of the blood. The fatty acids required by the liver are obtained directly from the bloodstream or by synthesis from sources such as glucose, amino acids, and alcohol. Liver-synthesized triglycerides are incorporated into lipoprotein packages before entering the bloodstream. There are three types of lipoprotein packages that transport lipids to and from the liver. Very-low-density lipoproteins (VLDLs) transport triglycerides to tissues; low-density lipoproteins (LDLs) transport the cholesterol from the liver to other cells; and high-density lipoproteins (HDLs) transport cholesterol from other tissues to the liver for destruction.

Disorders and Diseases

Lipid consumption is an important dietary concern. Lipid deficiency is rarely observed in adults but can occur in infants who are fed nonfat formulas. Since fatty acids are essential for growth, lipid consumption should not be restricted in individuals under two years of age. Excess lipid consumption is associated with health problems such as obesity and cardiovascular disease. Although excess calories from any dietary source can lead to obesity, the body must expend less energy to store dietary fat than to store dietary carbohydrate as body fat. Thus, high-fat diets produce more body fat than do high-carbohydrate, low-fat diets.

Atherosclerosis, or "hardening of the arteries," is the leading cause of cardiovascular disease. A strong correlation exists between diets high in saturated fats and the incidence of atherosclerosis. In this condition, deposits called plaques, which have a high cholesterol content, form on artery walls. Over time, these deposits narrow the artery and decrease its elasticity, resulting in reduced blood flow. Blockages can occur, resulting in heart attack or stroke. High serum cholesterol levels (total blood cholesterol content) often result in increased plaque formation. Since dietary cholesterol is not efficiently absorbed into the bloodstream and the serum cholesterol level is largely determined by the amount of cholesterol synthesized in the liver, high serum cholesterol levels are frequently related to high saturated fat intake.

Since the measurement of the serum cholesterol level gives the total cholesterol concentration of the blood, it can be a somewhat misleading predictor of atherosclerosis risk; cholesterol is not free in blood, but is encapsulated in lipoproteins. Since the cholesterol packaged in the LDL, cholesterol that can be deposited in plaques ("bad" cholesterol), has a very different fate from that in the HDL, which is transporting cholesterol for destruction ("good" cholesterol), measuring the ratio of LDL cholesterol to HDL cholesterol has been found to be a better indicator of atherosclerosis risk. Decreasing dietary intake of cholesterol and saturated fats, increasing water-soluble fibers in the diet, removing excess body weight, and increasing the amount of aerobic exercise will all serve to improve the LDL-C/HDL-C ratio.

A number of hereditary diseases are known that result from abnormal accumulation of the complex lipids utilized in membranes. These diseases are called lipid (or lysosomal) storage diseases, or lipidoses. In normal individuals, the amount of each complex lipid present in the body is relatively constant; in other words, the rate of formation equals the rate of destruction. The lipids are broken down by enzymes that attack specific bonds in the lipid structure. Lipid storage diseases occur when a lipid-degrading enzyme is defective or absent. In these cases, the lipid synthesis proceeds normally, but the degradation is impaired, causing the lipid or a partial degradation product to accumulate, with consequences such as an enlarged liver and spleen, mental disability, blindness, and death.

Niemann-Pick, Gaucher's, and Tay-Sachs diseases are examples of lipidoses. Niemann-Pick disease is caused by a defect in an enzyme that breaks down sphingomyelin. The disease becomes apparent in infancy, causing mental retardation and death normally by age four. Gaucher's disease, a more common disease involving the accumulation of a glycolipid, produces two different syndromes. The acute cerebral form affects infants, causing severe nervous system abnormalities, retardation, and death before age one. The chronic form, which may become evident at any age, causes enlargement of the spleen, anemia, and erosion of the bones. In Tay-Sachs disease, a partially degraded lipid accumulates in the tissues of the central nervous system. Symptoms include progressive loss of vision, paralysis, and death at three or four years of age. Although Tay-Sachs disease is relatively rare (1 in 300,000 births), it has a high incidence in individuals of Eastern European Jewish descent (1 in 3,600 births). This defect is a recessive genetic trait that is found in one of every twenty-eight members of this population. For two parents who are both carriers of this trait, there is a one in four chance that their child will develop Tay-Sachs disease. Tests have been developed to detect the presence of the defective gene in the parent, and the amniotic fluid of a developing fetus can be sampled using a technique called amniocentesis to detect Tay-Sachs disease. Lipid storage diseases have no known cures; however, they can be prevented through genetic counseling.

Perspective and Prospects

The ability of a cell to discriminate in its chemical exchanges with the environment is fundamental to life. How the cell membrane accomplishes this feat has been a subject of intense biochemical research since the beginning of the twentieth century.

In 1895, Ernst Overton observed that substances that are lipid-soluble enter cells more quickly than those that are lipid-insoluble. He reasoned that the membrane must be composed of lipids. About twenty years later, chemical analysis showed that membranes also contain proteins. Irwin Langmuir prepared the first artificial membrane in 1917 by mixing a phospholipid-containing hydrocarbon solution with water. Evaporation of the hydrocarbon left a phospholipid film on the surface of the water, which showed that only the hydrophilic heads contacted the water. When the Dutch biologists E. Gorter and F. Grendel deposited the lipids from red blood cell membranes on a water surface and decreased the occupied surface area with a movable barrier, a continuous film resulted that occupied an area approximately twice the surface area of the original red blood cells. In 1935, all these observations, along with the fact that the surfaces of artificial membranes containing only phospholipids are less water-absorbent than the surfaces of true biological membranes, were combined by Hugh Davson and James Danielli into a membrane model in which a phospholipid bilayer was sandwiched between two water-absorbent protein layers.

The technological advances of the 1950s in x-ray diffraction and electronmicroscopy allowed the structures of membranes to be probed directly. Such studies revealed that membranes are indeed composed of parallel orderly arrays of lipids, although many of the proteins are attached to one of the faces of the bilayer: The Davson-Danielli model was too simplistic. The freeze-fracture technique of preparing cells for electron microscopy has provided the most information about the nature of membrane proteins. In this technique, the two layers are separated so that the inner topography can be studied. Instead of the smooth surface predicted by the Davson-Danielli model, a cobblestone-like surface was observed that resulted from proteins penetrating into the interior of the membrane. All experimental evidence supports the fluid mosaic model for biological membranes, a model first proposed by Seymour Singer and Garth Nicholson in 1972. In this model, proteins are dispersed and embedded in a phospholipid bilayer that is in a fluid state. How membranes function was the next question to be considered.

Although most of the small molecules needed by cells cross the barrier via protein channels, some essential nutrients, such as cholesterol in its LDL package, are too large to pass through a small channel. In 1986, Michael Brown and Joseph Goldstein received the Nobel Prize for their discovery of specific protein receptors on the membranes of liver cells to which LDL molecules attach. These receptors move across the surface until they encounter a shallow indentation or pit. As the pit deepens, the membrane closes behind the LDL, forming a coating allowing transport across the hydrophobic membrane interior. The presence of insufficient numbers of these receptors causes abnormal LDL-cholesterol buildup in the blood.

Many questions remain unanswered concerning the roles of proteins and glycolipids in membranes. Membranes are involved in the movement, growth, and development of cells. How the membrane is involved in the uncontrolled multiplication and migration in cancer is one medically important question. Experiments that will answer questions about how membrane structure affects functioning should lead to the development of new medical treatments.

—*Arlene R. Courtney*

References

Dehghan, Mahshid, et al. "Associations of Fats and Carbohydrate Intake with Cardiovascular Disease and Mortality in 18 Countries from Five Continents (PURE): a Prospective Cohort Study." *The Lancet*, vol. 390, no. 10107, 2017, pp. 2050–2062., doi:10.1016/s0140-6736(17)32252-3.

Dinicolantonio, James J, and James H O'Keefe. "Effects of Dietary Fats on Blood Lipids: a Review of Direct Comparison Trials." *Open Heart*, vol. 5, no. 2, 2018, doi:10.1136/openhrt-2018-000871.

Dubroff, Robert. "A Reappraisal of the Lipid Hypothesis." *The American Journal of Medicine*, vol. 131, no. 9, 2018, pp. 993–997., doi:10.1016/j.amjmed.2018.04.027.

Meynier, Anne, and Claude Genot. "Molecular and Structural Organization of Lipids in Foods: Their Fate during Digestion and Impact in Nutrition." *Ocl*, vol. 24, no. 2, 2017, doi:10.1051/ocl/2017006.

Wang, Shiming, and Xianyi Bao. "Hyperlipidemia, Blood Lipid Level, and the Risk of Glaucoma: A Meta-Analysis." *Investigative Opthalmology & Visual Science*, vol. 60, no. 4, 21 Mar. 2019, p. 1028., doi:10.1167/iovs.18-25845.

■ Menopause

CATEGORY: Biology

The risk for weight gain and obesity is increased in women after menopause, which is likely due to a combination of factors that include changes in levels of reproductive hormones and age-related changes in body composition and metabolism of carbohydrates and fats.

Causes of Menopausal Obesity

Multiple factors influence the development of obesity in adults, including caloric intake, eating habits, and the level of energy expenditure and physical activity. Glucose levels, lipid levels, and hormones, including estradiol, testosterone, and inhibin B, which is an ovarian hormone that controls follicle-stimulating hormone (FSH) secretion, modify energy intake and expenditure.

Although the role of estrogens in the development of obesity is not understood, there is evidence that the metabolic changes that occur during midlife and menopause are associated with obesity and metabolic syndrome (MetS; i.e., a condition that is characterized by insulin resistance, hyperglycemia, and dyslipidemia, which are risk factors for cardiovascular disease [CVD]).

Low levels of estradiol, which is the primary sex hormone produced by ovaries, and sex hormone binding globulin (SHBG), which is a protein that binds sex hormones, have been found in women who are obese and premenopausal. Although estradiol may be synthesized by adipose tissue, where it may play a significant role in the development of obesity in postmenopausal women, total levels of circulating estradiol remain low after menopause.

Additional factors that have been associated with weight gain in menopausal women include:

- menstruation that began in the early adolescence, late maternal age at first birth, low number of births, high weight gain during pregnancy, and/or a short duration of breast-feeding
- the aging process, which induces lower basal metabolic rate, decreased sympathetic nervous system activity, and reduced levels of human growth hormone
- changing lifestyle factors that affect energy balance (i.e., equilibrium between energy expenditure and energy intake), which may include a decrease in physical activity and/or a change in diet that increases consumed fat, carbohydrates, and/or protein
- genetic susceptibility for weight gain
- difficulty maintaining a healthy weight during childhood and/or adolescence
- certain races/ethnicities; Chinese and Japanese women are relatively protected from menopause-related weight gain compared with women who are White, Black, or Hispanic

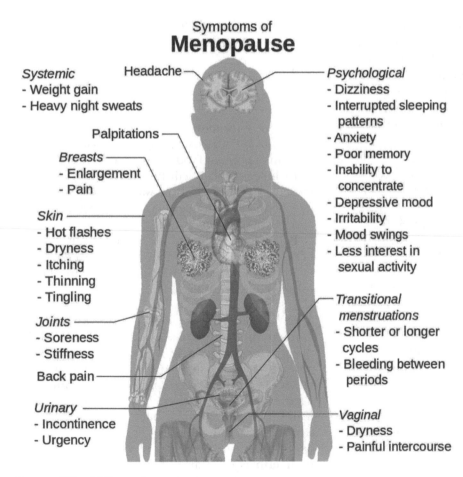

Symptoms of
Menopause

Systemic
- Weight gain
- Heavy night sweats

Headache

Palpitations

Breasts
- Enlargement
- Pain

Skin
- Hot flashes
- Dryness
- Itching
- Thinning
- Tingling

Joints
- Soreness
- Stiffness

Back pain

Urinary
- Incontinence
- Urgency

Psychological
- Dizziness
- Interrupted sleeping patterns
- Anxiety
- Poor memory
- Inability to concentrate
- Depressive mood
- Irritability
- Mood swings
- Less interest in sexual activity

Transitional menstruations
- Shorter or longer cycles
- Bleeding between periods

Vaginal
- Dryness
- Painful intercourse

Source: Mikael Häggström

- surgical menopause (i.e., menopause that occurs as a result of surgical removal of the ovaries), which is associated with a 78% increased risk of obesity and a 500% increased risk of severe obesity compared with natural menopause

Researchers who followed 15,920 postmenopausal women of normal weight who were enrolled in the Women's Health Initiative Clinical Trial during a period of 7 years reported that moderate alcohol intake was associated with reduced risk of becoming overweight or obese.

Menopausal Obesity Risk Factors

Changes in body composition in menopausal women include weight gain and central/abdominal adiposity due to decreased energy expenditure and a decline in estrogen levels, which normally promote fat deposition in the gluteofemoral region of the body (i.e., lower body, hips, and thighs). Central/abdominal obesity refers to a concentration of subcutaneous fat in the abdominal wall and visceral fat surrounding the abdominal organs. Central/abdominal obesity is defined by a waist-to-hip ratio > 0.85 for women (defined as > 0.9 for men).

Weight gain and abdominal obesity have been associated with atherosclerosis and resulting CVD, cerebrovascular disease, and increased severity of hot flashes in menopausal and postmenopausal women. It is also associated with type 2 diabetes mellitus (DM2) Obesity is the most predictive risk factor for developing DM2 because it is associated with hyperinsulinemia, which is a result of impaired insulin resistance and a precursor to DM.

There is also an increased risk of endometrial, breast, and renal cancer. Cancer risk is associated with increased extraovarian estrogen. Progesterone is prescribed to reduce the risk of cancer in women who receive estrogen supplementation.

Risk of postmenopausal breast cancer is increased by 3% for every 1-point increase in body mass index (BMI). By reducing obesity rates, it has been estimated that breast cancer rates can be reduced by one-tenth.

Treatment for Menopausal Obesity

Treating obesity varies according to the underlying cause. Significant reduction in weight can be achieved through changes in diet and lifestyle.

Balancing calorie intake and physical activity to achieve a healthy body weight. Calculate the patient's body mass index (BMI) by dividing body weight (kilograms) by height (meters squared); or 703 multiplied by weight (pounds) and divided by height (inches squared). In patients over 65 years of age, evidence suggests that a slightly higher BMI (25–27) may help prevent bone deterioration and is associated with a lower risk of mortality. In some cases, body composition testing (e.g., dual-energy x-ray absorptiometry scan, skin calipers) may be necessary.

BODY MASS INDEX	
Underweight	< 18.5
Normal	18.5–24.9
Overweight	25–29.9
Obese	>30.

Patient education is recommended to increase awareness and understanding of food labels, calorie content of popular food items, and portion control.

Include physical activity lasting 30–60 minutes most days of the week. Brisk walking 3 days per week may be the best strategy because of its accessibility and low risk for injury.

Bariatric surgery may be considered after failure of other treatment in women who have a BMI > 40 or women who have a BMI of 35–40 with obesity-related complications.

Summary

Women should learn about the risk of obesity during menopause. Risk factors include hormonal, body composition and metabolism changes. Eating a well-rounded diet that includes a variety of fruits, vegetables, whole grains, and lean proteins may help reduce risk factors of obesity. Clinicians may educate and encourage the development of strategies to support women in their efforts to attain a healthy weight by referring to appropriate disciplines (e.g., internal

DIETARY RECOMMENDATIONS FOR WOMEN IN MENOPAUSE

Consume a diet rich in fruits and vegetables.	• Choose a variety of deeply colored fruits and vegetables (e.g., spinach, carrots, berries). • Drinking fruit juice is not encouraged because it does not provide the fiber of whole fruit and has a higher calorie content per serving.
Include whole-grain, high-fiber foods.	• At least half of the grains consumed should be whole grains.
Consume oily fish at least twice a week.	• Fish are a good source of omega-3, an unsaturated fatty acid that has many health benefits, including reducing risk for CVD.

Limit intake of saturated fat, trans fat, and cholesterol.	• It is currently recommended that dietary fat and cholesterol intake should be limited as follows:
	
	  ◦ Total dietary fat < 35% of total caloric intake but not less than 20%
	
	  ◦ Saturated fat < 7% of total caloric intake
	
	  ◦ Trans fat < 1% of total caloric intake
	
	  ◦ Cholesterol < 300 mg/day

Choose and prepare foods with little or no salt.	• Sodium intake should not exceed 2,300 mg/day.
For those who consume alcohol, do so in moderation.	• It is recommended that men limit alcohol to 2 drinks/day and women limit alcohol to 1 drink/day, preferably to be consumed with meals. • A drink = 12 oz of beer, 4 oz of wine, or 1 ½ oz of 80-proof liquor.
Maintain adequate calcium intake to prevent osteoporosis and cardiac disease.	• The recommended daily intake of calcium is at least 1,200 mg/day. • Good sources of calcium include dairy products, fish with bones, broccoli, and legumes.
Include adequate vitamin D in the diet to promote calcium absorption.	• It is recommended that adults aged 51–70 years receive 400 international units (IU)/day and adults over age 70 receive 600 IU/day.

medicine, endocrinology, mental health specialists, and registered dietitians). A healthy lifestyle to improve stress management skills and increase physical activity is beneficial in reducing menopausal obesity.

—*Carita Caple, Tanja Schub*

References

Al-Safi, Zain A., and Alex J. Polotsky. "Obesity and Menopause." *Best Practice & Research Clinical Obstetrics & Gynaecology*, vol. 29, no. 4, 2015, pp. 548–553., doi:10.1016/j.bpobgyn.2014.12.002.

Atapattu, Piyusha M. "Obesity at Menopause: An Expanding Problem." *Journal of Patient Care*, vol. 01, no. 01, 2015, doi:10.4172/2573-4598.1000103.

Avraham, Yosefa, and Sapir Nachum. "Management of Obesity in Menopause: Lifestyle Modification, Medication, Bariatric Surgery and Personalized Treatment." *Current Topics in Menopause*, 2013, pp. 143–162., doi:10.2174/9781608054534113010010.

Richard-Davis, Gloria A. "Obesity and Menopause: A Growing Concern." *The North American Menopause Society*, 14 Dec. 2016, www.menopause.org/for-women/menopause-take-time-to-think-about-it/consumers/2016/12/14/obesity-and-menopause-a-growing-concern.

Rubin, Rita. "Postmenopausal Women With a 'Normal' BMI Might Be Overweight or Even Obese." *JAMA*, vol. 319, no. 12, 27 Mar. 2018, p. 1185., doi:10.1001/jama.2018.0423.

■ Mental Health

CATEGORY: Psychology

Good mental health is often described as having a state of sound cognitive, emotional, and perceptual functioning. A healthy brain and nervous system provide the foundation for good mental health. The notion that diet affects our physical health is evidence-based and commonly accepted; although it makes sense that diet is able to affect mental health through the action of nutrients on the brain and nervous system, the relationship between diet and mental health is complex.

Results of studies indicate that persons with poor mental health tend to engage in unhealthy dietary practices, are more likely to be overweight, and have significantly poorer nutrient intake than persons with good mental health. Certain nutrient deficiencies can result in cognitive decline, suggesting a causative role on the part of dietary intake. Mental illness can result in having less motivation, or ability, to shop for groceries and prepare healthy meals, suggesting that the poor diet is a result of cognitive impairment.

Other factors associated with mental illness and poor dietary intake include age, gender, environment, and genetics, although the mechanism of causation regarding these factors is unclear. There is evidence, however, that diet can contribute to the prevention, progression, and management of mental health conditions such as depression, anxiety, schizophrenia, attention deficit/hyperactivity disorder (ADHD), and Alzheimer's disease (AD).

Carbohydrates

Carbohydrates metabolize to glucose, which is the body's primary source of fuel. At rest, the brain uses 20–30% of a person's energy consumption. If caloric intake is inadequate to meet basic energy requirements, cognitive function decreases.

Intake of carbohydrates results in the release of insulin. Insulin stimulates the uptake of large neutral amino acids (LNAAs) into muscle, but insulin has no effect on the amino acid tryptophan, resulting in an increased ratio of tryptophan to LNAAs, and elevated levels of tryptophan in the brain. Tryptophan contributes to the synthesis of serotonin, which is a neurotransmitter that calms mood, improves sleep patterns, increases pain tolerance, and reduces food cravings. Low levels of serotonin in the brain are associated with depression, ADHD, anxiety, obsessive-compulsive disorder (OCD), and panic disorder.

Simple carbohydrates (also called simple sugars; e.g., low-fiber, sweet breads and cereals) break down rapidly, and provide a quick dose of high energy for only a short period of time. High intake of simple carbohydrates can cause spikes and drops in insulin and blood glucose levels, which results in fluctuating moods. Hit is also associated with a higher likelihood of depression in adults and disturbed emotional function in children.

Complex carbohydrates (e.g., high-fiber, whole grains) take longer to metabolize and provide the body with a slower release of energy over a longer period of time, which maintains normal blood glucose levels and stabilizes mood.

Protein

Protein-rich foods (e.g., eggs, lean meat, dairy products, beans) provide the amino acids tyrosine and tryptophan, which are vital for the production of important neurotransmitters (i.e., chemicals that facilitate the transmission of signals between cells). In combination with folate, magnesium, and vitamin B12, tyrosine manufactures the neurotransmitters norepinephrine and dopamine, which increase mental energy and alertness.

Tryptophan is the precursor to the neurotransmitter serotonin, which stabilizes mood. Eating meals that are high in protein results in a high number of amino acids competing with tryptophan for entry into the brain. Eating meals that contain a balance of protein and carbohydrates results in the necessary release of insulin to facilitate the redistribution of the competing amino acids, allowing tryptophan to cross the blood-brain barrier.

Fat

The brain is largely composed of fat, especially the essential fatty acids (EFAs) omega-3 and omega-6. EFAs are considered essential because they cannot be produced by the body, and must be provided through the diet. Both omega-6 and omega-3 EFAs are vital to the development and normal function of the brain and peripheral nervous system.

Traditional Western diets tend to include more omega-6 EFA, which is found in red meat, poultry, eggs, nuts, and seeds, than omega-3 EFA, which is primarily found in fish and seafood; results of research indicate that increasing the ratio of omega-3 EFA intake to be at least equal to intake of omega-6 EFA reduces the risk of developing many chronic diseases (e.g., cardiovascular disease [CVA], inflammatory bowel disease [IBD], cancer), and is associated with a reduction in cognitive decline and a reduced risk of developing AD.

Antioxidants and Vitamins

Antioxidants in fruits and vegetables protect brain cells from the damaging effects of free radicals. Many nutrients exhibit antioxidant activity, including vitamins C, E, and A; selenium; and the phytonutrients (i.e., beneficial plant-derived substances) beta-carotene and lycopene. By protecting brain cells from oxidation, antioxidants are thought to aid in the prevention of AD, other types of dementia, and depression.

B-complex vitamins are found in green leafy vegetables, eggs, milk, chicken, and fortified cereals, and play a significant role in sustaining mental health. Researchers report that persons with deficiencies in niacin, riboflavin, and/or folate are more likely to experience anxiety, depression, memory loss, insomnia, and fatigue.

Caffeine

Caffeine is found in coffee, tea, chocolate, certain soft drinks, and certain medications (e.g., analgesics, cold medications, diet pills). Study results show that caffeine boosts energy, awakens and clears the mind, and reduces the risk for depression. The primary action of caffeine is antagonism of the adenosine receptor. Adenosine dilates blood vessels and facilitates sleep. By binding with the adenosine receptor, caffeine interferes with the action of adenosine in slowing the body down. The result is increased neural activity (e.g., alertness, wakefulness).

Although most persons experience no adverse effects from drinking 3–4 8 oz. cups of coffee a day, which contains 250–350 mg of caffeine, there is some evidence that caffeine consumption can amplify feelings of anxiety in certain persons.

Regular consumption of caffeine can create a chemical dependence. For individuals who consume caffeine habitually, sudden elimination of caffeine from the diet can result in signs and symptoms of withdrawal, including irritability, agitation, and lethargy.

Medical Nutrition Therapy

- Eat a balanced diet that includes lean sources of protein, unsaturated fats, complex carbohydrates, and a variety of fruits and vegetables.
- Choose complex carbohydrates (e.g., whole grain cereals and breads) to stimulate the production of serotonin, a mood-boosting hormone, and maintain normal blood levels of glucose.
- Avoid simple carbohydrates (e.g., cookies, chips, ice cream), which can increase the risk for high levels of blood glucose and stimulate hunger.
- Regularly consume foods that provide dietary omega-3 EFAs such as fish and seafood, or take omega-3 EFA supplements.
- Regularly consume foods rich in B-complex vitamins (e.g., leafy greens, meat), vitamin C (e.g., orange and red fruits and vegetables), magnesium (e.g., beans, leafy greens), and protein (e.g., lean meat, beans, nuts), which are important for rapid energy during times of stress.
- Keep healthier snack choices (e.g., unsalted nuts, fresh fruit, dried fruit) on hand to prevent impulsive snacking of junk foods.
- Avoid consuming a large amount of caffeine (e.g., coffee, caffeinated sodas, tea), which increases signs and symptoms of anxiety and agitation.
- Avoid alcohol, which has a depressant effect on the brain and can impact mood.
- Engage in daily physical activity. Exercise reduces stress hormones, increases a sense of well-being, and improves sleep and overall health.

Research Findings

Results of clinical studies show lower levels of omega-3 EFAs in psychiatric patients (e.g., patients with AD or schizophrenia), and researchers have suggested that difficulty with lipid metabolism may play a role in schizophrenia and bipolar disorder. Supplementation with omega-3 EFAs has also been shown to improve the manifestations of ADHD and borderline personality disorder, and to reduce behaviors of impulsivity, deliberate self-harm, and violent aggression.

Researchers have reported that women increase their intake of saturated fatty acids and sugar during times of stress; this increased intake has been attributed to an increase in the stress hormone cortisol.

With the clear association between increased stress and poor dietary choices, future study is needed regarding cognitive/behavioral therapies to reduce stress-induced dietary changes.

Researchers have reported a strong link between insulin resistance in the brain and the development of early AD, suggesting that AD could be considered a neuroendocrine disorder of the brain or type 3 diabetes mellitus (T3DM).

Summary

Individuals suffering from mental health conditions (and their family members/caregivers) should learn about the role of diet in mental health based on personal characteristics and health needs. Individuals should be assessed for the risk for mental health conditions, such as chronic stress, depression and anxiety, and be referred to a mental health clinician for counseling and education, as appropriate. Individuals suffering from (or at risk of developing) mental health conditions should be encouraged to eat a nutrient-dense diet that includes fatty fish and lean proteins, unsaturated fats (including omega-3), complex carbohydrates (e.g., whole unrefined grains), legumes, and a variety of fruits and vegetables. Research suggests supplementation with omega-3 EFAs may reduce erratic behaviors, as well as improve the manifestations of ADHD and borderline personality disorder.
—*Cherie Marcel*

References

Aubrey, Allison, and Rhitu Chatterjee. "Changing Your Diet Can Help Tamp Down Depression, Boost Mood." *National Public Radio*, 9 Oct. 2019, www.npr.org/sections/thesalt/2019/10/09/768665411/changing-your-diet-can-help-tamp-down-depression-boost-mood.

Chattu, Vijayk, et al. "Nutritional Aspects of Depression in Adolescents - A Systematic Review." *International Journal of Preventive Medicine*, vol. 10, no. 1, 2019, p. 42., doi:10.4103/ijpvm.ijpvm_400_18.

Davies, Nicola. "Mental Illness and Obesity." *Psychiatry Advisor*, 17 Dec. 2018, www.psychiatryadvisor.com/home/conference-highlights/aaic-2015-coverage/mental-illness-and-obesity/.

Dunne, Annette. "Food and Mood: Evidence for Diet-Related Changes in Mental Health." *British Journal of Community Nursing*, vol. 17, no. Sup11, 2012, doi:10.12968/bjcn.2012.17.sup11.s20.

Korn, Leslie E. *Nutrition Essentials for Mental Health: a Complete Guide to the Food-Mood Connection.* W.W. Norton & Company, 2016.

LaChance, Laura R., and Drew Ramsey. "Food, Mood, and Brain Health: Implications for the Modern Clinician." *Missouri Medicine*, vol. 112, no. 2, Mar. 2015, pp. 111–115.

Mayer, Emeran A. *The Mind-Gut Connection: How the Hidden Conversation within Our Bodies Impacts Our Mood, Our Choices, and Our Overall Health.* HarperWave, 2018.

Selhub, Eva. "Nutritional Psychiatry: Your Brain on Food." *Harvard Health Blog*, Harvard Medical School, 5 Apr. 2018, www.health.harvard.edu/blog/nutritional-psychiatry-your-brain-on-food-201511168626.

■ Metabolism

CATEGORY: Biology

Structure and Functions

Metabolism is an ongoing process in living organisms. It is fundamentally concerned with the chemistry of life. An organism's metabolic rate is the rate at which it consumes the energy it derives from the nutrients that sustain it. Organisms consume energy by converting chemical energy to heat and external work; most of the latter is converted to heat also, as external work, such as walking or moving in any way, overcomes friction. A workable measure of metabolic rate, therefore, is the rate at which an organism produces heat. The food that organisms ingest is measured in calories, each calorie being the measure of what is required to raise the temperature of one kilogram of water by one degree Celsius.

Metabolism consists of two essential underlying processes, anabolism and catabolism. In vertebrates, the food ingested is immediately mixed with digestive enzymes in the mouth. These enzymes are produced by the salivary glands. As a ball of food, a bolus, passes through the digestive system, additional enzymes found in the stomach, the pancreas, and the small intestine work upon it, accelerating the digestive process.

Some nonenzymes are also vital to the digestive process. Most notable are hydrochloric acid, which, in the stomach, is a necessary ingredient for the efficient use of the stomach's pepsin, and bile salts in the small intestine, nonenzymes essential to the digestive process. The action of the digestive apparatus results in catabolism, or the breaking down of the components of food, notably lipids, carbohydrates, and proteins, into small molecules used to build and repair cells. Such molecules, through absorption, traverse the wall of the small intestine to enter the blood or the lymph so that they can be distributed throughout the body to meet its immediate requirements.

Amino acids break down protein, permitting it to enter the bloodstream, whereas glucose and other enzymes act to break down the large carbohydrates into small molecules that are absorbed into the bloodstream. After they are catabolized into smaller molecules, the lipids or fats, unlike proteins and carbohydrates, enter the lymphatic system rather than the bloodstream, which they can enter only after they have passed through the lymphatic system.

Organisms typically cannot digest all the types of nutrients they ingest. Most vertebrates, for example, are incapable of digesting cellulose, the major carbohydrate component of most plants. This material, therefore, simply passes through the digestive system and is excreted. Fiber, which passes through the digestive tract essentially undigested, performs a valuable function in keeping the colon clear and, over the long term, in preventing colon cancer.

A remarkably complex biochemical process occurs when the circulatory system delivers its absorbed sugars, lipids, and amino acids to the parts of the body where they are needed to build new cells and repair existing cells. Sometimes, this process requires the conversion of sugar molecules to fat molecules or amino acids. For a cell to construct a protein, it must connect in a specific, complex order the many amino acid molecules that the process requires. While some of the requisite amino acids result directly from ingesting nutrients, others are not available in this way and must be obtained through the synthesis of sugar molecules.

Molecules that an organism need for survival but that it cannot manufacture itself are obtained through ingestion. Such molecules are called essential nutrients. It takes twenty different kinds of amino acids, for example, to manufacture protein, but the body is capable of producing only half of these. Because green plants can synthesize all twenty forms of amino acids, they are a major and ready source of the essential nutrients required to sustain life.

Also, as part of a nutritional chain, one can note that although neither humans nor chickens can synthesize valine, a vital amino acid, chickens obtain valine by eating grain that is rich in it. Humans, in turn, eat chickens, through which they obtain valine. This amino acid is also available to humans through the green vegetables they eat.

The food that organisms ingest is used both to provide the necessary building blocks for the synthesis of membranes, enzymes, and other parts of cells and to provide energy. If the nutrients ingested are greater than the body's requirements for such synthesis and for the production of energy, then food molecules may be husbanded for future use in storage compounds within the organism. The excess stored in this way is usually in the form of lipids. In humans, such excesses are stored essentially around the abdomen and buttocks, where they can accumulate in considerable quantity.

If a human's food supply is severely reduced or completely cut off, the body draws on these reserves, using the stored fat cells until they have been completely depleted. Afterward, nutrients, mostly proteins, will be drawn from muscle mass, the sudden reduction of which can quickly eventuate in death.

The survival of organisms is usually dependent upon the work that they perform. Energy to carry out this work is derived through the splitting of the chemical bonds of adenosine triphosphate (ATP) and the splitting of the bonds of food molecules. Highly sophisticated and refined series of biochemical reactions called cellular respiration and aerobic catabolism permit most animals to transfer energy from the chemical bonds of nutrient molecules to the bonds of ATP.

Every cell in the body has the enzymes and cellular equipment to carry out aerobic catabolism and to manufacture its own ATP. Oxygen, carried through the blood, is the essential ingredient in aerobic catabolism, which results in the oxidization of nutrient molecules and their being broken up into small molecules composed largely of carbon dioxide and water. In this process, energy is released, some of it lost as heat and some of it conserved in the bonds of ATP.

As amino acids, lipids, and carbohydrates are catabolized in humans, the lipids and carbohydrates are used by the muscles, whereas the brain gains its energy almost exclusively through the glucose that catabolized carbohydrates produce. Excess amino acids are converted by the liver and, to a smaller extent, by the kidneys to carbohydrates or lipids.

In a process called anaerobic glycolysis, which involves the creation of ATP without the presence of oxygen, energy is produced by converting glucose or glycogen into lactic acid. The body cannot excrete lactic acid, thereby making impossible its accumulation in its original form in the body. Lactic acid is released into the bloodstream after exercise and, subjected to oxygen, is metabolized by the liver and either converted to glucose or oxidized aerobically in order to release additional energy.

As vertebrates age, their metabolic rate often decreases. In humans, a decreased metabolic rate, reduced activity in old age, and a failure to reduce caloric intake can result in substantial weight gain. Therefore, as humans age, their physicians usually encourage them to engage in physical activity and to reduce the overall number of calories that they consume. Physical activity generally helps to sustain the basal metabolism at levels higher than those found among the sedentary.

Disorders and Diseases

All metabolic disorders stem either from genetic or environmental origins, or from a combination of the two. For example, a person with a predisposition for diabetes, an inherited genetic disorder, may exacerbate this predisposition by indulging in a diet high in fats and carbohydrates, by overindulging in alcoholic beverages, and by engaging in little physical activity.

Environmental factors such as diet and exercise can hasten the onset of a disease that lurks in one's genes. People with this predisposition who control diet and alcohol consumption and who make strenuous exercise regular parts of their daily activity, however, may forestall the onset of the disease, possibly keeping it at bay for their entire lifetimes.

Significant advances were first made in the 1960s in tracing the genetic origins of diseases. The discovery that deoxyribonucleic acid (DNA), the molecular basis of heredity, exists in the nucleus of every cell of living organisms was a major biochemical discovery. It has led to vastly increased insights into heredity and into metabolic disorders of genetic origin, certainly the overwhelming majority of all such disorders. Among the many metabolic disorders attributable to inheritance are diabetes, arthritis, gout, phenylketonuria (PKU), Tay-Sachs disease, Niemann-Pick disease, and hemochromatosis.

Microbiologists can detect a number of abnormalities in fetuses by analyzing the amniotic fluid that surrounds them in the womb. This process, known as amniocentesis, can identify more than twenty inherited metabolic disorders before an infant is born. Genetic manipulation in utero can alter some metabolic disorders, thereby bypassing or modifying faulty or abnormal genes. The genes of a person carrying a predisposition for a metabolic defect usually do not carry the information required for the synthesizing of a particular protein, usually an enzyme. This deficiency inhibits catalytic activity and blocks a metabolic pathway, resulting in a genetic abnormality.

In a minority of cases, the protein serves a role in transport or acts as a cell-surface receptor. Whatever role the protein in question serves, a delicate balance exists within the cells. When this balance is disturbed, metabolic problems ensue. For example, a gene may be responsible for producing an enzyme that converts one substance to another substance. If this gene is defective, the enzyme derived from it may be deficient and may fail to carry out the conversion or carry it out so slowly as to result in an inefficient conversion. While the first substance, a protein, accumulates in the cell, causing a surplus, it will be in short supply in the cell involved in the conversion, resulting in a deficiency. The surplus or the shortage may eventuate in a metabolic disorder, the genetic disbalance often revealing itself in overt symptoms.

Evidence of metabolic disorders can occur at any time in a person's life. They sometimes are detectable prenatally, but they may occur in early childhood, adolescence, adult life, or old age. In some cases, the onset of a serious metabolic disorder will be followed quickly by death. Many people suffering from such disorders, however, live long, active, full lives, many of them exceeding the average life span. Some metabolic disorders, such as diabetes, are manageable over long periods through diet and medication.

Some types of metabolic disorders can be treated successfully with massive doses of vitamins. At least twenty fairly common disorders respond favorably to such treatment. For example, Wilson disease, which results in excessive amounts of copper being accumulated in the tissues, is generally treated successfully with D-penicillamine, a compound that removes copper from the tissues and deposits it into the urinary system for excretion as urine.

Certain nutrients trigger metabolic disorders in some organisms. The avoidance of these nutrients can prevent the triggering of the disorder on a permanent basis. Also, where the disorder results from a deficiency of an end product in a reaction, the disorder may be forestalled by replacing the end product.

Perspective and Prospects

Metabolism was scarcely understood until the 1770s, when Joseph Priestley discovered oxygen and set other researchers on the path to understanding its role in the biochemical aspects of all life. In the next decade, Antoine-Laurent Lavoisier and Adair Crawford were the first researchers to measure the heat produced by animals and to suggest convincingly that animal catabolism is a form of combustion.

These early, tentative steps toward understanding how organisms derive energy and how they expend it led to further research that, in 1828, resulted in Friedrich Wohler's synthesis of an organic compound, urea, from inorganic substances, demonstrating that the compounds that living organisms produce can be converted from inorganic to organic through metabolism.

It was not until 1842 that Justus von Liebig categorized foods as falling into three essential types: carbohydrates, lipids, and proteins. He measured the caloric values of nutrients and advanced considerably what was known about nutrition and its role in metabolism. At about the same time, Julius Robert von Mayer and James Joule discovered that motion, heat, and electricity are all forms of the same thing, energy. It was not until the 1890s, however, that Max Rubner and Wilbur Atwater demonstrated conclusively through empirical data that animals release energy according to thermodynamic and biochemical principles established through studies of inanimate systems.

Landmark discoveries about metabolism proceeded into the twentieth century. In 1907, Walter Fletcher and Frederick Gowland Hopkins

discovered that lactic acid results when glucose is subjected to the anaerobic contraction of muscles. Five years later, Hopkins discovered substances that are now recognized as vitamins, a term invented in 1912 by Casimir Funk. Ten years later, Frederick Banting and others pinpointed insulin as a substance that could be synthesized and used to reduce levels of blood sugar in humans, thereby making diabetes a manageable rather than a clearly fatal disorder.

A turning point in the understanding of metabolism and especially of metabolic disorders came in 1926 when James B. Sumner purified the first enzyme, showing it to be a protein, clearly leading to the realization that metabolic disorders result from a faulty protein in the genes. In 1941, Fritz Lipmann established the central role of ATP as a carrier of energy in living organisms, and the following year, Rudolf Schoenheimer demonstrated that the adult body's chemical constituents are in constant flux, suggesting that normal, healthy organisms are constantly renewing themselves.

As one surveys the future in terms of the rapidly increasing knowledge of metabolism and genetics, it is clear that genetic engineering offers daunting biological challenges. Birth defects can be detected well before birth, and many of them, through genetic manipulation, can be prevented. It is now within the capability of genetic engineering to predetermine the sex of a fetus and to control matters of gender. Amniocentesis can reveal abnormalities by the second trimester of pregnancy, revealing such conditions as metabolic disorders.

The capabilities that currently lie within reach pose substantial ethical problems and challenges. For example, if a fetus clearly shows evidence of being afflicted with a metabolic disorder, what use should be made of this information? Some parents would elect to terminate the pregnancy, given the challenges of raising such a child.

—R. Baird Shuman

References

"Does Metabolism Matter in Weight Loss?" *Harvard Health Blog*, Harvard Medical School, July 2015, www.health.harvard.edu/diet-and-weight-loss/does-metabolism-matter-in-weight-loss.

Galgani, Jose E., et al. "Carbohydrate, Fat, and Protein Metabolism in Obesity." *Metabolic Syndrome*, 2016, pp. 327–346., doi:10.1007/978-3-319-11251-0_21.

Hensrud, Donald. "The Truth about Slow Metabolism." *Mayo Clinic*, Mayo Foundation for Medical Education and Research, 21 Feb. 2019, www.mayoclinic.org/healthy-lifestyle/weight-loss/expert-answers/slow-metabolism/faq-20058480.

Knight, Helen. "A Metabolic Master Switch Underlying Human Obesity." *MIT News*, 19 Aug. 2015, news.mit.edu/2015/pathway-controls-metabolism-underlying-obesity-0819.

Oussaada, Sabrina M., et al. "The Pathogenesis of Obesity." *Metabolism*, vol. 92, 2019, pp. 26–36., doi:10.1016/j.metabol.2018.12.012.

Scripps Research Institute. "Little-Known Protein Appears to Play Important Role in Obesity and Metabolic Disease." *ScienceDaily*, 20 Nov. 2019.

Uranga, Romina María, and Jeffrey Neil Keller. "The Complex Interactions Between Obesity, Metabolism and the Brain." *Frontiers in Neuroscience*, vol. 13, 24 May 2019, doi:10.3389/fnins.2019.00513.

■ Race, ethnicity, culture and socioeconomic status

CATEGORY: Physiology

Obesity in the United States has traditionally been oversimplified as a disorder caused by physical inactivity and the unhealthy nature of the typical Western diet (i.e., a diet that consists mainly of processed and fast foods high in sodium, sugar, and fat). However, although obesity rates are increasing across all sociocultural groups, the overall incidence of obesity and related diseases is not equal among all Americans. Data show that rates of obesity and related diseases are significantly higher among Blacks, Hispanics, Pacific Islanders, and Native Americans than among Whites and Asians; higher among persons of low socioeconomic status (SES); and differ between individuals within the same ethnic/cultural groups. Thus, obesity is now recognized as a complex disorder caused by the interplay of multiple contributing factors.

Ethnic, racial, and cultural factors have been found to influence obesity in the following ways: through genetic predisposition, by affecting socioeconomic level and geographic location, through traditional cultural attitudes and beliefs, and by influencing activity level and dietary behaviors. By gaining understanding about how a patient's sociocultural background can affect risk for obesity and obesity-related behaviors, registered dietitians can be better prepared to offer effective, culturally sensitive care.

For the purposes of this article, the following definitions apply: Obesity in adulthood is defined as a body mass index (BMI; a measure of weight in relation to height) ≥ 30; childhood overweight and obesity are defined as weight ≥ 85th and 95th percentiles on CDC growth charts, respectively; Hispanic is used to describe Spanish-speaking persons; Black and White are used to describe members of those racial groups who are non-Hispanic; Pacific Islander is used to describe individuals whose families originated in the Polynesian, Melanesian, and Micronesian islands, including native Hawaiians; Asian is used to describe persons who are of Filipino, Taiwanese, Chinese, Japanese, Vietnamese, Korean, and Indian descent; and Native American is used to describe persons indigenous to North America, including Alaska Natives.

Because vast differences in attitudes and behaviors can exist within any one ethnic or racial group, the following information is provided as a general overview and is not intended to describe the characteristics of any group in absolute terms.

Genetic/Racial Influences

Genetic variation appears to influence variation in obesity rates between racial/ethnic groups. Obesity-related complications are more prevalent in all minority populations, except Asians, than in Whites, regardless of the presence of other contributing factors (e.g., socioeconomic status, education level).

Blacks appear to be genetically predisposed to obesity and obesity-related HTN; Hispanics, Native Americans, and Pacific Islanders appear to be genetically predisposed to obesity-relatedDM2. The increased rate of obesity among Blacks in comparison to persons of other ethnicities may be due in part to high insulin sensitivity among Black persons, a quality that may predispose to adiposity. Blacks report higher chronic stressors, total stress, and discrimination than Whites, which may be related to faster weight gain and slower weight loss among Blacks.

FACTS AND FIGURES

- Currently, an estimated 36.5% of Americans over the age of 20 are obese, including about 29.7% of Whites, 35.2% of Pacific Islanders, 39.8% of Blacks, 42.9% of Native Americans, 31.8% of Hispanics, and 10.7% of Asians

- Of all demographic groups, Black women (54.8%) are most likely to be obese

- In 2019, 17% of American youth aged 2 through 19, were overweight or obese, with rates of overweight and obesity highest in Black girls

- Obese individuals are 4 times more likely than non-obese individuals to have type 2 diabetes (DM2), hypertension (HTN), and cardiovascular disease (CVD)

- Rates of diagnosed DM2 among adults in the United States are 7.5% in Whites, 9.2% in Asian Americans, 12.5% in Hispanics, 11.7% in Blacks, and 14.7% in Native Americans

- HTN is more common in Blacks (54%) than in Whites (46%), Asians (39%), or Hispanics (36%)

- Rates of morbidity and mortality secondary to obesity-related diseases are highest in Black women

- Whites (23.7%) and Blacks (23.5%) are about equally at risk of death from CVD, and both experience higher rates than Asians and Pacific Islanders (21.4% - combined statistic), Hispanics (20.3%) and Native Americans (18.3%)

Hispanic children with a family history of diabetes may be biologically predisposed to development of metabolic syndrome (i.e., a combination of medical disorders that increases the risk of developing CVD and DM2) regardless of their degree of overweight.

Type 2 diabetes mellitus, dyslipidemia, and other cardiovascular risk factors occur at significantly lower BMI and waist circumference among Asian Indians compared to Whites. For this reason, consensus guidelines in India recommend that cut-offs for both measures should be lower for Indians compared to White populations.

Racial discrimination may serve as a psychosocial stressor that contributes to higher rates of obesity. In a study on obesity and discrimination, Irish, Jewish, Polish, and Italian Whites who perceived chronic racial discrimination were 2–6 times more likely to have a high waist circumference than Irish, Jewish, Polish, and Italian Whites who did not perceive chronic discrimination.

Cultural Beliefs and Attitudes

Although obese individuals are often discriminated against, members of certain minority groups are more likely than Whites to perceive overweight and obesity in childhood as healthy, normal, or harmless.

Among Hispanics, chubby children often are perceived as healthy and a manifestation of their parents' prosperity. Among Blacks, overweight children typically are not considered overweight but are described as "thick," "big-boned," or "carrying baby fat." When Blacks do identify their children as being overweight, they are less likely to associate the extra weight with risk factors for co-occurring disorders. Hispanic and Black women are more likely to accept or embrace being overweight or obese, and more likely to associate being overweight or "curvy" with being desirable than women of other races or ethnic groups.

Among Native Americans, only 15% of obese children with a BMI greater than the 99th percentile are correctly identified as obese by their family members.

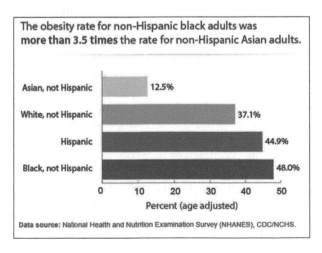

The obesity rate for non-Hispanic black adults was more than 3.5 times the rate for non-Hispanic Asian adults.

	Percent (age adjusted)
Asian, not Hispanic	12.5%
White, not Hispanic	37.1%
Hispanic	44.9%
Black, not Hispanic	48.0%

Data source: National Health and Nutrition Examination Survey (NHANES), CDC/NCHS.

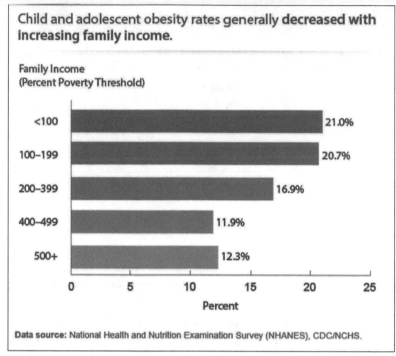

Child and adolescent obesity rates generally decreased with increasing family income.

Family Income
(Percent Poverty Threshold)

Family Income	Percent
<100	21.0%
100–199	20.7%
200–399	16.9%
400–499	11.9%
500+	12.3%

Percent

Data source: National Health and Nutrition Examination Survey (NHANES), CDC/NCHS.

Socioeconomic/Geographical Influences

Hispanic and Black children living in low socioeconomic households are more likely than White children or children in higher socioeconomic households to be overweight or obese, due to the abundance of fast food restaurants in poorer neighborhoods and the higher cost of nutrient-rich foods. Low income Black mothers sometimes hold misconceptions about nutrition during pregnancy that can promote obesity, with potential elevation of risk for adverse pregnancy outcomes.

Persons of all races may refrain from outdoor physical exercise because of threats to their physical safety (e.g., snakes or packs of dogs in rural areas, gangs and violence in urban areas). Individuals of low socioeconomic status may also lack access to affordable, convenient exercise facilities.

Americans living in southern states are more likely to be obese than those living in northern states. In the southeastern region of the United States, 71% of Black women are obese. Black adolescents living in both urban and rural areas are more likely than their White counterparts to be obese.

Activity Level and Dietary Behaviors

Physical inactivity is highest among women, members of ethnic or racial minority groups, and persons with lower education levels and lower SES; in total, 38% of women and 34% of men do not engage in any physical activity.

American children and adolescents spend a great deal of time in sedentary activities such as watching television, and many do so in their bedroom. The 2013 Healthy Habits, Happy Homes study, which examined the effects implementing healthy household habits found that in racial and ethnic minority families with young children, aged 2 to 5 years, BMI was reduced and sleep time increased in children when television time was limited.

Among many racial and ethnic minority families and communities, consuming great quantities of food during celebrations is an expectation and to refrain from excessive consumption can be perceived as insulting to family, friends, or the culture itself.

Ethnic minorities and persons of low SES are more likely to attempt unproven methods of dieting (e.g., fad diets, diet pills, non-prescribed diuretics) than Whites, but neither Whites nor members of ethnic and racial minority groups are likely to achieve lasting weight loss from diets that are not medically supervised.

Effect of Immigration and Acculturation

Acculturation (i.e., changes in behavior of an immigrant group as a result of contact with the new dominant culture) increases the likelihood of obesity in members of some racial and ethnic groups. Although immigrants of most ethnicities exhibit increases in obesity rates as their stay in the United States lengthens, Asian and White immigrants do not show any statistically significant increase in obesity.

Second- and third-generation immigrants are more likely to be obese than first-generation immigrants. Hispanic children born outside the United States are less overweight than those born in the United States of immigrant parents. First-generation Blacks of Caribbean descent are more likely than Blacks who immigrate from other nations to maintain the highly nutritious diets of their countries of origin (e.g., fresh fish, fruits, and vegetables) as a way of preserving their heritage and the healthy lifestyle of their ancestors.

—*Tanja Schub, Nathalie Smith*

References

Bentley, R. Alexander, et al. "Recent Origin and Evolution of Obesity-Income Correlation across the United States." *Palgrave Communications*, vol. 4, no. 1, 2018, doi:10.1057/s41599-018-0201-x.

Byrd, Angel S., et al. "Racial Disparities in Obesity Treatment." *Current Obesity Reports*, vol. 7, no. 2, 31 July 2018, pp. 130–138., doi:10.1007/s13679-018-0301-3.

Krueger, Patrick M., and Eric N. Reither. "Mind the Gap: Race/Ethnic and Socioeconomic Disparities in Obesity." *Current Diabetes Reports*, vol. 15, no. 11, 16 Nov. 2015, doi:10.1007/s11892-015-0666-6.

McIntosh, James. "How Do Race and Ethnicity Influence Childhood Obesity?" *Medical News Today*, 23 Apr. 2013, www.medicalnewstoday.com/articles/292913.

McQuillan, Susan. "How Your Culture Affects Your Weight." *Psychology Today*, 12 May 2016, www.psychologytoday.com/us/blog/cravings/201605/how-your-culture-affects-your-weight.

Newton, Suzy, et al. "Socio-Economic Status over the Life Course and Obesity: Systematic Review and Meta-Analysis." *Plos One*, vol. 12, no. 5, 16 May 2017, doi:10.1371/journal.pone.0177151.

Petersen, Ruth, et al. "Racial and Ethnic Disparities in Adult Obesity in the United States: CDC's Tracking to Inform State and Local Action." *Preventing Chronic Disease*, vol. 16, 11 Apr. 2019, doi:10.5888/pcd16.180579.

Wang, Liang, et al. "Ethnic Differences in Risk Factors for Obesity among Adults in California, the United States." *Journal of Obesity*, vol. 2017, 2017, pp. 1–10., doi:10.1155/2017/2427483.

■ Stress

CATEGORY: Disorder

Causes and Symptoms

Stress is a psychophysiological response, within an individual, to a perceived danger. Stress involves a complex interplay of nervous and hormonal reactions to internal and external stimuli. All living organisms respond to stimuli, usually by means of gene-regulating chemical messengers called hormones. The nervous system detects danger; such as predators, competitors, or life-threatening events.

Increased electrical conductivity along millions of nerve cells targets various tissues to prepare the body for maximum physical activity. Among the tissues affected will be the skeletal muscles, the heart muscle, the hormone-secreting glands of the endocrine system, the immune system, the stomach, and blood vessels. Under nerve-activated stress, skeletal muscles will be poised for contraction.

Heightened nerve activity also will trigger the production of various hormones from the immune system, specifically hormones that influence bodily metabolism such as thyroxine and epinephrine (adrenaline). These hormones target body tissue cells to prepare the body for increased output in the face of danger. Massive production of epinephrine will trigger maximum physical readiness and extraordinary muscular output, a phenomenon often referred to as the fight-or-flight response.

These physiological changes are important survival adaptations that evolved very early in the history of animal life on earth. Stress is a fact of life for animals because they must eat to survive. Competition for available food resources and avoidance of predators must be faced by all animals, including humans. While predation by larger animals is of little worry to current-day modern humans, the struggle for available resources remains. Furthermore, human technology has created stresses of an entirely different character.

The fight-or-flight stress response and other evolutionary stress adaptations endure within the individual for only seconds or minutes. Such natural stresses are to an individual's advantage, ensuring survival. The stresses that humans face are based on these behavioral adaptations. Much human stress is artificial, however, and lasts not for minutes but for hours, days, weeks, months, and years. Such stresses involve the same nervous and endocrine system responses, but they are usually brought about by perceived danger, not true danger.

Human societies impose norms and rules for the behavior of the individuals who compose the society. People must adhere to the societal norms or face punishment. In fast-paced technological societies, increasing bureaucratization and organization place less emphasis on the individual and more emphasis on process and productivity. People must face deadlines, be on time, produce quotas, generate company profit, and meet the demands of family, colleagues, and administration simultaneously. The result is a continuous fight-or-flight response in which individuals fear losing their jobs and thus the means of supporting themselves and their families.

The physiological manifestations of prolonged stress are devastating. Continued hyperactivity of nerve impulses and overproduction of hormones at incorrect developmental stages lead to the abnormal functioning of internal organs. The stomach undersecretes mucus, thereby leading to ulcers.

The heart muscle contracts too rapidly, leading to higher pulse and respiration rates. The blood vessels constrict for lengthy periods of time, thereby causing the heart to pump harder and leading to high blood pressure and heart disease. Hormone overproduction leads to incorrect cell instructions and gene activation/inactivation, causing abnormal tissue functioning and cellular transformation leading to cancer. The immune system weakens under abnormal signaling by hormones, thereby decreasing the body's ability to defend itself from disease.

Stress and Disease

A wide variety of human illnesses and disorders have been associated with stress. Heart disease, obesity, cancer, stroke, mental illness, allergies, accidents, asthma, chronic fatigue, depression, suicide, and deviant behavior are among the many illnesses and disorders that are considered by scientists to be stress-related illnesses. These stress-related diseases and disorders are responsible for the majority of deaths, hospitalizations, and visits to physicians by people in highly technological societies such as the United States, Japan, and Western Europe. In the United States alone, several billion dollars are spent each year for medications to treat stress-related illnesses that otherwise could be prevented by anti-stress methodologies.

Before the advent of industrialization in Europe and North America, the leading killers of humans were bacterial and viral diseases, which continue to be the principal killers of humans in the pretechnological and emerging technological countries of the Middle East, Asia, Africa, Latin America, and Oceania. European and North American industrialization has been accompanied by prodigious advances in medical science and the eradication or control of many microorganismal diseases. The psychological demands of fast-paced living and the dehumanized expectations of technological societies, however,

have produced a plethora of stress-generated diseases and disorders, some of which had been masked by microorganismal diseases.

There still is some debate concerning the causal relationship between stress and illness, despite overwhelming scientific evidence demonstrating bodily responses to stressful situations. Abnormal nerve hyperactivity and prolonged, abnormal secretions of gene regulatory hormones from various endocrine glands disrupt the balanced homeostasis of many different body systems. Immune system reduction often occurs during stress, thereby making a stressed individual more susceptible to contracting infectious bacterial and viral diseases.

A clear linkage exists between the occurrence of stress in people and their subsequent susceptibility to infectious disease. Furthermore, there is a tendency for strokes, heart attacks, cancer, and sudden death to occur in individuals who recently have experienced major traumatic events in their lives. Too little attention has been given to the effects of everyday living upon the physical well-being of people. Environmental stimuli, nervous and endocrine systems, and physiological rhythms within the body are intricately connected.

Treatment and Therapy

Psychologists, psychiatrists, physicians, and other medical professionals are becoming more aware of the physiological effects of stress. Through this awareness, professionals have sought to examine whether there are any characteristic styles of stress response. In response, psychologists have identified two principal behavioral types when it comes to stress among humans: type A behavior pattern and type B behavior pattern. Type A individuals are highly anxious, task-oriented, time-conscious, constantly in a rush to accomplish their jobs and other objectives, and somewhat prone to hostility. Research indicates that type A individuals may have a higher incidence of heart disease. Increasingly, the hostility component of type A behavior is seen as a very important contributing factor. On the other hand, type B individuals are more relaxed and experience less stress. Nevertheless, it should be emphasized that behavior is a continuum: Different people may exhibit varying degrees of type A and B behavior patterns. Given this discovery, it is not uncommon for professionals to recommend to their stressed clients to monitor their participation in type A behavior and to try behaving more in kind with type B behavior patterns.

Another important focus for health care has become the prevention, management, and treatment of stress itself. Health education programs emphasize the importance of physical fitness and stress reduction in everyday living. Stress-reducing methodologies for the individual include time management, peer counseling and support, spending longer amounts of time relaxing, strengthening family bonds, improving self-esteem, exercise, and learning to reframe how daily life events are interpreted, such as may be done through cognitive behavior therapy. These approaches greatly enhance an individual's quality of life and help the individual to cope positively with stressful events. All these stress reduction techniques emphasize an individual's personality and the more efficient use of an individual's free time. Relaxation, social interaction, and physical activity help the body to return to normal physiological rhythms following the numerous stressful events that every person faces daily. Individuals in American and Western societies are coming to realize that a slower, more relaxed living pace is essential for reducing stress and the millions of cases of stress-related disease that occur each year.

Perspective and Prospects

Because stress is a major contributor to illness and disease in American and Western societies, a major objective of health care professionals in these countries is the identification of stress initiators and the reduction of stress in the general population. Stress cannot be eliminated entirely in any individual. Humans always will experience stress as a result of their continuous interactions with one another and with the environment. Stress is an important survival adaptation for animal life on earth. Nevertheless, stressful events in an individual's life serve as negative environmental stimuli that hyperactivate the human nervous and endocrine systems to create a fight-or-flight response. When this fight-or-flight response is maintained for abnormally long periods of times, prolonged elevations in nervous and hormonal activity modify body tissues and the developmental gene expression within cells to produce abnormal growths (such as cancers) and abnormal system functioning (such as diabetes mellitus). Breakdown of the human immune system under stress makes the body less capable of fighting spontaneous tumors, cancers,

and infectious disease. The net result from physiological stress is illness, poor weight maintenance, disease, rapid aging, and death.

Stress reduction should be a prime focus of medical research and education. The simplicity of educating the public with respect to stress can yield incredible savings in terms of lives saved, quality of lives improved, length of human life spans increased, and money saved. Some researchers propose that stress reduction not only can yield enormous health benefits but also can produce greater industrial productivity, happier people, and considerably less crime. It is expected that additional research into oxytocin, the tend-and-befriend response, and yet undiscovered mechanisms of stress response will contribute meaningfully to decreased stress and increased mental and physical well-being.

—*David Wason Hollar Jr., Nancy A. Piotrowski*

References

Creagan, Edward T. "How to Manage Stress and Avoid Overeating When Stressed." *Mayo Clinic,* Mayo Foundation for Medical Education and Research, 20 July 2017, www.mayoclinic.org/healthy-lifestyle/stress-management/expert-answers/stress/faq-20058497.

Koski, Marja, and Hannu Naukkarinen. "The Relationship between Stress and Severe Obesity: A Case-Control Study." *Biomedicine Hub,* vol. 2, no. 1, 3 Mar. 2017, pp. 1–13., doi:10.1159/000458771.

Rapaport, Lisa. "More Evidence Linking Stress to Obesity." *Reuters,* 30 Mar. 2017, www.reuters.com/article/us-health-stress-cortisol-obesity/more-evidence-linking-stress-to-obesity-idUSKBN17130P.

Valk, Eline S. Van Der, et al. "Stress and Obesity: Are There More Susceptible Individuals?" *Current Obesity Reports,* vol. 7, no. 2, 16 Apr. 2018, pp. 193–203., doi:10.1007/s13679-018-0306-y.

Whiteman, Honor. "Chronic Stress May Raise Obesity Risk." *Medical News Today,* 27 Feb. 2017, www.medicalnewstoday.com/articles/316074.

"Why Stress Causes People to Overeat." *Harvard Health Blog,* Harvard Medical School, 18 July 2018, www.health.harvard.edu/staying-healthy/why-stress-causes-people-to-overeat.

Xenaki, Niovi, et al. "Impact of a Stress Management Program on Weight Loss, Mental Health and Lifestyle in Adults with Obesity: a Randomized Controlled Trial." *Journal of Molecular Biochemistry,* vol. 7, no. 2, 3 Oct. 2018, pp. 78–84.

■ Sugar

CATEGORY: Nutrition

Causes and Symptoms

Island inhabitants of New Guinea were the first to notice that chewing a piece of raw sugar cane caused the release of a sudden sweet taste in the mouth. Eventually sugar was transported to other islands and to Asia. Muslim warriors carried it to the lands where they fought. Europeans were introduced to sugar during the Crusades. European explorers sailed for new lands, carrying sugar plants to establish crops. Soon, sugar was in high demand.

The white crystalline substance familiar as sugar has been processed from the sugar plant for centuries. However, these plants only grow in certain climates, limiting sugar's availability. Later, it was discovered that sugar beets could be processed to produce sugar, and growers learned ways to increase sugar cane crops. The availability of sugar expanded, but demand continued to grow. Industrialization added to the number and types of food produced commercially, many of which included sugar. Where people once had to take time to make cookies, cakes, or candy, commercially packaged versions became readily available. This, along with sweetened beverages such as soda, increased the amount of processed sugar people consumed.

Sugar is not necessarily bad. The human body needs glucose to generate energy and glucose is the most important fuel source for the brain and a key nutrient for the rest of the body. However, processed sugar contains sixteen calories per teaspoon and has no other nutritional value. Sugar from fruit contains the same number of calories and provides the same energy, but also contains other beneficial nutrients such as fiber, vitamins, and minerals. Experts have raised concerns about what happens to the body when a large portion one's daily calories come from sugar in processed foods as opposed to natural sugar sources. Two concerns include the negative effects of excess sugar on the body, and that a person eating sugary foods may not consume foods with greater nutritional value.

Disorders and Diseases

Connections between sugar and health were first made in the seventeenth century when, in the absence of sophisticated medical tests, British physician Thomas Willis (1621-1675) noticed the sweet taste of the urine of people with diabetes. During the nineteenth century, physicians noticed that people who ate more sugar had a greater chance of being overweight and had high blood pressure and diabetes. Subsequent research has indicated the extent to which sugar may play a role in health.

A study published in 2014 in the *Journal of the American Medical Association* (JAMA) reported that the average American eats more sugar than the recommended daily amount, which is 5 to 15 percent of daily calories. Assuming an average calorie intake of two thousand calories a day, this means about one hundred to three hundred calories a day, less than the amount of sugar in one-to-two cans of soda. According to the researchers, most Americans, from 2005-2010, derived about one tenth of their calories from "added" sugar, which refers to sugar added to foods during processing or preparation. However, the study found about 10 percent of the population, during the same time period, consumed an average of 25 percent or more of their calories from added sugar. Sugar comes from obvious sources, such as sugar-sweetened sodas and energy drinks. Other inconspicuous dietary sugar sources may include breads, sauces, condiments, processed meats, and vitamins. Consumers must read labels for names like corn syrup, sucrose, maltose, and dextrose, among others.

Many studies have shown a correlation between sugar consumption and negative health effects, such as increased weight and elevated blood sugar, blood pressure, and serum cholesterol. One study showed dramatic drops in levels of these important health measures in as few as nine days when children were put on a diet that reduced sugar without reducing calories. Other conditions linked to ingesting too much sugar include obesity and non-alcoholic fatty liver as well as increased risk for metabolic disease, type 2 diabetes, cardiovascular disease, oral cavities, inflammation, rheumatoid arthritis, sexual dysfunction, and even cancer. Continued research on the impact of sugar on health is needed.

The 2014 JAMA study found that people who consumed 21 percent or more of their daily calories from sugar had twice the chance of dying from

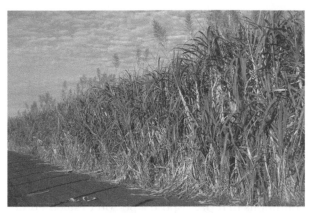

Sugar cane plantation ready for harvest. (Mariordo)

heart disease than someone who did not. This held true even if the person ate mostly healthy food. The study did not determine exactly why sugar had such a negative effect, but researchers noted that sugar causes arteries to grow thicker and more dense, which raises blood pressure, a known risk factor for heart disease. They theorized that excessive amounts of sugar might cause the liver to release more fat into the blood stream, another known risk factor.

Sugar is known to increase the amount of fat that accumulates around the internal organs, especially the liver. A high-sugar diet increases the likelihood of diabetes by straining the metabolic systems the body uses to process and remove sugar from the body. The way the body processes sugar can lead to energy crashes, when the body quickly burns through sugar in a candy bar or soda and becomes tired from the decrease in easily accessible fuel.

Researchers have found some evidence that sugar acts as an addictive substance. Sugar affects the release of dopamine and natural opioids in the body, chemicals that increase feelings of well-being. People can come to crave this feeling and build a tolerance for sugar so that it takes more sugar to reach this state. It is thought that sugar interferes with the body's natural system for regulating appetite, causing the body to not release enough leptin, an appetite-regulating hormone. The body continues to send out hunger signals even when enough food has been consumed. This can lead to excess weight, a risk factor for heart disease and diabetes.

—*Janine Ungvarsky, Marylane Wade Koch*

References

Bentley, R. Alexander, et al. "U.S. Obesity as Delayed Effect of Excess Sugar." *Economics & Human Biology*, vol. 36, 2020, p. 100818., doi:10.1016/j.ehb.2019.100818.

Bray, George A., and Barry M. Popkin. "Dietary Sugar and Body Weight: Have We Reached a Crisis in the Epidemic of Obesity and Diabetes?" *Diabetes Care*, vol. 37, no. 4, 20 Apr. 2014, pp. 950–956., doi:10.2337/dc13-2085.

Carmel, Molly. *Breaking up with Sugar: a Plan to Divorce the Diets, Drop the Pounds, and Live Your Best Life.* Avery, 2019.

Corliss, Julie. "Eating Too Much Added Sugar Increases the Risk of Dying with Heart Disease." *Harvard Health Blog*, Harvard Medical School, 27 Aug. 2019, www.health.harvard.edu/blog/eating-too-much-added-sugar-increases-the-risk-of-dying-with-heart-disease-201402067021.

European Association for the Study of Obesity. "Analysis of New Studies Including 250,000 People Confirms Sugar-Sweetened Drinks Are Linked to Overweight and Obesity in Children and Adults." *ScienceDaily*, 23 Dec. 2017.

Fox, Maggie. "Cutting Processed Sugar for Just 9 Days May Improve Health." *Today*, NBC Universal, 4 Oct. 2016, www.today.com/health/cutting-processed-sugar-just-9-days-has-striking-effect-health-t52516.

Luger, Maria, et al. "Sugar-Sweetened Beverages and Weight Gain in Children and Adults: A Systematic Review from 2013 to 2015 and a Comparison with Previous Studies." *Obesity Facts*, vol. 10, no. 6, 2017, pp. 674–693., doi:10.1159/000484566.

Nordqvist, Joseph. "How Much Sugar Is in Your Food and Drink?" *Medical News Today*, 7 July 2013, www.medicalnewstoday.com/articles/262978.php.

Ruanpeng, D., et al. "Sugar and Artificially Sweetened Beverages Linked to Obesity: a Systematic Review and Meta-Analysis." *QJM: An International Journal of Medicine*, vol. 110, no. 8, 11 Apr. 2017, pp. 513–520., doi:10.1093/qjmed/hcx068.

Stanhope, Kimber L. "Sugar Consumption, Metabolic Disease and Obesity: The State of the Controversy." *Critical Reviews in Clinical Laboratory Sciences*, vol. 53, no. 1, 17 Sept. 2015, pp. 52–67., doi:10.3109/10408363.2015.1084990.

■ Sugar addiction

CATEGORY: Nutrition

Sugar addiction is the compulsive physiological need for sugar. This compulsive need constitutes a behavioral addiction, an interpretation that is reinforced when sugar addicts, long habituated to large amounts of sugar, experience classic withdrawal symptoms when their sugar intake is reduced.

Causes

Just as the search for explanations of addiction to alcohol and other drugs has been complicated by the nature-nurture debate, so too have been the controversies over sugar addiction. Some medical researchers and physicians believe that sugar addiction might be genetic, that is, that the biological nature of certain humans or, more specifically, the information programmed into their deoxyribonucleic acid (DNA), can explain why some people become addicted to sugar (in a way similar to how others become addicted to, for example, alcohol, nicotine, or heroin).

Other researchers have traced the pleasurable physiological state (popularly known as a sugar high) induced by an intake of sugar to the activation of certain receptors in the brain. Sugar is said to affect the same neurotransmitters in the brain associated with the pleasure produced by such substances as nicotine in cigarette smoke.

Those who emphasize the cultural rather than the genetic causes of physiological addiction to sugar point out that refined sugar (or sucrose, largely derived from sugar cane and sugar beets) has been a relatively recent addition to the human diet. Throughout most of the evolution of Homo sapiens and the early history of civilized humans, the dietary need for glucose was satisfied by the ingestion of fruits, vegetables, and fats, which could, as needed, be metabolized into glucose.

Even after techniques were discovered allowing sugar to be extracted from plants, most humans were unable to use this sugar because of its expense. Sugar did not become an inexpensive commodity until the eighteenth century, when doctors began to discover some of its negative effects on the human body. For some historians, the origin of sugar addiction can be traced to this period, when laborers could be inexpensively fed with sweetened

foods and drinks rather than with costly meats, fruits, and vegetables.

Contemporary analysts now believe that sugar addiction has both genetic and cultural causes. However, because of the uniqueness of every person's biochemistry, it is difficult if not impossible to precisely divide causality for this relatively recent medical phenomenon into its biological and environmental sources.

Risk Factors

Scientists have discovered a number of medical conditions that predispose a person to sugar addiction. For example, a weak adrenal gland results in an insufficient quantity of glucocorticoid hormones to properly regulate glucose levels in the blood, leading to an intense craving for sugar. Furthermore, persons with a penchant for overeating are often susceptible to sugar addiction.

Cultural factors also can pose risks. For instance, in many advanced societies the processed food industries add massive amounts of refined sugar to numerous products, thus allowing for large numbers of suitably predisposed persons to become sugar addicts.

Symptoms

A common symptom of sugar addiction is the overpowering urge, several times a day, to consume something sweet. If afflicted persons are unable to satisfy these urges, they often feel weak, apathetic, and dizzy. These symptoms may be relieved by the ingestion of sugar-containing foods and sweetened beverages, but continued dependence on sugar results in tolerance with increased consumption needed to relieve symptoms and re-experience the pleasurable feelings that sugar consumption initially created.

With the removal of sugar from the addict's diet, withdrawal symptoms often occur, such as tremors of the extremities, painful headaches, and digestive difficulties, including nausea. Psychological symptoms include irritability, depression, and drastic mood changes.

Researchers have noted numerous long-term health problems associated with sugar addiction, including such well-known consequences as obesity and dental decay. The American Diabetes Association regards the overconsumption of sugar as a major cause of degenerative diseases in the United

States, including diabetes, heart disease, and cancer. Sugar also has a negative effect on the body's immune system by depleting white blood cells, thus reducing this system's ability to fight infectious agents.

Screening and Diagnosis

Screening for sugar addiction has not been a part of most routine physical examinations, with the exception of physical exams of the obese and of persons showing clear symptoms. For those who believe that sugar addiction is endemic to Western society, this neglect to screen for the addiction imperils the health of many people.

This lack of monitoring for sugar addiction has led to numerous books on this disorder, many of which contain guidelines for self-diagnosis. However, self-diagnoses can be inaccurate, even dangerous. Blood tests exist to monitor symptoms before and after the ingestion of sugar, and these tests can provide reliable evidence leading to a diagnosis of sugar addiction.

Treatment and Therapy

According to some advocates, the world is facing a crisis centered on the treatment of sugar addiction that faces several cultural barriers. Sugar has become "a legalized recreational drug" that is "socially acceptable to consume." Sugar addiction is considered an acceptable addiction, one wholly separate from other addictions; this is an alarming perspective to those calling for prevention and treatment of sugar addiction.

The treatment of sugar addicts is also hindered by the denial of their dependence in a manner reminiscent of classic drug addicts. Also, similar to another addictive product—tobacco—countries frequently subsidize sugar production because of its importance to their economies. Furthermore, it is common for sugar and its presence in numerous foods and drinks to receive much more legal immunity than tobacco.

Therapy for sugar addiction can be a long and difficult process. Sugar addicts should not expect their sugar cravings to vanish in a few weeks or months. Most physicians and nutritionists begin treatment with diet modification. After tests, doctors generally attempt to stabilize blood sugar levels by getting their sugar-addicted patients to eat modest meals rich in protein. A nutritious breakfast is especially important, as is the elimination of sugar and artificial sweeteners from all meals and snacks.

Some doctors insist on treating sugar addiction the way they treat alcohol and other drug addictions, that is, by insisting their patients avoid all refined sugars and sugar-containing foods and drinks from their diet. This can be daunting because so many processed foods contain fructose, dextrose, maltose, and other sugary additives such as corn syrup. Some nutritionists even suggest a drastic reduction in the consumption of fresh fruits and fruit juices, which contain sugar. Others, though, allow some fruit in the diet during the transition to a totally sugar-free diet.

Doctors also can prescribe medicines that may help reduce the craving for sugar, and nutritionists may advise recovering sugar addicts to take amino acids, such as glutamine and tyrosine, to help reduce cravings. Others have found that chromium supplements help to balance blood sugar.

Orthomolecular physicians believe that good health can be achieved by balancing substances normally present in the body or by adding essential vitamins and minerals to the diet. These practitioners tend to agree with believers in sugar addiction that this sweet substance is alien to the body and poses a danger to health. For orthomolecular physicians, megavitamin therapy, along with the elimination of sugars and other processed foods that are incompatible with the body's normal and natural array of molecules, is optimum for health.

Other therapies add behavioral modifications for the treatment of sugar addiction. These therapies include exercise, especially relaxed walking, and eight hours of sleep every night. For serious cases, some professionals recommend psychotherapy, because certain patients become addicted to sugar to assuage feelings of loneliness or self-hatred. Therapists often try to discover why patients crave sugar; oftentimes, this craving is caused by past trauma.

With increasing awareness of sugar addiction, many treatment options have become available. Professionals now promote their services in treating this disorder. Treatment centers that include group therapy for sugar addiction also are available.

Prevention

Curbing sugar addiction involves both the individual and society. Even those skeptical of this addiction agree that most persons consume far too much sugar and that this overconsumption contributes to many health problems. Evolution has not prepared the human body to handle an average intake of 150 to 300 pounds of sugar each year. Several states in the United States have failed in their attempts to put a tax on sugary soft drinks. In concept, the prevention of sugar addiction is simple: Drastically reduce sugar consumption. In reality, though, individuals and societies rarely are willing to accomplish this.

—*Robert J. Paradowski*

References

Bray, George A. "Is Sugar Addictive?" Diabetes, vol. 65, no. 7, 2016, pp. 1797–1799., doi:10.2337/dbi16-0022.

Bray, George A., and Barry M. Popkin. "Dietary Sugar and Body Weight: Have We Reached a Crisis in the Epidemic of Obesity and Diabetes?" Diabetes Care, vol. 37, no. 4, 2014, pp. 950–956., doi:10.2337/dc13-2085.

Lerma-Cabrera, Jose Manuel, et al. "Food Addiction as a New Piece of the Obesity Framework." Nutrition Journal, vol. 15, no. 1, 2015, doi:10.1186/s12937-016-0124-6.

"The Sweet Danger of Sugar." Harvard Health Publishing, Harvard Medical School, 6 Nov. 2015, www.health.harvard.edu/heart-health/the-sweet-danger-of-sugar.

Westwater, Margaret L., et al. "Sugar Addiction: the State of the Science." European Journal of Nutrition, vol. 55, no. S2, 2016, pp. 55–69., doi:10.1007/s00394-016-1229-6.

Wiss, David A., et al. "Sugar Addiction: From Evolution to Revolution." Frontiers in Psychiatry, vol. 9, 2018, doi:10.3389/fpsyt.2018.00545.

■ Sugar-sweetened soft drinks

CATEGORY: Nutrition

Soft drinks (commonly called soda) are carbonated beverages that are sweetened with either a caloric sugar sweetener or a noncaloric sweetener. Many soft drinks also contain caffeine. The caloric sweetener that is typically used to sweeten soft drinks is high-fructose corn syrup (HFCS). Soft drinks that are sweetened with a noncaloric sweetener are commonly referred to as diet soft drinks, and are typically sweetened with the artificial sweetener aspartame. Global soft drink sales have increased in recent decades.

With an estimated increase of 300% in soft drink consumption in the past 20 years, sugar-sweetened soft drinks are now considered the leading source of added sugar in the traditional Western diet, particularly in younger persons (i.e., persons under 40 years of age). This increase in consumption of sugar-sweetened soft drinks parallels the dramatic increase in rates of obesity over the past 2 decades. Researchers believe that the increased consumption of sugar-sweetened soft drinks and the high prevalence of obesity are intimately connected. However, drinking diet soft drinks instead of sugar-sweetened soft drinks does not appear to prevent obesity. In fact, researchers report that when compared with persons who do not consume diet soft drinks, consumers of diet soft drinks have a 70% larger waist circumference; researchers also report that intake of 1 or more diet soft drinks a day is linked to an increased risk for stroke.

The HFCS in sugar-sweetened soft drinks contains the monosaccharide (i.e., simple sugar) fructose, glucose, and processed starches, which accelerate the absorption of fructose. Unlike glucose, fructose cannot be stored as glycogen to be used as energy; if consumed in large amounts, fructose is likely to be converted to fat by the liver. Fat that is synthesized by the liver is released into the bloodstream as very low density lipoproteins (VLDLs), which is a form of cholesterol that is known to contribute to coronary artery disease (CAD).

Many soft drinks (e.g., Coke, Pepsi, Dr. Pepper, Mountain Dew) contain caffeine. Results of studies show that caffeine increases energy, awakens and clears the mind, and reduces the risk for depression. The primary action of caffeine is antagonism of the adenosine receptor. Adenosine dilates blood vessels and facilitates sleep. By binding with the adenosine receptor, caffeine interferes with the ability of adenosine to slow the body down. The result is increased neural activity (e.g., alertness, wakefulness). Caffeine is readily absorbed, and its effects last 4–6 hours. If consumed too close to bedtime, caffeine can interfere with the ability to fall asleep, and negatively affect sleep patterns.

The consumption of both sugar-sweetened and diet soft drinks is associated with poor dietary and

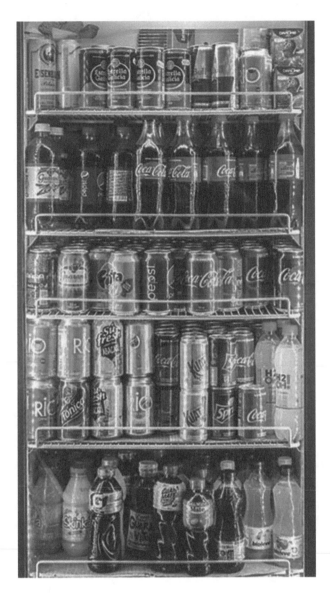

Researchers report that large amounts of fructose consumption can result in visceral fat accumulation (i.e., in the abdominal cavity) and insulin resistance. Because fructose is converted to fat and stored in the liver, researchers are concerned that excessive intake of HFCS-sweetened soft drinks can contribute to non-alcoholic fatty liver disease (NAFLD).

Summary

Consumers should become knowledgeable about the physiologic risks of sugar-sweetened soft drink consumption, specifically those with risk factors for obesity, DM2, and heart disease. Consumers should also be aware of the benefits of limiting sugar-sweetened soft drink consumption, and eating a balanced diet that includes unsaturated fats, lean proteins, complex carbohydrates, and a wide variety of fresh fruits and vegetables. Research suggests that drinking diet soft drinks instead of sugar-sweetened soft drinks does not appear to prevent obesity, and that consuming 1 or more diet soft drinks a day is associated with an increased risk for stroke.

References

Bleich, Sara N., and Kelsey A. Vercammen. "The Negative Impact of Sugar-Sweetened Beverages on Children's Health: an Update of the Literature." BMC Obesity, vol. 5, no. 1, 2018, doi:10.1186/s40608-017-0178-9.

"Get the Facts: Sugar-Sweetened Beverages and Consumption." Centers for Disease Control and Prevention, 27 Feb. 2017, www.cdc.gov/nutrition/data-statistics/sugar-sweetened-beverages-intake.html.

Keller, Amélie, and Sophie Bucher Della Torre. "Sugar-Sweetened Beverages and Obesity among Children and Adolescents: A Review of Systematic Literature Reviews." Childhood Obesity, vol. 11, no. 4, 2015, pp. 338–346., doi:10.1089/chi.2014.0117.

"Sugary Drinks." The Nutrition Source, Harvard School of Public Health, 16 Oct. 2019, www.hsph.harvard.edu/nutritionsource/healthy-drinks/sugary-drinks/.

Torre, Sophie Bucher Della, et al. "Sugar-Sweetened Beverages and Obesity Risk in Children and Adolescents: A Systematic Analysis on How Methodological Quality May Influence Conclusions." Journal of the Academy of Nutrition and Dietetics, vol. 116, no. 4, 2016, pp. 638–659., doi:10.1016/j.jand.2015.05.020.

lifestyle choices, including higher intake of fast foods, unhealthy snacks, and sugary desserts; as well as lower intake of fruits and vegetables, less night-time sleep, and less regular exercise.

Research Findings

The intake of sugar-sweetened soft drinks has been shown to increase postprandial (i.e., after meals) blood glucose levels, decrease insulin sensitivity, and reduce the sensation of fullness, which results in overeating. Results of studies have linked the consumption of sugar-sweetened soft drinks to excessive weight gain, increased risk for type 2 diabetes mellitus (DM2), and increased triglycerides.

■ Trans Fat

CATEGORY: Nutrition

Trans fats exist naturally in many foods (e.g., fat in dairy products, lamb, and beef) in small amounts, but most are the result of hydrogenation (i.e., a process that involves adding hydrogen to the double bond of unsaturated fatty acids). Because unsaturated fats are generally liquid at room temperature, some food manufacturers hydrogenate fats to form a solid. Hydrogenation is also used to increase the shelf-life and stability of fatty acids.

Most food sources of trans fats are processed and packaged foods (e.g., cookies, potato chips, fast foods). Although trans fats exist naturally in many foods in small amounts, most are found in processed foods such as margarine, fast foods, packaged cookies, crackers, and potato chips, fried foods, foods that contain "partially hydrogenated fat," "hydrogenated fat," or "shortening" in the list of labeled ingredients.

Trans fats have been shown to increase the risk of heart disease by increasing blood levels of low-density lipoprotein (LDL) cholesterol, lowering high-density lipoprotein (HDL) cholesterol levels, and increasing platelet coagulation (i.e., blood clotting). Additionally, the consumption of trans fats has been associated with a significant increase in the risk for type 2 diabetes mellitus (DM2) and cancer of the breast and colon.

It is currently recommended that dietary intake of trans fat be limited to less than 1% of total daily caloric consumption. Trans fats are not nutritionally necessary and a recent review of available literature found no information on trans fat deficiency.

Research Findings

In addition to certain health risks (e.g., heart disease, cancer, DM2) associated with trans fat consumption, researchers report a connection between trans fat intake and mental health. Results of a study conducted on older adults without dementia showed that high blood levels of trans fats are strongly linked with poor overall cognitive function. Results indicated that high consumption of trans fats has a detrimental impact on memory, language, attention, and mental processing speed. Researchers who conducted a separate study, which included 5,038 men and 7,021 women with an

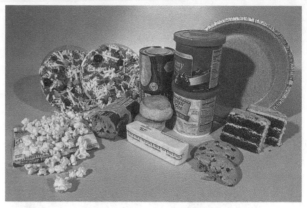

A variety of processed foods, including frozen, canned and baked goods, containing trans fat. (U.S. Food and Drug Administration)

average age of 37.5, reported that individuals with the highest trans fat intake were at a significantly elevated risk for developing depression.

Summary

Individuals should learn about the physiologic effects of trans fat consumption. High trans fat intake is associated with increased risk for heart disease, heart attack, stroke, DM2, dementia, gallstones, infertility, and certain cancers (e.g., colon cancer, breast cancer). Avoiding foods that contain "partially hydrogenated fat," "hydrogenated fat," or "shortening" in the list of labeled ingredients; margarine; fast foods; fried foods; and packaged cookies, crackers, and potato chips is recommended. Dietary intake of trans fat should be limited to less than 1% of total daily caloric consumption. Research suggests that trans fat may be have a negative impact on cognitive ability.

—Cherie Marcel

References

Cunningham, Aimee. "Ban on Artificial Trans Fats in NYC Restaurants Seems to Be Working." *Science News*, 8 Aug. 2019, www.sciencenews.org/article/ban-artificial-trans-fats-nyc-restaurants-appears-be-working.

Liu, Ann G., et al. "A Healthy Approach to Dietary Fats: Understanding the Science and Taking Action to Reduce Consumer Confusion." *Nutrition Journal*, vol. 16, no. 1, 30 Aug. 2017, doi:10.1186/s12937-017-0271-4.

Parziale, Andrea, and Gorik Ooms. "The Global Fight against Trans-Fat: the Potential Role of

International Trade and Law." *Globalization and Health*, vol. 15, no. 1, 11 July 2019, doi:10.1186/s12992-019-0488-4.

Souza, Russell J De, et al. "Intake of Saturated and Trans Unsaturated Fatty Acids and Risk of All Cause Mortality, Cardiovascular Disease, and Type 2 Diabetes: Systematic Review and Meta-Analysis of Observational Studies." *BMJ*, 11 Aug. 2015, doi:10.1136/bmj.h3978.

Wanders, Anne, et al. "Trans Fat Intake and Its Dietary Sources in General Populations Worldwide: A Systematic Review." *Nutrients*, vol. 9, no. 8, 5 Aug. 2017, p. 840, doi:10.3390/nu9080840.

Related Conditions, Diseases, and Comorbidities

◼ Angina

CATEGORY: Disorder

Causes and Symptoms

Usually located below the sternum, angina may radiate down the left arm and/or left jaw, or down both arms and jaws. It is ischemic in nature, meaning that the pain is produced by a variety of conditions that result in insufficient supply of oxygen-rich blood to the heart. Some examples include arteriosclerosis (hardening of the arteries), atherosclerosis (arteries clogged with deposits of fat, cholesterol, and other substances), coronary artery spasms, low blood pressure, low blood volume, vasoconstriction (a narrowing of the arteries), anemia, and chronic lung disease.

Precipitating factors for angina include physical exertion, strong emotions, consumption of a heavy meal, temperature extremes, cigarette smoking, and sexual activity. These factors can cause angina because they may increase heart rate, cause vasoconstriction, or divert blood from the heart to other areas, such as the gastrointestinal system. Angina usually lasts from three to five minutes and commonly subsides when the precipitating factors are relieved. Typically, it should not last more than twenty minutes after rest or treatment.

Diagnosis consists of a physical examination which includes a chest X ray to determine any obvious lung or structural cardiac abnormalities; blood tests to screen risk factors such as lipids or to detect enzymes that can indicate if a heart attack has occurred; electrocardiography (ECG or EKG) to look at the electrical activity of the heart for evidence of damage or insufficient blood flow; nuclear studies such as thallium stress tests, which measure myocardial perfusion; and cardiac catheterization and coronary angiography to evaluate the anatomy of the coronary arteries, the location and nature of artery narrowing or constriction, and to assess the muscular function of the heart, including cardiac output.

Treatment depends on the specific cause of the angina. Three types of drugs are the most common form of treatment: nitrates, to increase the supply of oxygen to the heart by dilating the coronary arteries; beta-blockers, to lower oxygen demand during exercise and improve oxygen supply and demand; and calcium blockers, to decrease the work of the heart by decreasing cardiac contractility. A study published in March 2013 found that the drug Ranexa (ranolazine) might reduce symptoms of angina in patients with type 2 diabetes.

—*John A. Bavaro*

References

Kloner, Robert A., and Bernard Chaitman. "Angina and Its Management." *Journal of Cardiovascular Pharmacology and Therapeutics*, vol. 22, no. 3, 14 Dec. 2016, pp. 199–209.

Kreatsoulas, Catherine, et al. "Interpreting Angina: Symptoms along a Gender Continuum." *Open Heart*, vol. 3, no. 1, 2016, doi:10.1136/openhrt-2015-000376.

Luca, Leonardo De, et al. "Characteristics, Treatment and Quality of Life of Stable Coronary Artery Disease Patients with or without Angina: Insights from the START Study." *Plos One*, vol. 13, no. 7, 12 July 2018, doi:10.1371/journal.pone.0199770.

Nall, Rachel. "Unstable Angina." *Healthline*, 30 May 2017, www.healthline.com/health/unstable-angina.

Wee, Yong, et al. "Medical Management of Chronic Stable Angina." *Australian Prescriber*, vol. 38, no. 4, 1 Aug. 2015, pp. 131–136., doi:10.18773/austprescr.2015.042.

■ Arterial plaque

CATEGORY: Disorder
ALSO KNOWN AS: Atheroma, atheromatous plaque

Causes and Symptoms

Arterial plaques are caused by a buildup of cholesterol and cell debris within arterial walls. This process occurs over a period of decades, starting at local sites of arterial inflammation. Low-density lipoproteins carrying cholesterol (LDL-C) that infiltrate these sites are highly susceptible to oxidation, which activates another inflammatory response that summons macrophages (part of the immune system). The macrophages engulf the oxidized LDL-C and accumulate as bloated foam cells along with some other cells to become a fatty streak. A tug-of-war ensues in which cholesterol continues to accumulate while other processes remove it. When too much cholesterol accumulates, a scablike cap is formed, while other processes slowly calcify the plaque from the bottom up. This strategy works well as long as the cap does not crack; a cracked cap leaks debris into the artery, which triggers thrombosis (clotting). Blockage of a large coronary artery causes a heart attack; blockage of arteries feeding the brain causes a stroke. Clots that are not fully occlusive get degraded, but repeated rounds of plaque rupturing and recapping eventually cause stenosis (narrowing of the artery) and ischemia (oxygen starvation).

Treatment and Therapy

Treatment begins with lifestyle changes-exercising, managing stress, stopping smoking, lowering blood pressure, eating more fruits and vegetables. The next step is reducing high levels of LDL-C using statins, which also provide antioxidant, anti-inflammatory, and plaque-stabilizing benefits. Bile acid sequestrants and cholesterol absorption inhibitors are sometimes used as well. Fibrates and niacin are used to counteract LDL-C by boosting HDL-C, the high-density lipoprotein or "good" cholesterol. High blood pressure is typically treated using diuretics, beta blockers, or angiotensin-converting enzyme (ACE) inhibitors. Thrombosis risk is reduced using low-dose aspirin or drugs such as warfarin, clopidogrel, and prasugrel. Stenosis can be treated using nitroglycerin, ranolazine, and calcium-channel inhibitors to help arteries dilate. A common surgical procedure is to physically open the artery using a catheter, often done in conjunction with implanting a stent to keep the artery propped open. Surgery can also be used to scrape out arteries or replace them.

Perspective and Prospects

Once plaques reach their later stages of development, they are extremely difficult, if not impossible, to remove. Prospects are best when lifestyle changes are initiated early in adulthood. Blood tests for assessing risk factors are invaluable; the most useful ones measure fasting levels of glucose, total cholesterol, LDL-C, HDL-C, triglycerides, homocysteine, and C-reactive protein (a marker of inflammation). Monitoring and controlling blood pressure is also vitally important.

—*Brad Rikke, Ph.D.*

References

Csige, Imre, et al. "The Impact of Obesity on the Cardiovascular System." *Journal of Diabetes Research*, vol. 2018, 4 Nov. 2018, pp. 1–12., doi:10.1155/2018/3407306.

King, Rhodri J, and Ramzi A Ajjan. "Vascular Risk in Obesity: Facts, Misconceptions and the Unknown." *Diabetes and Vascular Disease Research*, vol. 14, no. 1, 14 Nov. 2016, pp. 2–13., doi:10.1177/1479164116675488.

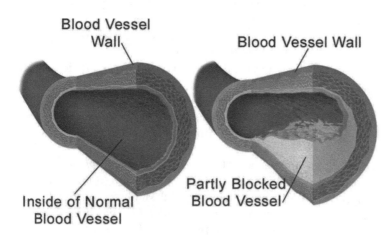

Normal and Partly Blocked Blood Vessel

Source: BruceBlaus

Mendizábal, Brenda, and Elaine M. Urbina. "Subclinical Atherosclerosis in Youth: Relation to Obesity, Insulin Resistance, and Polycystic Ovary Syndrome." *The Journal of Pediatrics*, vol. 190, 2017, pp. 14–20., doi:10.1016/j.jpeds.2017.06.043.

Roever, Leonardo S., et al. "Abdominal Obesity and Association With Atherosclerosis Risk Factors." *Medicine*, vol. 95, no. 11, 2016, doi:10.1097/md.0000000000001357.

■ Bipolar disorder

CATEGORY: Psychology

Bipolar disorder (BD; also called manic-depressive disorder) refers to a mental health condition that is characterized by episodes of mania and depression and dramatic fluctuations in energy, activity, and mental clarity. BD can greatly disable the affected person's ability to function in relationships, school, work, and normal daily activities (e.g., grocery shopping, paying bills, preparing meals).Risk of suicide is significantly higher in individuals with BD than in persons with good mental health. According to the *Diagnostic and Statistical Manual of Mental Disorders, 5th Edition (DSM-5)*, there are several types of BD that are classified based on the duration and severity of manic-depressive episodes, including BD type I, BD type II, rapid cycling BD, cyclothymic BD, mixed affective BD, and BD not otherwise specified).

Treatment of BD with Medication

BD is a lifelong illness that requires continuous treatment, including medication (e.g., mood stabilizers, antidepressants), psychotherapy, and lifestyle modifications (e.g., adequate sleep, healthy diet, exercise).

Many types of medication (e.g., mood stabilizers [e.g., lithium], anticonvulsants [e.g., valproic acid], anti-psychotics [e.g., Seroquel]) are prescribed singly or in combination to treat BD. These medications can have adverse effects that impact appetite, nutrient intake, and weight. Adverse effects that affect diet include weight gain, stomach pain, thyroid abnormalities, weakness, fatigue, and drowsiness, diarrhea or constipation, and nausea and vertigo.

It is important to note whether or not the prescribed medication should be taken with meals because food can affect the bioavailability of certain medications. For example, the medication ziprasidone should be taken with a meal containing at least 500 calories in order to achieve optimal bioavailability; absorption of ziprasidone is decreased by half if taken in a fasting state

Dietary Considerations for BD

Diet affects mental health through the action of nutrients on the brain and nervous system, and the relationship between diet and mental health is complex and cyclical. Mental illness can impair one's ability to prepare and consume a healthy meal, and nutrient deficiencies can result in

SIGNS AND SYMPTOMS OF BD	
Manic Episodes	**Depressive Episodes**
◦ Elevated energy and activity	◦ Depressed mood
◦ Inflated self-image and a sense of grandiosity	◦ Lack of interest in activity
◦ Reckless behavior with a lack of self-control (e.g., excessive spending, promiscuity, binge eating, substance abuse)	◦ Fatigue
	◦ Feelings of hopelessness and worthlessness, or inappropriate guilt
◦ Easily agitated and highly irritable	◦ Inability to concentrate or make decision s
◦ Racing thoughts but easily distracted	◦ Suicidal thoughts, plans, or attempts
◦ Little desire for sleep	◦ Significant change in weight (e.g., weight gain or loss)
	◦ Change in appetite (e.g., excessive eating or lack of interest in food)

cognitive decline. Results of studies indicate that persons with a mental health disorder are more likely to be overweight and have significantly poorer nutrient intake than persons with good mental health. Persons with BD tend to be erratic in their dietary patterns. During manic-depressive episodes they can experience appetite changes, loss of interest in food, poor self-control, and/or inability to procure or prepare food due to mental instability. Additionally, many of the medications prescribed for the treatment of BD can have a dramatic affect on appetite and weight.

Carbohydrates (CHOs) metabolize to glucose, the body's primary source of energy. At rest, the brain uses 20–30% of a person's energy consumption. If caloric intake is inadequate to fuel basic energy requirements, cognition decreases. CHO intake results in the release of insulin. Insulin stimulates the uptake of large neutral amino acids (LNAAs) in muscle, but it has no effect on the amino acid tryptophan (TRP), which results in an increased ratio of TRP to LNAAs and elevated levels of TRP in the brain. TRP contributes to the synthesis of serotonin, which is a neurotransmitter that calms mood, improves sleep patterns, increases pain tolerance, and reduces food cravings. Low levels of serotonin in the brain are associated with depression, anxiety, panic disorder, obsessive-compulsive disorder (OCD), and attention deficit hyperactivity disorder (ADHD), all of which are commonly associated with BD.

Simple CHOs, or simple sugars (e.g., low-fiber breads and cereals, sugary foods), break down quickly, giving the body a rapid dose of energy, but only for a short duration. Eating a high amount of simple CHOs can produce spikes and drops in insulin and glucose levels, resulting in fluctuating moods. High consumption of simple CHOs has been associated with increased depression in adults and mood swings in children with otherwise good mental health.

Complex CHOs (e.g., high-fiber, whole grain breads and cereals) take longer to metabolize than simple CHOs, providing the body with a slower release of energy over a longer period of time. This helps to maintain normal glucose levels and stabilize mood.

Protein-rich foods (e.g., eggs, lean meats, dairy products, beans) provide the amino acids, tyrosine (TYR) and TRP, both of which are vital for the production of important neurotransmitters (i.e., chemicals that facilitate the transmission of signals between cells). Mental energy and alertness are increased by the neurotransmitters norepinephrine and dopamine, which are manufactured from TYR with the help of folate, magnesium, and vitamin B12. TRP is the precursor to the neurotransmitter serotonin, which stabilizes mood. Eating meals that are high in protein results in a high amount of amino acids competing with TRP for entry to the brain. Eating meals that contain a balance of protein and CHO results in normal release of insulin to facilitate the redistribution of the competing amino acids, allowing TRP to cross the blood-brain barrier.

The brain is largely composed of fat, especially the essential fatty acids (EFAs) omega-3 and omega-6. EFAs are considered essential because they are necessary for physiologic function, cannot be produced by the body, and must be consumed in the diet. Omega-6 and omega-3 EFAs are both important in the development and normal functioning of the brain and peripheral nervous system. The typical Western diet tends to include more omega-6 EFAs (found in red meat, poultry, eggs, nuts, and seeds) than omega-3 EFAs (found in fish and seafood). Results of research indicate that increasing the ratio of omega-3 intake to be at least equal to that of omega-6 can reduce the risk of developing many chronic diseases (e.g., cardiovascular disease [CVD], inflammatory bowel disease [IBD], cancer) and has been associated with a reduction in cognitive decline.

Antioxidants, found abundantly in fruits and vegetables, protect brain cells from the damaging effects of free radicals. Many nutrients exhibit antioxidant activity, including vitamins C, E, and A; selenium; and the phytonutrients (i.e., beneficial, plant-derived chemicals) beta-carotene and lycopene. By protecting the brain cells from oxidation, antioxidants aid in the prevention of dementia and depression.

B-complex vitamins (found in green leafy vegetables, eggs, milk, chicken, and fortified cereals) are necessary for sustaining mental health. Deficiencies in the B-complex vitamins niacin, riboflavin, and folate are associated with an increased likelihood of developing anxiety, depression, memory loss, insomnia, and fatigue

MEDICAL NUTRITION THERAPY FOR BD

- Eat a balanced diet that includes lean proteins, unsaturated fats, complex CHOs, and a variety of fruits and vegetables

- Choose complex CHOs, which stimulate the production of serotonin and maintain normal insulin and glucose levels, stabilizing mood

- Avoid simple CHOs, which can increase the risk of mood swings and depression

- Include foods that provide omega-3 EFAs in the diet to support healthy cognitive function

- Include foods that are rich in B-complex vitamins (e.g., green leafy vegetables), vitamin C (e.g., orange and red fruits and vegetables), magnesium (e.g., beans, leafy greens), and protein (e.g., lean meats, beans, nuts), which are quickly used up during times of stress

- Maintain a supply of healthy snacks (e.g., unsalted nuts, fresh fruit, dried fruit) to prevent impulse snacking of junk foods

- Avoid alcohol, which has a depressant effect on the brain, resulting in impaired mood

- Avoid excessive intake of caffeine (e.g., coffee, tea, caffeinated soda), which increases anxiety and agitation and can interfere with healthy sleep patterns

- Participate in daily physical activity. Exercise reduces stress hormones, increases the sense of well-being, improves sleep, and improves overall health

- Recruit the help of family and friends to assist in meal planning, grocery shopping, and food preparation during manic or depressive episodes or during stressful, life-altering events that may trigger mood shifts

Research Findings

Results of clinical studies have shown lower levels of omega-3 EFAs in psychiatric patients. Researchers have suggested that problems with lipid metabolism may play a role in BD and schizophrenia. Supplementation with omega-3 EFAs has been shown to reduce behaviors of impulsivity, deliberate self-harm, and violent aggression.

Researchers are investigating the complex interconnections among the gut, brain, and immune and hormonal systems in order to better understand how to effectively intervene in depression-related mental health conditions. Improving the microbiome (i.e., our microbes' genes) within the gut appears to play a significant role in improving the health of all the connected biological systems by reducing proinflammatory and stress hormone signals (known as cytokines). Steps toward improving intestinal health include avoiding overuse of antibiotics and nonsteroidal anti-inflammatory drugs (NSAIDs) and including probiotics and omega-3–rich foods in the diet.

Researchers have observed a potential relationship between relapse in patients with BD and excessive consumption of energy drinks by individuals with BD and comorbid substance abuse disorder.

Summary

Individuals diagnosed with this disorder (and their family members) should learn about the role diet plays in BD based on personal characteristics and health needs. Individuals should understand the importance of consuming a diet that is high in nutrition and contains a variety of fruits, vegetables, whole grains, and lean meats, as appropriate to individualized characteristics. Individuals should meet with a registered dietitian (RD) and a mental health clinician to discuss diet-related complications associated with BD or adverse effects of medications used to treat BD that affect diet.

Individuals should also be aware of the potential risks of erratic eating patterns during manic or depressive episodes, and the importance of maintaining healthy dietary habits and enlisting the help of family and/or friends for food purchase and preparation. Research suggests that supplementation with omega-3 EFAs has been shown to reduce erratic behaviors of BD.

—Cherie Marcel

References

"Biobank Research Identifies Bipolar-Obesity Link." *Mayo Clinic*, Mayo Foundation for Medical

Education and Research, 11 Nov. 2016, www.mayoclinic.org/medical-professionals/psychiatry-psychology/news/biobank-research-identifies-bipolar-obesity-link/mac-20429510.

Brogan, Kelly. "The Role of the Microbiome in Mental Health: A Psychoneuroimmunologic Perspective." *Alternative and Complementary Therapies*, vol. 21, no. 2, 2015, pp. 61–67., doi:10.1089/act.2015.21204.

Mangge, Harald, et al. "Weight Gain During Treatment of Bipolar Disorder (BD)—Facts and Therapeutic Options." *Frontiers in Nutrition*, vol. 6, 11 June 2019, doi:10.3389/fnut.2019.00076.

Strassler, Douglas. "Greater Cognitive Decline in Individuals at Risk for Bipolar Disorder With Obesity." *Psychiatry Advisor*, 17 Dec. 2018, www.psychiatryadvisor.com/home/topics/mood-disorders/bipolar-disorder/greater-cognitive-decline-in-individuals-at-risk-for-bipolar-disorder-with-obesity/.

Strassnig, Martin, et al. "Obesity Rates Higher in Schizophrenia, Bipolar Disorder." *Bipolar Disorders*, vol. 19, no. 5, 29 Aug. 2017, pp. 336–343., doi:10.1111/bdi.12505.

Tully, Agnes, et al. "Interventions for the Management of Obesity in People with Bipolar Disorder." *Cochrane Database of Systematic Reviews*, 12 Apr. 2018, doi:10.1002/14651858.cd013006.

Zhao, Zhuoxian, et al. "The Potential Association between Obesity and Bipolar Disorder: A Meta-Analysis." *Journal of Affective Disorders*, vol. 202, 2016, pp. 120–123., doi:10.1016/j.jad.2016.05.059.

■ Body dysmorphic disorder

CATEGORY: Disorder
ALSO KNOWN AS: Dysmorphobia, imagined ugliness syndrome

Causes and Symptoms

Body dysmorphic disorder (BDD) may be related to, though distinct from, other psychiatric disorders such as obsessive-compulsive disorder, eating disorders, and depression. No definitive cause has been identified, though proposed models suggest an interaction of societal overemphasis on physical appearance, low self-esteem, and brain neurotransmitter abnormalities. There is increasing evidence of a genetic predisposition to anxiety-related disorders.

Patients have an overblown concern about one or more perceived body defects, commonly of the face, hair, or skin. Some patients may fixate on muscles, penis, breasts, or buttocks. Individuals suffer extreme distress as a result, which interferes with social and occupational functioning. Diagnostic criteria determined by the American Psychiatric Association include preoccupation with an imagined or minor defect in physical appearance that causes significant interruption of social functioning and is not explained by another mental disorder, such as anorexia nervosa.

Patients are often embarrassed or ashamed of the problem. They may become housebound and have difficulty maintaining interpersonal relationships. They may spend hours each day checking their appearance in mirrors and attempting to correct or hide the defect with excessive grooming rituals. Poor school and job performance are common, and approximately three-quarters of patients are unmarried.

Sufferers will often seek help from plastic surgeons or dermatologists to correct their perceived defect. This approach is most often unsuccessful, as the change in appearance is rarely enough to satisfy the patient. This may lead to repeated attempts at corrective surgery, which continue to result in disappointment, as they address only a symptom rather than the underlying disordered thinking.

Approximately 1 percent of the general adult population is thought to suffer from body dysmorphic disorder, with men and women being equally affected. The typical onset is in late adolescence or early adulthood. Patients are at increased risk for major depression. It is estimated that 60 percent of these patients also suffer from depression, and this combination places them at significant risk of suicide. Coexisting obsessive-compulsive disorder is also common.

Treatment and Therapy

The disorder is not uncommon, but it is frequently missed or misdiagnosed. Patients are most likely to be identified during visits to family practitioners, internists, dermatologists, or plastic surgeons where they describe physical features that they wish to change. Often they are seeking referral to a specialist for correction of the imagined defect.

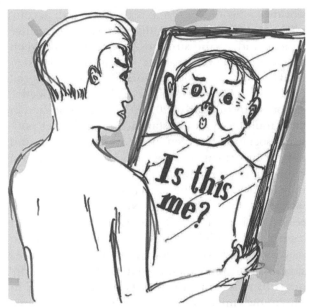

A cartoon of a patient looking into the mirror, seeing body dysmorphia. (Chainwit via Wikimedia Commons)

When BDD is suspected, referral to a psychiatrist for evaluation and treatment is most appropriate. Definitive treatment is unknown, but pharmacologic treatment with high-dose selective serotonin reuptake inhibitors (SSRIs) combined with nonpharmacologic cognitive behavior psychotherapy is the most effective approach currently. It is important to avoid attempted cosmetic correction, which does not treat the underlying disorder and is rarely effective.

SSRIs are thought to reduce symptoms by regulating neurotransmitters in the brain. Their use has been shown to decrease the frequency of disturbing thoughts and ritualistic behaviors related to the perceived physical flaw. This treatment is more effective when combined with cognitive behavior psychotherapy to address the patient's low self-esteem and negative body image. Therapy that educates and includes family members, spouses, and other close individuals may improve outcome.

Body dysmorphic disorder is typically a chronic condition requiring ongoing care. Relapse following discontinuation of therapy is common. The prognosis is good with continued treatment and follow-up.

Perspective and Prospects

Italian physician Enrique Morselli coined the term *dysmorphobia* in 1891 to describe patients who were tortured by their fear of an imagined physical deformity that was not noticeable to others. The condition was recognized by the American Psychiatric Association in 1987, renamed body dysmorphic disorder, and classified as a distinct somatoform disorder in the *Diagnostic and Statistical Manual of Mental Disorders, Fourth Edition* (DSM-IV; 1994). Among other updates, the *DSM-5*, published in 2013, adds the diagnostic criterion of repetitive behavior, feelings, or thoughts in response to a preoccupation with a perceived flaw.

The disorder has received significant attention and is now the subject of ongoing clinical research. Additional data are needed to pinpoint causes and evaluate new treatment approaches.

—Rachel Zahn

References

Davis, Kathleen. "What's to Know about Body Dysmorphic Disorder." *Medical News Today*, 12 Mar. 2019, www.medicalnewstoday.com/articles/309254.

Geliebter, Allan, et al. "Physiological and Psychological Changes Following Liposuction of Large Volumes of Fat in Overweight and Obese Women." *Journal of Diabetes and Obesity*, vol. 2, no. 4, 2015, pp. 1–7., doi:10.15436/2376-0494.15.032.

Heerden, Ingrid van. "Body Dysmorphic Disorder Can Lead to Obsessive Dieting." *Health24*, 19 Mar. 2015, www.health24.com/Diet-and-nutrition/Healthy-foods/Body-dysmorphic-disorder-can-lead-to-obsessive-dieting-20150319.

Littleberry, Merrill. "Beyond the Looking Glass: An Honest View of Body Dysmorphic Disorder." *Obesity Action Coalition*, 2019, www.obesityaction.org/community/article-library/beyond-the-looking-glass-an-honest-view-of-body-dysmorphic-disorder/.

McConville, Sharon. "Body Dysmorphia and Its Link to Eating Disorders: How Do They Relate?" *Eating Disorder Hope*, 10 June 2019, www.eatingdisorderhope.com/information/body-image/body-dysmorphia.

McGuire, Jane. "Binge Eating Disorder & Body Dysmorphic Disorder Connection." *Eating Disorder Hope*, 12 Oct. 2017, www.eatingdisorderhope.com/blog/bed-bdd-connection.

Ueland, Venke, et al. "Living with Obesity — Existential Experiences." *International Journal of Qualitative Studies on Health and Well-Being*, vol. 14, no. 1, 1 Aug. 2019, p. 1651171., doi:10.1080/17482631.2019.1651171.

■ Breast cancer recurrence

CATEGORY: Disorder

Researchers report that breast cancer (BC) survivors frequently revert to their former lifestyle habits, such as being sedentary, smoking cigarettes, and making poor dietary choices. Researchers also report that there are long-term nutritional implications for cancer survivors that increase their chances of developing cardiovascular disease, diabetes mellitus, hypertension, osteoporosis, and obesity. It is well known that overweight and obese individuals are at greater risk for cancers of the breast; excess body fat is associated with about 17% of BC incidences. Achieving and maintaining a healthy weight, participating in regular physical activity, and consuming a healthy diet are effective in reducing the risk of developing cancer. In addition, obesity is associated with increased risk of BC recurrence. The best diet recommendation for preventing BC and for reducing risk of BC recurrence is to consume a diet that is low in saturated fat and high in fiber, includes fish and other lean proteins, and is rich in a wide variety of fruits and vegetables.

Research Findings

Understanding the effect of diet on risk for breast cancer, the most common cancer in women

MEDICAL NUTRITION THERAPY FOR BREAST CANCER

Achieve and maintain a healthy weight.

Participate in regular physical activity for at least 150 minutes/week, including strength training at least 2 days/week.

Eat a diet high in fiber and low in fat (less than 30% of total calorie intake) that includes fish and other lean proteins, whole grains, and a wide variety of fruits and vegetables (at least 5 servings/day).

Choose unprocessed, unrefined foods.

Avoid saturated fats and trans fats (i.e., fats with added hydrogen to make them solid at room temperature); limit fat intake to unsaturated fats such as those found in vegetable oils, avocado, and nuts and seeds.

Limit alcohol consumption to 1 drink/day for women and 2 drinks/day for men.

Stop using tobacco if currently using.

worldwide, would be a major public health accomplishment. Based on results of large prospective cohort studies, the strongest associations between dietary fat and breast cancer appear to be related to intake of saturated fat and animal fat, not to overall fat intake. Investigators in a large prospective cohort study of nearly 320,000 women published in 2008 found a weak but statistically significant positive association between intake of saturated fat and risk for breast cancer. The association was greatest in postmenopausal women who never received hormone-replacement therapy (HRT).

Results from the large Nurses' Health Study cohort indicated a 50% increased risk for breast cancer with a higher intake of animal fat and no increase in risk with overall fat intake. The authors suggest that rather than the fat itself, other components of fatty animal products (e.g., hormones in whole cow's milk) could play a role in increased risk.

Researchers report that lower dietary fat intake, higher soy protein intake, and consumption of 3 or more cups of green tea per day may be associated with reduced risk of BC recurrence.

Researchers in studies of breast and colon cancer survivors have shown that those who adopt a physically active lifestyle after diagnosis have a 26–50% lower risk of cancer recurrence, cancer mortality, and all-cause mortality.

BC survivors who received dietary counseling and adopted a low-fat diet for 5 years lost an average of 6 lbs. and had a 24% lower risk for BC recurrence at 5 years than BC survivors who did not receive dietary counseling and who did not adopt a low-fat diet.

The risk of BC recurrence may be influenced by factors that are associated with diet, such as weight gain and higher body mass index (BMI). Researchers report that being overweight at the time of BC diagnosis and gaining weight after diagnosis are both associated with a higher risk of recurrence after treatment-induced remission.

Summary

Breast cancer survivors should become knowledgeable about the latest research on diet and BC recurrence. Adopting the recommended dietary and lifestyle modifications may help reduce the risk of BC recurrence. Educational materials on local nutrition programs and on eating a healthy diet that emphasizes adequate nutrition and low-fat food choices, including a variety of vegetables, fruits, whole grains, and fiber may help prevent BC recurrence. BC survivors should continue their medical surveillance and promptly report any health-related changes to their treating clinician. Research suggests maintaining a healthy weight, and consuming soy protein and green tea may help reduce BC recurrence.

—Cherie Marcel, Tanja Schub

References

Blair, Cindy K., et al. "Obesity and Survival among a Cohort of Breast Cancer Patients Is Partially Mediated by Tumor Characteristics." *Npj Breast Cancer*, vol. 5, no. 1, 2 Oct. 2019, doi:10.1038/s41523-019-0128-4.

Ecker, Brett L., et al. "Impact of Obesity on Breast Cancer Recurrence and Minimal Residual Disease." *Breast Cancer Research*, vol. 21, no. 1, 13 Mar. 2019, doi:10.1186/s13058-018-1087-7.

Lee, Kyuwan, et al. "The Impact of Obesity on Breast Cancer Diagnosis and Treatment." *Current Oncology Reports*, vol. 21, no. 5, 27 Mar. 2019, doi:10.1007/s11912-019-0787-1.

Picon-Ruiz, Manuel, et al. "Obesity and Adverse Breast Cancer Risk and Outcome: Mechanistic Insights and Strategies for Intervention." *CA: A Cancer Journal for Clinicians*, vol. 67, no. 5, 1 Aug. 2017, pp. 378–397., doi:10.3322/caac.21405.

Sattler, Elisabeth Lilian Pia. "Weight Management in Overweight and Obese Breast Cancer Survivors." *Advances in Obesity, Weight Management & Control*, vol. 7, no. 3, 2017, doi:10.15406/aowmc.2017.07.00200.

Sun, Li, et al. "Body Mass Index and Prognosis of Breast Cancer." *Medicine*, vol. 97, no. 26, 2018, doi:10.1097/md.0000000000011220.

■ Bulimia

CATEGORY: Disorder
ALSO KNOWN AS: Bulimia nervosa

Causes and Symptoms

Bulimia is typically regarded as a psychologically based disorder caused by childhood experiences, family influences, and social pressures, particularly on young women to be thinner than natural. Many people who develop bulimia have been overweight in the past and suffer from poor self-image and depression. Body weight is often within normal limits, but persons with bulimia perceive themselves as fat and are often obsessed with their body image. Others may have a history of sexual or physical abuse or of alcohol or drug abuse. Medical research suggests that bulimia may be partially caused by impaired secretion of cholecystokinin (CKK), a hormone that normally induces a feeling of fullness after a meal, or by depletion of the chemical serotonin in the brain, which contributes to a craving for carbohydrates.

Intense preoccupation with food and weight are invariably present, and eating binges are followed with self-induced vomiting or the ingestion of laxatives to rid the body of the consumed food. Depression and suicidal feelings sometimes accompany bulimia. The disorder can cause nutritional deficiencies, dehydration, hormonal changes, gastrointestinal problems, changes in metabolism and blood chemistry, heart disorders, persistent sore throat, and teeth and gum damage as a result of the acidic nature of regurgitated food.

Treatment and Therapy

Treatment of bulimia requires a combination of nutritional counseling, medication, and psychotherapy. Psychotherapists try to get to the root of any underlying psychological problems and resolve them. Various modes of group and cognitive behavioral therapy have proven effective.

Cognitive therapy usually includes confronting people with bulimia about their inaccurate perceptions of body weight and making contracts with them to shift their focus to nutrition rather than weight gain in exchange for rewards. Group therapy has helped many bulimics stop their binge eating, while treatment with antidepressant drugs, especially fluoxetine (Prozac), has helped many bulimic patients gain partial or full relief from their symptoms. Hospitalization is common treatment and is virtually always necessary if body weight is more than 30 percent below ideal.

Perspective and Prospects

Bulimia was classified as a distinct disorder by the American Psychiatric Association in 1980; the name was officially changed to bulimia nervosa in 1987. The disorder occurs mostly in adolescent and young adult females, with only about

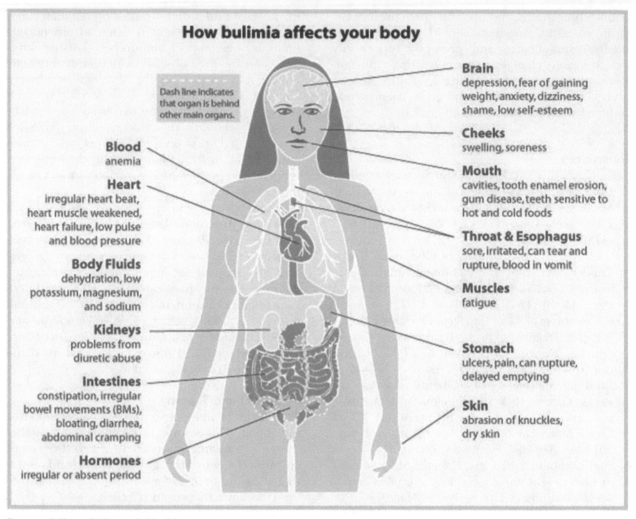

How bulimia affects your body

Dash line indicates that organ is behind other main organs.

Brain
depression, fear of gaining weight, anxiety, dizziness, shame, low self-esteem

Cheeks
swelling, soreness

Mouth
cavities, tooth enamel erosion, gum disease, teeth sensitive to hot and cold foods

Throat & Esophagus
sore, irritated, can tear and rupture, blood in vomit

Muscles
fatigue

Stomach
ulcers, pain, can rupture, delayed emptying

Skin
abrasion of knuckles, dry skin

Blood
anemia

Heart
irregular heart beat, heart muscle weakened, heart failure, low pulse and blood pressure

Body Fluids
dehydration, low potassium, magnesium, and sodium

Kidneys
problems from diuretic abuse

Intestines
constipation, irregular bowel movements (BMs), bloating, diarrhea, abdominal cramping

Hormones
irregular or absent period

Source: Office of Women's Health

10 percent of cases in males. Many cases of bulimia end after a few weeks or months but may reoccur. Other cases last for years without interruption.

In 2006, researchers developed a new test that analyzes carbon and nitrogen in hair, which is suggestive of eating disorders. This technique is beneficial because eating disorders are difficult to diagnose, in part because sufferers sometimes do not know that they have an eating disorder or do not want to be honest. By analyzing just five strands of hair, researchers were able to diagnose anorexia and bulimia accurately 80 percent of the time. This test may hasten treatment and prove an effective and objective method of monitoring recovery.

—*Alvin K. Benson, LeAnna DeAngelo*

References

Anonymous. "I'm a Fat Bulimic – Here's Why the Idea of Loving My Body Feels Impossible for Me." *Everyday Feminism*, 17 Sept. 2015, everydayfeminism.com/2015/09/im-a-fat-bulimic/.

Castillo, Michelle. "Doctors Warn Obese Teens May Be at Higher Risk for Anorexia, Bulimia." *CBS News*, 9 Sept. 2013, www.cbsnews.com/news/doctors-warn-obese-teens-may-be-at-higher-risk-for-anorexia-bulimia/.

Eenfeldt, Andreas. "FDA Approves Bulimia Device as Treatment of Obesity." *Diet Doctor*, 15 June 2016, www.dietdoctor.com/fda-approves-bulimia-device-treatment-obesity.

Gander, Kashmira. "This Revolutionary Weightloss Aid Is Extremely Controversial." *The Independent*, Independent Digital News and Media, 15 Dec.

2016, www.independent.co.uk/life-style/health-and-families/health-news/medical-bulimia-aspireassist-weight-obesity-crisis-quick-fix-eating-disorders-diets-health-a7475161.html.

Habibzadeh, Nasim, and Hassn Daneshmandi. "The Effects of Exercise in Obese Women with Bulimia Nervosa." *Asian Journal of Sports Medicine*, vol. 1, no. 4, 2010, doi:10.5812/asjsm.34829.

Howard, Jacqueline. "How Bulimics' Brains Are Different." *CNN*, Cable News Network, 24 July 2017, www.cnn.com/2017/07/18/health/bulimia-brain-stress-food-study/index.html.

Luz, Felipe Da, et al. "Obesity with Comorbid Eating Disorders: Associated Health Risks and Treatment Approaches." *Nutrients*, vol. 10, no. 7, 27 June 2018, p. 829., doi:10.3390/nu10070829.

Masheb, Robin, and Marney A. White. "Bulimia Nervosa in Overweight and Normal-Weight Women." *Comprehensive Psychiatry*, vol. 53, no. 2, 2012, pp. 181–186., doi:10.1016/j.comppsych.2011.03.005.

McGuire, Jane. "Teens, Eating Disorders, and Obesity." *Eating Disorder Hope*, 25 Apr. 2018, www.eatingdisorderhope.com/blog/teens-eating-disorders-obesity.

Schwartz, Allan. "Obesity, An Addiction?" *MentalHelp.net*, American Addiction Centers, 2019, www.mentalhelp.net/blogs/obesity-an-addiction/.

Chronic fatigue syndrome

CATEGORY: Disorder

Chronic fatigue syndrome (CFS) refers to a syndrome characterized by profound mental and physical fatigue along with a combination of other disabling symptoms, including cognitive impairment, persistent musculoskeletal pain, post-exertional malaise (PEM) (i.e., a worsening of CFS symptoms following mental or physical exertion), headaches, sore throat, and sleep disturbance. Also known as chronic fatigue immune dysfunction syndrome (CFIDS) and myalgic encephalomyelitis (ME), CFS is a complex and debilitating condition with unclear etiology and debated treatment strategies. Evidence is clear that early intervention is vital to symptom improvement; however, due to the confusing nature of CFS and lack of a consistently successful treatment protocol, many patients experience gross delays in diagnosis and treatment. It is not uncommon for individuals with CFS to spend years visiting many different practitioners, undergoing invasive testing procedures and treatments, and ultimately adopting a daily regimen of complicating, and often addictive, pharmaceutical medications and supplements. Research has demonstrated that individuals with CFS have abnormalities in their immune, endocrine, musculoskeletal, neurological, and central nervous systems; however, researchers have not determined whether these abnormalities are caused by the primary disease process or are a secondary result of CFS. There is no cure for CFS. Treatment of CFS is focused primarily on changes in lifestyle (e.g., diet and exercise) and cognitive behavioral therapy (CBT; e.g., for depression or anxiety), with only minimal pharmaceutical therapy to target specific symptoms (e.g., pain, headaches, sleep deprivation).

Treatment of CFS with Medication

Many types of medication (e.g., antidepressants, anti-anxiety medications, pain relievers) are prescribed singly or in combination to treat the symptoms of CFS. These medications can have adverse effects that impact appetite, nutrient intake, and weight. Adverse effects that affect diet include weight gain, stomach pain, weakness, fatigue, and drowsiness, diarrhea or constipation, and nausea and vertigo

While medication can treat symptoms, it is considered to be of little value to actual improvement of the condition. It can, however, be used to reduce symptom load so that individuals with CFS are more able to implement lifestyle and behavioral changes.

Response to treatment tends to fluctuate and is typically slow, with gradual improvement over a period of months to years. It is estimated that only 5% of individuals with CFS ever fully recover.

Because traditional medicine has not yet established a consistently effective treatment plan for CFS, patients frequently turn to complementary and alternative treatment options. There are several diet- and supplement-centered protocols that are advertised to treat CFS; unfortunately, no specific diet plan has been proven effective in the treatment of CFS. Rigid treatment protocols that have not been adequately studied carry the risk of causing further harm to patients with CFS. Extreme dietary changes and increases in activity can result in weight fluctuations, headaches, intestinal distress, and PEM.

Medical Nutrition Therapy for CFS

Morbid obesity is associated with profound fatigue regardless of the presence of CFS, and a body mass index (BMI) > 45 is among the exclusion criteria for a CFS diagnosis. Research is lacking to determine whether or not weight loss can improve CFS symptoms in obese patients.

There is no officially recognized diet plan that is specific to the needs of patients with CFS. The best dietary approach is to follow a healthy, well-rounded diet to support the body's systems in combating the complicated disease process of CFS.

Because the dominant symptom of CFS is debilitating fatigue, persons with CFS can find meal planning and food procurement and preparation to be overwhelming. Participate in physician-directed, graded physical activity (i.e., a gradual increase in activity not beyond a level of individual tolerance). Exercise reduces stress hormones, increases the sense of well-being, improves sleep, and improves overall health.

Many individuals who have CFS present with other comorbidities, which should be addressed with appropriate dietary recommendations. Some commonly associated comorbidities and symptoms that can require dietary management include irritable bowel syndrome (IBS), intolerance to gluten or dairy products, chewing/swallowing difficulties, and unexplained weight changes.

Summary

Individuals diagnosed with CFS (and their family members) should learn about the role of diet in alleviating symptoms of CFS based on personal characteristics and health needs. Individuals should seek the guidance of a healthcare professional to have their dietary habits assessed, and to receive education regarding the importance of consuming a diet that is high in nutrition and contains a variety of fruits, vegetables, whole grains, and lean proteins. Individuals should also understand the importance of maintaining healthy dietary habits by keeping healthy snack foods available and enlisting the help of family and/or friends for food purchase and preparation. Individuals should be assessed for diet-related complications associated with CFS or adverse effects of medications used to treat CFS that affect diet. Referral to a mental health clinician for counseling and to a registered dietitian (RD) for nutrition evaluation and education may be necessary.

Individuals and their family members should discuss treatment plans with a medical practitioner that is trained in the treatment of CFS, and should also be cautioned against rigid treatment protocols that have not been adequately studied.

—_Cherie Marcel_

References

Bozzini, Sara, et al. "Cardiovascular Characteristics of Chronic Fatigue Syndrome." _Biomedical Reports_, 28 Nov. 2017, doi:10.3892/br.2017.1024.

Brazier, Yvette. "What Causes Fatigue, and How Can I Treat It?" _Medical News Today_, 15 Aug. 2017, www.medicalnewstoday.com/articles/248002.

Norris, T, et al. "Obesity in Adolescents with Chronic Fatigue Syndrome: an Observational Study." _Archives of Disease in Childhood_, vol. 102, no. 1, 21 Sept. 2016, pp. 35–39., doi:10.1136/archdischild-2016-311293.

■ Colorectal cancer

CATEGORY: Disorder

In the United States, cancer is second only to heart disease as a cause of mortality. Colorectal cancer (also called colon cancer) is a neoplasm that originates in the large intestine or the rectum. Most colorectal neoplasms develop from a benign polyp. Screening (e.g., colonoscopy or sigmoidoscopy) can detect colon cancer early, frequently before the onset of signs and symptoms (e.g., diarrhea, constipation, unexplained weight loss). Although colorectal cancer is highly curable when diagnosed early, it is currently the second leading cause of cancer-related death in the U.S. each year. In the U.S. there are over 145,000 new cases of colorectal cancer and more than 56,000 colorectal cancer-related deaths. Ninety percent of new colorectal cancer cases are diagnosed in individuals who are over 50 years of age. Treatment depends on the stage of the cancer and the age and health of the patient, and can involve surgery, chemotherapy, and/or radiation therapy.

Dietary Considerations for Colorectal Cancer

Overweight and obese individuals are at higher risk for colorectal cancer. High intake of fats is a risk factor for overweight and obesity, and is also associated with increased incidence of colorectal cancer. The contribution of fat intake to cancer risk involves many variables, including the type of fat (e.g., saturated, unsaturated, polyunsaturated), preparation of fat (e.g., heating, hydrogenating), and source of fat (e.g., animal or plant). Multiple study results show a correlation between animal fat intake and increased cancer risk, although fat from plant sources has not proven to be as significant a risk. Because unsaturated fats are generally in liquid form at room temperature, food manufacturers hydrogenate (i.e., add hydrogen) these fats to change them into a solid form of fat (e.g., vegetable oil processed to be a butter-like spread). This process results in the production of trans fats, which raise low-density lipoproteins (LDLs; commonly called "bad" cholesterol) levels in the blood and have exhibited carcinogenic properties

Regular intake of fruits and vegetables can help prevent colorectal cancer. Results of studies show a definite protective benefit in folate intake and strong evidence for the existence of anti-cancer properties in raw, green, and cruciferous vegetables. The antioxidant vitamins (e.g., E, C, and A), vitamin D, magnesium, and calcium have been shown to exhibit anticancer activity but are still being investigated. Regardless of whether a direct preventative relationship exists, higher fruit and vegetable consumption is usually associated with higher fiber intake, lower fat intake, and lower body weight, all of which are associated with cancer prevention.

Research Findings

Evidence suggests that lifestyle behaviors such as achieving and maintaining a healthy weight,

regular physical activity, and consuming a healthy diet are effective in reducing the risk for colorectal cancer. Results of studies on survivors of breast and colorectal cancer show that those who adopt a physically active lifestyle after diagnosis have a 26–50% lower risk for cancer recurrence, cancer mortality, and all-cause mortality.

Results of many studies have reported an association between red meat consumption and increased risk for colorectal cancer. The exact cause for the increased cancer risk is not completely understood, but the saturated fat and cholesterol content of red meat is thought to be partly responsible. Researchers believe that the cooking method of red meat plays a significant role in its affect on cancer risk. Cooking red meats at high temperatures (e.g., frying, broiling) results in the formation of heterocyclic amines (HCAs), which are known to be carcinogenic. Educating individuals to cut the fat off their meat and grill instead of frying can reduce the amount of fat consumed and reduce potential carcinogenic effects.

Although the consumption of red meat and saturated fats can increase the risk for colorectal cancer, results of studies indicate that the inclusion of fish and foods rich in monounsaturated fats (e.g., olive oil and avocado) in the diet can reduce cancer risk. The omega-3 fatty acids docosahexaenoic acid (DHA) and eicosapentaenoic acid (EPA), found in fish, have been shown to play a protective role against inflammatory bowel disease and colorectal cancer, which is likely the result of their anti-inflammatory activity. Researchers also report that individuals who consume greater quantities of fish than other forms of

RISK FACTORS	SIGNS AND SYMPTOMS
Age over 60 years	Abdominal pain
Family history of colorectal cancer	Diarrhea
Black or eastern European ancestry	Constipation
Inflammatory bowel disease (IBS), colorectal polyps, or cancer at another site	Unexplained weight loss
Overweight and obesity	Stools that are narrow in diameter
Increased alcohol intake	Blood in the stool
High-fat diet, especially high levels of fat from red and processed meats	
History of breast cancer	

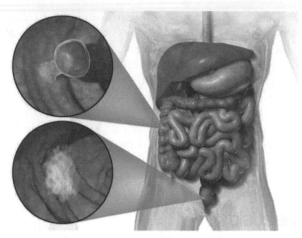

Location and appearance of two example colorectal tumors. (BruceBlaus)

meat in their regular diet are more likely to make healthy dietary choices overall. For example, they tend to consume higher amounts of whole grains, fruits, and vegetables.

Summary

Individuals diagnosed with colorectal cancer (and their family members/caregivers) should learn about dietary recommendations based on personal characteristics and health needs. Patients should eat a high-fiber diet that includes a wide variety of fruits, vegetables, lean proteins, and unsaturated fats. It is important to report any health-related changes to the treating clinician as soon as possible to prevent worsening health status. Patients and their family members should understand and adhere to the prescribed treatment regimen, while continuing medical surveillance to monitor health status. Research suggests that reducing red meat and saturated fats consumption may help reduce risk of colorectal cancer.

—*Cherie Marcel*

References

Liu, Po-Hong, et al. "Association of Obesity With Risk of Early-Onset Colorectal Cancer Among Women." *JAMA Oncology*, vol. 5, no. 1, 11 Oct. 2018, p. 37., doi:10.1001/jamaoncol.2018.4280.

Martinez-Useros, Javier, and Jesus Garcia-Foncillas. "Obesity and Colorectal Cancer: Molecular Features of Adipose Tissue." *Journal of Translational Medicine*, vol. 14, no. 1, 22 Jan. 2016, doi:10.1186/s12967-016-0772-5.

Soltani, Ghodratollah, et al. "Obesity, Diabetes and the Risk of Colorectal Adenoma and Cancer." *BMC Endocrine Disorders*, vol. 19, no. 1, 29 Oct. 2019, doi:10.1186/s12902-019-0444-6.

Whitlock, Kevin, et al. "The Association between Obesity and Colorectal Cancer." *Gastroenterology Research and Practice*, 2012, pp. 1–6., doi:10.1155/2012/768247.

■ Deep vein thrombosis

CATEGORY: Disorder
ALSO KNOWN AS: Blood clots, hypercoagulation

Causes and Symptoms

Deep vein or venous thrombosis (DVT) is a blood clot (thrombus) in a deep vein. In vessels that transport blood toward the heart, various disorders including skin infections or phlebitis (inflammation of the vein) can occur; however, specific tests are required to diagnose the existence of DVT. While phlebitis afflicts superficial veins, DVT occurs in deep veins, usually in the legs.

Because of the possibility of its breaking loose, lodging in the lungs, and creating a potentially fatal pulmonary embolism (blockage of blood to the lungs), a clot in the leg is highly dangerous. Clots in veins in the legs generally form following long periods of inactivity or lengthy bed rest, pregnancy, obesity, smoking, estrogen therapy, oral contraceptive medication, or surgery.

With DVT, the afflicted leg begins to swell, turn red, become warm, and throb. Occasionally, the area is tender to touch or movement. However, about one-half of the instances of DVT produce no symptoms, and it is frequently referred to as a silent killer.

Treatment and Therapy

Treatment for deep vein thrombosis begins with anticoagulants (blood thinners), specifically heparin, administered intravenously in the hospital, or through self-injections given at home. The anticoagulant warfarin (Coumadin), given as pills, are then prescribed daily to prevent clots from becoming larger. Frequent check-ups with a physician are mandatory to maintain a certain level of medication effectiveness; depending upon the risk of further clotting, Coumadin can be required

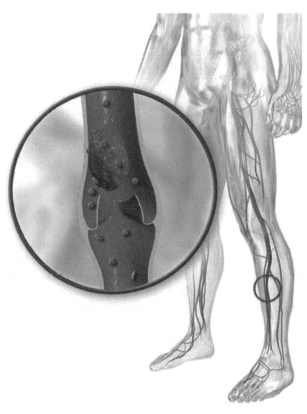

Depiction of a deep vein thrombosis. (BruceBlaus)

anywhere from three months to the remainder of the patient's life. Patients may also be advised to elevate the afflicted leg or apply a heating pad to the area. Walking is sometimes recommended, as is wearing tight-fitting stockings or compression stockings to reduce pain and swelling. In the event that Coumadin is unable to prevent blood clots, a filter may be surgically placed into the vena cava, the large vein carrying blood from the lower body to the heart, to prevent clots from entering the lungs. Also, a large clot may be removed through surgery or may be treated with powerful clot-destroying drugs.

Perspective and Prospects

Inquiries into the mysteries of blood coagulation have existed since 400 BCE, when Hippocrates observed that blood appeared to congeal as it cooled. By the nineteenth century, Pierre Andral, the founder of hematology (the branch of biology that deals with the blood and the blood-forming organs) and one of the first physicians to study the chemistry of the blood, formulated the classical hypothesis of blood coagulation. He found that the process of

blood coagulation follows two pathways: the intrinsic, wherein, within seconds, platelets form a hemostatic plug at the site of the injury (primary hemostasis, or stoppage of bleeding); and the extrinsic, wherein fibrin molecules react in a complex cascade or network (secondary hemostasis) that ultimately moves into a third stage, wherein protein factors combine with the enzyme thrombin and contribute to the clotting of blood. Twentieth-century research determined, however, that the tissue pathway (formerly known as the extrinsic) is a series of enzymes generated to participate with thrombin and catalyze fibrinogen into fibrin, which is essential to blood clotting. These factors are responsible for any abnormalities in the clotting of blood.

While the most commonly known blood clotting disorder is hemophilia, or uncontrolled bleeding, its opposite condition, hypercoagulation, specifically the formation of abnormal clots in veins, can also be life-threatening. In 1994, the clotting disorder factor V Leiden (named for the Dutch city in which it was discovered) was identified as a hereditary resistance to activated protein C. An estimated 30 percent of those individuals who suffer from hypercoagulation are afflicted by this enzyme mutation that encourages the overproduction of thrombin and, consequently, causes excessive clotting. Most of these persons are unaware of their condition or its dangers. Treatment and control of this disorder depends largely on antiplatelet medication, such as aspirin or clopidogrel (Plavix), that is designed to prevent platelets from sticking together. Maintaining a heart-healthy lifestyle by getting regular caradiovascular exercise, maintaining a healthy weight, avoiding smoking, and controlling blood pressure and cholesterol levels can significantly reduce an individual's risk of developing lethal blood clots.

Continued research into the complexities of coagulation account for new developments in medications, including thrombin inhibitors or molecular products that target enzymes controlling specific coagulation factors.

—*Mary Hurd*

References

Blokhin, Ilya O., and Steven R. Lentz. "Mechanisms of Thrombosis in Obesity." *Current Opinion in Hematology*, vol. 20, no. 5, 2013, pp. 437–444., doi:10.1097/moh.0b013e3283634443.

El-Menyar, Ayman, et al. "Role of Overweight and Obesity in Occurrence and Outcomes of Venous Thromboembolism." *Journal of the American College of Surgeons*, vol. 223, no. 4, 2016, doi:10.1016/j.jamcollsurg.2016.08.167.

Mandal, Ananya. "Obesity and Deep Vein Thrombosis (DVT)." *News-Medical.Net*, 14 June 2019, www.news-medical.net/health/Obesity-and-deep-vein-thrombosis-(DVT).aspx.

Sundbøll, Jens, et al. "Changes in Childhood Body Mass Index and Risk of Venous Thromboembolism in Adulthood." *Journal of the American Heart Association*, vol. 8, no. 6, 19 Mar. 2019, doi:10.1161/jaha.118.011407.

Yang, Genyan, et al. "The Effects of Obesity on Venous Thromboembolism: A Review." *Open Journal of Preventive Medicine*, vol. 02, no. 04, 2012, pp. 499–509., doi:10.4236/ojpm.2012.24069.

◼ Depression

CATEGORY: Disorder

Causes and Symptoms

The word "depression" is used to describe many different things. For some, it defines a fleeting mood, for others an outward physical appearance of sadness, and for others a diagnosable clinical disorder. In any year, millions of adults suffer from a clinically diagnosed depression, a mood disorder that often affects personal, vocational, social, and health functioning. The *Diagnostic and Statistical Manual of Mental Disorders: DSM-5* (5th ed., 2013) of the American Psychiatric Association delineates a number of mood disorders that include clinical depression, known as major depression. A major depressive episode is a syndrome of symptoms, present during a two-week period and representing a change from previous functioning. The symptoms include at least five of the following: depressed or irritable mood, diminished interest in previously pleasurable activities, significant weight loss or weight gain, insomnia or hypersomnia, physical excitation or slowness, loss of energy, feelings of worthlessness or guilt, indecisiveness or a diminished ability to concentrate, and recurrent thoughts of death. The clinical depression cannot be initiated or maintained by another illness or condition, and it cannot be a normal reaction to the death of a loved one

(some symptoms of depression are a normal part of the grief reaction).

In major depressive disorder, the patient experiences a major depressive episode and does not have a history of mania or hypomania. Major depressive disorder is often first recognized in the patient's late twenties, while a major depressive episode can occur at any age, including infancy. Women are twice as likely to suffer from the disorder than are men. There are several potential causes of major depressive disorder. Genetic studies suggest a familial link with higher rates of clinical depression in first-degree relatives. There also appears to be a relationship between clinical depression and levels of the brain's neurochemicals, specifically norepinephrine and serotonin, as well as hormones. It is important to keep in mind, however, that anywhere from 15 to 40 percent of adults will experience depression in their lifetimes. Furthermore, not everyone has a biological cause for this depression. Common causes of clinical depression also include psychosocial stressors such as the death of a loved one, financial stress, loss of a job, interpersonal problems, or world events. It is unclear, however, why some people respond to a specific psychosocial stressor with a clinical depression and others do not.

Finally, certain prescription medications have been noted to cause or be related to clinical depression. These drugs include muscle relaxants, heart medications, hypertensive medications, ulcer medications, oral contraceptives, painkillers, narcotics, and steroids. Thus there are many causes of clinical depression, and no single cause is sufficient to explain all clinical depressions.

Another category of depressive disorder is bipolar disorders. Bipolar disorders occur in about 1 percent of the population as a whole. In persons over the age of eighteen, about two to three persons out of one hundred are diagnosed. Bipolar I disorder is characterized by one or more manic episodes along with persisting symptoms of depression. A manic episode is defined as a distinct period of abnormally and persistently elevated, expansive, or irritable mood. Three of the following symptoms must occur during the period of mood disturbance: inflated self-esteem, decreased need for sleep, unusual talkativeness or pressure to keep talking, racing thoughts, distractibility, excessive goal-oriented activities (especially in work, school, or social areas), and reckless activities with a high potential for negative consequences (such as buying sprees or risky business ventures). For a diagnosis of bipolar disorder, the symptoms must be sufficiently severe to cause impairment in functioning and/or concern regarding the person's danger to himself/herself or to others, must not be superimposed on another psychotic disorder, and must not be initiated or maintained by another illness or condition.

Bipolar II disorder is characterized by symptoms of a history of a major depressive episode and symptoms of hypomania. Cyclothymia is another cyclic mood disorder related to depression. Considered a mild form of bipolar disorder, it involves symptoms of both depression and mania. However, the manic symptoms are without marked social or occupational impairment and are known as hypomanic episodes. Similarly, the symptoms of major depressive episodes do not meet the clinical criteria (less than five of the nine symptoms described above), but the symptoms must be present for at least two years. Cyclothymia cannot be superimposed on another psychotic disorder and cannot be initiated or maintained by another illness or condition. This mood disorder is a particularly persistent and chronic disorder with an identified familial pattern.

Dysthymia is another chronic mood disorder affecting approximately 6 percent of the population in a lifetime. Dysthymia is characterized by at least a two-year history of depressed mood and at least two of the following symptoms: poor appetite, insomnia or hypersomnia, low energy or fatigue, low self-esteem, poor concentration or decision making, or feelings of hopelessness. There cannot be evidence of a major depressive episode during the first two years of the dysthymia or a history of manic episodes or hypomanic episodes. The individual cannot be without the symptoms for more than two months at a time, the disorder cannot be superimposed on another psychotic disorder, and it cannot be initiated or maintained by another illness or condition. Dysthymia is more common in adult females, equally common in both sexes of children, and with a greater prevalence in families. The causes of dysthymia are believed to be similar to those listed for major depressive disorder, but the disorder is less well understood than is depression. A final variant of clinical depression is known as seasonal affective disorder. Patients with this illness demonstrate a pattern of clinical depression during the winter, when there is a reduction in the amount of daylight hours. For these patients, the reduction in available light is thought to be the cause of the depression.

Treatment and Therapy
Crucial to the choice of treatment for clinical depression is determining the variant of depression being experienced. Each of the diagnostic categories has associated treatment approaches that are more effective for a particular diagnosis. Multiple assessment techniques are available to the health care professional to determine the type of clinical depression. The most valid and reliable is the clinical interview. The health care provider may conduct either an informal interview or a structured, formal clinical interview assessing the symptoms that would confirm the diagnosis of clinical depression. If the patient meets the criteria set forth in the DSM-5, then the patient is considered for depression treatments. Patients who meet many but not all diagnostic criteria are sometimes diagnosed with a "subclinical" depression. These patients might also be considered appropriate for the treatment of depression, at the discretion of their health care providers.

Another assessment technique involves using a questionnaire to determine the degree and severity of depression. A variety of questionnaires have proven useful in confirming the diagnosis of clinical depression. Questionnaires such as the Beck Depression Inventory, Hamilton Depression Rating Scale, Zung Self-Rating Depression Scale, and the Center for Epidemiologic Studies Depression Scale are used to identify persons with clinical depression and to document changes with treatment. This technique is often used as an adjunct to the clinical interview and rarely stands alone as the definitive assessment approach to diagnosing clinical depression.

Laboratory tests, most notably the dexamethasone suppression test, have also been used in the diagnosis of depression. The dexamethasone suppression test involves injecting a steroid (dexamethasone) into the patient and measuring the production levels of another steroid (cortisol) in response. Studies have demonstrated, however, that certain severely depressed patients do not reveal the suppression of cortisol production that would be expected following the administration of dexamethasone. The test has also failed to identify some patients who were depressed and has mistakenly identified others as depressed. Research continues to determine the efficacy of other measures of brain activity, including computed tomography (CT) scanning, positron emission tomography (PET) scanning, and functional magnetic resonance imaging (fMRI). However, laboratory and imaging tests are not a reliable diagnostic strategy for depression.

Once a clinical depression (or a subclinical depression) is identified, several types of treatment options are available. These options are dependent on the subtype and severity of the depression. They include psychopharmacology (drug therapy), individual and group psychotherapy, light therapy, family therapy, electroconvulsive therapy (ECT), and other less traditional treatments. These treatment options can be provided to the patient as part of an outpatient program or, in certain severe cases of clinical depression in which the person is a danger to himself/herself or others, as part of a hospitalization.

Clinical depression often affects the patient physically, emotionally, and socially. Therefore, prior to beginning any treatment with a clinically depressed individual, the health care provider will attempt to develop an open and communicative relationship with the patient. This relationship will allow the health care provider to provide patient education on the illness and to solicit the collaboration of the patient in treatment. Supportiveness, understanding, and collaboration are all necessary components of any treatment approach. Three primary types of medications are used in the treatment of clinical depression: cyclic anti-depressants, monoamine oxidase inhibitors (MAOIs), and lithium salts. These medications are considered equally effective in decreasing the symptoms of depression, which begin to resolve in several weeks after initiating treatment. The health care professional will select an antidepressant based on side effects, dosing convenience (once daily versus three times a day), and cost.

The cyclic antidepressants are the largest class of antidepressant medications. As the name implies, the chemical makeup of the medication contains chemical rings, or "cycles." There are unicyclic (buproprion and fluoxetine, or Prozac), bicyclic (sertraline and trazodone), tricyclic (amitriptyline,

desipramine, and nortriptyline), and tetracyclic (maprotiline) antidepressants. These antidepressants function to either block the reuptake of neurotransmitters by the neurons, allowing more of the neurotransmitter to be available at a receptor site, or increase the amount of neurotransmitter produced. The side effects associated with the cyclic antidepressants—dry mouth, blurred vision, constipation, urinary difficulties, palpitations, sexual dysfunction and sleep disturbance—vary and can be quite problematic. Some of these antidepressants have deadly toxic effects at high levels, so they are not prescribed to patients who are at risk of suicide. Some drugs are more specific in terms of the drug action. For instance, fluoxetine is a selective serotonin reuptake inhibitor (SSRI) and works specifically on the neurotransmitter serotonin by making more of it available in the synaptic cleft. Similarly, buproprion is a norepinephrine and dopamine reuptake inhibitor (NDRI) and works specifically on the neurotransmitters norepinephrine and dopamine. More specific drugs generally create fewer side effects. Fewer side effects can be associated with greater medication compliance, potentially making these drugs a more effective treatment.

Monoamine oxidase inhibitors (isocarboxazid, phenelzine, and tranylcypromine) are the second class of antidepressants. They function by slowing the production of the enzyme monoamine oxidase. This enzyme is responsible for breaking down the neurotransmitters norepinephrine and serotonin, which are believed to be responsible for depression. By slowing the decomposition of these transmitters, more of them are available to the receptors for a longer period of time. Restlessness, dizziness, weight gain, insomnia, and sexual dysfunction are common side effects of the MAOIs. MAOIs are most notable because of the dangerous adverse reaction (severely high blood pressure) that can occur if the patient consumes large quantities of foods high in tyramine (such as aged cheeses, fermented sausages, red wine, foods with a heavy yeast content, and pickled fish). Because of this potentially dangerous reaction, MAOIs are not usually the first choice of medication and are more commonly reserved for depressed patients who do not respond to the cyclic antidepressants.

A third class of medication used in the treatment of mood disorders are mood stabilizers, the most notable being lithium carbonate, which is used primarily for bipolar disorder. Lithium is a chemical salt that is believed to affect mood stabilization by influencing the production, storage, release, and reuptake of certain neurotransmitters. It is particularly useful in stabilizing and preventing manic episodes and preventing depressive episodes in patients with bipolar disorder. Psychotherapy refers to a number of different treatment techniques used to deal with the psychosocial contributors and consequences of clinical depression. Psychotherapy is a common supplement to drug therapy. In psychotherapy, the patients develop knowledge and insight into the causes and treatment for their clinical depression. In cognitive psychotherapy, symptom relief comes from assisting patients in modifying maladaptive, irrational, or automatic beliefs that can lead to clinical depression. In behavioral psychotherapy, patients modify their environment such that social or personal rewards are more forthcoming. This process might involve being more assertive, reducing isolation by becoming more socially active, increasing physical activities or exercise, or learning relaxation techniques. Research on the effectiveness of these and other psychotherapy techniques indicates that psychotherapy is as effective as certain antidepressants for many patients and, in combination with certain medications, is more effective than either treatment alone.

Electroconvulsive (or "shock") therapy is the single most effective treatment for severe and persistent depression. If the clinically depressed patient fails to respond to medications or psychotherapy and the depression is life-threatening, electroconvulsive therapy is considered. It is also considered if the patient cannot physically tolerate antidepressants, as with elders who have other medical conditions. This therapy involves inducing a seizure in the patient by administering an electrical current to specific parts of the brain. The therapy has become quite sophisticated and much safer than it was in the mid-twentieth century, and it involves fewer risks to the patient. Patients undergo several treatments over a period of time, such as a week, and show marked treatment benefit. Some temporary memory impairment is a common side effect of this treatment. In the past, however, more memory impairment, of lasting duration for some, was more common.

A special treatment used for individuals with seasonal affective disorder is light therapy, or phototherapy. Light therapy involves exposing patients to bright light for a period of time each day during seasons of the year when there is decreased light. This may be done as a preventive measure and also during depressive episodes. The manner in which this treatment approach modifies the depression is unclear and awaits further research, but some believe it affects the internal clock of the body, or circadian rhythm. Studies of the effectiveness of light therapy have been mixed, but interest in this promising treatment is strong, as it may prove useful for working with nonseasonal mood disorders as well. It should be noted, however, that light therapy does have some risks associated with it. Caution must be used to protect the eyes and use the light as directed. Additionally, the intensity of light must be correct so as to achieve therapeutic effects and not cause other problems. Finally, some individuals can experience manic episodes if they are exposed to too much light, so caution must be exercised in terms of the length of time for light exposure treatment sessions.

Psychosurgery, the final treatment option, is quite rare. It refers to surgical removal or destruction of certain portions of the brain believed to be responsible for causing severe depression. Psychosurgery is used only after all treatment options have failed and the clinical depression is life-threatening. Approximately 50 percent of patients who undergo psychosurgery benefit from the procedure. A newer surgical procedure called deep brain stimulation involves the implantation of electrodes that fire a continuous yet weak electrical current to a localized area of brain tissue. The electrodes are connected to a subcutaneous implantable pulse generator that is mounted in the chest and provides power for the system. Although deep brain stimulation has Food and Drug Administration approval (FDA) for several movement disorders (e.g., Parkinson's disease), it has not received approval for the treatment of depression. The procedure is used experimentally for those who suffer from drug-resistant depression.

Perspective and Prospects

Depression, or the more historical term "melancholy," has had a history predating modern medicine. Writings from the time of the ancient Greek physician Hippocrates refer to patients with a symptom complex similar to the present-day definition of clinical depression.

The rates of clinical depression have increased since the early twentieth century, while the age of onset of clinical depression has decreased. Women appear to be at least twice as likely as men to suffer from clinical depression, and people who are happily married have a lower risk for clinical depression than those who are separated, divorced, or dissatisfied in their marital relationship. This data, along with recurrence rates of 50 to 70 percent, indicate the importance of this psychiatric disorder.

While most psychiatric disorders are nonfatal, clinical depression can lead to death. About 60 percent of individuals who commit suicide have a mood disorder such as depression at the time. In a lifetime, however, only about 7 percent of men and 1 percent of women with lifetime histories of depression will commit suicide. Though these numbers are very high, what this means is that not everyone who is depressed will commit suicide. In fact, many receive help and recover from this illness. There are, however, other costs of clinical depression. Billions of dollars are spent on clinical depression, divided among the following areas: treatment, suicide, and absenteeism (the largest). Clinical depression obviously has a significant economic impact on a society.

The future of clinical depression lies in early identification and treatment. Identification will involve two areas. The first is improving the social awareness of mental health issues to include clinical depression. By eliminating the negative social stigma associated with mental illness and mental health treatment, there will be an increased level of the reporting of depression symptoms and thereby an improved opportunity for early intervention, preventing the progression of the disorder to the point of suicide. The second approach to identification involves the development of reliable assessment strategies for clinical depression. Data suggests that the majority of those who commit suicide see a physician within thirty days of the suicide. The field will continue to strive to identify biological markers and other methods to predict and/or identify clinical depression more accurately. Treatment advances will focus on further development of pharmacological strategies and drugs with more specific actions and fewer side effects. Adjuncts to traditional drug therapies need continued development and refinement to maximize the success of integrated treatments.

—*Oliver Oyama, Bryan C. Auday*

References

Carey, Mariko, et al. "Prevalence of Comorbid Depression and Obesity in General Practice: a Cross-Sectional Survey." *British Journal of General Practice*, vól. 64, no. 620, 24 Mar. 2014, doi:10.3399/bjgp14x677482.

Gibson-Smith, Deborah, et al. "The Relation between Obesity and Depressed Mood in a Multi-Ethnic Population. The HELIUS Study." *Social Psychiatry and Psychiatric Epidemiology*, vol. 53, no. 6, 11 Apr. 2018, pp. 629–638., doi:10.1007/s00127-018-1512-3.

Mannan, Munim, et al. "Prospective Associations between Depression and Obesity for Adolescent Males and Females- A Systematic Review and Meta-Analysis of Longitudinal Studies." *Plos One*, vol. 11, no. 6, 10 June 2016, doi:10.1371/journal.pone.0157240.

Mulugeta, Anwar, et al. "Obesity and Depressive Symptoms in Mid-Life: a Population-Based Cohort Study." *BMC Psychiatry*, vol. 18, no. 1, 17 Sept. 2018, doi:10.1186/s12888-018-1877-6.

Nemiary, Deina, et al. "The Relationship Between Obesity and Depression Among Adolescents." *Psychiatric Annals*, vol. 42, no. 8, 1 Aug. 2012, pp. 305–308., doi:10.3928/00485713-20120806-09.

Newman, Tim. "Does Depression Cause Obesity or Does Obesity Cause Depression?" *Medical News Today*, 13 Nov. 2018, www.medicalnewstoday.com/articles/323668.

University of South Australia. "'Strongest Evidence Yet' That Being Obese Causes Depression." *ScienceDaily*, 12 Nov. 2018, www.sciencedaily.com/releases/2018/11/181112095951.htm.

■ Diabetes mellitus

CATEGORY: Disorder

Causes and Symptoms

Diabetes mellitus is by far the most common of all endocrine (hormonal) disorders. The disorder's name is derived from the Greek word *diabetes*, meaning "siphon" or "running through," a reference to the potentially large urine volume that can accompany the condition. The Latin word *mellitus*, meaning "honey," was added to the name when physicians began to make the diagnosis of diabetes mellitus based on the sweet taste of the patient's urine. The disease has been depicted as a state of starvation in the midst of plenty. Although there is plenty of sugar in the blood, without proper insulin action the sugar does not reach the cells that need it for energy. Glucose, the simplest form of sugar, is the primary source of energy for many vital functions. Deprived of glucose, cells starve and tissues begin to degenerate. The unused glucose builds up in the bloodstream, which leads to a series of secondary complications.

The most common symptoms of diabetes mellitus are related to hyperglycemia, glycosuria, and ketoacidosis. The acute symptoms of diabetes mellitus are all attributable to inadequate insulin action. The immediate consequence of an insulin insufficiency is a marked decrease in the ability of muscle, liver, and adipose (fat) tissue to remove glucose from the blood. In the presence of inadequate insulin action, a second problem manifests itself. People with diabetes continue to make the hormone glucagon. Glucagon, which raises the level of blood sugar, can be considered insulin's biological opposite. Like insulin, glucagon is released from the pancreatic islets. The release of glucagon is normally inhibited by insulin; therefore, in the absence of insulin, glucagon action elevates concentrations of glucose. For this reason, diabetes may be considered a two-hormone disease. With a reduction in the conversion of glucose into its storage forms of glycogen in liver and muscle tissue and lipids in adipose cells, concentrations of glucose in the blood steadily increase (hyperglycemia). When the amount of glucose in the blood exceeds the capacity of the kidney to reabsorb this nutrient, glucose begins to spill into the urine (glucosuria). Glucose in the urine then drags additional body water along with it so that the volume of urine dramatically increases. In the absence of adequate fluid intake, the loss of body water and accompanying electrolytes (sodium) leads to dehydration and, ultimately, death caused by the failure of the peripheral circulatory system.

Insulin deficiency also results in a decrease in the synthesis of triglycerides (storage forms of fatty acids) and stimulates the breakdown of fats in adipose tissue. Although glucose cannot enter the cells and be used as an energy source, the body can use its supply of lipids from the fat cells as an alternate source of energy. Fatty acids increase in the blood, causing hyperlipidemia. With large amounts of circulating free fatty acids available for processing by the liver, the production and release of ketone bodies (breakdown products of fatty acids) into the circulation are accelerated, causing both ketonemia and an increase in the acidity of the blood. Since the ketone levels soon also exceed the capacity of the kidney to reabsorb them, ketone bodies soon appear in the urine (ketonuria).

Insulin deficiency and glucagon excess also cause pronounced effects on protein metabolism and result in an overall increase in the breakdown of proteins and a reduction in the uptake of amino acid precursors into muscle protein. This leads to the wasting and weakening of skeletal muscles and, in children who are diabetics, results in a reduction in overall growth. The increased level of amino acids in the blood provides an additional source of material for glucose production (gluconeogenesis) by the liver. All these acute metabolic changes in carbohydrates, lipids, and protein metabolism can be prevented or reversed by the administration of insulin.

There are three distinct types of diabetes mellitus. Type 1, or insulin-dependent diabetes mellitus (IDDM), is an absolute deficiency of insulin that accounts for approximately 5 to 10 percent of all cases of diabetes. Until the discovery of insulin, people stricken with type 1 diabetes faced certain death within about a year of diagnosis. In type 2, or non-insulin-dependent diabetes mellitus (NIDDM), the most common form of the disorder, insulin secretion may be normal or even increased, but the target cells for insulin are less responsive than normal (insulin resistance); therefore, insulin is not as effective in lowering blood glucose concentrations. Although either type can be manifested at any age, type 1 diabetes has a greater prevalence in children, whereas the incidence of type 2 diabetes increases markedly after the age of forty. Genetic and environmental factors are important in the expression of both of these types of diabetes mellitus. The third type is gestational diabetes, which is characterized by high blood glucose during pregnancy in a person who did not previously have diabetes.

Type 1 diabetes is an autoimmune process that involves the selective destruction of the insulin-producing beta cells in the islets of Langerhans (insulitis). The triggering event that initiates this process in genetically susceptible persons is linked to environmental factors that result from an infection, a virus, or, more likely, the presence of toxins in the diet. The body's own T lymphocytes progressively attack the beta cells but leave the other hormone-producing cell types intact. T lymphocytes are white blood cells that normally attack virus-invaded cells and cancer cells. For up to ten years, there remains a sufficient number of insulin-producing cells to respond effectively to a glucose load, but when approximately 80 percent of the beta cells are destroyed, there is insufficient insulin release in response to a meal and the deadly spiral of the consequences of diabetes mellitus is triggered. Insulin injection can halt this lethal process and prevent it from recurring but cannot mimic the normal pattern of insulin release from the pancreas. It is interesting that not everyone who has insulitis actually progresses to experience overt symptoms of the disease.

Type 2 diabetes is normally associated with obesity and lack of exercise. Recently, with the reported increased rates of obesity and inactivity in children, there has also been an increase of type 2 diabetes at younger and younger ages. Genetic factors also play a key role in the development of the disorder. Research has shown that individuals who have a sibling or parent with type 2 diabetes are about three times as likely to develop diabetes themselves.

Because there is a reduction in the sensitivity of the target cells to insulin, people with type 2 diabetes must secrete more insulin to maintain blood glucose at normal levels. Because insulin is a storage, or anabolic, hormone, this increased secretion further contributes to obesity. In response to the elevated insulin concentrations, the number of insulin receptors on the target cell gradually decreases, which triggers an even greater secretion of insulin. In this way, the excess glucose is stored despite the decreased availability of insulin binding sites on the cell. Over time, the demands for insulin eventually exceed even the reserve capacity of the "genetically weakened" beta cells, and symptoms of insulin deficiency develop as the plasma glucose concentrations remain high for increasingly longer periods of time. This phenomenon is known as

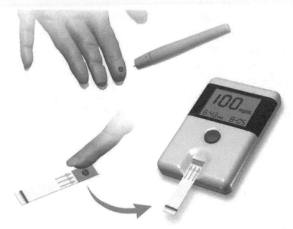

Glucometer. (BruceBlaus)

beta-cell burn out. Because the symptoms of type 2 diabetes are usually less severe than those of type 1 diabetes, many persons have the disease but remain unaware of it. By the time the diagnosis of diabetes is made in these individuals, they also exhibit symptoms of long-term complications that include atherosclerosis and nerve damage. Hence, type 2 diabetes has been called the silent killer.

Gestational diabetes develops during pregnancy in a person who did not have diabetes before becoming pregnant. It occurs in 3 to 8 percent of all pregnancies. Women with gestational diabetes have an increased risk of developing diabetes after pregnancy. Children of women with gestational diabetes have a higher risk of obesity, glucose intolerance, and diabetes in adolescence.

Prediabetes is a condition in which individuals have blood glucose levels that are high, but not high enough for them to be diagnosed with type 2 diabetes. Persons with prediabetes are at higher risk to develop diabetes in the future.

Treatment and Therapy

Insulin is the only treatment available for type 1 diabetes, and in many cases it is used to treat individuals with type 2 diabetes. Insulin is available in many formulations, which differ in respect to the time of onset of action, activity, and duration of action. Insulin preparations are classified as fast acting, intermediate acting, and long acting; the effects of fast-acting insulin last for thirty minutes to twenty-four hours, while those of long-acting preparations last from four to thirty-six hours. Some of the factors that affect the rate of insulin absorption include the site of injection, the patient's age and health status, and the patient's level of physical activity. For a person with diabetes, however, insulin is a reprieve, not a cure.

Because of the complications that arise from chronic exposure to glucose, it is recommended that glucose concentrations in the blood be maintained as close to physiologically normal levels as possible. For this reason, it is preferable to administer multiple doses of insulin during the day. By monitoring plasma glucose concentrations, the diabetic person can adjust the dosage of insulin administered and thus mimic normal concentrations of glucose relatively closely. Basal concentrations of plasma insulin can also be maintained throughout the day by means of electromechanical insulin delivery systems. Whether internal or external, such insulin pumps can be programmed to deliver a constant infusion of insulin at a rate designed to meet minimum requirements. The infusion can then be supplemented by a bolus injection prior to a meal. Increasingly sophisticated systems automatically monitor blood glucose concentrations and adjust the delivery rate of insulin accordingly. These alternative delivery systems are intended to prevent the development of long-term tissue complications.

There are a number of chronic complications that account for the shorter life expectancy of diabetic persons. These include atherosclerotic changes throughout the entire vascular system. The thickening of basement membranes that surround the capillaries can affect their ability to exchange nutrients. Cardiovascular lesions are the most common cause of premature death in diabetic persons. Kidney disease, which is commonly found in longtime diabetics, can ultimately lead to kidney failure. For these persons, expensive medical care, including dialysis and the possibility of a kidney transplant, overshadows their lives. Diabetes is the leading cause of new blindness in the United States. Delayed gastric emptying

(gastroparesis) occurs when the stomach takes too long to empty its contents; it results from damage to the vagus nerve from long-term exposure to high glucose levels. In addition, diabetes leads to a gradual decline in the ability of nerves to conduct sensory information to the brain. For example, the feet of some diabetics feel more like stumps of wood than living tissue. Consequently, weight is not distributed properly; in concert with

the reduction in blood flow, this problem can lead to pressure ulcers. If not properly cared for, areas of the foot can develop gangrene, which may then lead to amputation of the foot. Finally, in male patients, there are problems with reproductive function that generally result in impotence.

The mechanism responsible for the development of these long-term complications of diabetes is genetic in origin and dependent on the amount of time the tissues are exposed to the elevated plasma glucose concentrations. What, then, is the link between glucose concentrations and diabetic complications?

As an animal ages, most of its cells become less efficient in replacing damaged material, while its tissues lose their elasticity and gradually stiffen. For example, the lungs and heart muscle expand less successfully, blood vessels become increasingly rigid, and ligaments begin to tighten. These apparently diverse age-related changes are accelerated in diabetes, and the causative agent is glucose. Glucose becomes chemically attached to proteins and deoxyribonucleic acid (DNA) in the body without the aid of enzymes to speed the reaction along. What is important is the duration of exposure to the elevated glucose concentrations. Once glucose is bound to tissue proteins, a series of chemical reactions is triggered that, over the passage of months and years, can result in the formation and eventual accumulation of cross-links between adjacent proteins. The higher glucose concentrations in diabetics accelerate this process, and the effects become evident in specific tissues throughout the body.

Understanding the chemical basis of protein cross-linking in diabetes has permitted the development and study of compounds that can intervene in this process. Certain compounds, when added to the diet, can limit the glucose-induced cross-linking of proteins by preventing their formation. One of the best-studied compounds, aminoguanidine, can help prevent the cross-linking of collagen; this fact is shown in a decrease in the accumulation of trapped lipoproteins on artery walls. Aminoguanidine also prevents thickening of the capillary basement membrane in the kidney. Aminoguanidine acts by blocking glucose's ability to react with neighboring proteins. Vitamins C and B6 are also effective in reducing cross-linking. Aminoguanidine and vitamins C and B6 are thought to have antiaging properties and may also improve the complications resulting from the high blood-glucose levels seen in diabetes mellitus.

Alternatively, transplantation of the entire pancreas is an effective means of achieving an insulin-independent state in persons with type 1 diabetes mellitus. Both the technical problems of pancreas transplantation and the possible rejection of the foreign tissue, however, have limited this procedure as a treatment for diabetes. Diabetes is usually manageable; therefore, a pancreas transplant is not necessarily lifesaving. Success in treating diabetes has been achieved by transplanting only the insulin-producing islet cells from the pancreas or grafts from fetal pancreas tissue. It may one day be possible to use genetic engineering to permit cells of the liver to self-regulate glucose concentrations by synthesizing and releasing their own insulin into the blood.

Some of the less severe forms of type 2 diabetes mellitus can be controlled by the use of oral hypoglycemic agents that bring about a reduction in blood glucose. These drugs can be taken orally to drive the beta cells to release even more insulin than usual. These drugs also increase the ability of insulin to act on the target cells, which ultimately reduces the insulin requirement. The use of these agents remains controversial, because they overwork the already strained beta cells. If a diabetic person is reliant on these drugs for extended periods of time, the insulin cells could "burn out" and completely lose their ability to synthesize insulin. In this situation, the previously non-insulin-dependent person would have to be placed on insulin therapy for life. Other hypoglycemic agents lower blood glucose by decreasing hepatic glucose output, reducing insulin resistance, and delaying the absorption of glucose from the gastrointestinal tract.

If obesity is a factor in the expression of type 2 diabetes, as it is in most cases, the best therapy is a combination of a reduction of calorie intake and an increase in activity. More than any other disease, type 2 diabetes is related to lifestyle. It is often the case that people prefer having an injection or taking a pill to improving their quality of life by changing their diet and level of activity. Attention to diet and exercise results in a dramatic decrease in the need for drug therapy in most diabetics. In some cases, the loss of only a small percentage of body weight results in an increased sensitivity to insulin. Exercise is particularly helpful in the management of both types of diabetes, because working muscle does not require insulin to metabolize glucose. Thus, exercising muscles take up and use some of the excess glucose in the blood, which reduces the overall need for insulin. Permanent weight reduction and exercise also help to prevent long-term complications and permit a healthier and more active lifestyle.

Perspective and Prospects

Diabetes mellitus is a disease of ancient origin. The first written reference to diabetes, which was discovered in the tomb of Thebes in Egypt (1500 BCE), described an illness associated with the passage of vast quantities of sweet urine and an excessive thirst.

The study of diabetes owes much to the Franco-Prussian War. In 1870, during the siege of Paris, it was noted by French physicians that the widespread famine in the besieged city had a curative influence on diabetic patients. Their glycosuria decreased or disappeared. These observations supported the view of clinicians at the time who had previously prescribed periods of fasting and increased muscular work for the treatment of the overweight diabetic individual.

It was Oscar Minkowski of Germany who, in 1889, accidentally traced the origin of diabetes to the pancreas. Following the complete removal of the pancreas from a dog, Minkowski's technician noted the animal's subsequent copious urine production. Acting on the basis of a hunch, Minkowski tested the urine and determined that its sugar content was greater than 10 percent.

In 1921, Frederick Banting and Charles Best, at the University of Toronto in Canada, successfully extracted the antidiabetic substance insulin using a cold alcohol-hydrochloric acid mixture to inactivate the harsh digestive enzymes of the pancreas. Using this substance, they first controlled the disease in a depancreatized dog and then, a few months later, successfully treated the first human diabetic patient. The clinical application of a discovery normally takes a long time, but in this case a mere twenty weeks had passed between the first injection of insulin into the diabetic dog and the first trial with a diabetic human. Three years later, in 1923, Banting and Best were awarded the Nobel

Prize in physiology or medicine for their remarkable achievement.

Although insulin, when combined with an appropriate diet and exercise, alleviates the symptoms of diabetes to such an extent that a diabetic can lead an essentially normal life, insulin therapy is not a cure. The complications that arise in diabetics are typical of those found in the general population, except that they happen much earlier in the diabetic. With regard to these glucose-induced complications, it was first postulated in 1908 that sugars could react with proteins. In 1912, Louis Camille Maillard further characterized this reaction at the Sorbonne and realized that the consequences of this reaction were relevant to diabetics. Maillard suggested that sugars were destroying the body's amino acids, which then led to increased excretion in diabetics. It was not until the mid-1970s, however, that Anthony Cerami in New York introduced the concept of the nonenzymatic attachment of glucose to protein and recognized its potential role in diabetic complications. A decade later, this development led to the discovery of aminoguanidine, the first compound to limit the cross-linking of tissue proteins and thus delay the development of certain diabetic complications.

In 1974, Josiah Brown published the first report showing that diabetes could be reversed by transplanting fetal pancreatic tissue. By the mid-1980s, procedures had been devised for the isolation of massive numbers of human islets that could then be transplanted into diabetics. For persons with diabetes, both procedures represent more than a treatment; they may offer a cure for the disease.

By the turn of the twenty-first century, there was a noticeable rise in the prevalence of type 2 diabetes in both developing and developed countries. According to the World Health Organization (WHO), an estimated 347 million people worldwide have diabetes, a number expected to rise. Although the incidence of type 2 diabetes typically increases with age, the first decades of the twenty-first century have seen a dramatic rise in the number of cases in younger people.

Obesity is clearly linked to the increase of type 2 diabetes. The growing sedentary lifestyle and increase in energy-dense food intake are significant risk factors. The WHO reported that worldwide obesity nearly doubled between 1980 and 2013. By 2008, about 35 percent of adults were overweight, and 11 percent were obese. Due in large part to these factors, the WHO has predicted that diabetes will become the seventh leading cause of death by 2030.

—*Hillar Klandorf, Sharon W. Stark*

References

Algoblan, Abdullah, et al. "Mechanism Linking Diabetes Mellitus and Obesity." *Diabetes, Metabolic Syndrome and Obesity: Targets and Therapy*, 2014, p. 587., doi:10.2147/dmso.s67400.

Bramante, Carolyn T., et al. "Treatment of Obesity in Patients With Diabetes." *Diabetes Spectrum*, vol. 30, no. 4, 2017, pp. 237–243., doi:10.2337/ds17-0030.

Corbin, Karen D, et al. "Obesity in Type 1 Diabetes: Pathophysiology, Clinical Impact, and Mechanisms." *Endocrine Reviews*, vol. 39, no. 5, 27 July 2018, pp. 629–663., doi:10.1210/er.2017-00191.

Leitner, Deborah R., et al. "Obesity and Type 2 Diabetes: Two Diseases with a Need for Combined Treatment Strategies - EASO Can Lead the Way." *Obesity Facts*, vol. 10, no. 5, 2017, pp. 483–492., doi:10.1159/000480525.

Minges, Karl E., et al. "Overweight and Obesity in Youth With Type 1 Diabetes." *Annual Review of Nursing Research*, vol. 31, no. 1, 2013, pp. 47–69., doi:10.1891/0739-6686.31.47.

Mottalib, Adham, et al. "Weight Management in Patients with Type 1 Diabetes and Obesity." *Current Diabetes Reports*, vol. 17, no. 10, 23 Aug. 2017, doi:10.1007/s11892-017-0918-8.

Wooton, Angela Kaye, and Lynne M. Melchior. "Obesity and Type 2 Diabetes in Our Youth: A Recipe for Cardiovascular Disease." *The Journal for Nurse Practitioners*, vol. 13, no. 3, 2017, pp. 222–227., doi:10.1016/j.nurpra.2016.08.035.

◼ Diabetic nephropathy

CATEGORY: Disorder

Causes and Symptoms

Diabetes mellitus is a disease in which the body's ability to produce the hormone *insulin* is impaired (type 1 diabetes mellitus) or the body's ability to respond to insulin is impaired (type 2 diabetes mellitus). Insulin regulates the concentration of *glucose*, or sugar, in the blood. Prolonged exposure to high levels of glucose in the blood damages the blood vessels, eyes, heart, nerves, and kidneys.

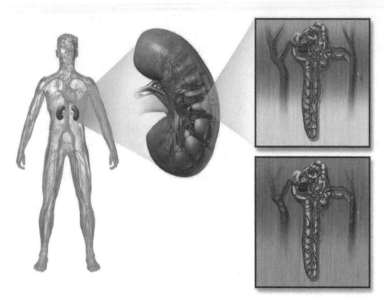

Diabetic nephropathy. (BruceBlaus)

Kidneys consists about one million of tiny functional units called *nephrons*. Nephrons filter the blood to remove the byproducts of metabolism and foreign molecules that are left over after the body burns food for energy and convert them into urine, which is excreted from the body. In diabetics, especially those who might not know they are diabetic and are therefore untreated, the excess glucose in the blood is excreted into the urine (glycosuria) and can cause damage to the nephrons, especially the *glomeruli*, the tiny knot of blood vessels that are covered by the podocytes in the Bowman's capsule where the blood is filtered. As damage to the glomeruli accumulates, the glomeruli become scarred, which limits their ability to participate in blood filtration. Such a condition is known as diabetic nephropathy (DN). If the damage becomes severe, it can severely limit the ability of the kidneys to filter blood, and the patient will require *dialysis*. In this process, the blood is removed from the body by a tube, filtered by a special machine, and returned to the body via another tube.

All diabetics are at risk for DN, including those who do not know they have diabetes. It is estimated that more than six million people in the United States alone may have type 2 diabetes without knowing it. These people are at greater risk for developing DN. Other risk factors include high blood pressure, a family history of kidney disease or diabetes with kidney disease, and smoking. In addition, certain ethnic groups have an increased risk of developing diabetes and DN, including African Americans, Native Americans, and Hispanics.

In the early stages of diabetic neuropathy, there may be no symptoms. The disease comes on slowly, and damage to the kidneys can begin ten years before any symptoms present. When the damage becomes severe enough, the patient will likely experience fatigue, headaches, digestive issues, frequent nighttime urination, swelling or cramping in the lower extremities, and itchy skin.

Because DN occurs so frequently in diabetics, comes on slowly, and may be present for years without any symptoms, physicians routinely screen patients for higher levels of albumin in the urine. This condition, known as *albuminuria*, indicates that there is kidney damage. DN is diagnosed when a patient has albuminuria with protein levels greater than 300 milligrams in a 24-hour urine collection accompanied by damage to the glomeruli and high blood pressure. Physicians use blood tests and urine tests as part of the diagnosis and may use ultrasound technology to image the kidneys. In some cases, a kidney biopsy may be ordered.

Patients newly diagnosed with type 2 diabetes are generally tested immediately for DN because their condition may have existed without detection for some time. In these patients, kidney disease may have begun even before they were aware of their diabetes.

Kidney disease caused by DN is categorized by five stages. These stages are based on the ability of the glomeruli to continue filtering the blood, known as the *glomerular filtrationrate*, or GFR. Stage 1 indicates kidney damage with continued normal GFR. Stage 2 is kidney damage with mild decrease in GFR. Stage 3 indicates moderate decrease in GFR, while Stage 4 is characterized by a severe decrease in GFR. Stage 5 is kidney failure, necessitating medical intervention such as dialysis or a kidney transplant.

Treatment and Therapy

The first step in treatment is to minimize the impact of diabetic nephropathy by ensuring blood sugar levels are under control. This may require medication changes or adjustments, exercise, and/ or weight loss. Adequate diabetic control will minimize the amount of blood glucose and reduce the chances of it causing damage to other parts of the body, including the kidneys. Adequate blood pressure control is also important, so medication and other steps to reduce high blood pressure are part of the treatment for DN. Pharmacological agents that inhibit the renin-angiotensinaldosterone system (RAAS) are of particular efficacy.

The RAAS is used by the kidney to maintain blood flow to the kidney and thereby assure relatively constant blood filtration rates. In response to decreased blood flow rates through the kidney, the kidney responds by secreting an enzyme called renin into the blood. Renin acts upon a small blood-based protein made by the liver called angiotensin ogen. Renin cleaves angiotensinogen into the smaller peptide angiotensin I. While circulating through the bloodstream, angiotensin I encounters the enzyme angiotensin converting enzyme (ACE) in the capillaries of the lung, which cleaves angiotensin I to the smaller peptide angiotensin II. Angiotensin II is a potent blood vessel constrictor that cinches down blood vessels everywhere else and leave most of the blood flowing to the kidney. Angiotensin II, therefore, substantially raises blood pressure, and is a prime target for blood pressure medicine (antihypertensives).

Angiotensin Converting Enzyme (ACE) inhibitors, such as captopril, enalapril, lisinopril, and others, prevent the conversion of angiotensin I into the potent vasoconstrictor angiotensin II. Angiotensin Receptor Blockers (ARBs) such as irbesartan, telmisartan, valsartan, and others, prevent angiotensin II from binding to its main receptor an eliciting its biological response. Both class of drugs have been shown in many clinical trials to preserve renal function in patients with DN. Avoiding dietary sodium is often recommended. Considerable uncertainty remains regarding the efficacy of a low protein diet in DN patients and the disadvantages of such a diet may outweigh the benefits.

In addition, patients are often advised to avoid medications known to adversely affect the kidneys, including nonsteroidal anti-inflammatory drugs (NSAIDs) and higher doses of aspirin. Diuretics, which increase urine output, can also cause problems, as can the radiocontrast agents used in some imaging tests.

In severe cases, a patient will be placed on dialysis. Stage 5 patients may also require a kidney transplant, where the damaged kidney or kidneys are surgically removed and replaced by a donor kidney. Because a person can live with one kidney, a kidney donation may come from a living person, such as a relative or another individual who is medically compatible with the patient.

—*Janine Ungvarsky, Michael A. Buratovich*

References

Batuman, Vecihi. "Diabetic Nephropathy." *Medscape*, 9 Oct. 2019, emedicine.medscape.com/ article/238946-overview.

Chao, Anthony Tl, et al. "Effect of Bariatric Surgery on Diabetic Nephropathy in Obese Type 2 Diabetes Patients in a Retrospective 2-Year Study: A Local Pilot." *Diabetes and Vascular Disease Research*, vol. 15, no. 2, 18 Nov. 2017, pp. 139–144., doi:10.1177/1479164117742315.

Maric-Bilkan, Christine. "Obesity and Diabetic Kidney Disease." *Medical Clinics of North America*, vol. 97, no. 1, 2013, pp. 59–74., doi:10.1016/j. mcna.2012.10.010.

Todd, Jennifer N., et al. "Genetic Evidence for a Causal Role of Obesity in Diabetic Kidney Disease." *Diabetes*, vol. 64, no. 12, 25 Dec. 2015, pp. 4238–4246., doi:10.2337/db15-0254.

■ Diabetic neuropathy

CATEGORY: Disorder

Causes and Symptoms

It has been reported that diabetic neuropathy, one of the most common consequences of long-standing diabetes mellitus, occurs at rates as high as 49% according to a community-based study of 15,692 people with confirmed diagnoses. Symptomatic neuropathy, defined as impairment of pain, light touch, and temperature, is reported as high as 35% in the same population. The risk for diabetic neuropathy increases as the duration of the disease increases, and the disease prevalence has reached epidemic proportions.

Diabetes mellitus, Types I and II, is a disease that is caused by the body's inability to handle ingested sugar. In the juvenile, or congenital, form of diabetes mellitus Type I, a lack of -cells in the pancreas, which normally produce insulin, the primary hormone that handles glucose, leads to the disease. In diabetes mellitus Type II, there is typically a lifestyle component that contributes to an overload of glucose, overworking the insulin receptors and creating insulin resistance. In both types, the high circulating blood glucose content (hyperglycemia) damages many different cells and can cause four major forms of neuropathy: peripheral, autonomic, proximal, and focal.

Peripheral neuropathy is the most common form, affecting the toes, feet, and legs. It can also involve the arms and hands, but primarily affects the lower extremities due their distance from the central circulation of the heart. This is also caused by blood pooling within the extremities. In a healthy, ambulatory person, skeletal muscle contraction pumps blood from the legs back to the heart through via a network of veins that contain one-way valves. This system is named the veno-muscular pump and acts as the primary source of venous blood movement. If the person is non-ambulatory or their valves are disrupted, the blood pools, thereby exposing the vessel and nerve cells to large amounts of stagnant glucose that can cause damage. This type of neuropathy is experienced as loss of feeling or as painful sensations in the affected body parts. Patients with peripheral neuropathy describe the sensations as tingling or burning and can feel as if something is crawling over their limbs or stabbing them with a pin. The pain can be mild or severe and typically is worse following a high sugar meal or periods of immobility such as at night. Some patients experience peripheral neuropathy at the opposite extreme of sensation and are unable to sense pain or temperature changes. This form of neuropathy makes foot care critical for diabetics, who may sustain a significant injury or infection to the foot without realizing it due to a lack of sensation. Patients with peripheral neuropathy are at increased risk of requiring amputation because of poor healing and infections, particularly to the foot and lower extremities. Some patients might also experience cramping, have extreme sensitivity to touch, or suffer loss of coordination and balance because of the nerve damage in advanced cases.

Autonomic neuropathy can affect the heart and blood vessels, the lungs, the digestive system, the urinary tract, reproductive organs, sweat glands, and the eyes. It can result in changes to blood pressure, lung function, and vision. This form of neuropathy can also cause changes to digestion, leading to difficulty swallowing, constipation, and diarrhea. Bladder function can be impaired and lead to retained urine, which can cause urinary tract infections. If the nerves that alert a person to a full bladder are affected, the opposite problem can occur resulting in incontinent. The condition can also cause decreased sexual responsiveness due to a lack of nerve sensitivity. When the sweat glands are affected, the patient may sweat profusely or be unable to sweat, both of which impair the body's ability to regulate its temperature efficiently. Some diabetics will also experience a condition known as hypoglycemic unawareness, in which they become unable to detect the warning signs of low blood sugar levels, such as irregular heartbeat, shakiness, weakness, and blurred vision. This condition of hypoglycemia can result in seizures and even death if left untreated.

Proximal neuropathy affects the upper portions of the legs, including the thighs, hips, and buttocks. It can cause weakness and subsequent difficulty in transitioning from a seated position to a standing position, and visa versa. Proximal neuropathy is also known as diabetic amyotrophy, lumbosacral plexus neuropathy, or femoral neuropathy.

Focal neuropathy affects nerves in a specific area, usually in the head, torso, or legs. It can cause vision problems, such as double vision or difficulty focusing. When the nerves on one side of the face are affected, it can cause a paralytic condition known as Bell's palsy. Focal neuropathy can also cause severe pain in the chest, stomach, lower back or pelvis, thighs, lower legs, or the feet.

Although each patient's symptomatology can be different and onset may be delayed for some and acute in others, the foremost concern for these individuals is undergoing an injury that they cannot feel. Ulcer formation is one of the most common ailments affecting people with neuropathy because they simply cannot feel a wound beginning to form. It is not uncommon for these individuals to undergo a puncture wound to their foot and only notice a discoloration on their sock at the end of the day. That is how infection starts and how the path to more serious injuries begins. This also acts as the source for chronic wounds of such severity that they may warrant amputation before more harm befalls the patient such as major bacterial infection and

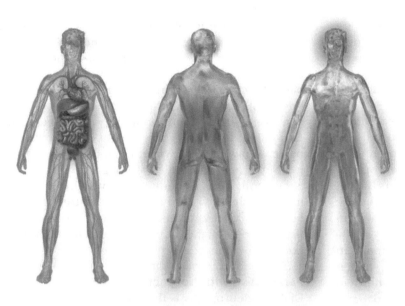

Illustration depicting areas affected by diabetic neuropathy. (BruceBlaus)

sepsis. Early prevention is key in all cases of neuropathy due to the dire consequences implicit within its untreated form, and often accomplished with a skilled team of physicians from primary care, endocrinology, and podiatric services.

With the high number of symptoms and complications associated with diabetic neuropathy, the sequence of diagnosis is done frequently and by a skilled physician. This is indicated due to the direct correlation between severity of symptoms and duration of the disease. Several neurological tests are employed to help inform the treatment of the patient, the most common of which are discussed below.

Protective sensation is one of the most ubiquitous examinations to determine neuropathic numbness in a patient. It is assessed on the extremities in two primary ways. The "Semmes Weinstein Monofilament" is a tool that exerts a standard force to various points on the hands and feet. With eyes closed, the patient is asked if they are able to feel the device. Related to this exam is the Ipswitch Touch Test, which also assesses protective sensation. This is performed in a similar fashion, but the physician's fingertips are used in lieu of a device. Both versions of the assessment have been deemed reliable, sensitive, and specific to symptomatic neuropathy and are standard practice in many physician offices if neuropathy is suspected. Sharp and dull discrimination testing is done with standard

devices and is also performed with the patients eyes closed, testing whether or not an individual can determine the correct sensation.

Muscle strength testing is used to assess the ability of the patients own body to adequately perform activities and to protect from abnormal movement that can lead to injury. This is done by testing force exerted on the practitioner, and is often examined according to individual muscles or muscle groups. Related to this is proprioception, or the body's ability to sense where it is in space and in relation to itself. One common way this is assessed is by moving the toes or the foot up and down while the patient's eyes are closed and having the patient determine the movement. Vibratory sensation is also related to the same neurological mechanisms that dictate proprioception and pain, and is assessed by placing a standard vibrating device on a bony prominence and assessing the patient's ability to feel when the vibration has ceased.

In a similar vein, deep tendon reflexes are a good determinant for assessing if certain nervous system structures are intact and healthy, namely the communication between the brain and the spinal cord. Many people have experienced this exam as part of their regular physical exam and entails lightly tapping several areas, namely the patellar tendon, the Achilles tendon, the biceps and triceps tendons to assess the corresponding movement. Implicit within the aforementioned brain and spinal cord communication is the patient's ability to ambulate with coordinated movement. This is assessed with a standing gait exam performed by a trained physician and often can employ devices that can record gait, weight balance, base of gait, cadence, and other factors that may be adversely affected by neuropathy.

Treatment and Therapy
Lifestyle modification, mainly the incorporation of diet and exercise into a person's daily regimen, may lead to decreases in symptomatic neuropathy. This stems from the benefits gained with proper glycemic control, or control of your body's sugar

intake and processing, as well as lowers the likelihood of vascular compromise to the extremities. Additionally, people with lower incidence of obesity tend to have a decreased chance of developing diabetes mellitus type II, thereby preventing the most common cause of neuropathy before it begins.

Beginning from the most conservative end of the spectrum, barring lifestyle modifications such as diet and exercise which have been proven to be the most efficacious ways of preventing neuropathy, is the use of vitamin supplements. Vitamins B6 and B12 have shown to protectively impact the structure of the myelin sheath, or the protective coating surrounding nerve cells, thereby preventing breakdown and subsequent neuropathic symptoms. In paradoxical contrast, longstanding use of Vitamin B6, greater than 500mg per day, has been shown to increase the chances of neuropathy in patients already susceptible to the condition. In addition, there are a myriad of pharmacological therapies that can also lower the body's sugar tolerance, the most common of which is Metformin. This drug is considered a "first line treatment" therapy for diabetes mellitus type II, acting to inhibit the liver's ability to break down and release sugar into the bloodstream, effectively preventing high latent sugar levels from causing nerve damage.

In cases of painful neuropathy, there are several pharmacological agents aimed at decreasing the most common symptoms associated with nerve damage and associated pain. Tricyclic anti-depressants and anticonvulsants have shown promise in decreasing the body's ability to sense pain in the extremities, namely Gabapentin. Capsaicin cream, derived from a naturally occurring compound found in hot peppers, can also be used as a topical agent to effectively overload the mechanism that would normally sense pain. Topical anesthetic drugs such as lidocaine patches have also been used as adjunctive therapy for pain localized to one particular area. Overall, a combination of pharmacologic agents and lifestyle modification with goals of increasing glucose control have been shown to be the most efficacious route in quelling neuropathic pain in the diabetic population.

Future studies have shed light on possible therapies that can decrease painful neuropathic symptoms. Electric nerve stimulation, a procedure often performed within the field of physical therapy,

augments the normal nerve activation system by essentially turning off pain signaling within the peripheral nerve being targeted. Another possible treatment with still limited research is the use of cannabis and cannabinoid derivatives to treat painful neuropathy. These agents, namely Nabilone and Dronabinol, have already been in use for decreasing nausea and vomiting associated with chemotherapy. They have also been shown to decrease pain associated with diabetic neuropathy in several reported studies, although more research is currently being conducted. Overall, there are many possibilities on the horizon for treating diabetic neuropathy, and new research is consistently being used to further mitigate its painful effect on a population of increasing incidence.

Perspective and Prospects

Diabetic neuropathy is the most common neuropathy in the western world, more prevalent than neuropathy associated with alcoholism or chemotherapeutic agents combined. The prevalence of its precursor and namesake, diabetes, affects approximately 9.4% of the US population and its incidence is on the rise. This number may also be falsely decreased with a large population that remains undiagnosed but fail to seek medical attention until symptoms require them. The increased occurrence of this disease is, in part, due to a failure in proper nutrition and emphasis on exercise within the general population. Years of smoking, eating large amounts of fatty and sugar-laden foods, and being sedentary are all contributing factors.

Recently there have been efforts to educate and inform the general public about the consequences of not eating right and maintaining a regular exercise regimen, although the effects are still not leading to a decrease in new reports of the disease. Pharmacologic efforts have shown great promise in slowing the harmful effects of heightened sugar on neuropathic symptoms. New studies on the benefits of exercise have also shown to improve the efficacy of these medications, with some anecdotal evidence even suggests that the symptoms of neuropathy can be reversed. There are numerous approaches to combating this disease, namely stopping it before it occurs with proper diet and exercise, and more treatments remain forthcoming. Perhaps with continued efforts and an emphasis on educating people about diet and lifestyle modification, the ravaging effects of diabetes, and the disease itself, will be a thing of the past.

—*Zachary Sax*

References

Callaghan, Brian C., et al. "Diabetes and Obesity Are the Main Metabolic Drivers of Peripheral Neuropathy." *Annals of Clinical and Translational Neurology*, vol. 5, no. 4, 14 Feb. 2018, pp. 397–405., doi:10.1002/acn3.531.

Hozumi, Jun, et al. "Relationship between Neuropathic Pain and Obesity." *Pain Research and Management*, vol. 2016, 2016, pp. 1–6., doi:10.1155/2016/2487924.

Look AHEAD Research Group. "Effects of a Long-Term Lifestyle Modification Programme on Peripheral Neuropathy in Overweight or Obese Adults with Type 2 Diabetes: the Look AHEAD Study." *Diabetologia*, vol. 60, no. 6, 27 Mar. 2017, pp. 980–988., doi:10.1007/s00125-017-4253-z.

Stiles, Laura. "Prediabetes, Obesity May Impact Risk of Polyneuropathy." *Neurology Advisor*, 15 Feb. 2020, www.neurologyadvisor.com/topics/neuropathy/prediabetes-obesity-may-impact-risk-of-polyneuropathy/.

Wyne, Kathleen l. "The Lesser-Known Consequences of Obesity." *EmPower*, 2014, pp. 7–9.

■ Dietary fat and risk of cancer

CATEGORY: Disorder; Nutrition

An individual's risk of developing cancer is influenced by a combination of genetic, environmental, and lifestyle factors. Some lifestyle practices are well-established risk factors for cancer, such as cigarette smoking in the development of lung cancer. The role of other practices, such as diet, is less clear in the evidence-based research. One focus of current cancer research is the effect that specific components of the diet, including dietary fat, have on a person's risk of developing cancer.

The term dietary fat encompasses two types of fat: saturated fat and unsaturated fat. The unsaturated fatty acids are further classified as monounsaturated fatty acids (MUFAs), polyunsaturated fatty acids (PUFAs), and trans fat.

Saturated fat is found mainly in animal-based foods, including red meat, dairy products, and eggs, but is also found in coconut, palm, and palm kernel oils. Saturated fat intake raises low-density lipoprotein (LDL) cholesterol, is associated with insulin resistance (i.e., decreased effect of insulin in lowering blood glucose levels), and is potentially linked to increased cancer risk.

Unsaturated fat is found in a variety of vegetables, vegetable oils (e.g., olive oil), and fatty fish (e.g., salmon, herring, and mackerel). The essential fatty acids linoleic acid and linolenic acid are types of PUFAs. MUFAs and PUFAs are considered "good" fats; consumption of these unsaturated fats can help maintain healthy blood cholesterol levels and lower risk for cardiovascular disease. MUFAs and PUFAs are not generally thought to increase cancer risk; results of some studies actually suggest that high intake of some unsaturated fats lowers risk for some types of cancer. Researchers report that omega-3 PUFAs inhibit the growth of premalignant and malignant bladder cancer lesions in a rat model. Results of a New England case-control study revealed that omega-3 PUFA's are protective against epithelial ovarian cancer, particularly against endometrioid tumors, while trans fats are associated with an increase in epithelial ovarian cancer risk.

Trans fats occur naturally in small amounts in meat and dairy products but are primarily consumed in margarine, fried foods, and other processed foods that contain partially hydrogenated oils. Food manufacturers purposely hydrogenate oils that are desired to be solid at room temperature by adding hydrogen. Trans fat intake of any quantity is widely discouraged, as trans fats have no known health benefits and are associated with an increased risk for heart disease and diabetes mellitus, type 2 (DM2); the role of trans fats in the development of cancer is unclear.

Research Findings

Dietary fat was first implicated as a risk factor for cancer based on results of animal studies conducted prior to 1950. In the second half of the 20th century, the link between dietary fat intake and cancer risk was strengthened when investigators of ecologic studies attributed the wide disparity in worldwide cancer incidence to population-specific differences in dietary fat intake. The association that was made between the intake of dietary fat and cancer risk led to the development of public health guidelines in the 1980s regarding reducing dietary fat intake to 30% of calories to prevent cancer.

Investigators in large prospective cohort studies and authors of meta-analyses have published data that do not consistently support the hypothesis that high dietary fat intake increases cancer risk. This supports the ongoing need to differentiate fat subtypes (e.g., saturated versus unsaturated fats) and fat sources (e.g., animal versus non-animal sources) when examining the potential role of dietary fat in the development of or protection against specific types of cancer.

Researchers evaluated the relationship between dietary fat intake and the risk of non-Hodgkin lymphoma (NHL) and concluded that diets high in trans fats, processed meats, and high-fat dairy are associated with an increased risk for NHL, while high intake of omega-3 PUFA's is associated with a lower risk of NHL.

Previous associations have been drawn between higher intake of red meat and dairy products and increased risk for prostate cancer. Recently, researchers have added to these findings by reporting that the connection between intake of dairy products and increased rate of death from prostate cancer was limited to intake of whole milk.

Summary
Individuals should learn about the association of dietary fat and risk for cancer. The current public health recommendations for cancer prevention include maintaining a healthy body weight, exercising regularly, and eating well. It is important to not restrict unsaturated fat intake because unsaturated fats (with the exception of trans fats) can actually reduce risk for cardiovascular disease. Limiting red meat consumption to small, lean portions and getting adequate physical activity may also reduce cancer risk. Although a definitive link between dietary fat and cancer risk has not been established, a clear link does exist between having a high percentage of body fat and increased risk for cancer. It is beneficial to stay current on recent research regarding the effects of dietary components on cancer risk.

—*Gilberto Cabrera, Cherie Marcel*

References
Forouhi, Nita G, et al. "Dietary Fat and Cardiometabolic Health: Evidence, Controversies, and Consensus for Guidance." *BMJ*, 13 June 2018, doi:10.1136/bmj.k2139.

Liu, Ann G., et al. "A Healthy Approach to Dietary Fats: Understanding the Science and Taking Action to Reduce Consumer Confusion." *Nutrition Journal*, vol. 16, no. 1, 2017, doi:10.1186/s12937-017-0271-4.

Sackner-Bernstein, Jonathan, et al. "Dietary Intervention for Overweight and Obese Adults: Comparison of Low-Carbohydrate and Low-Fat Diets. A Meta-Analysis." *Plos One*, vol. 10, no. 10, 20 Oct. 2015, doi:10.1371/journal.pone.0139817.

■ Eating disorders

CATEGORY: Disorder

Causes and Symptoms
Identified eating disorders include anorexia nervosa, bulimia nervosa, and binge-eating disorder. These disorders are not always distinct, and many individuals exhibit symptoms of more than one. Their prevalence has increased during the past several decades. Anorexia nervosa and bulimia nervosa predominantly affect adolescent and young adult females. However, they can also occur in males and the elderly, and binge-eating disorder occurs more frequently in males. Approximately 4 percent of females have eating disorders, although the number of those who do not meet the full criteria for diagnosing any specific disorder is much higher. There is an approximately nine to one ratio of females to males with eating disorders. The incidence of eating disorders in males is rising, however, and they are most commonly associated with sports (such as wrestling), bodybuilding, and the performing arts (such as dance). The disorders can be chronic and recur across the life span of an individual. Recognition of eating disorders in the elderly has increased, as have the negative health affects of the conditions on this population.

Anorexia nervosa is characterized by refusal to maintain normal body weight (less than 85 percent of expected weight), extreme fear of becoming fat, and relentless pursuit of thinness. Individuals with anorexia nervosa have a distorted perception of body weight and size and consider themselves to be overweight even when the opposite is true. Their view of themselves is heavily dependent on factors such as their level of adherence to a restrictive diet or the fit of their clothes. They often deny the negative aspects of low weight even in the face of serious health problems.

Two types of anorexia nervosa have been identified: the restricting type, involving dieting, fasting, or skipping meals, but not bingeing/purging; and the binge-eating/purging type, involving binge eating and purging (self-induced vomiting or misusing laxatives, enemas, or diuretics). The latter type is primarily distinguished from bulimia nervosa by refusal to maintain 85 percent of normal body weight. Dieting regimens may be severe, with intake reduced to between three hundred and six hundred kilocalories (Calories) per day and strict habits regarding food selection and eating.

Individuals with anorexia nervosa commonly display a set of personality and behavioral characteristics including being goal driven, perfectionistic, and overtly competent at school or work. Underlying these tendencies is often a lack of confidence and low sense of self-worth. As dieting increases, individuals may become depressed and fatigued, causing school or work to suffer and further eroding self-perception. Rigid "all or nothing" thinking influences the severity of dieting. Thus, anorexic people might believe that if they permit themselves even one lapse in dieting, then they will become obese. As starvation develops, focus on food and weight increases, and behaviors such as hoarding food, gazing in mirrors, or seeking reassurance about appearance may be observed. Significant energy is expended to keep secret the severity of weight loss efforts. Consequently, exercise may be conducted privately, family meals and public eating avoided, or food disposed of surreptitiously. In some cases, anorexia nervosa is not discovered until after a health problem has developed consequent to malnutrition.

A number of serious health problems stemming from starvation and malnutrition are seen in people with anorexia nervosa. Among the most serious are those associated with cardiac functioning, including cardiomyopathy, arrhythmias, and altered heart rates. In rare cases, sudden death can occur as a result of irregular heart muscle contractions. Other health problems caused by anorexia nervosa involve the gastrointestinal system (bloating and constipation), the reproductive system (amenorrhea, hormonal abnormalities, and infertility), and the

skeletal system (osteoporosis and osteopenia). Additional complications include lowered metabolism, cold intolerance, weakness, loss of muscle mass, low body temperature, and growth suppression. While elderly individuals with anorexia nervosa may not exhibit a drive for thinness, behaviors such as food refusal, the hoarding or hiding of food, and distorted body image are often observed. The health effects of anorexia nervosa in this population are significant and worsen coexisting illnesses, sometimes hastening death. A very serious condition known as the "female athlete triad" is a combination of factors involving athletic training: disordered eating, amenorrhea, and osteoporosis. Permanent damage to bone strength can result from this condition. Despite the numerous medical problems caused by anorexia nervosa, many with the disorder appear superficially healthy even after significant weight loss.

Bulimia nervosa is characterized by recurrent episodes of binge eating followed by purging or other inappropriate efforts to avoid weight gain. The episodes are accompanied by feelings of being out of control and subsequent self-disgust, guilt, and depression. Bingeing involves eating over a limited period of time an amount of food that is markedly larger than most people would under similar circumstances. Caloric intake during binges may range from two thousand to ten thousand. Social interruption, fear of discovery, or physical discomfort (nausea or abdominal pain) typically terminates the binge episode. The binge-purge cycle may occur several times per day, with considerable effort directed toward keeping the episodes secret. Typically, bulimics recognize that their behavior is abnormal and desire to change (as opposed to those with anorexia nervosa). The disorder is divided into two types. The purging type involves self-induced vomiting or laxative, diuretic, or enema misuse as methods to avoid weight gain. The nonpurging type involves fasting or excessive exercise to prevent weight gain.

Self-induced vomiting is the most frequent method of purging and is typically accomplished by initiating the gag reflex by placing fingers down the throat. Over time, many bulimics are able to vomit reflexively without the need to use their fingers. Though employed less frequently as the sole methods of purging, laxatives, enemas, and rarely diuretics may be used in conjunction with vomiting. Abuse of laxatives is more common among the elderly.

Individuals with nonpurging bulimia nervosa, especially males, engage in hours of exercise every day or fast following bingeing. Typically, the fast is broken by another binge episode and the cycle continues.

Those with bulimia nervosa place strong emphasis on appearance, and their mood and view of themselves are highly dependent on their weight and body shape. Most are at a normal weight, but some are underweight or overweight. Often bulimia nervosa is initiated by a restrictive diet that appears to cause many of the unusual behaviors and thinking patterns associated with anorexia nervosa, such as secretive behavior, food hoarding, and extreme focus on food and eating. There may be signs of depression and anxiety as well as compulsive behavior. As opposed to anorexia nervosa, those with bulimia nervosa are more likely to be interested in social relations and to worry more about how others perceive them. Some engage in impulsive behaviors such as substance abuse or shoplifting.

Serious medical complications can result from bulimia nervosa. Chronic vomiting or laxative abuse and consequent loss of body fluids may cause dizziness, cardiac abnormalities, dehydration, and weakness. Tooth decay caused by repeated exposure to gastric acids from vomiting may occur. Erosion or tearing of the esophagus can result from chronic vomiting. Bingeing is associated with a variety of gastrointestinal disturbances including bloating, diarrhea, and constipation.

Binge-eating disorder is a relatively newly identified condition, and less is known about it. The disorder is similar to bulimia nervosa but does not involve efforts to avoid weight gain (such as purging). Individuals with the disorder regularly engage in binges lasting up to several hours, during which from two thousand to ten thousand Calories may be consumed. Eating during binges is typically at a rapid pace and continues in spite of feeling discomfort or pain. Bingeing may occur when an individual is not very hungry, after attempting to keep a strict diet, or as a means to reduce stress. It is usually done in private and kept secret. Feeling out of control during binges is common, followed by feelings of self-disgust and shame. Preoccupation with food and unusual food-related behaviors (such as hiding food) are common. Individuals with binge-eating disorder are typically overweight and unhappy with their body shape and size. General mood and self-perception may be dependent on their weight and size. Depression and anxiety are common coexisting conditions. Distorted body image is less likely than with anorexia nervosa and bulimia nervosa. The health problems related to obesity are seen in those with binge-eating disorder. They include high blood pressure, diabetes, high cholesterol, and heart disease. Gastrointestinal problems may also result from bingeing.

The precise causes of eating disorders are unknown; however, a number of factors involving biological, psychological, and social variables have been identified as contributing to the conditions. The primary biological influences on all eating disorders are related to hunger and starvation. Research indicates that in healthy individuals, severe dieting produces moodiness, irritability, depression, food obsessions, social isolation, and apathy. These symptoms are also found in eating disorders and become more pronounced as starvation emerges. Thus, anorexia nervosa, bulimia nervosa, or binge-eating disorder may develop after food deprivation has occurred as a result of purposeful dieting in order to lose weight or enhance athletic performance, or consequent to food restriction resulting from illness (especially in the elderly) or stress. Hunger resulting from restrictive dieting is the major stimulus for bingeing. Because a majority of those who diet do not develop eating disorders, there is likely some as yet unidentified biological or genetic predisposition in some individuals. Biological abnormalities associated with the hypothalamus and thyroid gland have been identified in some individuals with anorexia nervosa, while other research points to neurochemical or hormonal imbalances. In the elderly, medications, coexisting health problems, and even poorly fitting dentures may initiate restricted eating, leading to anorexia nervosa. Irregular levels of the neurotransmitter serotonin may influence bingeing in bulimia nervosa and binge-eating disorder since it is associated with triggering signals of satiety to the brain. Knowledge of the causes of binge-eating disorder is limited; however, as with bulimia nervosa, there often is a history of being overweight or obese prior to developing the disorder.

A number of psychological factors have been identified as causing eating disorders. Most of these are not mutually exclusive, and none has been universally accepted as the primary causative factor for the conditions. Factors proposed to account for anorexia nervosa include phobic responses to food and weight gain, conflicted feelings over adolescent development and sexual maturity, and reactions to feelings of personal ineffectiveness by "controlling" hunger and the body. Faulty thinking, known as cognitive distortions, may cause misperceptions in body image and undue emphasis on the importance of appearance. Powerful needs to demonstrate self-discipline and to develop feelings of uniqueness and independence may also contribute to anorexia nervosa. Individuals with bulimia nervosa often exhibit mood fluctuations as well as impulsive behaviors. Bulimia nervosa is thought by some to be a variant of obsessive-compulsive disorder (OCD) in which bingeing results from irresistible urges to eat and purging is engaged in to alleviate overwhelming anxiety. Fewer psychological causes have been identified in binge-eating disorder. Some research suggests that characteristics seen in bulimia nervosa such as impulsivity and mood changes are also associated with this disorder. Depression, especially in the elderly population, appears to play a role in all eating disorders. Middle-aged and elderly individuals may employ behaviors such as extreme dieting, bingeing, and purging to reduce anxiety or to exert control in their lives.

Societal factors appear to also contribute to eating disorders. Popular media increasingly promotes physical appearance, and thinness is held up as the ideal body type. Since the 1950s, there have been steady decreases in the weights of influential persons such as actors, fashion models, and musicians. Many popular role models for females and males are underweight. Significant social approval is often associated with weight loss and disapproval with weight gain. Thus, females and males may feel pressured to attain an unhealthy weight or unrealistic body shape. A number of Web sites are devoted to promoting anorexia nervosa and bulimia nervosa as a means of personal choice and self-expression and minimizing the medical and psychological damage caused by these disorders. No reliable family characteristics have been conclusively associated with eating disorders; however, some families appear to have higher than usual levels of depression, difficulties in communication, conflict, and focus on weight and appearance.

Treatment and Therapy

Treatment of eating disorders incorporates medical, behavioral, and psychological interventions. Typically, those with anorexia nervosa believe that their diet is justified, and resistance to treatment is the norm. Males may be especially resistant. Weight restoration is the central focus of initial treatment. Hospitalization is recommended for persons with more serious medical complications or who have less than 75 percent of expected weight. During hospitalization, daily monitoring of weight and caloric intake occurs, as well as any other necessary medical management. Behavioral therapy is employed to facilitate eating habits, and privileges such as social activity or family visits are made dependent upon increased eating and daily weight gains. Individual and family therapy are introduced as malnutrition eases and irritability, depression, and preoccupation with diet diminishes. Lengths of hospital stays vary from weeks to months depending on severity of illness and treatment progress.

Outpatient treatment may be recommended with individuals who have less severe medical complications, who are motivated to cooperate with treatment, and who have families that can independently monitor diet and health status. Weight restoration is facilitated by supervision of caloric intake and regular measurements as well as behavioral therapy techniques. Individual therapy focuses on altering cognitive distortions and assumptions about diet, weight, and body image and developing more effective means of dealing with stress. Family therapy aims to improve communication patterns, eating habits, and supportive behaviors.

No medications have been identified as effective agents in treating the core symptoms of anorexia nervosa. Medications that promote hunger may be used during the initial stages of treatment to facilitate eating. Also, medications to treat coexisting conditions such as depression and anxiety are often employed in the treatment regimen.

Most patients with bulimia nervosa do not require hospitalization unless medical complications are severe. Outpatient treatment involves individual psychotherapy, family therapy, and pharmacotherapy. Individual psychotherapy addresses cognitive distortions involving appearance and body image as well as behaviors, thoughts, and emotions that lead to binge episodes. Skills for problem solving and stress reduction are also taught. Treatment methods used for obsessive-compulsive disorder may also be employed, involving exposure to stimuli that usually trigger binge-purge behaviors while preventing them from occurring. Family therapy for bulimia nervosa aims at strengthening support and communication and developing healthy eating habits. With adolescents, impulsive behaviors associated with bulimia nervosa may be addressed by helping parents develop more effective methods of discipline and behavior management.

Antidepressant medications that regulate the neurotransmitter serotonin have been found to reduce bingeing, improve mood, and lesson preoccupation with weight and size. These same medications are useful in treating depression and anxiety, which are also commonly seen in those with bulimia nervosa.

Treatment of binge-eating disorder is similar to that of bulimia nervosa. Psychotherapy aims toward identifying and altering behaviors and feelings that lead to bingeing and developing effective methods of dealing with stress. Group therapy and weight loss programs with medical management may also be utilized. Antidepressants have also been found effective with binge-eating disorder.

Perspective and Prospects

Behaviors associated with eating disorders have been identified in the earliest writings of Western civilization, including those by the ancient Greeks and early Christians. Formal identification of eating disorders as medical illnesses occurred in the nineteenth century when case studies were first recorded. Treatment methods at that time were limited and often involved "mental hygiene" measures such as rest, fresh air, and cold or hot baths.

In the early to mid-twentieth century, psychological theories influenced by Sigmund Freud, an Austrian psychiatrist, dominated treatment methods for eating disorders. These conditions were viewed as resulting from early childhood experiences that caused problems with psychological and sexual development. Treatment involved psychoanalysis, a form of psychotherapy, often lasting several years. Limited evidence for the success of this approach caused its decline in use.

More recent and successful treatment approaches involve cognitive and behavioral therapy that aims to alter thinking and behavior contributing to eating disorders. Medications have

increasingly been used in treating eating disorders since the 1980s. Identifying biological causes of the conditions and refining pharmacotherapy may offer the best hope for improving treatment in the future.

Eating disorders were once thought to occur exclusively among young Caucasian females from middle- and upper-class families. Consequently, research into the disorders has historically focused on this population. Increased awareness of the illnesses has revealed that they occur in all socioeconomic classes and races, as well as in males and the elderly. Additional research into these groups is needed.

Awareness of eating disorders and their dangers has expanded among the general public since the 1970s. Nevertheless, rates of these disorders are rising. The media publicizes celebrities' struggles with these conditions, which may glamorize the illnesses even when negative aspects are reported. Establishing healthy eating habits and identifying potential problems early constitute the current focus of prevention efforts in medicine and education.

—*Paul F. Bell*

References

Alberga, Angela S., et al. "Weight Bias: a Call to Action." *Journal of Eating Disorders*, vol. 4, no. 1, 7 Nov. 2016, doi:10.1186/s40337-016-0112-4.

Brownell, Kelly D., and B. Timothy Walsh. *Eating Disorders and Obesity a Comprehensive Handbook.* 3rd ed., The Guilford Press, 2017.

Giuseppe, Rachele De, et al. "Pediatric Obesity and Eating Disorders Symptoms: The Role of the Multidisciplinary Treatment. A Systematic Review." *Frontiers in Pediatrics*, vol. 7, 3 Apr. 2019, doi:10.3389/fped.2019.00123.

Hayes, Jacqueline F., et al. "Disordered Eating Attitudes and Behaviors in Youth with Overweight and Obesity: Implications for Treatment." *Current Obesity Reports*, vol. 7, no. 3, 1 Sept. 2018, pp. 235–246., doi:10.1007/s13679-018-0316-9.

Luz, Felipe Da, et al. "Obesity with Comorbid Eating Disorders: Associated Health Risks and Treatment Approaches." *Nutrients*, vol. 10, no. 7, 27 June 2018, p. 829., doi:10.3390/nu10070829.

Neumark-Sztainer, Dianne. "Higher Weight Status and Restrictive Eating Disorders: An Overlooked Concern." *Journal of Adolescent Health*, vol. 56, no. 1, 2015, pp. 1–2., doi:10.1016/j.jadohealth.2014.10.261.

Endometrial cancer

CATEGORY: Disorder

In the United States and other developed countries cancer is second only to heart disease as a cause of mortality. Endometrial cancer (also called uterine cancer) is a neoplasm that originates in the endometrial lining of the uterus. Endometrial cancer is the fourth most common cancer among women and the most common form of gynecologic cancer. Treatment depends on the stage of the cancer and on the age and health of the patient. Surgical hysterectomy is the most successful form of treatment for endometrial cancer. Other treatment options include chemotherapy, radiation therapy, and hormone therapy.

Diet-Related Risk Factors for Endometrial Cancer

Overweight and obese individuals are at greater risk for endometrial cancer. It has been estimated that 49% of endometrial cancer incidence is linked to excess body fat. High intake of fat is a risk factor for excessive weight gain and has been associated with an increased incidence of cancer.

Women who have hypertension have a higher incidence of endometrial cancer.

Individuals with type 2 diabetes mellitus (DM2) are more likely to develop endometrial cancer than persons who do not have DM2.

SIGNS AND SYMPTOMS
Postmenopausal vaginal bleeding Irregular menstrual bleeding Pelvic pain Pain during intercourse

Research Findings

Results of several studies have noted potential benefits from increased intake of fruits and vegetables for the prevention of endometrial, breast, lung and colorectal cancers. Researchers have reported that women who consume a primarily plant-based diet have a lower likelihood of developing endometrial cancer. Soybeans appear to be particularly protective against gynecological cancers. This is most likely due to the wealth of phytoestrogens found in soybeans. Phytoestrogens are plant-derived estrogens, which have been shown to reduce endogenous estrogen levels.

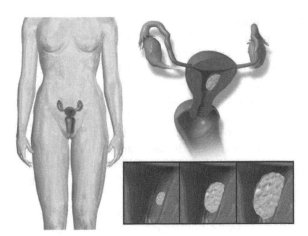

The location and development of endometrial cancer. (Blausen Medical Communications, Inc.)

Results of animal and lab studies suggest that omega-3 fatty acids may protect against cancer. A population-based case-control study found fish oil supplement use was significantly associated with reduced risk of endometrial cancer. In addition, there was a suggested, but not significant, inverse association between fish intake, especially dark fish, and endometrial cancer.

Summary

Individuals diagnosed with endometrial cancer (and their family members/caregivers) should learn about dietary recommendations based on personal characteristics and health needs. Patients should eat a high-fiber diet that includes a wide variety of fruits, vegetables, lean proteins, and unsaturated fats. Patients undergoing treatment for endometrial cancer need to be monitored for weight loss, signs of malnutrition, vitamin/ mineral deficiencies and electrolyte imbalances. It is important to report any health-related changes to the treating clinician as soon as possible to prevent worsening health status. A registered dietitian may provide appropriate nutrition support and counsel patients on appropriate foods or supplements to prevent weight loss or nutrient deficiencies. Patients and their family members should understand and adhere to the prescribed treatment regimen, while continuing medical surveillance to monitor health status. Research suggests that a plant based diet and consumption of soybeans, omega-3 fatty acids and coffee may help reduce the risk endometrial cancer.

—*Cherie Marcel*

References

Cusimano, Maria C, et al. "Barriers to Care for Women with Low-Grade Endometrial Cancer and Morbid Obesity: a Qualitative Study." *BMJ Open*, vol. 9, no. 6, 2019, doi:10.1136/bmjopen-2018-026872.

Laskey, R. A., et al. "Obesity-Related Endometrial Cancer: an Update on Survivorship Approaches to Reducing Cardiovascular Death." *BJOG: An International Journal of Obstetrics & Gynaecology*, vol. 123, no. 2, 29 Dec. 2015, pp. 293–298., doi:10.1111/1471-0528.13684.

Onstad, Michaela A., et al. "Addressing the Role of Obesity in Endometrial Cancer Risk, Prevention, and Treatment." *Journal of Clinical Oncology*, vol. 34, no. 35, 2016, pp. 4225–4230., doi:10.1200/jco.2016.69.4638.

Renehan, A. G., et al. "Obesity and Endometrial Cancer: Unanswered Epidemiological Questions." *BJOG: An International Journal of Obstetrics & Gynaecology*, vol. 123, no. 2, 2015, pp. 175–178., doi:10.1111/1471-0528.13731.

Sponholtz, Todd R., et al. "Body Size, Metabolic Factors, and Risk of Endometrial Cancer in Black Women." *American Journal of Epidemiology*, vol. 183, no. 4, 2016, pp. 259–268., doi:10.1093/aje/kwv186.

■ Esophageal cancer

CATEGORY: Disorder

Esophageal cancer is a malignant neoplasm (i.e., tumor) that originates in the lining of the esophagus, the organ which extends from the throat to the stomach, through which food passes. Esophageal cancer is categorized as squamous cell carcinoma when it originates in the flat cells of the esophageal lining and as adenocarcinoma when it originates in cells that produce mucus and fluids. Although relatively rare in the Unites States, esophageal cancer is quite prevalent in Asia and parts of Africa, particularly in men aged 45–70 years. It is currently believed that esophageal cancer is most likely caused by persistent irritation of the cells of the esophageal lining, which results in mutations in cellular deoxyribonucleic acid (DNA). Early-stage esophageal cancer is usually asymptomatic, but as the cancer grows it can produce symptoms of dysphagia (i.e., difficulty swallowing), unplanned weight loss, and fatigue.

Research Findings

Evidence indicates that lifestyle behaviors such as achieving and maintaining a healthy weight, performing regular physical activity, consuming a diet that is rich in a variety of fruits and vegetables and low in saturated fat, limiting alcohol intake, and avoiding chewing or smoking tobacco can significantly reduce risk for developing esophageal cancer. Researchers have reported that persons who consume a diet high in fiber demonstrate a tendency to practice healthier lifestyle habits overall. These persons are more physically active, follow a diet that is lower in fat and higher in fruits and vegetables, abstain from smoking, and consume less alcohol.

Results of many studies show a strong positive association between high intake of red and processed meats and risk for developing esophageal cancer. The exact cause for the increased cancer risk is not completely understood, but the saturated fat and cholesterol content of red meat is believed to be at least partially responsible.

Researchers have reported that dietary inclusion of fish and foods that are rich in monounsaturated fats (e.g., olive oil, avocado) can reduce risk for esophageal cancer. The linolenic metabolites eicosapentaenoic acid (EPA) and docosahexaenoic acid (DHA), which are found in fatty fish (e.g., salmon, mackerel), walnuts, soybeans, and flax seeds, have been shown to play a protective role against cancer that may be attributed to their anti-inflammatory activity. The results of studies indicate that individuals who regularly consume more fish than other forms of meat are more likely to make healthy dietary choices overall. For example, they tend to consume higher amounts of whole grains, fruits, and vegetables.

Because patients who undergo esophagectomy for esophageal cancer are at significant risk for compromised nutritional status, early enteral nutrition (EN) support is often recommended. However, a retrospective study which examined 103 cases found no significant advantage for the postoperative course whether EN was initiated within 24 hours or up to 72 hours after surgery.

RISK FACTORS	SIGNS AND SYMPTOMS
Men who are 45–70 years of age	Dysphagia
Individuals who abuse alcohol	Unintentional weight loss
Persons who smoke or chew tobacco	Fatigue
Persons with gastroesophageal reflux disease (GERD)	Pain or pressure in the chest
	Heartburn or indigestion
Persons who regularly drink very hot liquids	Coughing or a hoarse voice
Persons who consume a diet that is low in fruits and vegetables	
Individuals who regularly eat foods that are preserved in lye (e.g., lutefisk)	
Individuals who are obese	
Persons who receive radiation treatment to the chest or abdomen	
Persons with a family history of esophageal cancer	

Researchers recommend scheduling EN within 24 to 72 hours after surgery, based on patient condition.

Summary

Individuals diagnosed with esophageal cancer (and their family members/caregivers) should learn about dietary recommendations based on personal characteristics and health needs. Lifestyle behaviors such as achieving and maintaining a healthy weight, performing regular physical activity, consuming a diet that is rich in a variety of fruits and vegetables and low in saturated fat, limiting alcohol intake, and avoiding chewing or smoking tobacco can significantly reduce risk for developing esophageal cancer.

Patients with esophageal cancer may be at risk for vitamin and mineral deficiencies, malnutrition, and other adverse effects of cancer and its treatment. Dietary and other treatments may be prescribed to improve patient health status and quality of life. A registered dietitian may provide recommendations for appropriate diet texture and consistency, or initiate or continue EN post esophageal surgery, if patient is anticipated to have difficulty maintaining nutritional status. It is important to report any health-related changes to the treating clinician as soon as possible to prevent worsening health status. Patients and their family members should understand and adhere to the prescribed treatment regimen, while continuing medical surveillance to monitor health status.

Research suggests that limiting red and processed meat consumption may help reduce risk of esophageal cancer.

—*Cherie Marcel*

References

Alexandre, Leo. "Pathophysiological Mechanisms Linking Obesity and Esophageal Adenocarcinoma." *World Journal of Gastrointestinal Pathophysiology*, vol. 5, no. 4, 2014, p. 534., doi:10.4291/wjgp.v5.i4.534.

Du, Xuan, et al. "Abdominal Obesity and Gastroesophageal Cancer Risk: Systematic Review and Meta-Analysis of Prospective Studies." *Bioscience Reports*, vol. 37, no. 3, 2017, doi:10.1042/bsr20160474.

Gupta, Arjun, et al. "Obesity and Mortality in Patients with Esophageal Cancer: A Systematic Review and Meta-Analysis." *Journal of Clinical Oncology*, vol. 34, no. 4_suppl, 2016, pp. 20–20., doi:10.1200/jco.2016.34.4_suppl.20.

Long, Elizabeth, and Ian L.p. Beales. "The Role of Obesity in Oesophageal Cancer Development." *Therapeutic Advances in Gastroenterology*, vol. 7, no. 6, 2014, pp. 247–268., doi:10.1177/1756283x14538689.

Masab, Muhammad. "How Does Obesity Affect the Risk for Esophageal Adenocarcinoma?" *Medscape*, 5 Aug. 2019, www.medscape.com/answers/277930-38122/how-does-obesity-affect-the-risk-for-esophageal-adenocarcinoma.

■ Fatty liver disease, nonalcoholic

CATEGORY: Disorder

Nonalcoholic fatty liver disease (NAFLD) is one of the leading causes of chronic liver disease, affecting an estimated 20–30% of the population of the United States, 2.5% of which are children. The primary risk factors for NAFLD are obesity, insulin resistance and diabetes mellitus, type 2 (DM2), and hypertriglyceridemia (i.e., elevated fat levels in blood). Men are affected by NAFLD more often than women, and the prevalence and severity of NAFLD increases with increased age and body weight. NAFLD is a spectrum disorder that ranges from steatosis (i.e., fatty liver) to cirrhosis (i.e., scarring and malfunction of liver tissue) and end-stage liver disease (ESLD). Steatosis develops when the liver is overloaded with fatty acids. As the liver cells become overwhelmed by the influx of fatty acids, they can become injured and die. As the damage progresses due to mitochondrial injury, stellate cell activation, microvascular injury, and/or oxidative stress, steatosis becomes steatohepatitis and eventually fibrosis and cirrhosis develop. Nonalcoholic steatohepatitis (NASH; i.e., inflammation caused by the build-up of fat in the liver) occurs within the spectrum of NAFLD manifestations and is similar to alcohol-induced liver disease, although persons with NASH are often asymptomatic. NASH is the primary cause of abnormal increases in the level of the liver enzyme aminotransferase. Untreated NASH is progressive and can lead to ESLD. Physical activity is effective in preventing NASH.

Signs and symptoms of NAFLD

Persons with NAFLD are usually asymptomatic, although in some cases patients report feeling discomfort in the upper right quadrant. Up to 75% of individuals with NAFLD have hepatomegaly (i.e., an abnormally large liver). Aminotransferase and alkaline phosphatase levels may become slightly elevated as NAFLD progresses, but laboratory test values are frequently normal in persons with hepatic steatosis. Histologic examination of biopsied liver tissue that identifies the presence of fibrosis and inflammation is diagnostic of NAFLD, and is also useful in identifying the degree of liver damage.

Treatment and Therapy

NAFLD is treated by personalized lifestyle interventions that resolve the causes, including weight loss, diet modification, and increased exercise. A hypocaloric diet is recommended if weight loss is indicated. Quality and quantity of carbohydrate intake is likely to influence the development of NAFLD.

Diet recommendations include moderate to low carbohydrate diets (40–45 percent of total calories), avoidance of products with high fructose corn syrup, and inclusion of high fiber, low glycemic-index carbohydrate foods.

Initiating prompt treatment of DM2, hypertension, metabolic syndrome, or any other coexisting medical conditions is imperative. In cases of morbid obesity, gastric bypass may be considered.

Research Findings

Study results overwhelmingly show that alteration in diet and exercise is the most effective treatment

---

RISK FACTORS FOR NAFLD

- Obesity: Factors considered predictive of NASH in persons with morbid obesity include high total and low-density lipoprotein (LDL) cholesterol levels, high intake of dietary cholesterol, hypertension, DM2, sleep apnea, elevated liver enzymes, and non-Black race.

- Insulin resistance and related conditions, including DM2, metabolic syndrome, and polycystic ovarian syndrome

- Disorders of lipid metabolism

- Total parenteral nutrition (i.e., intravenous nutrition)

- Severe weight loss due to jejunoileal bypass, gastric bypass, or severe starvation

- Refeeding syndrome (i.e., a metabolic imbalance which occurs when previously starved persons are fed too much and too rapidly)

- Certain medications such as steroids, amiodarone, diltiazem, tamoxifen, and highly active antiretroviral therapy (HAART) can induce NAFLD, which resolves when the causal medication is discontinued.

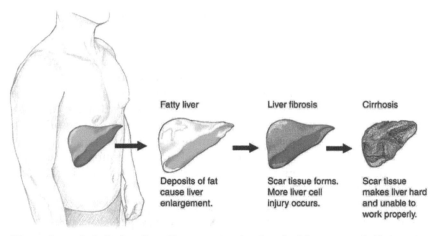

Fatty liver

Deposits of fat
cause liver
enlargement.

Liver fibrosis

Scar tissue forms.
More liver cell
injury occurs.

Cirrhosis

Scar tissue
makes liver hard
and unable to
work properly.

Stages of non-alcoholic fatty liver disease, progressing from healthy, to steatosis (fat accumulation), inflammation, fibrosis and cirrhosis. (National Institute of Diabetes and Digestive and Kidney Diseases)

for most individuals with NAFLD. Although calorie restriction is important, following a diet low in carbohydrates, and especially refined carbohydrates, appears to have the greatest effect. Researchers have also suggested that restricting iron intake may reduce oxidative stress on the liver. Increasing cardiorespiratory fitness alone—regardless of weight loss or diet—results in reduced liver fat, and including resistance training with aerobic exercise is more effective than aerobic training alone. These alterations in lifestyle also result in weight loss, improved insulin resistance, and reduced blood pressure, all of which contribute to improved liver health.

Researchers are studying the effects of certain medications for the treatment of NAFLD. Although lifestyle modification is the recommended method of treatment, inclusion of medications such as metformin for treatment of insulin resistance and metabolic syndrome or statin drugs for the lipid-lowering effect is a more aggressive approach that could be effective. In patients with NASH, supplementation with vitamin E to reduce oxidative stress has also been shown to be beneficial.

Summary

Individuals should become knowledgeable about the nutritional management of NAFLD to accurately assess personal characteristics and health needs. The treating clinician may provide emotional support and education about the

importance of making changes in diet and exercise. A registered dietitian may provide education about nutrition, meal planning, and dietary restrictions. Patients with NAFLD should follow the prescribed treatment regimen, monitor for and promptly report any health-related changes to the treating clinician, and continue medical and nutrition surveillance to monitor health and nutritional status. Research suggests diet and exercise are the most effective treatments for NAFLD.

—*Cherie Marcel*

References

Carvalhana, Sofia, and Helena Cortez-Pinto. "From Obesity to Fatty Liver/NASH: Two Parallel Epidemics." *World Gastroenterology Organisation*, July 2013, www.worldgastroenterology.org/publications/e-wgn/e-wgn-expert-point-of-view-articles-collection/from-obesity-to-fatty-liver-nash-two-parallel-epidemics.

Franceschelli, ennifer E. "The Skinny on 'Fatty' Liver Disease." *Obesity Action Coalition*, 2013, www.obesityaction.org/community/article-library/the-skinny-on-fatty-liver-disease/.

Polyzos, Stergios A., et al. "Obesity and Nonalcoholic Fatty Liver Disease: From Pathophysiology to Therapeutics." *Metabolism*, vol. 92, 2019, pp. 82–97., doi:10.1016/j.metabol.2018.11.014.

Sarwar, Raiya, et al. "Obesity and Nonalcoholic Fatty Liver Disease: Current Perspectives." *Diabetes, Metabolic Syndrome and Obesity: Targets and Therapy*, vol. 11, 2018, pp. 533–542., doi:10.2147/dmso.s146339.

■ Gout

CATEGORY: Disorder

Gout is an inflammatory arthritic condition associated with hyperuricemia due to overproduction or inadequate excretion of uric acid (i.e., a byproduct of purine metabolism). Gout results from the accumulation of monosodium urate (MSU) crystals in tissue. As MSU deposits increase, the initially asymptomatic gout can cause a seemingly sudden attack of acute arthritis, which can be followed by months or years without further attacks. The attack-free periods are referred to as intercritical gout. When the gouty arthritic attacks increase, patients can develop chronic tophaceous (i.e., referring to the development of tophi) gout. Tophi are the knobby deformations that develop in the joints from MSU deposits in patients with chronic gout. Gout causes extreme pain and decreases quality of life. Treatment of gout is typically initiated when the affected person seeks care during the first acute attack, and usually involves the use of nonsteroidal anti-inflammatory drugs (NSAIDs) such as naproxen or indomethacin. Follow-up care is focused on the management of gout through dietary changes and medication, if necessary. Dietary recommendations include reducing foods that are high in purine (i.e., naturally occurring, organic compounds that break down to uric acid; e.g., found in meat and shellfish), avoiding alcohol consumption, and increasing in take of dairy products that are low in fat.

Signs and Symptoms of Gout

Gout can remain asymptomatic for as long as 30 years while MSU crystal deposits accumulate in the tissues. The initial presentation of gout is usually a sudden, painful, arthritic attack, frequently at night. The initial attack can be followed by months or years of intercritical gout.

RISK FACTORS FOR GOUT

- Weight gain and obesity
- Diabetes
- Metabolic syndrome, which is characterized by abdominal obesity, hypertension, poor lipid profile (e.g., high triglycerides, low levels of high-density lipoproteins), and insulin resistance
- Consuming a diet high in purine, including meats and shellfish
- Glycogen storage diseases such as von Gierke disease, which are inherited metabolic disorders that result in the accumulation of glycogen and fat in the liver and kidneys

---

The chronic accumulation of MSU crystals can result in tophi. Rarely, tophi can develop around the heart and spine. More common locations for tophi build-up include the edge of the outer ear, forearms, elbows and knees, and hands and feet. Chronic tophaceous gout develops in untreated persons and those whose gout is refractory to treatment; it is characterized by constant low-grade pain and inflammation and tophaceous deformities.

Potential complications of gout include renal damage. Uric acid kidney stones occur in 5–10% of persons with gouty arthritis.

DIETARY RECOMMENDATIONS FOR GOUT

- Limit or avoid consumption of meat-based foods, especially organ meats and shellfish, which are high in purine
- Avoid alcohol consumption
- Increase intake of dairy products that are low in fat. Increased dairy intake is inversely associated with risk for gout
- Maintain adequate hydration to promote urate excretion

Research Findings

Gout and hyperuricemia have been associated with metabolic syndrome and cardiovascular disease (CVD). The implementation of dietary and lifestyle modifications and achieving and maintaining a healthy weight are of particular importance in the non-pharmacologic approach to the management of gout.

Although research results have shown that dietary and lifestyle modifications are effective in managing gout, the benefits are directly proportional to patient adherence to the prescribed treatment regimen. Researchers have reported that patients frequently show little evidence of adherence to dietary recommendations, particularly in regard to limiting alcohol intake, avoiding foods high in purine, taking vitamin C supplements, and increasing intake of dairy products that are low in fat.

It is important for the treating clinician to emphasize the importance of increased patient awareness regarding the benefits of dietary

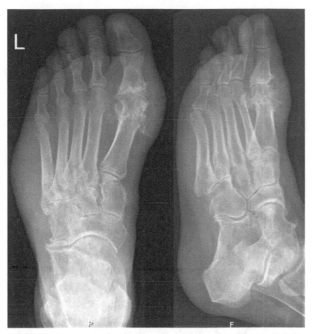

Gout on X-rays of a left foot in the metatarsal-phalangeal joint of the big toe. Note also the soft tissue swelling at the lateral border of the foot. (Hellerhoff via Wikimedia Commons)

management in treating gout. This can be done by providing appropriate, current promotional materials and by engaging the patient in a discussion of essential dietary recommendations. Allowing patients to share in decision making regarding lifestyle and dietary modifications helps to increase their sense of commitment and ownership of the treatment plan. Dietary interventions are more successful when simple guidelines are given for making healthy food choices (e.g., increase fiber and reduce purines by adding more vegetables and choosing grilled chicken instead of lobster) and minor modifications to food preparation practices (e.g., bake instead of fry) are presented. Presenting information on the need for major dietary changes that involve eliminating all familiar foods is often not successful. The focus of patient education should be on making gradual changes that involve retaining as many food preferences as possible while patients become comfortable with new dietary practices.

Summary

Individuals should become knowledgeable about diet therapy for gout to accurately assess personal characteristics and health needs. Medical history,

diet history, and risk factors for gout should be assessed by the treating clinician. A balanced diet designed to manage gout and achieve/maintain a healthy weight includes limiting or avoiding consumption of organ meats and shellfish, avoiding alcohol consumption, increasing intake of low fat dairy products, and maintaining adequate hydration to promote urate excretion. Patients and their family members should follow the prescribed treatment regimen and continue medical surveillance to monitor health status. Research suggests that medical nutrition therapy for gout is more successful when patients are given simple guidelines to make healthy food choices (e.g., increasing fiber and limiting high purine foods).

—*Cherie Marcel*

References

Kelly, Janis C. "Obesity Doubles Gout Risk, Reduces Age of Onset." *Medscape*, 12 Aug. 2011, www.medscape.com/viewarticle/747967.

Lee, Jennifer, et al. "Visceral Fat Obesity Is Highly Associated with Primary Gout in a Metabolically Obese but Normal Weighted Population: a Case Control Study." *Arthritis Research & Therapy*, vol. 17, no. 1, 24 Mar. 2015, doi:10.1186/s13075-015-0593-6.

Nielsen, Sabrina, et al. "Weight Loss for Overweight and Obese Individuals with Gout: a Systematic Review of Longitudinal Observational Studies." *Annals of the Rheumatic Diseases*, vol. 76, 2017, pp. 1870–1882., doi:10.1136/annrheumdis-2017-eular.2651.

Rapaport, Lisa. "Obesity, Drinking and Unhealthy Diet Add to Gout Risk." *Reuters*, 20 Sept. 2019, www.reuters.com/article/us-health-gout-prevention/obesity-drinking-and-unhealthy-diet-add-to-gout-risk-idUSKBN1W52AA.

■ Heart attack

CATEGORY: Disorder
ALSO KNOWN AS: Myocardial infarction

Causes and Symptoms

Although varied in origin and effect on the body, heart attacks (or myocardial infarctions) occur when there are interruptions in the delicately synchronized system either supplying blood to the heart or pumping blood from the heart to other vital organs. The heart is a highly specialized muscle whose function is to pump life-sustaining blood to all parts of the body. The heart's action involves the development of pressure to propel blood through arriving and departing channels-veins and arteries-that must maintain that pressure within their walls at critical levels throughout the system.

The highest level of pressure in the total cardiovascular system is to be found closest to the two "pumping" chambers on the right and left lower sections of the heart, called ventricles. Dark, bluish-colored blood, emptied of its oxygen content and laden with carbon dioxide waste instead of the oxygen in fresh blood, flows into the upper portion of the heart via the superior and inferior venae cavae. It then passes from the right atrium chamber into the right ventricle. Once in the ventricle, this blood cannot flow back because of one-way valves separating the "receiving" from the "pumping" sections of the total heart organ.

After this valve closes following a vitally synchronized timing system, constriction of the right ventricle by the myocardium muscle in the surrounding walls of the heart forces the blood from the heart, propelling it toward the oxygen-filled tissue of the lungs. Following reoxygenation, bright red blood that is still under pressure from the thrust of the right ventricle flows into the left atrium. Once channeled into the left ventricle, the pumping process that began in the right ventricle is then repeated on the left by muscular constriction, and oxygenated blood flows out of the aortic valve under pressure throughout the cardiovascular system to nourish the body's cells. Because the force needed to supply blood under pressure from the left ventricle for the entire body is greater than the first-phase pumping force needed to move blood into the lungs, the myocardium surrounding the left ventricle constitutes the thickest muscular layer in the heart's wall.

The efficiency of this process, as well as the origins of problems of fatigue in the heart that can lead to heart attacks and eventual heart failure, is tied to the maintenance of a reasonably constant level of blood pressure. If pulmonary problems (blockage caused by the effects of smoking or environmental pollution, for example) make it harder for the right ventricle to push blood through the lungs, the heart must expend more energy in the first stage of the cardiovascular process. Similarly, and often in addition to the added work for the heart because of pulmonary complications, the efficiency of the left ventricle in handling blood flow may be reduced by the presence of excessive fat in the body, causing this ventricle to expend more energy to propel oxygenated blood into vital tissues.

Although factors such as these may be responsible for overworking the heart and thus contributing to eventual heart failure, other causes of heart attacks are to be found much closer to the working apparatus of the heart, particularly in the coronary arteries. The coronary arteries begin at the top of the heart and fan out along its sides. They are responsible for providing large quantities of blood to the myocardium muscle, which needs continual nourishment to carry out the pumping that forces blood forward from the ventricles. The passageways inside these and other key arteries are vulnerable to the process known as atherosclerosis, which can affect the blood supply to other organs as well as to the heart. In the heart, atherosclerosis involves the accumulation, inside the coronary arteries, of fatty deposits called atheromas. If these deposits continue to collect, less blood can flow through the arteries. A narrowed artery also increases the possibility of a variant form of heart attack, in which a sudden and total blockage of blood flow follows the lodging of a blood clot in one of these vital passageways.

Asymptomatic condition called angina pectoris, characterized by intermittent chest pains, may develop if atherosclerosis reduces blood (and therefore oxygen) supply to the heart. These danger signs can continue over a number of years. If diagnosis reveals a problem that might be resolved by preventive medication, exercise, or recommendations for heart surgery, then this condition, known as myocardial ischemia, may not necessarily end in a full heart attack.

A full heart attack occurs when-for one of several possible reasons, including a vascular spasm suddenly constricting an already clogged artery or a blockage caused by a clot-the heart suddenly ceases to receive the necessary supply of blood. This brings almost immediate deterioration in some of the heart's tissue and causes the organ's consequent inability to perform its vital functions effectively.

Another form of attack and disruption of the heart's ability to deliver blood can come either

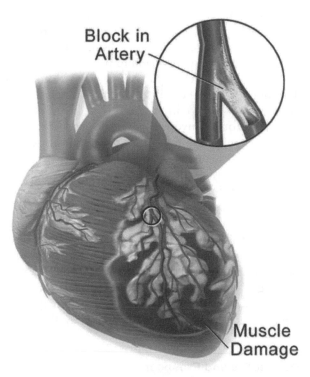

Heart Attack

Source: Blausen Medical Communications, Inc.

independently of or in conjunction with an arterially induced heart attack. This form of attack involves a sustained interruption in the rate of heartbeats. The necessary pace or rate of myocardial contractions, which can vary depending on the person's rate of physical exertion or age, is regulated in the sinoatrial node in the right atrium, which generates its own electrical impulses. The ultimate sources for the commands to the sinoatrial node are to be found in the network of nerves coming directly from the brain. There are, however, other so-called local pacemakers located in the atria and ventricles. If these sources of electrical charges begin giving commands to the myocardium that are not in rhythm with those coming from the sinoatrial node, then dysrhythmic or premature beats may confuse the heart muscle, causing it to beat wildly. In fact, the concentrated pattern of muscle contractions will not be coordinated and instead will be dispersed in different areas of the heart. The result is fibrillation, a series of uncoordinated contractions that cannot combine to propel blood out of the ventricles. This condition may occur either as the aftershock of an arterially induced heart attack or suddenly and on its own, caused by the deterioration of the electrical impulse system commanding the heart rate. In patients whose potential vulnerability to this form of heart attack has been diagnosed in advance, a heart physician may decide to surgically implant an electronic pacemaker to ensure coordination of the necessary electrical commands to the myocardium.

Treatment and Therapy

Extraordinary medical advances have helped reduce the high death rates formerly associated with heart attacks. Many of these advances have been in the field of preventive medicine. The most widely recognized medical findings are related to diet, smoking, and exercise. Although controversy remains, there is general agreement that cholesterol absorbed by the body from the ingestion of animal fats plays a key role in the dangerous buildup of platelets inside arterial passageways. It has been accepted that regular, although not necessarily strenuous, exercise is an essential longterm preventive strategy that can reduce the risk of heart attacks. Exercise also plays a role in therapy after a heart attack. In both preventive and postattack contexts, it has been medically proven that the entire cardiovascular system profits from the natural muscle-strengthening process (in the heart's case) and general cleansing effects (in the case of oxygen intake and stimulated blood flow) that result from controlled regular exercise.

The actual application of medical scientific knowledge to assist in the campaign against the deadly effects of heart disease involves multiple fields of specialization. These may range from the sophisticated use of electrocardiograms (ECGs) to monitor the regularity of heartbeats, to specialized drug therapies aimed at preventing heart attacks in people who have been diagnosed as high-risk cases, to coronary bypass surgery or even heart transplants. In the 1980s, highly specialized surgeons at several university and private hospitals began performing operations to implant artificial hearts in human patients.

In the case of ECGs, it has become possible, thanks to the use of portable units that record the heartbeat patterns of persons over an extended period of time, to gain a much more accurate impression of the actual functioning of the heart.

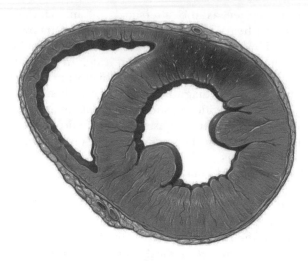

Drawing of the heart showing anterior left ventricle wall infarction. (Patrick J. Lynch, medical illustrator)

Previous dependence on electrocardiographic data gathered during an appointed and limited examination provided only minimal information to doctors.

The domains of preventive surgery and specialized drug treatment to prevent dangerous blood clotting are vast. Statistically, the most important and widely practiced operations that were developed in the later decades of the twentieth century were replacement of the aortic valve, the coronary bypass operation, and, with greater or lesser degrees of success, the actual transplantation of voluntary donors' hearts in the place of those belonging to heart disease patients. Coronary bypass operations involve the attachment to the myocardium of healthy arteries to carry the blood that can no longer pass through the patient's clogged arterial passageways; these healthy arteries are taken by the heart surgeon from other areas of the patient's own body.

Another sphere of medical technology, that of balloon angioplasty, held out a major nonsurgical promise of preventing deterioration of the arteries leading to the heart. This sophisticated form of treatment involves the careful, temporary introduction of inflatable devices inside clogged arteries, which are then stretched to increase the space within the arterial passageway for blood to flow. By the 1990s, however, doctors recognized one disadvantage of balloon angioplasty: By stretching the essential blood vessels being treated, this procedure

either stretches the plaque with the artery or breaks loose debris that remains behind, creating a danger of renewed clogging. Thus, although angioplasty remains a standard approach to treatment of heart disease, another technique, called atherectomy, was developed to clear certain coronary arteries, as well as arteries elsewhere in the body.

Atherectomy involves a motorized catheter device resembling a miniature drill that is inserted into clogged arteries. As the drill turns, material that is literally shaved off the interior walls of arteries is retrieved through a tiny collection receptacle. Early experimentation, especially to treat the large anterior descending coronary artery on the left side of the heart, showed that atherectomy was 87 percent effective, whereas, on the average, angioplasty removed only 63 percent of the blockage. In addition, similar efforts to provide internal, nonsurgical treatment of clogged arteries using laser beams were being made by the early 1990s.

Perspective and Prospects

The modern conception of cardiology dates from William Harvey's seventeenth-century discovery of the relationship between the heart's function as a pump and the circulatory "restoration" of blood. Harvey's much more scientific views replaced centuries-old conceptions of the heart as a blood-warming device only.

Although substantial anatomical advances were made over the next two centuries that helped explain most of the vital functions of the heart, it was not until the early decades of the twentieth century that science developed therapeutic methods to deal with problems that frequently cause heart attacks. Drugs that affect the liver's production of substances necessary for normal coagulation of blood, for example, were discovered in the 1930s. A large variety of such anticoagulants have since been developed to help thin the blood of patients vulnerable to blood clotting. Other drugs, including certain antibiotics, are used to treat persons whose susceptibility to infection is known to be high. In these cases, the simple action of dislodging bacteria from the teeth when brushing can cause an invasion of the vital parts of the heart by an infection. This bacterialendocarditis, the result of the actual destruction of heart tissue or the sudden release of clots of infectious residue, could lead to a heart attack in such individuals although they have no other symptoms of identifiable heart disease.

The most spectacular advance in the scientific treatment of potential heart attack victims, however, has been in the field of cardiac surgery. Many advances in open heart surgery date from the late 1950s, when the development of heart and lung replacement machines made it safe enough to substitute electronic monitors for some of the organism's normal body functions. Before the 1950s, operations had been limited to surgical treatment of the major blood vessels surrounding the heart.

Various technical methods have also been developed that help identify problems early enough for drug therapy to be attempted before the decision to perform surgery is made. The use of catheters, which are threaded into the coronary organ using the same vessels that transport blood, became the most effective way of locating problematic areas. The process known as angiography, which uses x-rays to trace the course of radiopaque dyes injected through a catheter into local heart areas under study, can actually tell doctors if drug therapy is having the desired effects. In cases where such tests show that preventive drug therapy is not effective, an early decision to perform surgery can be made, preventing the source of coronary trouble from multiplying the patient's chances of suffering a heart attack.

—*Byron D. Cannon*

References

Antipolis, Sophia. "Belly Fat Linked with Repeat Heart Attacks." *European Society of Cardiology*, 21 Jan. 2020, www.escardio.org/The-ESC/Press-Office/Press-releases/Belly-fat-linked-with-repeat-heart-attacks.

"Heart Attack." *National Heart Lung and Blood Institute*, U.S. Department of Health and Human Services, www.nhlbi.nih.gov/health-topics/heart-attack.

Mahajan, Rajiv, et al. "Complex Interaction of Obesity, Intentional Weight Loss and Heart Failure: a Systematic Review and Meta-Analysis." *Heart*, vol. 106, 17 Sept. 2019, pp. 58–68.

Moholdt, Trine, et al. "Sustained Physical Activity, Not Weight Loss, Associated With Improved Survival in Coronary Heart Disease." *Journal of the American College of Cardiology*, vol. 71, no. 10, 2018, pp. 1094–1101., doi:10.1016/j.jacc.2018.01.011.

"Your Weight History May Predict Your Heart Failure Risk." *Johns Hopkins Medicine*, 12 Dec. 2018, www.hopkinsmedicine.org/news/newsroom/news-releases/your-weight-history-may-predict-your-heart-failure-risk.

■ Heart disease

CATEGORY: Disorder

Causes and Symptoms

The heart is a fist-sized organ located in the lower left quarter of the chest. It consists of four chambers: the right and left atria on top and the right and left ventricles at the bottom. The chambers are enclosed in three layers of tissue: the outer layer (epicardium), the middle layer (myocardium), and the inner layer (endocardium). Surrounding the entire organ is the pericardium, a thin layer of tissue that forms a protective covering for the heart. The heart also contains various nodes that transmit electrochemical signals, causing heart muscle tissue to contract and relax in the pumping action that carries blood to organs and cells throughout the body.

Signals from the brain cause the heart to contract rhythmically in a sequence of motions that move the blood from the right atrium down through the tricuspid valve into the right ventricle. From here, blood is pushed through the pulmonary valve into the lungs, where it fulfills one of its major functions: to pick up oxygen in exchange for carbon dioxide. From the lungs, the blood is pumped back into the heart, entering the left atrium from which it is pumped down through the mitral valve into the left ventricle. Blood is then pushed through the aortic valve into the main artery of the body, the aorta, from which it starts its journey to the organs and cells. As it passes through the arteries of the gastrointestinal system, the blood picks up nutrients which, along with the oxygen that it has taken from the lungs, are brought to the cells and exchanged for waste products and carbon dioxide. The blood then enters the veins, through which it is eventually returned to the heart. The heart nourishes and supplies itself with oxygen through the coronary arteries, so called because they sit on top of the heart like a crown and extend down the sides.

The heart diseases collectively include all the disorders that can befall every part of the heart muscle: the pericardium, epicardium, myocardium, endocardium, atria, ventricles, valves, coronary arteries, and nodes. The most significant sites of heart diseases are the coronary arteries and the nodes; their malfunction can cause coronary artery disease and cardiac arrhythmias, respectively. These two disorders are responsible for the majority of heart disease cases.

Coronary artery disease occurs when matter such as cholesterol and fibrous material collects and stiffens on the inner walls of the coronary arteries. The plaque that forms may narrow the passage through which blood flows, reducing the amount of blood delivered to the heart, or may build up and clog the artery entirely, shutting off the flow of blood to the heart. In the former case, when the coronary artery is narrowed, the condition is called ischemic heart disease. Because the most common cause of ischemia is narrowing of the coronary arteries to the myocardium, another designation of the condition is myocardial ischemia, referring to the fact that blood flow to the myocardium is impeded. Accumulation of plaque within the coronary arteries is referred to as coronary atherosclerosis.

As the coronary arteries become clogged and then narrow, they can fail to deliver the required oxygen to the heart muscle, particularly during stress or physical effort. The heart's need for oxygen exceeds the arteries' ability to supply it. The patient usually feels a sharp, choking pain, called angina pectoris. Not all people who have coronary ischemia, however, experience anginal pain; these people are said to have silent ischemia.

The danger in coronary artery disease is that the accumulation of plaque will progress to the point where the coronary artery is clogged completely and no blood is delivered to the part of the heart serviced by that artery. The rough, uneven texture of the plaque instead may cause the formation of a blood clot, or thrombus, which closes the artery in a condition called coronary thrombosis. The result is a myocardial infarction (commonly called a heart attack), in which some myocardial cells die when they fail to receive blood.

Although coronary ischemia is usually thought of as a disease of middle and old age, in fact, it starts much earlier. Autopsies of accident victims in their teens and twenties, as well as young soldiers killed in battle, show that coronary atherosclerosis is often well advanced in young persons. Some reasons for these findings and for why the rates of coronary artery disease and death began to rise in the twentieth century have been proposed. While antibiotics and vaccines reduced the mortality of some bacterial and some viral infections, Western societies underwent significant changes in lifestyle and eating habits that contributed to the rise of coronary heart disease: high-fat diets, obesity, and the stressful pace of life in a modern industrial society. Furthermore, cigarette smoking, once almost a universal habit, has been shown to be highly pathogenic (disease-causing), contributing significantly to the development of heart disease, as well as lung cancer, emphysema, bronchitis, and other disorders. In the early and middle decades of the twentieth century, coronary heart disease was considered primarily an ailment of middle-aged and older men. As women began smoking, however, the incidence shifted so that coronary artery disease became almost equally prevalent, and equally lethal, among men and women.

Other conditions such as hypertension or diabetes mellitus are considered precursors of coronary artery disease. Hypertension, or high blood pressure, is an extremely common condition that, if unchecked, can contribute to both the development and the progression of coronary artery disease. Over the years, high blood pressure subjects arterial walls to constant stress. In response, the walls thicken and stiffen. This "hardening" of the arteries encourages the accumulation of fatty and fibrous plaque on inner artery walls. In patients with diabetes mellitus, blood sugar (glucose) levels rise either because the patient is deficient in insulin or because the insulin that the patient produces is inefficient at removing glucose from the blood. High glucose levels favor high fat levels in the blood, which can cause atherosclerosis.

Cardiac arrhythmias are the next major cause of morbidity and mortality among the heart diseases. Inside the heart, an electrochemical network regulates the contractions and relaxations that form the heartbeat. In the excitation or contraction phase, a chain of electrochemical impulses starts in the upper part of the right atrium in the heart's pacemaker, the sinoatrial or sinus node. The impulses travel through internodal tracts (pathways from one node to another) to an area between the atrium and the right ventricle called the atrioventricular node. The impulses then enter the bundle of His, which carries them to the left atrium and left ventricle. After the series of contractions is complete, the heart relaxes for a brief moment before another cycle is begun. On the average, the process is repeated sixty to eighty times a minute.

This is normal rhythm, the regular, healthy heartbeat. Dysfunction at any point along the electrochemical pathway, however, can cause an arrhythmia. Arrhythmias range greatly in their effects and their potential for bodily damage. They can be completely unnoticeable, merely annoying, debilitating, or frightening. They can cause blood clots to form in the heart, and they can cause sudden death.

The arrhythmic heart can beat too quickly (tachycardia) or too slowly (bradycardia). The contractions of the various chambers can become unsynchronized, or out of step with one another. For example, in atrial flutter or atrial fibrillation, the upper chambers of the heart beat faster, out of synchronization with the ventricles. In ventricular tachycardia, ventricular contractions increase, out of synchronization with the atria. In ventricular fibrillation, ventricular contractions lose all rhythmicity and become uncoordinated to the point at which the heart is no longer able to pump blood. Cardiac death can then occur unless the patient receives immediate treatment.

An arrhythmic disorder called heart block occurs when the impulse from the pacemaker is "blocked." Its progress through the atrioventricular node and the bundle of His may be slow or irregular, or the impulse may fail to reach its target tissues. The disorder is rated in three degrees. First-degree heart block is detectable only on an electrocardiogram (ECG or EKG), in which the movement of the impulse from the atria to the ventricles is seen to be slowed. In second-degree heart block, only some of the impulses generated reach from the atria to the ventricles; the pulse becomes irregular. Third-degree heart block is the most serious manifestation of this disorder: No impulses from the atria reach the ventricles. The heart rate may slow dramatically, and the blood flow to the brain can be reduced, causing dizziness or loss of consciousness.

Disorders that affect the heart valves usually involve stenosis (narrowing), which reduces the size of the valve opening; physical malfunction of the valve; or both. These disorders can be attributable to infection (such as rheumatic fever) or to tissue damage, or they can be congenital. If a valve has narrowed, the passage of blood from one heart chamber to another is impeded. In the case of mitral stenosis, the mitral valve between the left atrium and the left ventricle is narrowed. Blood flow to the left ventricle is reduced, and blood is retained in the left atrium, causing the atrium to enlarge as pressure builds in the chamber. This pressure forces blood back into the lungs, creating a condition called pulmonary edema, in which fluid collects in the air sacs of the lungs. Similarly, malfunctions of the heart valves that cause them to open and close inefficiently can interfere with the flow of blood into the heart, through it, and out of it. This impairment may cause structural changes in the heart that can be life-threatening.

Heart failure may be a consequence of many disease conditions. It occurs primarily in the elderly. In this condition, the heart becomes inefficient at pumping blood. If the failure is on the right side of the heart, blood is forced back into the body, causing edema in the lower legs. If the failure is on the left side of the heart, blood is forced back into the lungs, causing pulmonary edema. There are many manifestations of heart failure, including shortness of breath, fatigue, and weakness.

Numerous diseases afflict the tissues of the heart wall-the epicardium, myocardium, and endocardium, as well as the pericardium. They are often caused by bacterial or viral infection, but they may also result from tissue trauma or a variety of toxic agents.

Treatment and Therapy

The main tools for diagnosing heart disease are the stethoscope, the ECG, and the x ray. With the stethoscope the doctor listens to heart sounds, which provide information about many heart functions such as rhythm and the status of the valves. The doctor can determine whether the heart is functioning normally in pumping blood from one chamber into the other, into the lungs, and into the aorta. The ECG gives the doctor a graph representation of heart function. Twelve to fifteen electrodes are placed on various parts of the body, including the head, chest, legs, and arms. The activities of the heart are printed on a strip of paper as waves or tracings. The doctor analyzes the printout for evidence of heart abnormalities, changes in heart function, signs of a heart attack, or other problems. Generally, the electrocardiographic examination is conducted with the patient at rest. In some situations, however, the doctor wishes to view heart action during physical stress. In this case, the electrodes are attached to the patient and the patient is required to exercise on a treadmill or stationary bicycle. The physician can see what changes in heart function occur when the cardiac workload is increased. The x ray gives the doctor a visual picture of the heart. Any enlargements or abnormalities can be seen, as well as the status of the aorta, pulmonary arteries, and other structures.

Another standard diagnostic tool is the echocardiograph. High-frequency sound waves are pointed at the heart from outside the body. The sound waves bounce against heart tissue and are shown on a monitor. The general configuration of the heart can be seen, as well as the shape and thickness of the chamber walls, the valves, and the large blood vessels leading to and from the heart. Velocity and direction of blood flow through the valves can be determined.

Various procedures can help the doctor assess the degree of ischemia within the heart. In one test, a radioactive isotope is injected into a vein and its dispersion in the heart is read by a scanner. This procedure can show which parts of the heart are being deprived of oxygen. In another test using a radioactive isotope, the reading is made while the patient exercises, in order to detect any changes in expansion and contraction of the heart wall that would indicate impaired circulation. The coronary angiogram gives a picture of the blockage within the coronary arteries. A thin tube called a catheter is threaded into a coronary artery, and a dye that is opaque to x rays is released. The x-ray picture will reveal narrowings in the artery resulting from plaque buildup.

The main goals of therapy in treating heart diseases are to cure the condition, if possible, and otherwise help the patient live a normal life and prevent the condition from becoming worse. In coronary artery disease, the physician seeks to maintain blood flow to the heart and to prevent heart attack. Hundreds of medications are available for this purpose, including vasodilators (agents that relax blood vessel walls and increase their capacity

to carry blood). Chief among the coronary vasodilators are nitroglycerin and other drugs in the nitrate family. Also, calcium-channel blockers are often used to dilate blood vessels. Beta-blocking agents are used because they reduce the heart's need for oxygen and alleviate the symptoms of angina. In addition, various support measures are recommended by physicians to stop plaque buildup and halt the progress of the disease. These include losing weight, reducing fats in the diet, and stopping smoking. The physician also treats concomitant illnesses that can contribute to the progress of coronary artery disease, such as hypertension and diabetes.

Sometimes medications and diet are not fully successful, and the ischemia continues. The cardiologist can unblock a clogged artery by a procedure called angioplasty. The physician threads a catheter containing a tiny balloon to the point of the blockage. The balloon is inflated to widen the inner diameter of the artery, and blood flow is increased. This procedure is often successful, although it may have to be repeated. In atherectomy, a miniature drill shaves off the plaque, which is then removed. If neither procedure is successful, coronary bypass surgery may be indicated. In this procedure, clogged coronary arteries are replaced with healthy blood vessels from other parts of the body.

When coronary artery disease progresses to a heart attack, the patient should be treated in the hospital or similar facility. The possibility of sudden death is high during the attack and remains high until the patient is stabilized. Emergency measures are undertaken to minimize the extent of heart damage, reduce heart work, keep oxygen flowing to all parts of the body, and regulate blood pressure and heartbeat.

Cardiac arrhythmias can be managed by a variety of medications and procedures. Digitalis, guanidine, procainamide, tocanamide, and atropine are widely used to restore normal heart rhythm. In acute situations, the patient's heart rhythm can be restored by electrical cardioversion, in which an electrical stimulus is applied from outside the body to regulate the heartbeat. When a slowed heartbeat cannot be controlled by medication, a pacemaker may be implanted to regulate heart rhythm.

Treatment of heart valve disorders and disorders of the heart wall is directed at alleviating the individual condition. Antibiotics and/or valve replacement surgery may be required. In many cases, valve disorders can be completely corrected. Cardiac transplantation remains a possible treatment for some heart patients. This is an option for comparatively few patients because there are ten times as many candidates for heart transplants as there are available donor hearts.

Perspective and Prospects

Heart disease became a major killer in the United States in the twentieth century. In the early decades, the best that the medical community could do was to treat symptoms. Since then, the emphasis has shifted to prevention. Hundreds of investigative studies have been undertaken to determine the causes of the most prevalent heart dysfunction, coronary artery disease. Many of these studies have involved tens of thousands of subjects, and they point to a general consensus that coronary artery disease is a multifactorial disorder, the primary elements of which are cholesterol and other fatty substances circulating in the bloodstream, smoking, diabetes, high blood pressure, stress, and obesity.

The reasons that mortality from heart disease is declining include improved medications and treatment modalities, and much credit has to be given to the success of preventive measures. Millions of Americans have stopped smoking and have begun watching their diets. Entire industries are devoted to helping Americans eat more intelligently. While fast-food outlets continue to offer high-fat standards, such as hot dogs and hamburgers, they have also added salads and leaner selections.

Perhaps most important, medical and sociological authorities have turned their attention to children. Because advanced atherosclerosis has been detected in young men and women, cholesterol-watching has become a major preoccupation with parents and school dieticians. In addition, national programs have been instituted to discourage smoking among the young. Whether the rates of coronary heart disease will be lower in these individuals than in their parents remains to be seen, but the success of these measures in the older populations indicates that the prognosis is good.

The prognosis is also good for other heart diseases. New drugs continue to be licensed for the treatment of arrhythmias, and more versatile and reliable pacemakers increase the prospects of a normal life for many patients. Improvements in

heart surgery have been particularly impressive, especially those for managing congenital heart defects in neonates and infants. Heart transplants have been successfully performed on these patients, and numerous other procedures promise significant improvement in the prospects of young people with heart disease.

Rheumatic fever, however, one of the major causes of heart disease in children, remains a threat. No vaccine is available for immunization against the streptococcus strains that cause rheumatic fever, but fortunately there are effective antibiotics to control infection in these patients. Rheumatic fever usually develops subsequent to a streptococcal throat infection that has not been treated adequately with antibiotics. Careful evaluation of the child with a sore throat and prompt, complete antibiotic treatment of those with streptococcal infection can avoid progression of the infection to rheumatic fever.

—*C. Richard Falcon*

References

Carbone, Salvatore, et al. "Obesity Paradox in Cardiovascular Disease: Where Do We Stand?" *Vascular Health and Risk Management*, vol. 15, 2019, pp. 89–100., doi:10.2147/vhrm.s168946.

Cercato, C., and F. A. Fonseca. "Cardiovascular Risk and Obesity." *Diabetology & Metabolic Syndrome*, vol. 11, no. 1, 28 Aug. 2019, doi:10.1186/s13098-019-0468-0.

Daniel, Sunil. "Obesity and Heart Disease." *Obesity Action Coalition*, 2015, www.obesityaction.org/community/article-library/obesity-and-heart-disease/.

Kim, Seong Hwan, et al. "Obesity and Cardiovascular Disease: Friend or Foe?" *European Heart Journal*, vol. 37, no. 48, 18 Dec. 2015, pp. 3560–3568., doi:10.1093/eurheartj/chv509.

Koliaki, Chrysi, et al. "Obesity and Cardiovascular Disease: Revisiting an Old Relationship." *Metabolism*, vol. 92, 2019, pp. 98–107., doi:10.1016/j.metabol.2018.10.011.

"Obesity & Heart Disease." *Cleveland Clinic*, 2 Jan. 2019, my.clevelandclinic.org/health/articles/17308-obesity–heart-disease.

Riaz, Haris, et al. "Association Between Obesity and Cardiovascular Outcomes." *JAMA Network Open*, vol. 1, no. 7, 2018, doi:10.1001/jamanetworkopen.2018.3788.

■ Heart failure

CATEGORY: Disorder

Causes and Symptoms

The circulation of the blood has many functions. It is essential for the delivery of oxygen, nutrients, and elements of the immune system to tissues. It also contributes to regulation and communication between different parts of the body by moving chemical messengers from where they are produced to where they have a biological effect. The delivery of warm blood to the surface of the skin is one essential element in temperature control. The blood pressure determines how much water can move across the exchange surfaces in the kidneys, thus affecting water balance in the body. The movement of blood through the kidneys, the lungs, and all tissues is important for waste removal.

All these functions depend on the ability of the heart to contract and eject blood. Blood is pumped, in two serial circuits, from the right heart through the lungs into the left heart and from the left heart around the body back to the right heart. In each circuit, the blood travels through large arteries, then to smaller arterioles, to capillaries (where exchange takes place), and back via small venules and veins to the heart. Heart failure describes the situation in which heart function is reduced. While still able to beat, the heart is unable to meet the circulatory needs of the body. That is, the heart muscle is unable to contract enough to pump the blood adequately.

The severity of the heart failure can be gauged by the ejection fraction, a measure of the pumping capacity of the heart. It is the percentage calculated from the stroke volume (the volume of blood leaving a heart chamber with each beat) divided by the residual volume (the volume left in the heart chamber at the end of a heartbeat). Thus, the ejection fraction measures how much blood in the heart chamber can actually leave when the heartbeat occurs. In normal, healthy hearts, this value is 100 percent: the amount that stays in the heart is approximately equal to the amount that leaves it. In mild or moderate heart failure, it ranges approximately between 15 and 40 percent: Less blood leaves the heart with each beat, and more blood remains behind.

The pressure inside the heart at the end of a heartbeat is another index of heart performance. If the heart is failing and more blood is left behind in the heart at the end of a beat, the pressure inside the heart at the end of the beat will be increased. In cases of severe failure, the pressure in the arteries outside the heart will fall.

In failure, the heart cannot supply enough blood for all the functions of the circulation. This fact accounts for the variety of symptoms that accompany heart failure: labored breathing; light-headedness; generalized weakness; cold, pale, or even bluish skin tone; and accumulation of fluid in the extremities and/or lungs. Other possible symptoms include distended neck veins, accumulation of fluid in the abdomen, abnormal heart rate and rhythm, and chest pain.

The specific symptoms of the condition depend on the type of failure, its severity, its underlying causes, and the ways in which the body attempts to compensate. There are several ways to categorize types of heart failure: acute or chronic, forward or backward, and right-sided or left-sided.

Acute heart failure refers to a sudden decrease in heart function. It can be caused by toxic quantities of drugs, anesthetics, or metals or by certain disease states, such as infections. Most often, however, it is caused by a sudden blockage of the coronary arteries supplying the heart muscle. A sudden blockage caused by a blood clot can induce a heart attack and subsequent heart failure, causing chest pain and often abnormal heart rate or rhythm. These effects are sometimes so rapid that there is little time for the body to attempt compensation.

Chronic heart failure is a progressive reduction in heart function that develops over time. It can be caused by inherited or acquired diseases, allergic reactions, connective tissue or metabolic abnormalities, high blood pressure, and anatomical defects. The most common cause, however, is coronary artery disease. This disease narrows blood vessels and leads to a reduction in the amount of blood reaching the heart muscle. It causes reduced oxygen availability and, eventually, a reduction in the ability of the heart muscle to contract.

In the early stages of chronic failure, the hormone and nervous systems promote compensation in the heart, blood vessels, and kidneys to help the heart continue to pump enough blood. These systems stimulate the heart muscle directly to make it beat harder. They also take advantage of the fact that modest stretching of the heart muscle increases

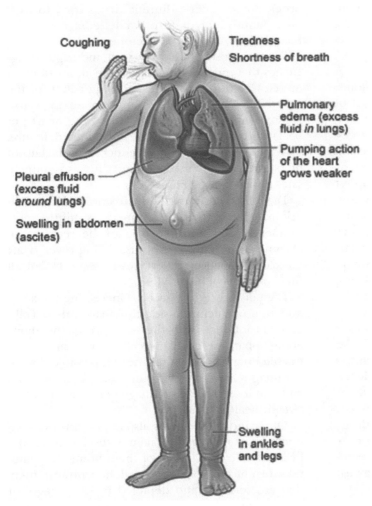

Coughing

Tiredness
Shortness of breath

Pulmonary edema (excess fluid *in* lungs)

Pumping action of the heart grows weaker

Pleural effusion (excess fluid *around* lungs)

Swelling in abdomen (ascites)

Swelling in ankles and legs

Signs and symptoms of severe heart failure. (National Heart, Lung, and Blood Institute)

pump hard enough to move the blood forward against the higher resistance caused by the contraction of the blood vessels. This condition is termed forward heart failure. Congestive heart failure is the stage that occurs when the backup of pressure is worsened by fluid retention and blood vessel contraction. The congestion, or accumulation of fluid, occurs in the veins and tissues.

Left-sided or right-sided heart failure can occur alone or together. The right side of the heart pumps blood to the lungs to be oxygenated, and the left side of the heart pumps oxygenated blood to the organs of the body. Normally, these two sides are well matched so that the same volume moves through each side. When the right heart cannot contract properly, however, blood accumulates upstream in the veins and somewhat less blood reaches the lungs to pick up oxygen, resulting in distended veins and shortness of breath. It is primarily a backward heart failure. Fluid can back up in the veins and increase pressure in the capillaries so that it starts to leak out of the circulation into the surrounding tissues. This leads to an accumulation of fluid (called edema), especially in the liver and lower extremities. In isolated right-sided heart failure, this pressure rarely backs up to such an extent that it causes problems through the rest of the circulation to the left side of the heart.

its ability to contract. By stimulating the blood vessels to contract, more blood moves back toward the heart, causing a cold, pale, or even bluish skin tone. Stimulation of the kidney to retain water and sodium results in an increase in blood volume, which also moves more blood back to the heart. In each case, the heart muscle is stretched by these increases and, therefore, can contract harder.

Yet these reactions do not constitute a long-term solution. The heart muscle can become fatigued from overwork and can become overstretched. A resulting accumulation of fluid in the heart reduces its ability to contract. Compensation fails, and the additional fluid in the blood starts to back up in the circulation. This condition is called backward heart failure. At the same time, the heart is unable to

In contrast, when the left side of the heart cannot contract properly, it can back up pressure so badly that it creates a pressure overload against which the right side of the heart must pump. This increase in the workload on the right side of the heart frequently leads to two-sided heart failure. This outcome is especially common since the disease conditions that exist in the left side are likely to exist on the right as well. In left-sided heart failure, blood accumulates upstream in the lungs, increasing pressure enough to cause a leakage of fluid into the lungs (pulmonary edema). This leakage interferes with oxygen uptake and therefore causes shortness of breath. It also results in inadequate blood flow to the body's tissues, including the muscles and brain, resulting in generalized weakness and light-headedness. Left-sided heart failure is thus both a backward and a forward failure.

Treatment and Therapy

Treatments for cardiac failure, like its symptoms, depend on a variety of factors. The first goal of treatment is to avoid any obvious precipitating causes of the failure, such as alcohol, drugs, the cessation of nonessential medications, acute stress, a salt-loaded diet, overexercise, infection, illness, or surgery. The next approach is to take the simplest measures to reduce distension of the heart by controlling salt and water retention and to decrease the workload of the heart by altering the circulatory needs of the tissues. The former can be achieved by dietary salt restriction, restriction of fluid consumption, or mechanical removal of fluid accumulating around the lungs or abdomen. The latter can be accomplished with bed rest and weight loss.

Typically, drug therapy is also required in order to treat heart failure. No single agent meets all the requirements for optimal treatment, which includes rapid relief of labored breathing and edema, enhanced heart performance, reduced mortality, reduced progression of the underlying disease, safety, and minimal side effects. Therefore, drugs are used in combination to achieve control over sodium and water retention, improve heart contraction, reduce heart work, and protect against blood clots.

The purpose of therapy with diuretic drugs (drugs that increase salt and water loss through the kidneys) is threefold: to reduce the pooling of fluid that can take place in the lungs, abdomen, and lower extremities; to minimize the buildup of back pressure from the accumulation of blood in the veins; and to reduce the circulating blood volume. All these things will lessen the overstretch of the heart muscle and bring it to a level of stretch that is closer to its optimum. Care must be taken, however, not to reduce severely the water content of the blood, which could reduce the stretch on the heart muscle to below the optimum and consequently impair heart contraction. One way to monitor how much water is lost or retained is for patients to empty their bladders and then weigh themselves each day before breakfast. If weight changes steadily or suddenly, then sodium and water loss may be too great or too little. In either case, an adjustment is in

order. Some generic diuretic drugs used to treat heart failure include furosemide, ethacrynic acid, the thiazides, and spironolactone.

The purpose of therapy with inotropic drugs (drugs that increase the contractile ability of heart muscle) is to improve the pumping action of the heart. This effect causes an increase in stroke volume (more blood moves out of the heart per beat) and helps compensate for forward failure. The increased output also reduces the backup of blood returning to the heart and thus also compensates for backward failure.

Digitalis, a derivative of the foxglove plant which originated as a Welsh folk remedy, is still the most frequently used inotropic drug for the treatment of chronic heart failure. Because it improves heart muscle contraction, it reverses to some extent all the symptoms of heart failure.

Digitalis exerts its effects by increasing the accumulation of calcium inside the heart muscle cells. Calcium interacts with the structure of the shortening apparatus inside the cell to make more contractile interactions within the cell possible. Its disadvantages are that it becomes toxic in high doses and that it can severely damage performance of an already healthy heart.

Other inotropic agents also act to improve contraction by increasing calcium levels within the heart muscle cells. Some of them mimic the naturally produced hormones and neurotransmitters that are released and depleted in early stages of heart failure. These are called the sympathomimetic drugs. They include drugs such as dopamine, terbutaline, and levodopa. While these drugs improve heart performance, they can have serious side effects: increased heart rate, palpitations, and nervousness. One group of inotropic agents improves cardiac contraction while relaxing blood vessels. These drugs, called phosphodiesterase inhibitors, stop the breakdown of an essential cellular messenger molecule which helps to manage calcium levels and other events inside both heart cells and blood vessel cells. Examples of these drugs include amrinone and milrinone. Their use is not common because they can cause stomach upset and fatigue and because they are not clearly superior to other treatments.

The purpose of therapy with vasodilator drugs (drugs that relax the blood vessels) is to decrease the work of the heart. The resulting expansion of the blood vessels makes it easier for blood to be pumped through them. It also leaves room for pooling some of the blood in the veins, decreasing the amount of blood returning to the heart and so reducing overstretching as well. Some of the vasodilators, such as hydralazine, pinacidil, dipyridamole, and the nitrates, act directly on the blood vessels. Other vasodilators, such as angiotensin-converting enzyme (ACE) inhibitors and adrenergic inhibitors, inhibit the release of naturally produced substances that would make the blood vessels contract. Sometimes it is hard to predict the effects of vasodilators because they may act differently in different blood vessels and the body may attempt to offset the effects of the drug by releasing substances that contract blood vessels. Vasodilator drug therapy is usually added to other treatments when the symptoms of heart failure persist after digitalis and diuretic therapy are used.

The purpose of therapy with antithrombotics (blood clot inhibitors) is to prevent any further obstruction of the circulation with blood clots. Because heart failure changes the mechanics of blood flow and is the result of damaged heart muscle, it can increase the formation of blood clots. When blood clots form an obstruction in the large blood vessels of the lungs, it is often fatal. Clots can also lodge in the heart, causing further damage to heart muscle, or in the brain, where they could cause a stroke. Both the short-acting clot inhibitor heparin and oral agents such as aspirin are used to prevent these effects.

The combination of all these drug therapies, while unable to reverse the permanent damage of heart failure, makes it possible to treat the condition. Individuals treated for heart failure can lead comfortable, productive lives.

If the heart failure progresses to acutely life-threatening proportions and the patient is in all other ways healthy, the next alternative is surgical replacement of the heart. Artificial hearts are sometimes used as a transition to heart transplant while a donor is sought. Yet transplantation is not a perfect solution. Transplanted hearts do not have the nervous system input of a normal heart and so their control from moment to moment is different. They are also subject to rejection. Nevertheless, they provide an enormous improvement in quality of life for severe heart failure patients.

Perspective and Prospects

The vital significance of the pulse and heartbeat have been part of human knowledge since long before recorded history. Pulse taking and herbal treatments for poor heartbeat have been recorded in ancient Chinese, Egyptian, and Greek histories. Digitalis has been used in treatment for at least two hundred years. It was first formally introduced to the medical community in 1785 by the English botanist and physician William Withering. He learned of it from a female folk healer named Hutton, who used it with other extracts to treat more than one kind of swelling. Withering identified the foxglove plant as the source of its active ingredient and characterized it as having effects on the pulse as well as on fluid retention. The plant is indigenous to both the United Kingdom and Europe and may well have been employed as a folk remedy for far longer.

The developments in physiology and medicine during the nineteenth century set the stage for greater understanding and further treatments of heart failure. It was then that the stethoscope and blood pressure cuff were created for diagnostic purposes. In basic science, cell theory, hormone theory, and kidney physiology led to a better understanding of how heart muscle contraction and fluid balance might be coordinated in the body. The concepts and techniques required to keep organs and tissues alive outside the body with an artificial circulation system were conceived and introduced. Anesthesia and sterile techniques essential for cardiac surgery were developed.

These ideas and accomplishments contributed to important discoveries in the early twentieth century that greatly enhanced the understanding of the early compensatory responses to heart failure. For example, it was found that when heart muscle is stretched, it will contract with greater force on the next beat and that heart muscle usually operates at a muscle length that is less than optimal. Thus, when the amount of blood returning to the heart increases and stretches the muscle in the walls of the heart, the heart will contract with greater force, ejecting a greater volume of blood. This phenomenon, called the Frank-Starling mechanism, was first demonstrated in isolated heart muscle by the German physiologist Otto Frank and in functional hearts by the British physiologist Ernest Henry Starling in 1914.

Subsequent developments in the second half of the twentieth century, such as more specific vasodilator and diuretic drugs as well as the heart-lung machine, have led to the options of more complete drug therapy, artificial hearts (first introduced to replace a human heart by William DeVries in 1982), and heart transplant (first performed by Christiaan Barnard in 1967) as options for the treatment of heart failure. Researchers have begun clinical trials to assess the viability of using gene therapy for increasing blood flow in patients with advanced heart failure. Though treating heart failure is an ongoing challenge for the medical profession, diagnosing the ailment is becoming easier than before through preventative methods such as annual blood tests and breath tests, findings for the latter of which were published in the *Journal of the American College of Cardiology* in 2013. Furthermore, ongoing stem-cell research may lead to greater advances in the treatment of heart failure.

—*Laura Gray Malloy*

References

Alpert, Martin A., et al. "Obesity and Heart Failure: Epidemiology, Pathophysiology, Clinical Manifestations, and Management." *Translational Research*, vol. 164, no. 4, 2014, pp. 345–356., doi:10.1016/j.trsl.2014.04.010.

Carbone, Salvatore, et al. "Obesity and Heart Failure: Focus on the Obesity Paradox." *Mayo Clinic Proceedings*, vol. 92, no. 2, 2017, pp. 266–279., doi:10.1016/j.mayocp.2016.11.001.

Finer, Nicholas. "Weight Loss for Patients with Obesity and Heart Failure." *European Heart Journal*, vol. 40, no. 26, 10 June 2019, pp. 2139–2141., doi:10.1093/eurheartj/ehz406.

Khalid, Mirza Umair, et al. "The Obesity Paradox in Heart Failure: Why Does It Clinically Matter?" *American College of Cardiology*, 7 May 2015, www.acc.org/latest-in-cardiology/articles/2015/05/06/10/22/the-obesity-paradox-in-heart-failure.

"Severe Obesity Revealed as a Stand-Alone High-Risk Factor for Heart Failure." *Johns Hopkins Medicine*, 22 Aug. 2016, www.hopkinsmedicine.org/news/media/releases/severe_obesity_revealed_as_a_stand_alone_high_risk_factor_for_heart_failure.

"Three Ways Obesity Contributes to Heart Disease." *Penn Medicine*, 25 Mar. 2019, www.pennmedicine.org/updates/blogs/metabolic-and-bariatric-surgery-blog/2019/march/obesity-and-heart-disease.

■ Hyperlipidemia

CATEGORY: Disorder

Causes and Symptoms

Although elevated triglyceride levels have been implicated in clinical ischemic diseases, most investigators believe that cholesterol-rich lipids are a more significant risk factor. Although measurements of bothcholesterol and triglyceride levels have been used to predict coronary disease, studies suggest that the determination of the alpha-lipoprotein/beta-lipoprotein ratio is a more reliable predictor. Because the alpha-lipoprotein has a higher density than the beta-lipoprotein, they are more often designated as high-density lipoprotein (HDL) and low-density lipoprotein (LDL), respectively. HDL is often referred to as "good cholesterol," and LDL is referred to as "bad cholesterol." The latter is implicated in the development of atherosclerosis.

Atherosclerosis is a disease that begins in the innermost lining of the arterial wall. Its lesions occur predominantly at arterial forks and branch openings, but they can also occur at sites where there is injury to the arterial lining. The initial lesion usually appears as fatty streaks or spots, which have been detected even at birth. With passing years, more of these lesions appear, and they may develop into elevated plaques that obstruct the flow of blood in the artery. The lesions are rich in cholesterol derived from beta-lipoproteins in the plasma. In addition to elevated blood lipids, other risk factors associated with atherosclerosis include hypertension, faulty arterial structure, obesity, smoking, and stress.

Treatment and Therapy

The treatment of hyperlipidemia involves both dietary and drug therapies. Although studies in nonhuman primates indicate that the reduction of hyperlipidemia results in decreased morbidity and mortality rates from arterial vascular disease, studies in humans are less conclusive. Initial treatment involves restricting the dietary intake of cholesterol and saturated fat. Drug therapy is instituted when further lowering of the serum lipids is desired. Among the drugs that have been used as antihyperlipidemic agents are lovastatin and its analogues, clofibrate and its analogues (particularly gemfibrozil), nicotinic acid, D-thyroxine, cholestyramine, probucol, and heparin.

Lovastatin blocks the synthesis of cholesterol by inhibiting the enzyme (HMGCoA reductase) that catalyzes the conversion of beta-hydroxy-beta-methyl glutaryl coenzyme A (HMGCoA) to mevalonic acid (MVA), the regulatory step in the biosynthesis of cholesterol. Both lovastatin and MVA are beta, delta-dihydroxy acids, but lovastatin has a much more lipophilic (fat-soluble) group attached to it. Clofibrate and gemfibrozil block the synthesis of cholesterol prior to the HMGCoA stage. For this reason, they are likely to inhibit triglyceride formation as well. Nicotinic acid inhibits the synthesis of acetyl coenzyme A (acetyl SCoA) and thus would be expected to block the synthesis of both cholesterol and the triglycerides. To be effective in lowering the serum level of lipids, nicotinic acid must be taken in large amounts, which often produces an unpleasant flushing sensation in the patient. A way to inhibit the synthesis of cholesterol at the post-MVA stages has also been sought. Agents such as triparanol, which inhibit biosynthesis near the end of the synthetic sequence, have been developed. Although they are effective in lowering serum cholesterol, they had to be withdrawn from clinical use because of their adverse side effects on the muscles and eyes. Moreover, the penultimate product in the biosynthesis of cholesterol proved to be atherogenic.

D-thyroxine promotes the metabolism of cholesterol in the liver, transforming it into the more hydrophilic (watersoluble) bile acids, thereby facilitating its elimination from the body. An approach to reducing the serum level of cholesterol by a process involving the sequestering of the bile acids utilizes the resin cholestyramine as the sequestrant. The sequestered bile acids cannot be reabsorbed into the enterohepatic system and are eliminated in the feces. Consequently, more cholesterol is oxidized to the bile acids, resulting in the reduction of the serum level of cholesterol. Unfortunately, a large quantity of cholestyramine is required. Sequestration of cholesterol with beta-sitosterol prevents both the absorption of dietary cholesterol and the reabsorption of endogenous cholesterol in the intestines. Here, too, a large quantity of the sequestrant needs to be administered.

Probucol is an antioxidant. Because, structurally, it is a sulfur analogue of a hindered hydroquinone, it acts as a free radical scavenger. Evidence suggests that the antihyperlipidemic effect of probucol is attributable to its ability to inhibit the oxygenation of LDL. The oxygenated LDL is believed to be the atherogenic form of LDL. Heparin promotes the hydrolysis of triglycerides as it activates lipoprotein lipase, thereby reducing lipidemia. Because of its potent anticoagulant properties, however, its use in therapy must be closely monitored. Cholesterol that is present in atherosclerotic plaques is acylated, generally by the more saturated fatty acids. The enzyme catalyzing the acylation process is acyl-CoA cholesterol acyl transferase (ACAT). The development of regulators of ACAT and the desirability of reducing the dietary intake of saturated fatty acids are based on this rationale.

Cholesterol within the cell is able to inhibit further synthesis of cholesterol by a feedback mechanism. Cholesterol that is associated with LDL is transported into the hepatic cell by means of the LDL receptor on the surface of the cell. In individuals who are afflicted with familial hypercholesterolemia, an inherited disorder that causes death at an early age, the gene that is responsible for the production of the LDL receptor is either absent or defective. Studies in gene therapy have shown that transplant of the normal LDL receptor gene to such an individual results in a dramatic decrease in the level of the "bad cholesterol" in the serum. Cholesterol derivatives that are oxygenated at various positions have also been found to regulate the serum level of cholesterol by either inhibiting its synthesis or promoting its catabolism.

—*Leland J. Chinn*

References

Chang, Chi-Jen, et al. "Evidence in Obese Children: Contribution of Hyperlipidemia, Obesity-Inflammation, and Insulin Sensitivity." *Plos One,* vol. 10, no. 5, 2015, doi:10.1371/journal.pone.0125935.

Davis, Kathleen. "What to Know about Hyperlipidemia." *Medical News Today,* 15 July 2019, www.medicalnewstoday.com/articles/295385.

Karr, Samantha. "Epidemiology and Management of Hyperlipidemia." *American Journal of Managed Care,* vol. 23, no. 9, 21 June 2017, pp. 139–148.

Shattat, Ghassan F. "A Review Article on Hyperlipidemia: Types, Treatments and New Drug Targets." *Biomedical and Pharmacology Journal,* vol. 7, no. 2, 2014, pp. 399–409., doi:10.13005/bpj/504.

■ Hypertension

CATEGORY: Disorder

Causes and Symptoms

Hypertension is a higher-than-normal blood pressure (either systolic or diastolic). Blood pressure is usually measured using a sphygmomanometer and a stethoscope. The stethoscope is used to hear when the air pressure within the cuff of the sphygmomanometer is equal to that in the artery. When taking a blood pressure, the cuff is pumped to inflate an air bladder secured around the arm; the pressure produced will collapse the blood vessels within. As cuff pressure decreases, a slight thump is heard as the artery snaps open to allow blood to flow. At this point, the cuff pressure equals the systolic blood pressure. As the cuff pressure continues to fall, the sound of blood being pumped will continue but become progressively softer. At the point where the last sound is heard, the cuff pressure equals the diastolic blood pressure.

Blood Pressure

Blood pressure is measured in two numbers: systolic pressure (the pressure of the blood as it flows out when the heart contracts) over diastolic pressure (the pressure of the blood within the artery as it flows in when the heart is at rest). Readings greater than 140 systolic over 90 diastolic indicate the presence of hypertension.

BLOOD PRESSURE AND HYPERTENSION	
Status	**Systolic/Diastolic**
Normal	>120/>80
Prehypertension	120-139/80-89
Stage I hypertension	140-159/90-99
Stage II hypertension	<160/100

In hypertension, both systolic and diastolic blood pressures are usually elevated. Blood pressures are reported as the systolic pressure over the diastolic pressure, such as 130/80 millimeters of mercury.

It is important to recognize there are degrees of seriousness for hypertension. The higher the blood pressure, the more rigorous the treatment may be. When systolic pressures are in the high normal range, the individual should be closely monitored with annual blood pressure checks. Persistently high blood pressures (greater than 140-159/90-99 millimeters of mercury) require closer monitoring and may result in a decision to treat the condition with medication or other types of intervention.

The blood pressure in an artery is determined by the relationship among three important controlling factors: the blood volume, the amount of blood pumped by the heart (cardiac output), and the contraction of smooth muscle within blood vessels (arterial tone). To illustrate the first point, if blood volume decreases, the result will be a fall in blood pressure. Conversely, the body cannot itself increase blood pressure by rapidly adding blood volume; fluid must be injected into the circulation to do so.

A second controlling factor of blood pressure is cardiac output (the volume of blood pumped by the heart in a given unit of time, usually reported as liters per minute). This output is determined by two factors: stroke volume (the volume of blood pumped with each heartbeat) and the heart rate (beats per minute). As heart rate increases, output generally increases, and blood pressure may rise as well. If blood volume is low, such as with excessive bleeding, the blood returning to the heart per beat is lower and could lead to decreased output. To compensate, the heart rate increases to prevent a drop in blood pressure. Therefore, as cardiac output changes, blood pressure does not necessarily change.

Last, a major controlling factor of blood pressure is arterial tone. Arteries are largely tubular, smooth muscles that can change their diameter based on the extent of contraction (tone). This contraction is largely under the control of a specialized branch of the nervous system called the sympathetic nervous system. An artery with high arterial tone (contracted) will squeeze the blood within and increase the pressure inside. There is also a relaxation phase that will allow expansion and a decrease in blood pressure. Along with relaxation, arteries are elastic to allow some stretching, which may further help reduce pressure or, more important, help prevent blood pressure from rising.

High Blood Pressure

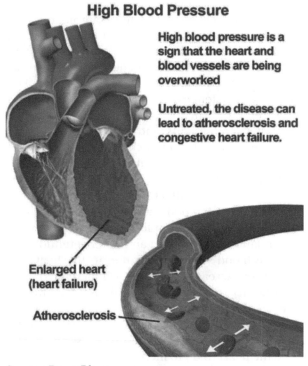

High blood pressure is a sign that the heart and blood vessels are being overworked

Untreated, the disease can lead to atherosclerosis and congestive heart failure.

Enlarged heart (heart failure)

Atherosclerosis

Source: BruceBlaus

There are two general types of hypertension: essential and secondary. Secondary hypertension is attributable to some underlying identifiable cause, such as a tumor or kidney disease, while essential hypertension has no identifiable cause. Therefore, essential hypertension is a defect that results in excessive arterial pressure secondary to poor regulation by any one of the three controlling factors discussed above. Each factor can serve as a focal point for treatment with medications.

The negative consequences of hypertension are mainly manifested in the deteriorating effect that this condition has on coronary heart disease (CHD). Cardiovascular risk factors for CHD are described as two types, unmodifiable and modifiable. Unmodifiable risk factors cannot be changed. This group includes gender, race, advanced age, and a family history of heart disease (hypertensive traits can be inherited). The modifiable risk factors are cigarette smoking (or other forms of tobacco abuse), high blood cholesterol levels, control over diabetes, and perhaps other factors not yet discovered. For example, additional factors are now recognized for their adverse effects on hypertension, including obesity, a lack of physical activity, and psychological factors.

There is no definitive blood pressure level at which a person is no longer at risk for CHD. While any elevation above the normal range places the person at increased risk for CHD, what are considered high normal blood pressures were previously defined as normal. (Looking back at older data, researchers noted that persons able to maintain pressures at or below 139/89 millimeters of mercury had less severe CHD.) The definition of normal blood pressure may change again in the future as new information is discovered. There is a practical limit as to how low pressure can be while maintaining day-to-day function.

In coronary heart disease, the blood supply to the heart is reduced, and the heart cannot function well. The common term for arteriosclerosis, "hardening of the arteries," indicates the symptom of reduced blood flow, which is a major component of CHD. When the heart cannot supply itself with the necessary amount of blood (a condition known as ischemia), a characteristic chest pain called angina may be produced. The hardening aspect of this disease is the result of cholesterol deposits in the vessel, which decrease elasticity and make the vessel wall stiff. This stiffness will force pressures in the vessel to increase if cardiac output rises. As pressures advance, the vessel may develop weak spots. These areas may rupture or lead to the development of small blood clots that may clog the vessel; either problem will disrupt blood flow, making the underlying CHD worse. Eventually, if the blood supply is significantly reduced, a myocardial infarction (heart attack) may occur. Where the blood supply to the heart muscle itself is functionally blocked, that part of the heart will die.

Besides contributing to an increased risk of heart attack and coronary heart disease, hypertension is a major risk for other vascular problems, such as stroke, kidney failure, heart failure, and visual disturbances secondary to the effects on the blood vessels within the eye. Hypertension is a major source of premature death in the United States and by all estimates affects more than sixty million Americans. Forty percent of all African Americans and more than half of those over the age of sixty are affected. Public awareness of hypertension is increasing, yet less than half of all patients diagnosed are treated. More important, only one in five identified hypertensives have the condition under control. This lack of control is particularly

113

important when one considers the organs influenced by hypertension, most notably the brain, eyes, kidneys, and heart.

Although causative factors of hypertension cannot be identified, many physiological factors contribute to hypertension. They include increased sympathetic nervous activity (part of the autonomic nervous system), which promotes arterial contraction; overproduction of an unidentified sodiumretaining hormone or chronic high sodium intake; inadequate dietary intake of potassium or calcium; an increased or inappropriate secretion of renin, a chemical made by the kidney; deficiencies of arterial dilators, such as prostaglandins; congenital abnormalities (birth defects) of resistance vessels; diabetes mellitus or resistance to the effects of insulin; obesity; increased activity of vascular growth factors; and altered cellular ion transport of electrolytes, such as potassium, sodium, chloride, and bicarbonate.

The kidneys are greatly responsible for blood pressure control. They have a key role in maintaining both blood volume and blood pressure. When kidney function declines, secondary to problems such as a decrease in renal blood flow, the kidney will release renin. High renin levels result in activation of the renin-angiotensin-aldosterone system. The resulting chemical cascade produces angiotensin II, a potent arterial constrictor. Another chemical released is aldosterone, an adrenal hormone which causes the kidney to retain water and sodium. These two actions add to blood volume and increase arterial tone, resulting in higher blood pressure. Normally, the renin-angiotensin-aldosterone system protects kidney function by raising blood pressure when it is low. In hypertensives, the controlling forces seem to be out of balance, so that the system does not respond appropriately. The renin-angiotensin-aldosterone system has a negative effect on bradykinin, a chemical that protects renal function by producing vasodilating prostaglandins that help maintain adequate renal blood flow. This protection is especially important in elderly individuals, who may depend on this system to maintain renal function. The system can be inhibited by medications such as aspirin or ibuprofen, resulting in a recurrence of hypertension or less control over the existing disease.

Arteries are largely smooth muscles under the control of the autonomic nervous system, which is responsible for organ function. Yet there is often no conscious control of organs; for example, one can tell the lungs to take a breath, but one cannot tell the heart to beat. The autonomic nervous system has two branches, sympathetic and parasympathetic, that essentially work against each other. The sympathetic system exerts much control over blood pressure. Many chemicals and medicines, such as caffeine, decongestants, and amphetamines, affect blood pressure by mimicking the effects of increased sympathetic stimulation of arteries.

Numerous factors associated with blood pressure elevations will affect one or more of the key determinants of blood pressure; they affect one another as well. An example will show the extent of their relationship. Sodium and water retention will increase blood volume returning to the heart. As this return increases, the heart will increase output (to a point) to prevent heart failure. This higher cardiac output may also raise blood pressure. If arterial vessels are constricted, pressures may be even higher. This elevated pressure (resistance) will force the heart to try to increase output to maintain blood flow to vital organs. Thus, a vicious cycle is started; hypertension can be perceived as a merry-go-round ride with no exit.

Treatment and Therapy
Blood pressure reduction has a protective effect against cardiovascular disease. Generally, as blood pressure decreases, arteries are less contracted and are able to deliver more blood to the tissues, maintaining their function. Furthermore, this decreased blood pressure will help reduce the risk of heart attack in the patient with heart disease. With lower pressures, the heart does not need to work as hard supplying blood to itself or the rest of the body. Therefore, the demand for cardiac output to supply blood flow is less. This reduced workload lowers the incidence of angina.

Treatment of hypertensive patients may involve using one to four different medications to achieve the goal of blood pressure reduction. There are many types of medications from which to choose: diuretics, sympatholytic agents (also known as antiadrenergic drugs), beta-blockers (along with one combined-action alpha-beta blocker), calcium-channel blockers, peripheral vasodilators, angiotensin-converting enzyme inhibitors, and the newest class, angiotension receptor inhibitors. The

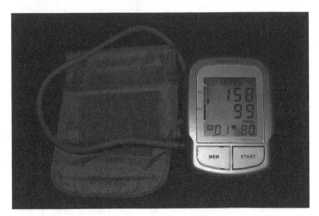

Automated arm blood pressure meter showing arterial hypertension (shown a systolic blood pressure 158 mmHg, diastolic blood pressure 99 mmHg and heart rate of 80 beats per minute). (Steven Fruitsmaak)

list of available drugs is extensive; for example, there are fourteen different thiazide-type diuretics and another six diuretics with different mechanisms of action.

Patients prone to sodium and water retention are treated with diuretics, agents that prevent the kidney from reabsorbing sodium and water from the urine. Diuretics are usually added to other medications to enhance those medications' activity. Research into thiazide-type diuretics has shown that these agents possess mild calcium-channel blocking activity, aiding their ability to reduce hypertension.

Beta-blocking agents are used less often than when they were first developed. They work by decreasing cardiac output through reducing the heart rate. Although they are highly effective, the heart rate reduction tends to produce side effects. Most commonly, patients complain of fatigue, sleepiness, and reduced exercise tolerance (the heart rate cannot increase to adapt to the increasing demand for blood in tissues and the heart itself). These agents are still a good choice for hypertensive patients who have suffered a heart attack. Their benefit is that they reduce the risk of a second heart attack by preventing the heart from overworking.

Calcium-channel blockers were originally intended to treat angina. These agents act primarily by decreasing arterial smooth muscle contraction. Relaxed coronary blood vessels can carry more blood, helping prevent the pain of angina. When calcium ions enter the smooth muscle, a more sustained contraction is produced; therefore, blocking this effect will produce relaxation. Physicians noted

that this relaxation also produced lower blood pressures. The distinct advantage to these agents is that they are well tolerated; however, some patients may require increasing their fiber intake to prevent some constipating effects.

Peripheral vasodilators have been a disappointment. Theoretically, they should be ideal since they work directly to cause arterial dilation. Unfortunately, blood pressure has many determinants, and patients seem to become immune to direct vasodilator effects. Peripheral vasodilators are useful, however, when added to other treatments such as beta-blockers or sympatholytic medications.

The sympatholytic agents are divided into two broad categories. The first group works within the brain to decrease the effects of nerves that would send signals to blood vessels to constrict (so-called constrict messages). They do this by increasing the relax signals coming out of the brain to offset the constrict messages. The net effect is that blood vessels dilate, reducing blood pressure. Many of these agents have fallen into disfavor because of adverse effects similar to those of beta-blockers. The second group of sympatholytics works directly at the nerve-muscle connection. These agents block the constrict messages of the nerve that would increase arterial smooth muscle tone. Overall, these agents are well tolerated. Some patients, especially the elderly, may be very susceptible to their effect and have problems with low blood pressure; this issue usually resolves itself shortly after the first dose.

The renin-angiotensin-aldosterone system is a key determinant of blood pressure. Angiotensin-converting enzyme inhibitors (ACE inhibitors) work by blocking angiotensin II and aldosterone and by preserving bradykinin. They have been found quite effective for reducing blood pressure and are usually well tolerated. Some patients will experience a first-dose effect, while others may develop a dry cough that can be corrected by dose reductions or discontinuation of the medication. The angiotension receptor inhibitors work, instead, by blocking the effects of this substance on the target cells of the arteries themselves. They are proving to be excellent substitutes for people who cannot tolerate the related class of ACE inhibitors.

Unfortunately, and contrary to popular belief, no one can reliably tell when his or her own blood pressure is elevated. Consequently, hypertension is called a "silent killer." It is extremely important to have regular blood pressure evaluations and, if diagnosed with hypertension, to receive treatment.

From 1950 through 1987, as advances in understanding and treating hypertension were made, the United States population enjoyed a 40 percent reduction in coronary heart disease and a more than 65 percent reduction in stroke deaths. (By comparison, noncardiovascular deaths during the same period were reduced little more than 20 percent.)

It is evident that blood pressure can be reduced without medications. Research in the 1980s led to a nonpharmacologic approach in the initial management of hypertension. This strategy includes weight reduction, alcohol restriction, regular exercise, dietary sodium restriction, dietary potassium and calcium supplementation, stopping of tobacco use (in any form), and caffeine restriction. Often, these methods can produce benefits without medication being prescribed. Stress is another common contributor to hypertension; therefore, stress reduction and management is another strategy to reduce blood pressure. This may be achieved through lifestyle changes, meditation, relaxation techniques, and exercise. Using this approach, medication is added to the therapy if blood pressure remains elevated despite good efforts at nonpharmacologic control.

Other aspects of hypertension and hypertensive patients have been identified to help guide the clinician to the proper choice of medication. With this approach, the clinician can focus therapy at the most likely cause of the hypertension: sodium and water retention, high cardiac output, or high vascular resistance. This pathophysiological approach led to the abandonment of the rigid step-care approach described in many texts covering hypertension. The pathophysiological approach to hypertension management is based on a series of steps that are taken if inadequate responses are seen.

The best strategy for controlling hypertension is to be informed. Each person needs to be aware of his or her personal risk for developing hypertension. One should have regular blood pressure evaluations, avoid eating excessive salt and sodium, increase exercise, and reduce fats in the diet. Maintaining ideal body weight may be a key control factor. Studies have shown that patients who have been successful at losing weight will require less

stringent treatment. The benefits could be a need for fewer medications, reduced doses of medications, or both.

—*Charles C. Marsh, Connie Rizzo*

References

Appel, Lawrence J. "Overweight, Obesity, and Weight Reduction in Hypertension." *UpToDate*, 24 Sept. 2018, www.uptodate.com/contents/overweight-obesity-and-weight-reduction-in-hypertension.

Gunta, Sujana S. "Hypertension in Children with Obesity." *World Journal of Hypertension*, vol. 4, no. 2, 2014, p. 15., doi:10.5494/wjh.v4.i2.15.

Hall, John E., et al. "Obesity-Induced Hypertension." *Circulation Research*, vol. 116, no. 6, 13 Mar. 2015, pp. 991–1006., doi:10.1161/circresaha.116.305697.

Jiang, Shu-Zhong, et al. "Obesity and Hypertension." *Experimental and Therapeutic Medicine*, vol. 12, no. 4, 6 Sept. 2016, pp. 2395–2399., doi:10.3892/etm.2016.3667.

Kotsis, Vasilios, et al. "Mechanisms of Obesity-Induced Hypertension." *Hypertension Research*, vol. 33, no. 5, 2010, pp. 386–393., doi:10.1038/hr.2010.9.

■ Hypoglycemia

CATEGORY: Disorder

Causes and Symptoms

The condition known as hypoglycemia exists when the concentration of glucose in the bloodstream is too low to meet bodily needs for fuel, particularly those of the brain. Ordinarily, physiological compensatory mechanisms are called into play when the circulating concentration of glucose falls below about 3.5 millimoles. Activation of the sympathetic nervous system and the secretion of glucagon are especially important in promoting glycogenolysis and gluconeogenesis. Symptoms of sympathetic nervous activation normally become apparent with glucose concentrations that are less than about 3 millimoles. Brain function is usually demonstrably abnormal at glucose concentrations below about 2 millimoles; sustained hypoglycemia in this range can lead to permanent brain damage.

Some of the symptoms of hypoglycemia occur as byproducts of activation of the sympathetic nervous system. These symptoms include trembling, pallor, palpitations and rapid heartbeat, sweating, abdominal discomfort, and feelings of anxiety and/or hunger. These symptoms are not dangerous in themselves; in fact, they may be considered to be beneficial, as they alert the individual of the need to obtain food. Meanwhile, the sympathetic nervous system signals compensatory mechanisms. The manifestations of abnormal brain function during hypoglycemia include blunting of higher cognitive functions, disturbed mentation, confusion, loss of normal control of behavior, headache, lethargy, impaired vision, abnormal speech, paralysis, neurologic deficits, coma, and epileptic seizures. The individual is usually unaware of the appearance of these symptoms, which can present real danger. For example, episodes of hypoglycemia have occurred while individuals were driving motor vehicles, which can lead to serious injury and death. After recovery from hypoglycemia, the patient may have no memory of the episode.

There are two major categories of hypoglycemia: fasting and reactive. The most serious, fasting hypoglycemia, represents impairment of the mechanisms responsible for the production of glucose when food is not available. These mechanisms include the functions of cells in the liver and brain that monitor the availability of circulating glucose. Additionally, there is a coordinated hormonal response involving the secretion of glucagon, growth hormone, and other hormones and the inhibition of the secretion of insulin. The normal consequences of these processes include the addition of glucose to the circulation, primarily from glycogenolysis, as well as a slowing of the rate of utilization of circulating glucose by many tissues of the body, especially the liver, skeletal and cardiac muscle, and fat. Even after days without food, the body normally avoids hypoglycemia through breakdown of stored proteins and activation of gluconeogenesis. There is considerable redundancy in the systems that maintain glucose concentration, so the occurrence of hypoglycemia often reflects the presence of defects in more than one of these mechanisms.

The other category of hypoglycemia, reactive hypoglycemia, includes disorders in which there is disproportionately prolonged and/or great activity of the physiologic systems that normally cause storage of the glucose derived from ingested foods. When a normal person eats a meal, the passage of food through the stomach and intestines elicits a complex and well-orchestrated neural and hormonal response, culminating in the secretion of insulin from the beta cells of the islets of Langerhans in the pancreas. The insulin signals the cells in muscle, adipose tissue, and the liver to stop producing glucose and to derive energy from glucose obtained from the circulation. Glucose in excess of the body's immediate needs for fuel is taken up and stored as glycogen or is utilized for the manufacture of proteins. Normally, the signals for the uptake and storage of glucose reach their peak of activity simultaneously with the entry into the circulation of glucose from the food undergoing digestion. As a result, the concentration of glucose in the circulation fluctuates only slightly. In individuals with reactive hypoglycemia, however, the entry of glucose from the digestive tract and the signals for its uptake and storage are not well synchronized. When signals for the cellular uptake of glucose persist after the intestinally derived glucose has dissipated, hypoglycemia can result. Although the degree of hypoglycemia may be severe and potentially dangerous, recovery can take place without assistance if the individual's general nutritional state is adequate and the systems for activation of glycogenolysis and gluconeogenesis are intact.

Diagnosis and Treatment

The diagnostic evaluation of an individual who is suspected of having hypoglycemia begins with verification of the condition. Evaluation of a patient's symptoms can be confusing. On one hand, the symptoms arising from the sympathetic nervous system and those of neuroglycopenia may occur in a variety of nonhypoglycemic conditions. On the other hand, persons with recurrent hypoglycemia may have few or no obvious symptoms. Therefore, it is most important to document the concentration of glucose in the blood.

To establish the diagnosis of fasting hypoglycemia, the patient is kept without food for periods of time, up to seventy-two hours, with frequent

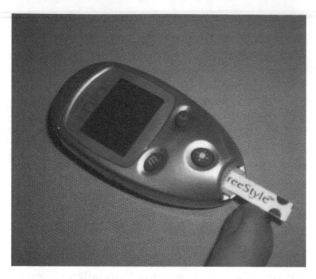

A glucose meter is used to test blood sugar levels. (Erik1980 via Wikimedia Commons)

monitoring of the blood glucose. Should hypoglycemia occur, blood is taken for measurements of the key regulatory neurosecretions and hormones, including insulin, glucagon, growth hormone, cortisol, and epinephrine, as well as general indices of the function of the liver and kidneys. If there is suspicion of an abnormality in an enzyme involved in glucose production, the diagnosis can be confirmed by measurement of the relevant enzymatic activity in circulating blood cells or, if necessary, in a biopsy specimen of the liver.

Fasting hypoglycemia may be caused by any condition that inhibits the production of glucose or that causes an inappropriately great utilization of circulating glucose when food is not available. Insulin produces hypoglycemia through both of these mechanisms. Excessive circulating insulin ranks as one of the most important causes of fasting hypoglycemia, most cases of which result from the treatment of diabetes mellitus with insulin or with an oral drug of the sulfonylurea class. If the patient is known to be taking insulin or a sulfonylurea drug for diabetes, the cause of hypoglycemia is obvious; appropriate modification of the treatment should be made. Hypoglycemia caused by oral sulfonylureas is particularly troublesome because of the prolonged retention of these drugs in the body. The passage of several days may be required for recovery, during which

time the patient needs continuous intravenous infusion of glucose.

Excessive insulin secretion may also result from increased numbers of pancreatic beta cells; the abnormal beta cells may be so numerous that they form benign or malignant tumors, called insulinomas. The preferred treatment of an insulinoma is surgery, if feasible. When the tumor can be removed surgically, the operation is often curative. Unfortunately, insulinomas are sometimes difficult for the surgeon to find. Magnetic resonance imaging (MRI), computed tomography (CT) scanning, ultrasonography, or angiography may help localize the tumor. Some insulinomas are multiple and/or malignant, rendering total removal impossible. In these circumstances, hypoglycemia can be relieved by drugs that inhibit the secretion of insulin.

Malignant tumors arising from various tissues of the body may produce hormones that act like insulin with respect to their effects on glucose metabolism. In some cases, these hormones are members of the family of insulin-like growth factors, which resemble insulin structurally. Malnutrition probably has an important role in predisposing patients with malignancy to hypoglycemia, which tends to occur when the cancer is far advanced.

Fasting hypoglycemia can be caused by disorders affecting various parts of the endocrine system. One such disorder is adrenal insufficiency; continued secretion of cortisol by the adrenal cortex is required for maintenance of normal glycogen stores and of the enzymes of glycogenolysis and gluconeogenesis. Severe hypothyroidism also may lead to hypoglycemia. Impairment in the function of the anterior pituitary gland predisposes a patient to hypoglycemia through several mechanisms, including reduced function of the thyroid gland and adrenal cortices (which depend on pituitary secretions for normal activity) and reduced secretion of growth hormone. Growth hormone plays an important physiologic role in the prevention of fasting hypoglycemia by signaling metabolic changes that allow heart and skeletal muscles to derive energy from stored fats, thereby sparing glucose for the brain. Specific replacement therapies are available for deficiencies of thyroxine, cortisol, and growth hormone.

Hypoglycemia has occasionally been reported as a side effect of treatment with medications other than those intended for treatment of diabetes. Drugs that have been implicated include sulfonamides, used for treatment of bacterial infections; quinine, used for treatment of falciparum malaria; pentamidine isethionate, given by injection for treatment of pneumocystosis; ritodrine, used for inhibition of premature labor; and propranolol or disopyramide, both of which are used for treatment of cardiac arrhythmias. Malnourished patients seem to be especially susceptible to the hypoglycemic effects of these medications, and management should consist of nutritional repletion in addition to discontinuation of the drug responsible. In children, aspirin or other medicines containing salicylates may produce hypoglycemia.

Alcohol hypoglycemia occurs in persons with low bodily stores of glycogen when there is no food in the intestine. In this circumstance, the only potential source of glucose for the brain is gluconeogenesis. When such an individual drinks alcohol, its metabolism within the liver prevents the precursors of glucose from entering the pathways of gluconeogenesis. This variety of fasting hypoglycemia can occur in persons who are not chronic alcoholics: It requires the ingestion of only a moderate amount of alcohol, on the order of three mixed drinks. Treatment involves the nutritional repletion of glycogen stores and the limitation of alcohol intake.

Severe infections, including overwhelming bacterial infection and malaria, can produce hypoglycemia by mechanisms that are not well understood. Patients with very severe liver damage can develop fasting hypoglycemia, because the pathways of glycogenolysis and gluconeogenesis in the liver are by far the major sources of circulating glucose in the fasted state. In such cases, the occurrence of hypoglycemia usually marks a near-terminal stage of liver disease. Uremia, the syndrome produced by kidney failure, can also lead to fasting hypoglycemia.

Some types of fasting hypoglycemia occur predominantly in infants and children. Babies in the first year of life may have an inappropriately high secretion of insulin. This problem occurs especially in newborn infants whose mothers had increased circulating glucose during pregnancy.

Children from two to ten years of age may develop ketotic hypoglycemia, which is probably related to insufficient gluconeogenesis. These disorders tend to improve with time. Fasting hypoglycemia is also an important manifestation of a variety of inherited disorders of metabolism characterized by the abnormality or absence of one of the necessary enzymes or cofactors of glycogenolysis and gluconeogenesis or of fat metabolism (which supplies the energy for gluconeogenesis). Most of these disorders become evident in infancy or childhood. If there is a hereditary or acquired deficiency of an enzyme of glucose production, the problem can be circumvented by provision of a continuous supply of glucose to the affected individual.

There are several other rare causes of fasting hypoglycemia. A few individuals have had circulating antibodies that caused hypoglycemia by interacting with the patient's own insulin or with receptors for insulin on the patient's cells. Although the autonomic (involuntary) nervous system has an important role in signaling recovery from hypoglycemia, diseases affecting this branch of the nervous system do not usually produce hypoglycemia; presumably, hormonal mechanisms can substitute for the missing neural signals.

Reactive hypoglycemia can occur with an unusually rapid passage of foodstuffs through the upper intestinal tract, such as may occur after partial or total removal of the stomach. Persons predisposed to maturity-onset diabetes may also have reactive hypoglycemia, probably because of the delay in the secretion of insulin in response to a meal. Finally, reactive hypoglycemia need not indicate the presence of any identifiable disease and may occur in otherwise normal individuals.

Diagnosis of reactive hypoglycemia is made difficult by the variability of symptoms and of glucose concentrations from day to day. Adding to the diagnostic uncertainty, circulating glucose normally rises and falls after meals, especially those rich in carbohydrates. Consequently, entirely normal and asymptomatic individuals may sometimes have glucose concentrations at or below the levels found in persons with reactive hypoglycemia. Therefore, the glucose tolerance test, in which blood samples are taken at intervals for several hours after the patient drinks a solution containing 50 to 100 grams of glucose, is quite unreliable and should not be employed for the diagnosis of reactive hypoglycemia. Proper diagnosis of reactive hypoglycemia depends on careful correlation of the patient's symptoms with the circulating glucose level, preferably measured on several occasions after ingestion of ordinary meals. Some persons develop symptoms such as weakness, nausea, sweating, and tremulousness after meals, but without a significant reduction of circulating glucose. This symptom complex should not be confused with hypoglycemia.

When rapid passage of food through the stomach and upper intestine causes reactive hypoglycemia, the administration of drugs that slow intestinal transit may be helpful. When reactive hypoglycemia has no evident pathological cause, the patient is usually advised to take multiple small meals throughout the day instead of the usual three meals and to avoid concentrated sweets. These dietary modifications can help avoid hypoglycemia by reducing the stimulus to secrete insulin.

Two rare inherited disorders of metabolism can produce reactive hypoglycemia after the ingestion of certain foods. In hereditary fructose intolerance, the offending nutrient is fructose, a sugar found in fruits as well as ordinary table sugar. In galactosemia, the sugar responsible for hypoglycemia is galactose, a major component of milk products. Management of these conditions, which usually become apparent in infancy or childhood, consists of avoidance of the foods responsible.

Perspective and Prospects

Fasting hypoglycemia is uncommon, except in the context of treatment of diabetes mellitus. The most serious public health problem associated with hypoglycemia is that it limits the therapeutic effectiveness of insulin and sulfonylurea drugs. Evidence suggests that elevation of the circulating glucose concentration (hyperglycemia) is responsible for much of the disability and premature death among patients with diabetes. In many of these patients, therapeutic regimens consisting of multiple daily injections of insulin

or continuous infusion of insulin through a small needle placed under the skin can reduce the average circulating glucose to normal. Frequent serious hypoglycemia is the most important adverse consequence of such regimens. Persons with diabetes seem to be at especially high risk for dangerous hypoglycemia for two reasons. First, there is often a failure of the warning systems that ordinarily cause uncomfortable symptoms when the circulating glucose concentration declines, a situation termed *hypoglycemic unawareness*. As a consequence, when a patient with diabetes attempts to control his or her blood sugar with more frequent injections of insulin, there may occur unheralded episodes of hypoglycemia that can lead to serious alterations in mental activity or even loss of consciousness. Many patients with diabetes also have hypoglycemic unresponsiveness, an impaired ability to recover from episodes of hypoglycemia. Also, diabetes can interfere with the normal physiologic responses that cause the secretion of glucagon in response to a reduction of circulating glucose, thus eliminating one of the most important defenses against hypoglycemia. If both hypoglycemic unawareness and hypoglycemic unresponsiveness could be reversed, intensive treatment of diabetes would become safer and more widely applicable.

Reactive hypoglycemia, although seldom a clue to serious disease, has attracted public attention because of its peculiarly annoying symptoms. These symptoms, which reflect activation of the sympathetic nervous system, resemble those of fear and anxiety. The symptoms are not specific, and many patients with these complaints do not have hypoglycemia.

In summary, hypoglycemia indicates defective regulation of the supply of energy to the body. When severe or persistent, hypoglycemia can lead to serious behavioral disorder, obtunded consciousness, and even brain damage. Fasting hypoglycemia may be a clue to significant endocrine disease. Reactive hypoglycemia, while annoying, usually responds to simple dietary measures. The study of hypoglycemia has led to many important insights into the regulation of energy metabolism.

—*Victor R. Lavis*

References

Cai, Xiaoling, et al. "Baseline Body Mass Index and the Efficacy of Hypoglycemic Treatment in Type 2 Diabetes: A Meta-Analysis." *Plos One*, vol. 11, no. 12, 9 Dec. 2016, doi:10.1371/journal.pone.0166625.

Carreau, Anne-Marie, et al. "Late Reactive Hypoglycemia (RHG) as a Common Early Sign of Glycemic Dysfunction in Obese Adolescent Girls." *Diabetes*, vol. 67, no. Supplement 1, 2018, doi:10.2337/db18-1361-p.

Thompson, Amy E. "Hypoglycemia." *Jama*, vol. 313, no. 12, 24 Mar. 2015, p. 1284., doi:10.1001/jama.2015.0876.

Tsai, Tsung-Cheng, et al. "Body Mass Index–Mortality Relationship in Severe Hypoglycemic Patients With Type 2 Diabetes." *The American Journal of the Medical Sciences*, vol. 349, no. 3, 2015, pp. 192–198., doi:10.1097/maj.0000000000000382.

■ Liver cancer

CATEGORY: Disorder

In the United States and other developed countries, cancer is second only to heart disease as a cause of mortality, and liver cancer is the most common cause of cancer-related death worldwide. Liver cancer is classified as primary or secondary (i.e., cancer that spreads to the liver from another site). Primary liver cancer is called hepatocellular carcinoma (HCC), which is a neoplasm that originates in the hepatocytes (i.e., cells in the liver). The liver is the largest organ in the abdominal cavity and performs many vital functions for processing and filtering blood. About 80% of HCC cases are associated with existing liver disease, most frequently cirrhosis. Cirrhosis refers to the scarring and resulting malfunction of the liver that is usually caused by hepatitis C, alcoholism, or nonalcoholic fatty liver disease (NAFLD). Treatment depends on the stage of the cancer as well as the age and health status of the patient. Surgical resection and liver transplantation are the most successful forms of treatment for HCC. Other treatment options include chemotherapy and radiation therapy. The information that follows focuses on HCC.

Diet-Related Risk Factors for HC

Cirrhosis secondary to alcoholism frequently precedes HCC. Alcohol is absorbed quickly and metabolized by the liver at a rate of one-half ounce of alcohol per hour. Alcohol is toxic to all human cells. If excessive amounts of alcohol are consumed, the hepatocytes are damaged and replaced by scar tissue

Persons with NAFLD are at greater risk of developing HCC. Risk factors associated with NAFLD include obesity, insulin resistance and related conditions, including DM2, metabolic syndrome, and polycystic ovarian syndrome (PCOS), and disorders of lipid metabolism (e.g., abetalipoproteinemia, hypobetalipoproteinemia, or Andersen disease).

SIGNS AND SYMPTOMS
Unintentional weight loss
Poor appetite
Discomfort in the upper right quadrant of the abdomen
Nausea and vomiting
Fatigue and generalized weakness
Hepatomegaly (i.e., enlarged liver)
Abdominal swelling
Jaundice (i.e., yellowing of the skin and eyes)
White, chalky stools

Research Findings

High intake of saturated fat and animal fat has been linked to increased risk for hepatocellular carcinoma (HCC), pancreatic cancer, prostate cancer, and colorectal cancer; investigators of these studies emphasize the need for further research to substantiate their findings.

Investigators of a large prospective cohort study published in 2010 found that high intake of saturated fat in red meat and other sources was associated with higher HCC risk. One possible reason for increased HCC risk is that fatty acid deposits in the liver can lead to nonalcoholic fatty liver disease, which increases risk for HCC. An explanation for the role of red meat consumption in HCC risk is that red meat contains large amounts of bioavailable heme iron; iron overload increases HCC risk. Nitrates formed during high-temperature cooking of meat increase risk for liver tumors.

Summary

Individuals at risk or diagnosed with HCC (and their family members/caregivers) should learn about dietary recommendations based on personal characteristics and health needs. Lifestyle behaviors such as achieving and maintaining a healthy weight, performing regular physical activity, consuming a diet that is rich in a variety of fruits and vegetables and low in saturated fat, limiting alcohol intake, and avoiding chewing or smoking tobacco can significantly reduce risk for developing liver cancer. Patients undergoing treatment for liver cancer need to be monitored for weight loss, signs of malnutrition, vitamin/mineral deficiencies and electrolyte imbalances. It is important to report any health-related changes to the treating clinician as soon as possible to prevent worsening health status. A registered dietitian may provide appropriate nutrition support and counsel patients on appropriate foods or supplements to prevent weight loss or nutrient deficiencies. Patients and their family members should understand and adhere to the prescribed treatment regimen, while continuing medical surveillance to monitor health status. Research suggests that foods rich in monounsaturated fats may help reduce risk of HCC.

—*Cherie Marcel*

References

Henry, Zachary H., and Stephen H. Caldwell. "Obesity and Hepatocellular Carcinoma: A Complex Relationship." *Gastroenterology*, vol. 149, no. 1, 2015, pp. 18–20., doi:10.1053/j.gastro.2015.05.024.

"Obesity Independently Drives NASH and Hepatocellular Carcinoma." *Cancer Discovery*, vol. 8, no. 12, 2018, doi:10.1158/2159-8290.cd-rw2018-190.

Ratziu, Vlad, and Giulio Marchesini. "When the Journey from Obesity to Cirrhosis Takes an Early Start." *Journal of Hepatology*, vol. 65, no. 2, 2016, pp. 249–251.

Saitta, Carlo, et al. "Obesity and Liver Cancer." *Annals of Hepatology*, vol. 18, no. 6, 2019, pp. 810–815.

Sun, Beicheng, and Michael Karin. "Obesity, Inflammation, and Liver Cancer." *Journal of Hepatology*, vol. 56, no. 3, 2012, pp. 704–713., doi:10.1016/j.jhep.2011.09.020.

■ Metabolic syndrome

CATEGORY: Disorder

ALSO KNOWN AS: Insulin resistance syndrome, Syndrome X, Deadly Quartet

Causes and Symptoms

Metabolic syndrome is a complex medical disorder. According to guidelines issued by the National Cholesterol Education Program/Adult Treatment Panel III (NCEP/ATP III), diagnosis of metabolic syndrome is made when an individual displays at least three of the following risk factors: abdominal obesity, elevated triglycerides, low levels of the high-density lipoprotein (HDL) type of cholesterol, high blood pressure, and the presence of more than 100 milligrams per deciliter (mg/dL) of glucose in the blood after fasting.

The National Heart, Lung, and Blood Institute (NHLBI) estimates that as many as forty-seven million adults in the United States suffer from metabolic syndrome, which is around 25 percent of the total adult population. A study published in *National Health Statistics Reports* in May 2009 reported that 34 percent of the study's 3,423 adults aged twenty and older met the criteria for metabolic syndrome. Age plays a large role in metabolic syndrome, with the likelihood of being diagnosed increasing as an individual gets older. Total body weight is also an indicator of the likelihood of the metabolic syndrome criteria being met. Males who are overweight are six times as likely as normal-weight males to be diagnosed with metabolic syndrome, and those who are obese are thirty-two times as likely.

In females, being overweight leads to a fivefold increase in the chances of being diagnosed with metabolic syndrome and obesity a seventeen-fold increase, compared to women of normal weight. Disturbingly, metabolic syndrome is now being recognized in children and adolescents; this is probably related to the increase in obesity and type 2 diabetes mellitus seen in this age group over recent years. There is also evidence to demonstrate a genetic component to metabolic syndrome; further research will clarify this.

Key aspects of the metabolic syndrome are an energy imbalance and resultant altered metabolic pathways. The abnormal metabolic reactions seen in metabolic syndrome confer an increased risk for type 2 diabetes mellitus and cardiovascular disease

(CVD). Several other diseases-colon cancer, nonalcoholic steatohepatitis (NASH), polycystic ovary disease, and chronic renal failure-can also be a consequence of this syndrome.

The National Health and Nutrition Examination Survey determined that the most prevalent risk factor displayed by individuals with metabolic syndrome is abdominal obesity. This is when fat is stored in the abdominal region of the body as opposed to in the buttocks and thighs. People with abdominally stored fat are often said to have "apple" type bodies; those with fat stored lower, in the buttocks and thighs, are said to be "pear" shaped. Men are typically apples and women are pears. Cortisol is a stress response hormone that promotes fat deposition in the abdominal area in individuals with chronic stress. Nearly all cases of overweight and obesity, including abdominal obesity, are due to excess calorific intake (overeating) combined with a sedentary lifestyle. In the United States, around one-third of the adult population is obese. Obesity greatly increases the risk for type 2 diabetes and cardiovascular disease.

Abnormal levels of fats in the blood is called dyslipidemia. In people who are overweight or obese, the levels of lipids in the body are so high that the pathways involved in fat synthesis and breakdown cannot keep up, and chronically high blood lipids are seen.

In addition, due to impaired insulin action and incorrect handling of glucose by their cells, individuals with type 2 diabetes tend to have high levels of blood triglyceride and low HDL cholesterol levels. This puts type 2 diabetics and obese individuals at high risk for CVD.

The second most prevalent factor seen in patients diagnosed with metabolic syndrome is hypertension, or high blood pressure. One in four Americans suffers from hypertension. If untreated, it can lead to CVD and kidney failure. The atherosclerotic process is accelerated in the metabolic syndrome and in type 2 diabetes because of the presence of multiple metabolic abnormalities. In insulin resistance, plaque formation may be enhanced because of the increased expression of adhesion molecules on endothelial cells and an increased rate of monocyte adhesion to endothelial cells. Circulating plasminogen is also more likely activated, which typically leads to increased clotting. In addition, hypertension may contribute to an increased risk of stroke in those with the metabolic syndrome.

The third most prevalent factor is hyperglycemia, or impaired fasting glucose. To satisfy the criterion for metabolic syndrome the glucose level in the blood after fasting must be over 100 mg/dl. A person with 100 to 125 mg/dl would be considered prediabetic, and diabetes is diagnosed when the fasting level of glucose is 126 mg/dl or above. Increases in blood glucose are indicative of a phenomenon called insulin resistance. Here, the cells of the body do not respond properly to insulin, and as a result glucose cannot enter the cells for use or storage so it remains in the circulating blood. Chronically elevated blood glucose concentration permits glucose molecules to combine with diverse proteins in the body, including hemoglobin within red blood cells, by a process known as glycation or glycosylation. Glycation also leads to blood vessels becoming rigid, a factor that contributes to CVD.

Treatment and Therapy

Treatment strategies for the metabolic syndrome focus on weight loss through a comprehensive program utilizing behavioral changes, including improved nutrition and an increase in physical activities. The long-term goal of therapy is a better balance between the intake of food energy sources and energy expenditure, so that a healthier body weight can be achieved. Dietary treatment typically requires the involvement of nutritionists and registered dieticians to provide educational information and institute changes in food selection.

Physicians provide overall care, and concomitant with lifestyle changes use the prescription of medications for one or more of the components of metabolic syndrome. Metformin is a drug used to treat type 2 diabetes mellitus; it works by improving insulin action, and has also been shown to stop the development of impaired fasting glucose to type 2 diabetes in patients with metabolic syndrome. Angiotensin-converting enzyme (ACE) inhibitors are used in the treatment of hypertension. They are successful in treating hypertension and, in addition, have a beneficial effect on insulin resistance in metabolic syndrome. Another class of drugs is the statins, which are used to improve cholesterol levels in people with metabolic syndrome. Statins also appear to cause a reduction in inflammation seen in metabolic syndrome, leading to a reduction in CVD.

Since the emerging epidemic of the metabolic syndrome is expected to continue, both preventive and treatment strategies are needed. Prevention aimed toward reducing the development of this syndrome in children and adolescents should involve schools and community agencies.

Perspective and Prospects
Recognition of the metabolic syndrome essentially paralleled the increases in overweight and obesity in the United States in the early 1990s. Physicians were diagnosing many overweight and obese patients with the major components of the metabolic syndrome without linking them to a major health trend. Other countries of affluence were also reporting cases.

The metabolic syndrome was first defined in 1998 by the World Health Organization (WHO). The WHO criteria included a BMI of more than thirty; a blood triglyceride level greater than or equal to 150 mg/dl; HDL cholesterol level under 35 mg/dl in men and 39 mg/dl in women; blood pressure over 140/90 mm Hg; impaired glucose tolerance, insulin tolerance or type 2 diabetes; insulin resistance; and microalbuminuria (protein in the urine). In 2001 the NCEP/ATP III released their guidelines for the diagnosis of metabolic syndrome, which quickly became the most widely accepted. These differed from the WHO guidelines in several ways. Firstly, BMI measurement was replaced with waist circumference measurement when it became clear that it was not necessarily the total body fat content, but the way in which it is deposited in the body that is important to pathogenesis. A waist circumference of over forty inches for men and over thirty-five inches for women is considered a risk factor for metabolic syndrome. Secondly, the HDL values were changed to less than 40 mg/dl for men and 50 mg/dl for women, and blood pressure limit was lowered to 130/85 mm Hg. A fasting glucose level of over 110 mg/dl was defined as a risk for metabolic syndrome. Finally, insulin resistance and microalbumiuria were removed from the criteria. In 2005 the guidelines were updated by American Heart Association (AHA) and NHLBI; the fasting blood glucose level was lowered to 100 mg/dl. These are the currently used criteria for the diagnosis of metabolic syndrome.

The metabolic syndrome has deadly consequences because of the nature of the chronic diseases that it spawns. This problem will worsen in the future in the United States because excessive calorific intake, eating the wrong kinds of food (for example highly processed food containing high

fructose corn syrup, trans fats, or too much salt), and too little physical activity continue to dominate society. The epidemic nature of this syndrome requires that new public health measures be initiated and implemented as soon as possible. Preventive strategies need to be instituted to reduce the enormous impact of this syndrome anticipated in the United States in the coming decades. The overall cost of treatment will be enormous.
—*Claire L. Standen, John J. B. Anderson*

References
Canale, Maria Paola, et al. "Obesity-Related Metabolic Syndrome: Mechanisms of Sympathetic Overactivity." *International Journal of Endocrinology*, vol. 2013, 2013, pp. 1–12., doi:10.1155/2013/865965.

Engin, Atilla. "The Definition and Prevalence of Obesity and Metabolic Syndrome." *Obesity and Lipotoxicity Advances in Experimental Medicine and Biology*, 2017, pp. 1–17., doi:10.1007/978-3-319-48382-5_1.

Gregory, John W. "Prevention of Obesity and Metabolic Syndrome in Children." *Frontiers in Endocrinology*, vol. 10, 1 Oct. 2019, doi:10.3389/fendo.2019.00669.

Mayo Clinic Staff. "Metabolic Syndrome." *Mayo Clinic*, Mayo Foundation for Medical Education and Research, 14 Mar. 2019, www.mayoclinic.org/diseases-conditions/metabolic-syndrome/symptoms-causes/syc-20351916?page=0&citems=10.

■ Osteoarthritis

CATEGORY: Disorder

Causes and Symptoms
There are several causes of osteoarthritis (OA), including traumatic injuries, joint overuse or repetitive movement of a joint, obesity, and genetic or metabolic diseases. The most commonly affected joints are in the hands, hips, knees, and spine. An inherited genetic defect in the production of collagen leads to defective cartilage and to more rapid joint deterioration. OA in the hands or hips may be hereditary. OA in the knees is linked to excess weight. X rays of more than half the population over sixty-five would show evidence of osteoarthritis in at least one joint.

Cartilage containing synovial fluid and elastic tissue reduces friction as joints move. Osteoarthritis

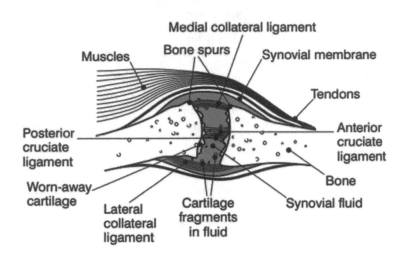

Muscles
Medial collateral ligament
Bone spurs
Synovial membrane
Tendons
Anterior cruciate ligament
Bone
Synovial fluid
Posterior cruciate ligament
Worn-away cartilage
Lateral collateral ligament
Cartilage fragments in fluid

With osteoarthritis, the cartilage becomes worn away. Spurs grow out from the edge of the bone, and synovial fluid increases. Altogether, the joint feels stiff and sore. (National Institute of Arthritis and Musculoskeletal and Skin Diseases)

develops when the cartilage wears away and bone rubs against bone. The most prominent symptom of osteoarthritis is joint pain. Other symptoms include morning stiffness or stiffness after long periods of immobility. Early in the disease, individuals may experience joint pain after strenuous exercise. As the disease progresses, joints stiffen and diminished joint mobility is experienced even with slight activity. As joint mobility decreases, the muscles surrounding the joint weaken, thereby increasing the likelihood of further injury to the joint. As the cartilage wears away, crepitus can often be heard as bone moves against bone. The development of Herberden's nodes on the distal interphalangeal joints and Bouchard's nodes on the proximal interphalangeal joints of the hands is not uncommon.

Confirmation of osteoarthritis is based on a history of joint pain and physical findings that indicate arthritic changes in the joints. An x-ray shows a loss of joint space, osteophytes, bone cysts, and sclerosis of subchondrial bone. Sometimes, a computed tomography (CT) scan or magnetic resonance imaging (MRI) may be helpful in confirming the presence of osteoarthritis.

Treatment and Therapy
The goal of treatment for OA is to preserve physical function and reduce pain. Education, physical therapy, and occupational therapy are instrumental in maintaining independence and improving

muscle strength around affected joints. Pacing activities to avoid over-exertion of the affected joints is an effective means to prevent further pain and injury. Heat therapies such as warm soaks, paraffin, and mud treatments may help to lessen the discomfort in tender joints. Moderate exercise such as walking, swimming, strength training, and stretching all may help to maintain mobility in arthritic joints and to improve posture and balance. Relaxation techniques, stress reduction activities, and biofeedback may also be helpful.

Topical analgesic ointments may help to reduce joint swelling and pain. Acetaminophen is very effective for controlling OA pain. However, persons who take blood-thinning medicines, have liver disease, or consume large amounts of alcohol should use acetaminophen with caution. Nonsteroidal anti-inflammatory drugs (NSAIDs) such as ibuprofen and naproxen are also effective for pain relief, but they may cause gastrointestinal bleeding. COX-2 selective inhibitors are the most recently introduced NSAIDs. This class of drugs selectively blocks the enzyme COX-2, thus controlling the production of prostaglandins, natural chemicals that contribute to body inflammation and cause the pain and swelling of arthritis. Since they do not block the COX-1 enzyme cyclooxygenase-1, which is present in the stomach and inflammation sites, the natural mucous linings of the stomach and intestine are protected, thereby reducing the incidence of upset, ulceration, or bleeding. This feature of blocking COX-2 but not COX-1 makes these drugs unique among traditional NSAIDs. COX-2 selective inhibitors include Celebrex (celecoxib), Vioxx (rofecoxib), and Bextra (valdecoxib); the latter two are no longer on the market, however. Other COX-2 inhibitors sold outside the United States include Prexige (lumiracoxib) and Arcoxia (etoricoxib). Any medication used to treat OA should be taken under the direction of a health care provider.

Glucosamine and chondroitin naturally occur in the body. Both have been promoted for the treatment of OA. Glucosamine may promote the formation and repair of cartilage, while chondroitin may promote water retention and elasticity in cartilage and prevent cartilage breakdown. However, recent studies indicate that taking glucosamine for arthritis may increase a patient's risk of developing glaucoma.

When interventions to relieve symptoms of OA no longer work, an orthopedic surgeon may inject cortisone or hyaluronic acid into joint spaces such as the knee. Hyaluronic acid is used to replace the synovial fluid that a joint has lost in order to maintain knee movement without pain. Cortisone may be injected into affected joint spaces to provide temporary relief of joint pain. Surgical intervention to trim torn and damaged cartilage from joint spaces, to partially or totally replace severely damaged joints in the knees and hips, or to fuse bones together are effective treatments in the most severe, debilitating stages of OA. Realignment of a joint (osteotomy) is another possible procedure.

Perspective and Prospects

Arthritis comprises more than one hundred diseases and conditions and is the major cause of disability in the United States. The incidence of OA increases with age, but it can affect individuals as young as eighteen. Almost 27 million people in the United States have OA, and it is the most common form of arthritis. OA is three times more common among women, although before forty-five years of age, it is more common in men. Costs for treatment of arthritis in the United States exceed $128 billion annually. There is no cure for OA, but a healthy diet, regular exercise, and weight control are measures that can slow its progress.

—*Sharon W. Stark, Victoria Price*

References

Doheny, Kathleen. "Osteoarthritis and Obesity: Anticipated Comorbidities with New Clues to Care." *EndocrineWeb*, 5 Feb. 2019, www.endocrineweb.com/professional/obesity/new-clues-obesity-osteoarthritis.

Kulkarni, Kunal, et al. "Obesity and Osteoarthritis." *Maturitas*, vol. 89, 2016, pp. 22–28., doi:10.1016/j.maturitas.2016.04.006.

Thijssen, E., et al. "Obesity and Osteoarthritis, More than Just Wear and Tear: Pivotal Roles for Inflamed Adipose Tissue and Dyslipidaemia in Obesity-Induced Osteoarthritis." *Rheumatology*, vol. 54, no. 4, 11 Dec. 2014, pp. 588–600., doi:10.1093/rheumatology/keu464.

■ Ovarian cancer

CATEGORY: Disorder

Ovarian cancer (OC) refers to several types of malignant neoplasms that originate in the cells of the ovary. Epithelial OC, found in the cells lining the surface of the ovary, is the most commonly diagnosed OC. The other types of OC are classified based on the type of cell in which they originate and include germ cell OC, which arises from the reproductive cells that produce eggs, and stromal OC, which originates in the cells of connective tissue that produce hormones and connective tissue cells that support ovarian structure. Because OC is usually asymptomatic in the early stages and there are no reliable screening tests for OC, it is frequently diagnosed late in the disease process, making it a particularly deadly cancer. Currently, OC is the fifth most common cause of cancer-related death among women.

Research Findings

Studies analyzing the relationship between diet and the risk or prognosis of OC have had mixed results. Some researchers have reported that high vegetable intake is inversely associated with OC risk, and others have reported that no relationship exists. Evidence that consuming a high-fat diet increases the risk for developing OC is conflictive. Researchers have reported an increased risk for OC in premenopausal women with obesity, and believe that risk could be related to increased estrogen levels.

Researchers have reported that higher intakes of cruciferous vegetables and black tea have been associated with reduced risk of OC. The relationship observed seems to be related to the phytonutrient content, with a specific OC preventive action noted with flavonoid intake.

High fat intake is a risk factor for becoming overweight or obese, which is a risk factor for OC. There are many variables associated with the contribution of fat intake to cancer risk, including the type of fat (e.g., saturated, unsaturated), preparation of fat (e.g., heating, hydrogenating), and source of fat (e.g., animal or plant). Although results of studies have repeatedly shown a correlation between animal fat intake and increased cancer risk, fat from plant sources has not proven to be a significant risk.

RISK FACTORS	SIGNS AND SYMPTOMS
Age: Women over the age of 60 are at greater risk for developing OC than younger women	Fatigue Sensation of fullness after eating a small amount of food
Obesity	Abdominal bloating or swelling
Early or later than average menopause	Abdominal pain
Use of estrogen replacement therapy after menopause	Back pain Swelling in the legs
Family history of OC or breast, endometrial, or colorectal cancer	Changes in bowel or bladder habits Shortness of breath
Personal history of breast or endometrial cancer	
Personal history of endometriosis	

Researchers report that omega-3 fatty acid consumption is inversely associated with the risk of epithelial OC, particularly endometrioid tumors. In contrast, the consumption of trans fat was observed to be positively associated with epithelial OC risk.

A study of obese and normal weight mice and the pathogenesis of OC revealed that biologically distinct cancers developed in the obese versus the nonobese mice. Researchers suggest that OC that arises in obese patients could require different treatment strategies than OC in normal weight patients.

Summary

Individuals at risk or diagnosed with OC (and their family members/caregivers) should learn about dietary recommendations based on personal characteristics and health needs. Patients should eat a high-fiber diet that includes a wide variety of fruits, vegetables, lean proteins, and unsaturated fats. Patients undergoing treatment for OC need to be monitored for weight loss, signs of malnutrition, vitamin/mineral deficiencies and electrolyte imbalances. It is important to report any health-related changes to the treating clinician as soon as possible to prevent worsening health status. A registered dietitian may provide appropriate nutrition support and counsel patients on appropriate foods or supplements to prevent weight loss or nutrient deficiencies. Patients and their family members should understand and adhere to the prescribed treatment regimen, while continuing medical surveillance to monitor health status. Research suggests consumption of cruciferous vegetables, black tea and omega-3 fatty acids may reduce risk of OC.

—*Cherie Marcel*

References

Aarestrup, Julie, et al. "Childhood Overweight, Tallness, and Growth Increase Risks of Ovarian Cancer." *Cancer Epidemiology Biomarkers & Prevention*, vol. 28, no. 1, Jan. 2019, pp. 183–188., doi:10.1158/1055-9965.epi-18-0024.

Bandera, Elisa V, et al. "Impact of Body Mass Index on Ovarian Cancer Survival Varies by Stage." *British Journal of Cancer*, vol. 117, no. 2, 6 June 2017, pp. 282–289., doi:10.1038/bjc.2017.162.

Foong, Ke Wei, and Helen Bolton. "Obesity and Ovarian Cancer Risk: A Systematic Review." *Post Reproductive Health*, vol. 23, no. 4, 18 July 2017, pp. 183–198., doi:10.1177/2053369117709225.

Leitzmann, Michael F., et al. "Body Mass Index and Risk of Ovarian Cancer." *Cancer*, vol. 115, no. 4, 2009, pp. 812–822., doi:10.1002/cncr.24086.

Liu, Zhen, et al. "The Association between Overweight, Obesity and Ovarian Cancer: a Meta-Analysis." *Japanese Journal of Clinical Oncology*, 21 Oct. 2015, doi:10.1093/jjco/hyv150.

Nagle, C M, et al. "Obesity and Survival among Women with Ovarian Cancer: Results from the Ovarian Cancer Association Consortium." *British Journal of Cancer*, vol. 113, no. 5, 7 July 2015, pp. 817–826., doi:10.1038/bjc.2015.245.

■ Pancreatic cancer

CATEGORY: Disorder

Pancreatic cancer is a malignant neoplasm that originates in the pancreas, a gland located between the stomach and the spine. The pancreas produces the enzymes and hormones necessary for food metabolism and control of blood glucose levels. Because of the relatively hidden location of the pancreas and the vagueness of signs and symptoms, pancreatic cancer is frequently identified at an advanced stage, and more than 95% of patients with pancreatic cancer die from it within 5 years. Treatment depends on the stage and type (i.e., exocrine or endocrine tumors) of the cancer as well as the age and health status of the patient, and can require the use of surgery, chemotherapy, radiation therapy, or nonchemotherapeutic, targeted therapies such as sunitinib malate or erlotinib hydrochloride.

Dietary and Lifestyle Recommendations for the Prevention of Pancreatic Cancer

According to researchers, obesity is directly responsible for up to 20% of all cancers. Overweight and obese individuals, particularly those with increased abdominal fat, are at significantly higher risk for developing pancreatic cancer and other gastrointestinal (GI) cancers (e.g., colon, gastric, esophageal) than healthy-weight persons.

The mechanisms of obesity complications that lead to carcinogenesis are varied in function and affect different tissues. Some of the obesity-related contributors that are implicated in cancer development include insulin and insulin-like growth factor (IGF) signaling pathways, adipokines, inflammation and immune responses, and microbiota of the GI tract.

Regular intake of fruits (especially citrus) and vegetables has shown potential to protect against pancreatic cancer in some but not all studies. The exact mechanism of the protective effect is not fully understood. The antioxidant vitamins A, C, and E; vitamin D; folate; magnesium; and calcium have demonstrated anticancer activity but are still being investigated. Regardless of whether a direct preventive relationship exists, higher fruit and vegetable consumption is associated with lifestyle habits such as higher fiber and lower fat intake, lower body weight, and increased physical activity, all of which are associated with cancer prevention.

Regular intake of whole grains has been demonstrated to reduce the risk of pancreatic cancer. There is some evidence that fortification of whole grain foods with folate can provide further protection against pancreatic cancer.

Research Findings

Evidence suggests that lifestyle behaviors such as achieving and maintaining a healthy weight, physical activity, consuming a diet rich in fruits and vegetables and low in saturated fat, limiting alcohol intake, and not smoking can reduce the risk of developing pancreatic cancer.

In a large prospective cohort study of over 500,000 adults, higher intakes of total, saturated, and monounsaturated (but not polyunsaturated)

RISK FACTORS	SIGNS AND SYMPTOMS
Age over 45 years with over 65% diagnosed over 65 years of age	Jaundice (i.e., yellowing of the eyes and skin)
Men are more likely to develop pancreatic cancer than women	Fatigue
Smoking	Abdominal and back pain
Long-term diabetes, type 1 (DM1) or diabetes, type 2 (DM2)	Unexplained weight loss
	Nausea and vomiting
Chronic pancreatitis	Blood clots
Cirrhosis of the liver	
Overweight and obesity	

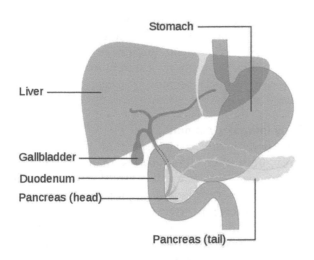

Diagram showing the position of the pancreas, behind the stomach. (Cancer Research UK)

fats from red meat and dairy products were found to increase risk for pancreatic cancer.

One possible explanation for this increased risk is that excessive secretion of digestive enzymes in response to high intake of dietary fat can lead to pancreatic hypertrophy and hyperplasia, which increase vulnerability to the effects of carcinogens. The link between saturated fat intake and pancreatic cancer risk may be due to the association between saturated fat and insulin resistance.

Summary

Individuals at risk and diagnosed with pancreatic cancer (and their family members/caregivers) should learn about dietary recommendations based on personal characteristics and health needs. Patients should eat a high-fiber diet that includes a wide variety of fruits, vegetables, lean proteins, and unsaturated fats. Patients undergoing treatment for pancreatic cancer need to be monitored for weight loss, signs of malnutrition, vitamin/mineral deficiencies and electrolyte imbalances. It is important to report any health-related changes to the treating clinician as soon as possible to prevent worsening health status. A registered dietitian may provide appropriate nutrition support and counsel patients on appropriate foods or supplements to prevent weight loss or nutrient deficiencies. Patients and their family members should understand and adhere to the prescribed treatment regimen, while

continuing medical surveillance to monitor health status. Research suggests that maintaining a healthy weight, physical activity, consuming a diet rich in fruits and vegetables and low in saturated fat, limiting alcohol intake, and not smoking can reduce the risk of developing pancreatic cancer.

—*Cherie Marcel*

References

American Association for Cancer Research. "Excess Body Weight before 50 Is Associated with Higher Risk of Dying from Pancreatic Cancer." *Science-Daily*, 31 Mar. 2019, www.sciencedaily.com/releases/2019/03/190331192525.htm.

Berger, Nathan A. "Obesity and Cancer Pathogenesis." *Annals of the New York Academy of Sciences*, vol. 1311, no. 1, 2014, pp. 57–76., doi:10.1111/nyas.12416.

Bracci, Paige M. "Obesity and Pancreatic Cancer: Overview of Epidemiologic Evidence and Biologic Mechanisms." *Molecular Carcinogenesis*, vol. 51, no. 1, 12 Jan. 2013, pp. 53–63., doi:10.1002/mc.20778.

Eibl, Guido, et al. "Diabetes Mellitus and Obesity as Risk Factors for Pancreatic Cancer." *Journal of the Academy of Nutrition and Dietetics*, vol. 118, no. 4, 2018, pp. 555–567., doi:10.1016/j.jand.2017.07.005.

Pothuraju, Ramesh, et al. "Pancreatic Cancer Associated with Obesity and Diabetes: an Alternative Approach for Its Targeting." *Journal of Experimental & Clinical Cancer Research*, vol. 37, no. 1, 2018, doi:10.1186/s13046-018-0963-4.

■ Poor body image

CATEGORY: Psychology

Body image refers to the way a person perceives his or her body; it encompasses various aspects of perception, including visual, mental, emotional, and physical. Although people frequently feel that their body image represents the "truth" about their bodies, it is important to recognize the distinction between one's perception and reality. Body image is shaped over time by past experiences, cultural context, and personality traits. It can also fluctuate considerably in response to a number of factors. Just a few of the many factors found to alter people's perceptions of their bodies include mood, recent television exposure, phase in the menstrual cycle, and whether or not one recently consumed junk food.

Introduction

Everyone develops a sense of identity. Part of one's sense of self is one's body image. Body image is how someone thinks and feels about his or her body. Someone might look in the mirror and have a thought about his or her body, or someone might have a mental picture of his or her body, or someone might just feel a certain way towards his or her body. All of this is part of body image. The concept of body image incorporates how a person feels inside his or her body and whether or not they are comfortable within their body. People often have multiple and complex feelings about bodies in general and one's own body, in particular. Body image can be positive or negative and it does not necessarily remain the same over time. One's opinion about his or her body can change within minutes or stay the same for several years.

People begin to develop an awareness of his or her body in early childhood. Babies can be seen feeling their toes or playing with their reflection in the mirror. As children grow up their bodies begin to change. During adolescence, puberty can be a time when children who never paid much attention to their bodies begin to notice changes. For children who have already been hyper focused on their bodies, adolescence can be particularly challenging. The pre-teen and teenage years can be difficult as one's body image continues to develop because it is normal for children to rely on the opinions of others around them. Peer groups during adolescence can make damaging comments about people's bodies that have long-lasting effects. Students begin to receive messages from all around them about what bodies are socially acceptable and which ones are not.

For a long time people focused only on females' body image. The general public felt that most men were unconcerned with how they looked and people assumed that men always felt good about their bodies. However, in the past twenty years research has started to focus more on male body image. Men are increasingly as likely as women to think about their body image, to be critical of their bodies, and to want their bodies to be "perfect."

There is a growing trend of widespread negative male body image. This could be due to changing attitudes towards male bodies in society. While some males have always cared about their body image, it seems to be more prevalent now than it once was.

Body Image in Women

Poor body image is an issue that affects women throughout their lifespan. As many as 80% of women over age 18 are dissatisfied with the image they see when they look in the mirror. And while it has been known for some time that individuals with eating disorders tend to overestimate their actual size, recent research suggests that this is true not only for women with eating disorders but for women in general. While the majority of women's dissatisfaction focuses on the size or shape of their bodies, more specifically their hips, thighs, and stomach, women's dissatisfaction with their appearance is by no means limited to these parts of their bodies.

Alarmingly, even very young girls worry about their appearance and about gaining weight, and they, too, have been found to overestimate their size. In a recent survey, 42% of girls in first to third grade felt they should lose weight, and more than half of normal weight girls aged 6 to 12 erroneously believed themselves to be overweight. Surveys have also found that as many as 25% of college-aged women binge in order to control their weight and up to 96% reported having opted out of activities because of anxiety about their appearance.

Body dissatisfaction does not seem to diminish with age; in a recent survey in which middle-aged women were asked what they would most want to change about their lives, more than half of the respondents replied that what they most wanted to change was their weight. Indeed, women's dissatisfaction with their bodies has been observed to be so commonplace that it has been termed "normative discontent" to signal how normal it has become for women in our society to be chronically dissatisfied with their bodies.

The proliferation of technology in recent years and the associated increase in media exposure has played a significant role in breeding body dissatisfaction by perpetuating rigid appearance-based ideals. The women featured in movies and advertisements are disproportionately young, white, tall, blonde, and thin. Women in the media are also routinely photo-shopped to have flawless skin or to appear even thinner than they already are. Because of the sheer quantity of images people are exposed to today, these unrealistic, often impossible-to-attain standards are so pervasive that they seem "normal". Young girls and women who consume these images compare their own bodies to this seemingly "normal" standard and feel inadequate by comparison.

Strong evidence of the link between media consumption and body image issues is provided by a study conducted in Fiji. As one of the last places in the world exposed to Western television, Fiji was an ideal place to study the impact of the media on body image. It was found that adolescent girls' body dissatisfaction dramatically increased after the introduction of television, with Fijians who had viewed television for an extended period of time suddenly reporting that they viewed themselves as "fat." After the introduction of television, a sharp rise in disordered eating was also observed among the girls in Fiji.

Further evidence for the impact of media on body image has been found in numerous studies. Experiments have shown that shortly after viewing images of models, women are more likely to be dissatisfied with their physical appearance. Similarly, frequent exposure to fashion magazines and television have been found to contribute to body shame and insecurity. These findings help to explain the pervasiveness of body dissatisfaction when one considers that adolescents interact with media (including television, advertisements, and social media) more than ever before and that adolescent girls spend an average of 4 hours each week reading fashion magazines.

Body Image in Men

While body image concerns have historically been associated with females, it is increasingly more common for males to also experience body image issues. It is normal for males to care about their bodies and most males begin dealing with body image issues during adolescence. Sometimes concerns about one's body can turn into body obsession and lead to a disorder or maladaptive behaviors.

Masculinity is the social phenomenon relating to acting, looking, and feeling "like a man."

Masculinity revolves around standards of strength, aggression, and independence. Masculinity shies away from dependence or from showing one's emotions, instead insisting that men are not often hurt and don't need to cry. It is this sense of masculinity that has pervaded the media and influenced portrayals of men in advertising. It is not surprising that the rise in male body image issues corresponds with the increase of advertisements showing lean, muscular, tan, and well-groomed male bodies. Just like women, men receive messages from the media about acceptable and non-acceptable bodies.

One example of the changing nature of the portrayal of male bodies in the media can be seen in the G. I. Joe action figure. From the 1960s to the 1990s, G. I. Joe's waist shrunk while his arms grew; mimicking what is represented as masculine in the media. If G. I. Joe were a real man, he would have the biggest biceps of any body builder in history.

For a long time, the thin ideal ruled in the world of body image. This meant that people with slender bodies were generally thought to be happier and more physically attractive than people with "chubby" or "fat" bodies. While this definitely still exists for males, often a more common phenomenon is the "muscular ideal." This ideal maintains that visibly muscular bodies are the best. This ideal is commonly seen on billboards, in magazines, on television, and in video game characters.

When males feel that they don't look like magazine cutouts or billboard models they often begin to feel shameful about their bodies. This can be taken to extremes in some instances when boys and men have distorted images of their bodies. This can include negative thoughts and feelings about one's body, engaging in negative self-talk, under-eating, excessive working out, or drug and steroid use.

It is important to understand that in some cases males may develop unhealthy self-images that can lead to psychological disorders. Males who are dissatisfied with their bodies are more likely to be depressed and suffer from low self-esteem. Furthermore, men with low body satisfaction are more likely to develop body dysmorphic disorder (BDD) or an eating disorder. Body dysmorphic disorder is when males have an excessive preoccupation with how their bodies look that becomes unhealthy. Both anorexia and bulimia have increased in the male population in recent decades. Anorexia is a disorder characterized by an extreme lack of eating to the point where the individual is excessively skinny and bones become visible underneath the skin. Bulimia is slightly more common in the male population and it is when individuals have cycles of binge eating (or consuming too much food) and then vomiting or using laxatives. Both of these disorders tend to occur when men have unrealistic ideas about their bodies.

Other possible negative consequences of body dissatisfaction include the use or abuse of substances such as steroids, illicit drugs, and alcohol. It has become commonplace for the news to report about famous sports players using steroids illegally. Males receive conflicting messages that they have to attain an excessively muscular or trim body, and some men end up overusing steroids or muscle enhancing drugs.

Clinicians may draw from strategies that have demonstrated efficacy in treating individuals suffering from body dysmorphic disorders and eating disorders. Psychoeducation regarding common symptoms associated with eating disorders (e.g. binge eating, vomiting, extreme food restriction) may be helpful during the initial phase of therapy. Developing a support system at home and among peer groups is also very helpful.

The Consequences of Poor Body Image

Although poor body image has become "normal," it is nevertheless detrimental to a woman's mental and physical health. A person with a poor body image is far more likely to engage in behaviors that may compromise their health. Some of these behaviors are frequently resorted to as a way to achieve weight loss, such as restrictive eating, self-induced vomiting, excessive exercising, smoking, and taking diet pills. It has also been found that people with poor body image are considerably less likely to exercise regularly or to eat a healthy diet. People with poor body image are also more likely to participate in risky sexual behaviors like engaging in sexual intercourse without a condom.

In addition to negative effects on physical health, poor body image has psychological consequences as well. It is linked to anxiety and depression as well as to diminished academic performance. Experiments have revealed that when young people are focused on their appearance, their performance declines; this has been found to be true for a variety of tasks ranging from athletic activities to math

tests. Poor body image is also the driving force behind several mental disorders, including body dysmorphic disorder, anorexia, bulimia, and binge eating disorder. These disorders can cause tremendous emotional and physical pain and can even be life-threatening.

Scientifically Supported Ways to Improve Body Image

Given how incredibly widespread the problem of body dissatisfaction is alongside the fact that body image can impact nearly every domain of a person's life, it is crucial to develop an understanding of how to combat poor body image. The first and most important thing to understand in seeking to improve body image is that body image is not improved by altering one's appearance. It may seem counterintuitive, but body image and appearance and not related to one another. While it is tempting to think that changing one's appearance will remedy body dissatisfaction, the underlying problems of shame, anxiety, and depression which fuel poor body image cannot be remedied by plastic surgery or by losing weight. On the contrary, it has been found that when people undergo cosmetic surgical procedures, though they may feel a temporary sense of relief, they almost always revert back to their pre-surgical levels of body dissatisfaction. Similarly, losing weight, despite what advertisements suggest, does not increase a person's level of happiness.

One strategy which has been found to immediately improve body image is physical activity. Exerting physical energy to participate in enjoyable activities has been shown to immediately boost women's mood and to increase body satisfaction and self-esteem. This is most true when the focus of the activity is on improving fitness levels or ability rather than on burning calories.

Another way to improve body image is to boost one's mood. While depression and anxiety may exacerbate poor body image, being in a good mood can have the opposite effect. Staying socially active, taking time to relax, and participating in meaningful activities, like volunteer work, all help to improve mood. Additionally, these activities can help to shift one's focus away from appearance and onto one's experiences or internal qualities.

Finally, several studies have revealed the importance of one's social interactions on body image. Comments from family members, friends, and peers all influence the way a woman thinks and feels about her own body. Studies have found that when a person makes a self-disparaging comment about appearance or weight, that leads to increased body anxiety and body dissatisfaction for everyone listening. It is therefore vital to surround oneself with others who are accepting towards their bodies and to refrain from making negative comments about one's body out loud.

Cultivating acceptance of one's body, regardless of its size or shape, can improve one's own physical and mental health and can make one a positive influence for family and friends. When more people can maintain a healthy body image they will be better able to pursue more important personal and professional goals that enable them to make meaningful contributions to society.

—*Cherie Oertel, Alyssa Tedder-King*

References

Baker, Amanda, and Céline Blanchard. "Men's Body Image: The Effects of an Unhealthy Body Image on Psychological, Behavioral, and Cognitive Health." *Weight Loss*, 5 Nov. 2018, doi:10.5772/intechopen.75187.

Lovejoy, Jessica. "Body Image Issues Are Not Just For Women." *The Huffington Post*, 26 May 2014, www.huffingtonpost.com/jessica-lovejoy/body-image-issues-are-not-just-for-women_b_5034285.html.

Ngo, Nealie Tan. "What Historical Ideals of Women's Shapes Teach Us About Women's Self-Perception and Body Decisions Today." *AMA Journal of Ethics*, vol. 21, no. 10, 1 Oct. 2019, doi:10.1001/amajethics.2019.879.

University of Texas Health Science Center at Houston. "Negative Body Image, Not Depression, Increases Adolescent Obesity Risk." *Science-Daily*, 9 Nov. 2015, www.sciencedaily.com/releases/2015/11/151109083418.htm.

Weinberger, Natascha-Alexandra, et al. "Body Dissatisfaction in Individuals with Obesity Compared to Normal-Weight Individuals: A Systematic Review and Meta-Analysis." *Obesity Facts*, vol. 9, no. 6, 2016, pp. 424–441., doi:10.1159/000454837.

Wolfram, Taylor. "Body Image and Young Women." *EatRight*, Academy of Nutrition and Dietetics, 31 May 2019, www.eatright.org/health/diseases-and-conditions/eating-disorders/body-image-and-young-women.

■ Schizophrenia

CATEGORY: Disorder; Psychology

According to the Diagnostic and Statistical Manual of Mental Disorders – 5 (DSM-5), schizophrenia refers to a psychiatric illness that is characterized by psychosis, apathy, social dysfunction, and cognitive impairment. Schizophrenia can negatively affect the ability to function in relationships, school, work, and normal daily activities (e.g., grocery shopping, paying bills, managing a home, preparing meals). Individuals with schizophrenia are at greater risk for comorbidities (e.g., cardiovascular disease [CVD], diabetes mellitus, type 2 [DM2], hypercholesterolemia), hospitalization, and early mortality compared with the general population. Most persons with schizophrenia develop normally during childhood, begin to experience social awkwardness, emotional bluntness, and cognitive decline during adolescence (referred to as the prodromal phase), and develop symptoms of psychosis (e.g., hallucinations and delusions) in early adulthood. Risk of suicide is significantly higher in individuals with schizophrenia than in persons with good mental health.

Risk Factors for Schizophrenia

The risk for developing schizophrenia is increased for individuals who have relatives with the disorder, although evidence indicates that environmental factors (e.g., exposure to viruses, fetal malnutrition, cannabis use) also influence risk.

Medical Nutrition Therapy for Schizophrenia

The relationship between diet and mental health is complex and cyclical. Mental illness can impair one's ability to prepare and consume healthy meals and nutrient deficiencies can result in further cognitive decline. Results of studies indicate that persons with schizophrenia tend to engage in unhealthy dietary practices, are more likely to be overweight, have poorer nutrient intake, are more sedentary, and are significantly more prone to the development of metabolic syndrome than persons with good mental health. Persons with schizophrenia can experience appetite changes (e.g., loss of interest in food or excessive hunger), poor self-control, and/or be unable to procure or prepare food due to mental instability.

Schizophrenia is a life-long, progressive mental illness that is frequently accompanied by complicating metabolic dysfunctions. Individuals with schizophrenia require continuous treatment, including with antipsychotic medications, psychotherapy, and education regarding the importance of making lifestyle modifications (e.g., changes in dietary intake and exercise).

The medications used to treat schizophrenia commonly result in side effects that affect appetite, nutrient intake, and weight. Adverse effects that can affect dietary intake include excessive hunger, weight gain, insulin resistance, glucose intolerance, sedation, fatigue, and drowsiness, and vertigo and nausea

It is important for patients to be aware whether or not the prescribed medication should be taken with meals because food can affect the bioavailability of certain medications. For example, ziprasidone should be taken with a meal that contains at least 500 calories in order to achieve optimal bioavailability. Absorption of ziprasidone is decreased by half if taken in a fasting state. Many of the medications prescribed for the treatment of schizophrenia can have a dramatic impact on appetite, weight, activity level, and metabolic processes.

Metabolic syndrome (also known as insulin resistance syndrome and syndrome X) is characterized by a cluster of risk factors for CVD, including abdominal obesity, hypertension, poor lipid profile (e.g., high triglycerides, low high-density lipoproteins), and insulin resistance. The existence of metabolic syndrome is predictive of heart attack, stroke, DM2, and all-cause mortality.

Dietary Considerations for Schizophrenia

Carbohydrates (CHOs) metabolize to glucose, which is the body's primary source of energy. At rest, the brain uses 20–30% of total energy consumption. If caloric intake is inadequate to fuel basic energy requirements, cognition declines.

CHO intake results in the release of insulin. Insulin stimulates the uptake of large neutral amino acids (LNAAs) in muscle, but it has no effect on the amino acid tryptophan (TRP), resulting in an increased ratio of TRP to LNAAs and elevated levels of TRP in the brain. TRP contributes to the

synthesis of serotonin, which is a neurotransmitter (i.e., a chemical that facilitates the transmission of signals between cells) that calms mood, improves sleep patterns, increases pain tolerance, and reduces food cravings.

Simple CHOs, or simple sugars (e.g., low-fiber breads and cereals, sugary foods), break down quickly, giving the body rapid energy, but only for a short duration. Eating a high amount of simple CHOs can produce spikes and drops in insulin and glucose levels, resulting in fluctuating moods and excessive feelings of hunger.

Complex CHOs (e.g., high-fiber, whole grain breads and cereals) take longer to metabolize than simple CHOs, and provide the body with a slower release of energy over a longer period of time. This helps to maintain normal glucose levels and stabilize mood.

Protein-rich foods (e.g., eggs, lean meats, dairy, beans) provide the amino acids tyrosine (TYR) and TRP, which are vital for the production of important neurotransmitters. Mental energy and alertness are increased by the neurotransmitters norepinephrine and dopamine, which are manufactured from TYR with the help of folate, magnesium, and vitamin B12. TRP is the precursor to serotonin, which stabilizes mood. Eating meals that are high in protein results in a high amount of amino acids competing with TRP for entry into the brain. Eating meals that are balanced with protein and CHOs results in the necessary release of insulin to facilitate the redistribution of the competing amino acids, allowing TRP to cross the blood-brain barrier.

The brain is largely composed of fat, especially the essential fatty acids (EFAs) omega-3 and omega-6. EFAs are considered essential because they are necessary for physiologic function, cannot be produced by the body, and must be consumed in the diet. Both omega-6 and omega-3 EFAs are important in the development and normal functioning of the brain and peripheral nervous system.

The typically Western diet tends to include more omega-6 EFA (found in red meat, poultry, eggs, nuts, and seeds) than omega-3 EFA (primarily found in fish and seafood). Results of research indicate that increasing the ratio of omega-3 intake such that it is at least equal to intake of omega-6 can reduce the risk of developing certain chronic diseases (e.g.,

CVD, inflammatory bowel disease [IBD], cancer) and has been associated with a reduction in cognitive decline. Evidence suggests thatomega-3 EFA supplementation can postpone the onset and/or slow the progression of schizophrenia.

Antioxidants, which are found abundantly in fruits and vegctables, protect brain cells from the damaging effects of free radicals. Many nutrients exhibit antioxidant activity, including vitamins A, C, and E; selenium; and the phytonutrients (i.e., beneficial, plant-derived chemicals) beta-carotene and lycopene. By protecting the brain cells from oxidation, antioxidants aid in the prevention of dementia and depression.B-complex vitamins (found in green, leafy vegetables, eggs, milk, chicken, and fortified cereals) are necessary for sustaining good mental health. Deficiencies in the B-complex vitamins niacin, riboflavin, and folate are associated with an increased likelihood of developing anxiety, depression, memory loss, insomnia, and/or fatigue.

Research Findings

Results of clinical studies show that there are lower levels of omega-3 EFAs in psychiatric patients. Researchers suggest that problems with lipid metabolism may play a role in schizophrenia and bipolar disorder. Supplementation with omega-3 EFAs has been shown to reduce behaviors of impulsivity, deliberate self-harm, and violent aggression.

Researchers have reported that babies born to mothers who were malnourished during pregnancy have a higher risk of developing schizophrenia later in life. Researchers have proposed that there is a causal relationship between vitamin D deficiency during pregnancy and the development of schizophrenia, which could explain the increased incidence of schizophrenia during winter at higher latitudes.

Summary

Individuals with schizophrenia (and their family members) should learn about dietary considerations based on personal characteristics and health needs. Individuals with schizophrenia should be assessed by a registered dietitian (RD) regarding dietary habits, and educated regarding the importance of consuming a diet that is high in nutrition and contains a variety of fruits, vegetables, whole grains, and lean meats. Individuals

should also be assessed for the risk for diet-related complications associated with schizophrenia and for adverse effects of medications used to treat schizophrenia that affect dietary intake. Individuals and their family members should be educated regarding dietary considerations to increase awareness and understanding of food labels, calorie content of popular food items, and portion control. Research suggests that supplementation with omega-3 EFAs has been shown to reduce erratic behaviors in individuals with schizophrenia.

—*Christen Miller*

References

Annamalai, Aniyizhai, et al. "Prevalence of Obesity and Diabetes in Patients with Schizophrenia." *World Journal of Diabetes*, vol. 8, no. 8, 2017, p. 390., doi:10.4239/wjd.v8.i8.390.

Davies, Nicola. "Mental Illness and Obesity." *Psychiatry Advisor*, 26 Feb. 2016, www.psychiatryadvisor. com/home/conference-highlights/aaic-2015-coverage/mental-illness-and-obesity/.

Franco, Viviane Carvalho, et al. "Obesity and Clozapine Use in Schizophrenia." *Obesity Research - Open Journal*, vol. 3, no. 2, 13 July 2016, pp. 24–29., doi:10.17140/oroj-3-124.

Pajk, Barbara. "Obesity among Patients with Schizophrenia: When We Fix One Problem and Create Another." *Clinical and Experimental Psychology*, vol. 2, no. 3, 2016, doi:10.4172/2471-2701.1000135.

Ventriglio, Antonio, et al. "Metabolic Issues in Patients Affected by Schizophrenia: Clinical Characteristics and Medical Management." *Frontiers in Neuroscience*, vol. 9, 3 Sept. 2015, doi:10.3389/fnins.2015.00297.

■ Sleep apnea

CATEGORY: Disorder
ALSO KNOWN AS: Obstructive sleep apnea

Causes and Symptoms

Obstructive sleep apnea (OSA) is caused by upper airway obstruction. Soft tissue in the back of the mouth collapses during sleep and temporarily obstructs airflow into the lungs. People with sleep apnea experience many periods of apnea and hypopnea. During such periods, the oxygen level in the bloodstream can decline significantly. Since these episodes happen throughout the night, the sleep pattern is interrupted, and the person will feel sleepy during the day. Symptoms of OSA may include morning headaches, fatigue, difficulty with concentration, and daytime sleepiness (somnolence). The person might doze off while watching television, reading, or, more dangerously, driving. The person may not be aware of apnea or the resultant snoring. However, a sleeping partner will frequently notice these symptoms. It should be noted, however, that snoring alone, without apnea, is very common and does not indicate sleep apnea.

Risk factors for the development of OSA include obesity, a small jaw, a deviated septum of the nose, a big tongue, or enlarged tonsils. Smokers are also at higher risk of developing sleep apnea.

If OSA is left untreated, then medical complications may occur, such as increased risks of hypertension, heart failure, strokes, and pulmonary hypertension. In pulmonary hypertension, the lungs become stiff and fail to provide normal oxygenation. Therefore, it is extremely important to recognize and treat sleep apnea.

The clinical triad of snoring, apneic episodes, and daytime somnolence suggests OSA. A diagnosis can be made by an overnight oximeter or by a formal sleep study (polysomnography). An oximeter is a noninvasive device worn over a finger that measures the oxygen level in the bloodstream. It can be worn overnight at home and is useful for detecting any drop in oxygen level caused by apneic or hypopneic episodes. A formal sleep study requires an overnight observation in a sleep center where multiple monitors record brain waves, heart rate, breathing rate, abdominal muscle movement, and oxygen level. Based on these measurements, an apnea-hypopnea index (AHI), the average number of apneic and hypopneic episodes in one hour, is reported. An AHI of 5 to 20 is considered mild sleep apnea. An AHI of 21 to 50 is moderate, and an AHI of greater than 50 is considered severe.

Treatment and Therapy

Obese individuals with OSA should lose weight, quit smoking, and avoid sedating medications and alcohol because they may impair breathing even further.

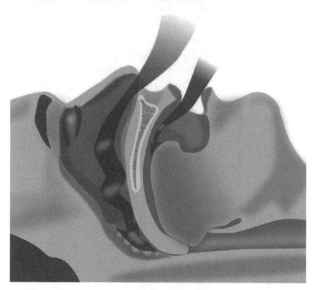

Obstructive sleep apnea. (Habib M'henni)

Initial OSA treatment consists of a nasal continuous positive airflow pressure (CPAP) machine. A triangular mask fits over the nose and is hooked up to a machine that pushes air under pressure into the upper airway to keep it open. A repeat sleep study using a CPAP machine can determine the level of pressure necessary to prevent apneic and hypopneic episodes. Such a device can be very effective in treating OSA. Side effects may include anxiety from using the mask, nasal congestion, nosebleeds, dry mouth, and irritation of the skin from the mask.

Some individuals require surgical treatment, especially those who cannot tolerate the use of a CPAP machine. The procedure called uvulopalatopharyngoplasty involves surgical removal of excess soft tissue including the tonsils in the back of the mouth. Laser-assisted uvulopalatoplasty, in which a laser is used to remove the soft tissue, can be performed in the office. Other surgeries can move the tongue and jaw forward in order to open up the airway in the back of the mouth. For very severe cases of sleep apnea, an opening can be made in the trachea (the windpipe in the upper neck) to bypass the obstruction in the mouth and nose.

Perspective and Prospects

Accounts of what may have been sleep apnea date back to 305 to 30 BCE and involve eleven members from seven generations of the Egyptian royal family. These individuals were obese and were reported by contemporary philosophers and historians to have a tendency toward falling asleep during social and political events.

Sleep apnea has sometimes made an appearance in literature. In the late sixteenth century, symptoms of OSA are suggested in characters created by William Shakespeare for this plays *Richard II* and *Henry IV*. In *Richard II*, the obese Sir John Falstaff snores and sleeps much of the day, interrupted by an apneic breathing pattern. In *Henry IV*, King Henry IV has trouble sleeping, with periods of not breathing in his sleep. Lewis Carroll described a character with sleep apnea in his book *Alice's Adventures in Wonderland* (1865). At the Mad Hatter's tea party, the Dormouse suffers from daytime sleepiness. The other characters try to help the Dormouse by putting him into a tight teapot, which would serve as a positive pressure to assist his breathing.

The famous composer Johannes Brahms (1833-1897) was thought to have developed sleep apnea in his later years when he gained weight. He was known to his friends to snore loudly at night. He also fell asleep during a performance by another famous composer, Franz Liszt.

—*Veronica N. Baptista*

References

Adelizzi, Angela. "Obesity and Obstructive Sleep Apnea." *Obesity Medicine Association*, 2 Aug. 2018, obesitymedicine.org/obesity-and-sleep-apnea/.

Hudgel, David W., et al. "The Role of Weight Management in the Treatment of Adult Obstructive Sleep Apnea. An Official American Thoracic Society Clinical Practice Guideline." *American Journal of Respiratory and Critical Care Medicine*, vol. 198, no. 6, 15 Sept. 2018, doi:10.1164/rccm.201807-1326st.

Mcfarlane, Samy I, et al. "Obstructive Sleep Apnea and Obesity: Implications for Public Health." *Sleep Medicine and Disorders: International Journal*, vol. 1, no. 4, 12 Dec. 2017, doi:10.15406/smdij.2017.01.00019.

Watson, Stephanie. "Weight Loss, Breathing Devices Still Best for Treating Obstructive Sleep Apnea." *Harvard Health Publishing*, Harvard Medical School, 18 Mar. 2019, www.health.harvard.edu/blog/weight-loss-breathing-devices-still-best-for-treating-obstructive-sleep-apnea-201310026713.

■ Stomach cancer

CATEGORY: Disorder

Stomach cancer (also called gastric cancer) is a neoplasm that originates in the tissue that lines the stomach. Currently, stomach cancer is the 4th most frequent cancer and the second leading cause of cancer-related death worldwide. Annually in the United States there are over 21,000 new cases of stomach cancer and over 10,000 stomach cancer-related deaths. Signs and symptoms of stomach cancer include fatigue, nausea, vomiting, a sensation of fullness or being bloated after eating very little, and weight loss. Treatment depends on the stage of the cancer as well as the age and health of the patient, and can require the use of surgery, chemotherapy, and/or radiation therapy.

RISK FACTORS	SIGNS AND SYMPTOMS
Men are more than twice as likely to develop stomach cancer as women.	Fatigue Abdominal pain and bloating
Consuming a diet that is low in fruits and vegetables	Fullness after eating very little Unexplained weight loss
Consuming a diet that is high in foods that are preserved with salt and smoked foods	Nausea and vomiting Heartburn
Being over 50 years of age	
A family history of stomach cancer	
Long-term stomach inflammation (e.g., gastritis) or the presence of stomach polyps	
Helicobacter pylori infection	

Dietary Recommendations for the Prevention of Stomach Cancer

Regular intake of fruits and vegetables can contribute to the prevention of stomach cancer. Results of studies show a definite protective benefit of the intake of fruits and strong evidence for anticancer properties in intake of raw, green, and cruciferous vegetables. The exact mechanisms of this protective effect are not fully understood. The antioxidant vitamins (e.g., E, C, and A), vitamin D, magnesium, and calcium have demonstrated anticancer activity but are still being investigated. Regardless of whether a direct preventative relationship exists, higher consumption of fruits and vegetables is usually associated with higher fiber and lower fat intake, as well as lower body weight; all of these are associated with cancer prevention.

In general, the best recommendation for a diet focused on cancer prevention is to eat a high-fiber diet, which includes a variety of fruits and vegetables, lean proteins, and unsaturated fats.

Summary

Individuals diagnosed with stomach cancer (and their family members) should become knowledgeable about stomach cancer and diet to accurately assess personal characteristics and health needs. To help prevent stomach cancer it is recommended to consume a high-fiber diet, which includes a variety of fruits and vegetables, lean proteins, and unsaturated fats. Stomach cancer patients should report any health-related changes to the treating clinician as soon as possible to prevent worsening health status. Patients and their family members should understand and adhere to the prescribed treatment regimen, while continuing medical surveillance to monitor health status. Research suggests that limiting red meat and poultry, high-fat, starchy and heavily processed foods, and salt-preserved and smoked meats may reduce the risk of stomach cancer.

—*Cherie Marcel*

References

Juo, Yen-Yi, et al. "Obesity Is Associated with Early Onset of Gastrointestinal Cancers in California." *Journal of Obesity*, vol. 2018, 19 Sept. 2018, pp. 1–6., doi:10.1155/2018/7014073.

Karczewski, Jacek, et al. "Obesity and the Risk of Gastrointestinal Cancers." *Digestive Diseases and Sciences*, vol. 64, no. 10, 9 Apr. 2019, pp. 2740–2749., doi:10.1007/s10620-019-05603-9.

Lin, X.-J., et al. "Body Mass Index and Risk of Gastric Cancer: A Meta-Analysis." *Japanese Journal of Clinical Oncology*, vol. 44, no. 9, 20 June 2014, pp. 783–791., doi:10.1093/jjco/hyu082.

Stone, Trevor W., et al. "Obesity and Cancer: Existing and New Hypotheses for a Causal Connection." *EBioMedicine*, vol. 30, 2018, pp. 14–28., doi:10.1016/j.ebiom.2018.02.022.

■ Stroke

CATEGORY: Disorder
ALSO KNOWN AS: Cerebrovascular accident (CVA)

Causes and Symptoms

Strokes produce damage to portions of the brain as a result of decreased blood supply due to occlusion or hemorrhage. Strokes are commonly known as cerebrovascular accidents (CVAs). Symptoms of strokes will vary depending on the part of the brain that is affected. Rapid intervention is critical to management of stroke. The American Stroke Association has developed a guide to recognizing stroke symptoms to encourage the public to seek immediate emergency care. Using the word "FAST" to represent facial drooping, arm weakness, speech difficulty and time to call 911, allows individuals to recognize the symptoms of stroke and seek immediate treatment. Other symptoms of stroke may include trouble speaking, confusion, difficulty understanding simple commands such as "raise your right arm", trouble walking and severe headache.

Resulting speech disorders may include aphasia (loss of the ability to speak) or dysarthria (difficulty in speaking). A sudden weakness or numbness of one side of the body is known as hemiparesis or hemiplegia. The eyes can also be involved. A dimness or transient loss of vision, particularly in one eye, is called amaurosis fugax. Occasionally, it can involve the same portion of the visual field in both eyes. Other symptoms of stroke may include dizziness, unsteadiness, sudden falls, headaches, confusion, or stupor. Coma is less commonly involved in a stroke.

Predisposing factors to strokes include hypertension (high blood pressure), diabetes, high cholesterol, smoking, atherosclerotic disease in other portions of the body (such as the heart or legs), and a previous or family history of strokes or transient ischemic attacks. Gender and age are also associated with the incidence of strokes.

In cerebrovascular disease, atherosclerosis affects the arteries that circulate blood to the brain. The brain receives blood from two major sets of arteries. The carotid arteries, in the front of the neck, supply the anterior (front) portions of the brain. The vertebral arteries travel through the transverse processes of the spine and join the basilar artery to provide blood to the posterior (back) portion of the brain. Both circulatory systems are joined within the brain in a structure known as the circle of Willis, a composite of arteries that join to form an anatomical circle. The various arteries supply the necessary blood flow to different areas of the brain. Only 25 to 50 percent of people have a complete circle of Willis; this anatomical variance may be a factor in the severity of the stroke.

In atherosclerotic disease, fat, cholesterol, and calcium deposits are laid down along the walls of the arteries, primarily at sites where arteries divide and natural turbulence tends to occur. These components build up to form plaques, which may cause stenosis (narrowing) and occlusion (closure) of the arterial lumen. Accumulation of platelets and other blood cells can form a thrombus (blood clot) along with plaque buildup, which also may obstruct the arteries. Pieces of plaque or thrombotic material may break off and cause emboli to lodge acutely in the main vessels or their more distant branches.

The most common components of cerebrovascular disease are transient ischemic attacks (TIAs), also referred to as ministrokes. By definition, TIA s last less than twenty-four hours; usually, they last only a few minutes or hours. Most TIAs are produced by emboli. An embolus occurs when a piece of plaque from the lining of a major artery breaks off and temporarily blocks the blood flow to a particular area of the brain. If the symptoms last for more than twenty-four hours, a cerebrovascular accident, cerebral infarct, or stroke has occurred. A reversible ischemic neurological deficit (RIND) is similar to a stroke in that it is an event that lasts for more than twenty-four hours but resolves in about seventy-two hours.

The majority of strokes in the United States (85 percent) are the result of impaired blood flow

(ischemia) to the brain. Atherosclerosis in the cerebrovascular system will cause similar symptoms of ischemia in other portions of the body. There is increasing narrowing, or stenosis, of blood vessels. Eventually, they will close off completely and become occluded. The development of new, small vessels that bypass a diseased artery is called collateralization. This process requires weeks or months to occur. Collateralization seems to be especially prominent in the cerebrovascular system, since the brain is an organ that requires constant blood flow at all times. Eventual occlusion or thrombosis of a major vessel causes the majority of CVAs, producing significant ischemia in a portion of the brain. In certain cases, the blockage is acute, having resulted from an embolus or thrombus that blocks an artery. If collateralization has not developed, the damage to an affected structure is more severe. A thrombus or embolus can also arise from the heart. This is most common in individuals who have had a recent heart attack, who have disease that involves the mitral valve, or who have atrial fibrillation, a variety of irregular heartbeat.

Another cause of stroke is cerebral hemorrhage, or bleeding into the brain, resulting in loss of consciousness or incapacity. An older term rarely used now for cerebral hemorrhage is apoplexy. Hypertension is the most common cause of intracranial bleeding and accounts for 10 to 15 percent of cases. Other causes of strokes are cerebral aneurysms (5 to 7 percent), tumors that have developed blood supplies (3 to 5 percent), and genetic bleeding tendencies (1 to 2 percent). A cerebral aneurysm occurs when the wall of an artery becomes weak and enlarges like a balloon. These aneurysms often rupture. With a ruptured cerebral aneurysm and subsequent hemorrhage, by-products of red blood cell degeneration may produce a condition called vasospasm, wherein the arteries will constrict. This often leads to ischemia. One or more thrombi are often formed in an aneurysm. If they break loose, they can become emboli, float until they become lodged in a small blood vessel, block the flow of blood, and cause ischemia. This can ultimately lead to a stroke.

Stroke refers to the disease process that is mainly produced by atherosclerotic changes in the arteries to the brain. Contributing or significant risk factors in the development of atherosclerosis include hypertension (high blood pressure), hyperlipidemia (high levels of cholesterol in the blood), smoking, diabetes mellitus, and a family history of similar incidents. Evidence of atherosclerotic disease in other portions of the body, such as the heart or legs, increases the risk of stroke. Atherosclerosis is a generalized disease process that affects arterial beds throughout the body.

Symptoms of TIAs in structures near the front of the brain, the area supplied by the carotid arteries, include hemiparesis, a numbness or loss of function in half of the body. Hemiplegia, a weakness of an arm or leg (or both), can be attributable to disease in the carotid artery on the side of the body opposite to the affected body part. Another relatively common problem usually caused by disease in the left carotid artery is aphasia, a speech disorder. Disease in either carotid artery can cause amaurosis fugax, or blindness in one eye. Victims often describe this condition as a shade being drawn over the eye.

Other, more generalized symptoms are the result of problems in the vertebral arteries or the blood vessels at the base of the brain, which supply the back portions of the brain. Associated symptoms include dizziness, a loss of orientation often produced by decreased blood flow to the brain. Dizziness is frequently caused by abrupt positional changes, in which blood pressure will suddenly fall with rapid standing or sitting, or by cardiac arrhythmias (irregular heartbeats), which prevent adequate amounts of blood flow from being delivered during certain cardiac cycles.

Vertigo is different from dizziness. Individuals suffering from vertigo experience a spinning sensation that may be accompanied by nausea. A common cause for vertigo is a condition known as subclavian steal, in which atherosclerotic disease affects the arteries of the arms just prior to the point where the vertebral arteries branch off. As an arm is used, or with abrupt changes in head position, blood will flow out of the vertebral arteries in a reverse manner (the so-called steal) to aid circulation in the arm (via the subclavian arteries) and vertigo will ensue. In addition, imbalance and other visual disturbances may be associated with problems in the vertebral arteries. These symptoms may also result from cerebrovascular disease in which inadequate blood supply to multiple areas of the brain can produce diverse symptoms. In the majority of strokes, symptoms last twenty-four to seventy-two hours. Approximately 25 percent of

patients will develop permanent deficits that will affect them for the rest of their lives. Approximately 20 percent of individuals who have strokes will experience no symptoms (be asymptomatic) and not know that they have had a stroke. They are unlikely to even develop TIAs. Such unheralded events result from occlusion or thrombosis of the blood vessels in the brain. This causes ischemia that leads to infarction or cell death in a particular section of the brain.

Asymptomatic cerebrovascular disease, however, can often be detected by the presence of a bruit, a French word meaning "noise." Stenosis in arteries can be compared to rapids in a river. Blood will flow very quickly through the narrow area and create turbulence, producing a bruit that can be heard with a stethoscope. Patients with narrowing in the carotid arteries ranging from 20 to 80 percent may possess a bruit. The absence of a bruit does not mean that the carotid arteries are disease-free. Once the stenosis reaches critical proportions, the flow is diminished and turbulence may be negligible, indicating a severe stenosis or an occluded artery. Often, doctors will recommend elective surgery to patients with coronary artery stenosis between 60 and 80 percent in an effort to reestablish blood flow and prevent eventual occlusion and possible stroke. About 75 percent of strokes are caused by ischemia that results from the above process. Crescendo TIAs, in which multiple TIAs occur in a brief period of time, and evolving strokes require immediate medical treatment. Appropriate diagnosis and treatment may prevent a stroke or decrease its severity.

Although disease caused by an aneurysm is a separate entity, it may be associated with atherosclerotic disease in certain cases. Most aneurysms within the brain produce no symptoms. As aneurysms increase in size, the probability of rupture increases; therefore, elective surgery may be recommended. Occasionally, diagnoses of cerebral aneurysms are made during investigations of other cerebral events, such as headaches. Acute onset of severe headaches or stiff neck should mandate immediate medical attention, since rupture of a cerebral aneurysm often manifests itself in this manner.

Treatment and Therapy

Strokes and TIAs often occur quickly and without warning. The best treatment for them is preventive behavior to avoid the atherosclerotic disease leading to such events.

Immediate medical care is critical to managing stroke and minimizing the long-term effects of the event, including the potential to prevent death. Medical advances in radiological imaging and stroke treatments have improved survival rates over the past decade. When a stroke is caused by a clot, Alteplase IV r-tPA may be administered in an attempt to dissolve the clot. As the only FDA-approved treatment for ischemic stroke, Alteplase IV r-tPA is a tissue plasminogen activator that works to improve blood flow by dissolving the clot and restoring blood flow to the brain. It must be administered within three hours of initial stroke symptoms, although certain patients may benefit up to 4 1/2 hours post symptoms. Often patients delay seeking hospital care resulting in permanent disability reflected by the tissues in the brain deprived of oxygen. If a patient experiences a stroke during the night or has no recollection of when symptoms began, the use of r-tPA is limited. Continued research may allow longer periods of time from onset to drug delivery. An endovascular procedure may be used to send a catheter to the site of blockage in an attempt to remove the clot and r-tPA may be injected intra-arterially into the clot in some instances. The best clinical protocols for endovascular procedures are still being researched.

When a stroke or TIA is suspected upon arrival to the Emergency Room, it is imperative to determine the time of onset of symptoms. A brief history and physical examination followed by a CT scan follows to determine the type of stroke and the patient's eligibility for r-tPA. Because of the three-hour time window for administration, determining symptoms and noting significant risk factors and findings upon physical examination will help a physician determine the primary area of the brain affected, schedule the appropriate tests for further diagnosis, and choose the best course of therapy. If the patient is documented to be well outside the three to 4 1/2 hour accepted window, a more comprehensive work-up may be acceptable. The National Institutes of Health Stroke Scale (NIHSS) was developed by national and international panels to provide a quantitative measure of stroke-related neurologic deficit. It provides baseline data for a comprehensive clinical assessment of stroke patients and may be a predictor of outcomes in stroke patients.

Stroke care has evolved over time and continues to be the focus of research due to the debilitating and costly impacts on the patient. Because of the high incidence of death and disability associated with strokes, a variety of diagnostic tests have been developed since the 1950s. One of the oldest noninvasive methods is the directional Doppler test. A Doppler device employs a probe with one or two piezoelectric crystals. An ultrasonic signal using a frequency of 2 to 5 megahertz (MHz) is sent into the body. Movement of red blood cells causes a shift in the frequency of the signal that is transmitted back. The amount of shift is proportional to the speed of blood flow. This device can also be used to determine the direction of blood flow. By listening with a continuous-wave Doppler over a branch of the ophthalmic artery at the corner of the eye and performing certain compression maneuvers on the arteries that supply the face, information regarding possible collateral pathways can be obtained concerning internal carotid artery blockages of greater than 75 percent.

The vascular surgeon William Gee developed another device, called an ocular pneumoplethysmograph (OPG). The OPG utilizes cups placed in the eye to measure the ocular pressure. A vacuum is applied to the eyes, effectively blocking the ophthalmic arteries, which are the first major branches of the internal carotid artery. As the vacuum is released, the blood flow is reestablished and the appearance of arterial pulsations is noted on a strip chart. These pulsations denote systolic blood pressure in the ophthalmic arteries. A pressure difference of 5 millimeters of mercury (mm Hg) between the two eyes or an index of less than 0.66 (comparing the systolic blood pressure in the ophthalmic artery with that in the brachial artery) is consistent with carotid artery blockage of more than 50 to 75 percent.

Both of these methods are indirect tests, in which significant internal carotid artery disease is implied if the test is positive. Deficiencies in the test procedures include quantification of the percentage of carotid artery disease or differentiation of significant stenosis from occlusions. They also may be wrong if the vertebral or basal arteries contribute significant collateral blood flow. The OPG is still used in certain situations as a quick screening tool, but the directional Doppler has lost favor as an accurate diagnostic test. Duplex ultrasound machines, first employed in the early 1980s, utilize B-mode (brightness-mode) ultrasound to visualize the vessels and type of plaque. In comparison, Doppler ultrasound can audibly evaluate the blood flow in the vessels. Using real-time spectrum analyzers, the Doppler signals are then analyzed in terms of velocity (speed of the blood flow) and waveform characteristics. The greater the velocity, the greater the amount of stenosis. Absence of blood flow will denote occlusions.

Much research has been done in evaluating plaque morphology and its association with the incidence of TIAs, but results have been controversial using the standard grayscale duplex devices. The use of color duplex ultrasound, in which the Doppler signals are color-coded in terms of flow direction and speed to denote the various flow patterns in normal and diseased vessels, has enhanced the diagnostic accuracies of the examinations. The use of color Doppler in many ultrasound machines is allowing more rapid detection of arterial lesions in blood vessels both inside and outside the skull. Transcranial Doppler uses a MHz pulsed Doppler probe through various normal anatomic windows (holes) in the skull. Measurements can be made through the side of the head (transtemporal), from the back of the head (transoccipital), and through the eye (transocular). The purpose of the examination is to assess the blood circulation in the circle ofWillis. The transcranial Doppler gives information concerning various collateral pathways established when significant disease is present in blood vessels outside the skull. It is also useful when there is stenosis of arteries inside the skull. It is extremely accurate in detecting and monitoring early vasospasm in individuals with bleeding inside the skull. Additional research with this device is ongoing in other areas, such as in the detection of cerebral aneurysms and arteriovenous malformations in which there is an abnormal connection between the arteries and the veins.

Computed tomography (CT) scanning is a radiological technique that provides a three-dimensional picture of the brain and its structures. Occasionally, a contrast medium is also used in this examination. CT scanning is especially useful in the diagnosis of cerebral aneurysms and areas of infarct. Magnetic resonance imaging (MRI) is a nonradiological technique that also provides exceptional three-dimensional images of the soft tissue structures of the brain. MRI can detect cerebral infarcts at an earlier stage than can CT scanning. Arteriography or angiography is an invasive procedure that is performed in a hospital setting. A catheter is placed in one of the arteries, and dye containing iodine is injected. Multiple X rays are then taken to visualize the circulation. Arteriograms are considered to be standard in diagnosis. The delineation of the blockages and collateral pathways is then used primarily to plan surgical procedures.

Aspirin is often prescribed to alleviate symptoms of TIAs and to help protect patients from strokes or heart attacks. Although it is a powerful drug in decreasing the incidence of embolus formation, a national study has demonstrated that patients with a history of TIAs and carotid artery stenosis of greater than 60 percent should undergo surgical revascularization to protect against major strokes. The chances of having a stroke after suffering a TIA are approximately 40 percent greater.

Endarterectomy is a surgical technique in which the inner wall and part of the middle wall of the carotid artery are excised, effectively scraping out atherosclerotic plaques. Although used in other arterial segments, endarterectomy is the most common surgical procedure used to revascularize the carotid arteries. Occasionally, procedures are performed to bypass diseased segments of the cerebral vessels. Long-term research has shown that they have limited effectiveness. Consequently, many have been abandoned.

Other techniques for intervention have been developed. Percutaneous balloon angioplasty involves placing a balloon catheter in the diseased segment during an angiogram. When the balloon catheter is inflated, it opens up the area of stenosis or small segment of occlusion. This method has been employed in the coronary arteries as well as in the vessels leaving the aorta, the iliac arteries, and arteries in the lower extremities. It is not used often in the treatment of atherosclerotic plaques in the cerebral circulation because of the possibility of emboli traveling to the more distant blood vessels of the brain or eye. Some success in the use of balloon angioplasty has been reported in the treatment of vasospasm.

Perspective and Prospects

Stroke is the third-leading cause of death in the United States, with approximately 158,000 deaths annually. There are 700,000 strokes annually, and about one-fourth of all nursing home patients are permanently impaired from strokes. These statistics have a great impact on the amount of money spent annually on care for victims of strokes.

Since the 1960s, the death rate from strokes in the United States has decreased significantly, by about 60 percent. Control of blood pressure and diet, the development of new drugs and diagnostic techniques, and the advent of cardiovascular surgery in the early 1950s have contributed to these results. Unfortunately, strokes are still prevalent given the extent of atherosclerotic disease in the American population, which is largely attributed to a high-fat diet. Autopsies of U.S. soldiers killed in the Korean and Vietnam Wars demonstrated evidence that atherosclerosis begins at a very early age, often by age eighteen. Atherosclerosis is more prevalent in males. Females have more protection until the onset of the menopause. Within five years of the menopause, however, the stroke and death rates of men and women tend to equalize.

High-salt diets, which contribute to hypertension, also contribute to the development and progression of atherosclerosis, as well as hemorrhagic strokes. Ethnic African and Asian populations appear to be at greater risk in this respect. Since the 1960s, however, extensive education of the American public concerning diet and the control of blood pressure has had a favorable impact. More recently, the increase in individuals who have stopped smoking and who have undertaken regular exercise has helped to lower stroke rates further.

Since the 1950s, a number of both noninvasive and invasive procedures have been developed to diagnose atherosclerotic disease. Cardiovascular surgical techniques were developed in the 1950s. The first bypass surgery (arterial autograft) probably occurred during the Korean War. The development of ultrasound devices in the 1950s initiated the research into using these noninvasive devices to diagnose cerebrovascular disease. The duplex devices introduced commercially in the late 1970s and early 1980s have spurred the development of new diagnostic devices for detecting atherosclerotic disease. These devices allow for visualization of plaque morphology (composition of the plaque, such as thrombus, calcium, hemorrhage, and other particulate matters) and blood flow characteristics for a better understanding of the disease process.

Future developments in the field of ultrasound include holographic imaging for the three-dimensional visualization of plaques. These noninvasive technologies will also allow physicians to monitor the effects of new drugs and techniques in the treatment of atherosclerosis. Advances in digital subtraction and computer enhancement of angiographic techniques, along with new contrast media, have made arteriograms safer and more accurate.

Color duplex devices are utilizing low-frequency probes to visualize and produce color scans of blood vessels that lie inside the skull. By analyzing the blood flow direction and velocity in the circle of Willis and within the blood vessels of the skull, physicians will come to a better understanding of the formation of collateral pathways and will learn how to detect other pathological conditions that lead to cerebrovascular disease. Magnetic resonance imaging (MRI) is also being utilized to measure actual flow in individual arterial segments of the body.

Carotid endarterectomies, which lost favor for a period of time, have become the preferred therapeutic treatment for individuals with episodes of TIAs and severe atherosclerotic plaques in the carotid arteries. Additional studies will further delineate which other patient populations may benefit from this surgery. Aspirin still remains a potent drug in the treatment of TIAs in patients with lesser degrees of disease and in post surgery patients. Recognition and prompt treatment of symptomatic cerebrovascular symptoms remain the key to better survival rates.

—*Silvia M. Berry, L. Fleming Fallon Jr., Bradley R.A. Wilson, Patricia Stanfill Edens*

References

Collier, Jasmin. "Being Overweight or Obese May Improve Stroke Survival." *Medical News Today*, 6 Mar. 2019, www.medicalnewstoday.com/articles/324628.

Guo, Yan, et al. "Overweight and Obesity in Young Adulthood and the Risk of Stroke: a Meta-Analysis." *Journal of Stroke and Cerebrovascular Diseases*, vol. 25, no. 12, 2016, pp. 2995–3004., doi:10.1016/j.jstrokecerebrovasdis.2016.08.018.

Mitchell, Andrew B., et al. "Obesity Increases Risk of Ischemic Stroke in Young Adults." *Stroke*, vol. 46, no. 6, 2015, pp. 1690–1692., doi:10.1161/strokeaha.115.008940.

Oesch, Lisa, et al. "Obesity Paradox in Stroke – Myth or Reality? A Systematic Review." *Plos One*, vol. 12, no. 3, 14 Mar. 2017, doi:10.1371/journal.pone.0171334.

Winter, Yaroslav, et al. "Obesity and Abdominal Fat Markers in Patients with a History of Stroke and Transient Ischemic Attacks." *Journal of Stroke and Cerebrovascular Diseases*, vol. 25, no. 5, 2016, pp. 1141–1147., doi:10.1016/j.jstrokecerebrovasdis.2015.12.026.

■ Thyroid cancer

CATEGORY: Disorder

Thyroid cancer is a malignant neoplasm that originates in the cells of the thyroid. The thyroid is a butterfly-shaped organ located at the base of the neck that produces hormones that regulate heart rate, respiration, blood pressure, body weight (by controlling fat and carbohydrate metabolism), and temperature. Thyroid cancer is categorized as papillary, follicular, medullary, or anaplastic depending on the appearance of the cancerous cells. Thyroid cancer tends to respond well to treatment and the 5-year survival rate is nearly 100% for stages I and II. Regardless of successful treatment, thyroid cancer can recur even if the thyroid was removed due to the spread of microscopic cancer cells prior to initial treatment. Recurrence can develop in the lymph nodes of the neck, remaining pieces of thyroid tissue, if present, the lungs, or bones.

Medical Nutrition Therapy for Thyroid Cancer

Cruciferous vegetables (e.g., broccoli, cauliflower, radish, turnip, Brussels sprouts) contain thioglucosides, which can be goitrogenic (i.e., goiter causing) because they block iodine uptake and can increase thyroid stimulating hormone (TSH) levels. However, large amounts of cruciferous vegetables would have to be consumed to induce a goitrogenic effect. Epidemiologic study results show no association between intake of cruciferous vegetables and elevated thyroid cancer risk in well nourished populations, and researchers report that a diet high in fruits and vegetables is associated with reduced risk of developing thyroid cancer.

In geographic locations where salt is not fortified with iodine and other iodine-containing foods (e.g., fish and seafood) are scarce, iodine deficiency can contribute to follicular thyroid cancer risk. However, excessive iodine consumption is associated with an increased risk for developing papillary thyroid carcinoma. Iodine supplementation is not recommended as a preventive strategy in the general population

Overweight and obese individuals are at a greater risk for developing thyroid cancer. High fat intake is a risk factor for becoming overweight or obese, and has been associated with an increased incidence of cancer. It has been estimated that diet

RISK FACTORS	SIGNS AND SYMPTOMS
Age: about two thirds of persons with thyroid cancer are diagnosed when they are younger than 55 years of age	Swollen lymph nodes in the neck A palpable lump in the neck Difficulty swallowing
Gender: women are three times more likely to develop thyroid cancer than men	Pain in the throat or neck that can radiate to the ears
A diet that is deficient in iodine	Difficulty breathing
Exposure to radiation	Persistent cough
Certain inherited conditions or a family history of thyroid cancer, including familial medullary thyroid carcinoma (FMTC), familial adenomatous polyposis (FAP), Cowden disease, and Carney complex, type I.	Fatigue
Personal or family history of goiter (i.e., a benign enlargement of the thyroid gland)	
Obesity is associated with an increased risk for thyroid cancer	

contributes to 35% of all human cancers. Additionally, it has been speculated that 10–70% of cancer-related deaths are preventable by alterations in the diet There are many variables to the contribution of fat intake on cancer risk, including the type of fat (e.g., saturated, unsaturated), preparation of fat (e.g., heating, hydrogenating), and source of fat (e.g., animal or plant). Results of many studies show a correlation between animal fat intake and increased cancer risk, and fat from plant sources has not proven to be a significant risk.

Summary

Individuals diagnosed with thyroid cancer (and their family members/caregivers) should learn about dietary recommendations based on personal characteristics and health needs Family history, maintaining a healthy weight and consuming a diet that is rich in a variety of fruits and vegetables and low in saturated fat may reduce risk for developing thyroid cancer. Patients with thyroid cancer may be at risk for vitamin and mineral deficiencies, malnutrition, and other adverse effects of cancer and its treatment. Dietary and other treatments may be prescribed to improve patient health status and quality of life. It is important to report any health-related changes to the treating clinician as soon as possible to prevent worsening health status. Patients and their family members should understand and adhere to the prescribed treatment regimen, while continuing medical surveillance to monitor health status. Research suggests that non-cruciferous fruits and vegetables may reduce thyroid cancer risk.

—*Cherie Marcel*

References

G sior-Perczak, Danuta, et al. "The Impact of BMI on Clinical Progress, Response to Treatment, and Disease Course in Patients with Differentiated Thyroid Cancer." *Plos One*, vol. 13, no. 10, 1 Oct. 2018, doi:10.1371/journal.pone.0204668.

Kitahara, Cari M, et al. "Impact of Overweight and Obesity on U.S. Papillary Thyroid Cancer Incidence Trends (1995-2015)." *JNCI: Journal of the National Cancer Institute*, 5 Dec. 2019, doi:10.1093/jnci/djz202.

Kwon, Hyemi, et al. "Weight Change Is Significantly Associated with Risk of Thyroid Cancer: A Nationwide Population-Based Cohort Study." *Scientific Reports*, vol. 9, no. 1, 7 Feb. 2019, doi:10.1038/s41598-018-38203-0.

Marcello, M. A., et al. "Obesity and Thyroid Cancer." *Endocrine Related Cancer*, vol. 21, no. 5, 16 Oct. 2014, doi:10.1530/erc-14-0070.

Zhao, Sitong, et al. "Association of Obesity with the Clinicopathological Features of Thyroid Cancer in a Large, Operative Population." *Medicine*, vol. 98, no. 50, 2019, doi:10.1097/md.0000000000018213.

Treatment and Weight Management

■ Aerobics

CATEGORY: Physiology

Aerobics, from the Greek words for air and life, is a term from the field of biology. It refers to sustained moderate physical activity during a specific period of time that requires an additional effort from the cardiovascular system—that is, heart and lungs—in order to increase the transport of oxygen to the muscles. Aerobic exercise is aimed at improving cardiovascular conditioning and lung function. Since its early days as a dance and exercise routine, aerobics has fueled a multibillion dollar industry and become a vital part of American culture.

Brief History

In biology, the word "aerobic" is used to describe organisms that need oxygen to live. Aerobics exercises, then, stimulate breathing are designed to improve how the body oxygenates. Aerobics as an exercise discipline began in the postwar years of the twentieth century, when a medical doctor and former military officer, Kenneth H. Cooper, authored the book *Aerobics* (1968). Cooper was already a respected exercise expert because of the studies he performed with the military. He worked not only to improve the physical condition of American soldiers but also to identify their individual limitations.

Cooper soon became known beyond military circles, as he expanded his research to better understand the benefits of intense physical activity called "cardiovascular workout." His research explored not only physical benefits, but also mental benefits. He continued to publish books on his findings, but it wasn't until 1982 that he could actually put into practice the overall techniques described in his work. In the beginning, however, aerobics lacked widespread acceptance. Some of the obstacles it faced in order to become universally popular were lack of adequate spaces to practice it and the tedium of repetitive exercise.

Cooper's first book has sold about 30 million copies worldwide. Nevertheless, the books and workout videos produced by actor Jane Fonda turned aerobics into an unprecedented mass phenomenon. By the 1990s, advances in the fields of biomechanics and physiology brought radical changes to the field of aerobics. These studies reduced the incidence of injuries incurred in doing aerobic exercise and helped increase the benefits to the body.

The addition of music, dance elements, and attractive gear made aerobic exercise more appealing and played a fundamental role in its widespread popularity. Other cardiovascular exercises were added to enhance aerobics, including boxing, martial arts, water exercises, and bicycling. Technology expanded apace, and gadgets meant to measure factors such as cardiovascular workout and calorie loss entered the market. Aerobics is the most practiced exercise worldwide.

Overview

What made aerobics different from other exercise routines, such as calisthenics, is the link to dance music. This novelty and the fact that it is usually practiced in groups increased its popularity. Eventually aerobics became a common household experience, as routines recorded on videocassettes by experts and celebrities, especially Jane Fonda and Richard Simmons, could be played at home. In time, fitness programs became incorporated into many workplaces.

Another factor that popularized aerobics is that practically everybody can practice some type of aerobics without being an athlete. A typical aerobics routine consists of warming and stretching exercises for about 20 to 30 minutes, to raise the cardiac rate to its target level. The appropriate level depends upon age and health conditions. Exercise intensity then decreases. Some exercise programs include a strength sequence for body-sculpting purposes. Merging aerobics with elements of other dance forms or

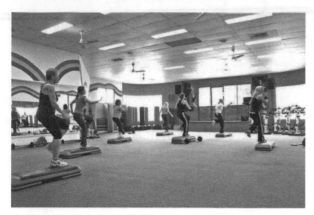

Step aerobics class at a gym. (Photo by www.localfitness.com. au)

sports has become commonplace, producing jazzercise, zumba, spinning, kickboxing, and many others.

Many social forces came together that helped spread the popularity of fitness by way of aerobic exercise. These included science, such as the studies on the health benefits of fitness, as well as government incentives, commercial interests, and national culture. In the United States, the cultivation of health and fitness had long been a cultural factor. The benefits of a healthy lifestyle had been touted by experts and popular periodicals since the nineteenth century. Nevertheless, prior to World War II, to be overly concerned with physical prowess and health was considered strange.

Decades prior to the success of aerobics trailblazer Jane Fonda, strongman Charles Atlas (1892-1972) and exercise guru Jack LaLanne (1914-2011) ran extremely successful marketing campaigns touting the benefits of proper nutrition and exercise. In 1956, President Dwight Eisenhower created the President's Council on Youth Fitness, with the main objective of raising public awareness across the nation. It developed a plan of action and a nationwide pilot program that studied the fitness level of more than eight thousand children between the ages of 5 and 12. In 1965, under President Lyndon B. Johnson, another nationwide fitness study took place with children ages 10 to 17 years of age.

These government studies highlighted a concern, specific to the Cold War period, with the health and fitness of the young. They heralded not only the eventual popularity of aerobics, but also of other new fitness sports such as jogging, which became a craze in the 1970s. Jogging, however, is a mostly solitary sport, and in the 1980s, a preference for the shared experience of health clubs and gyms prevailed.

In the second decade of the twenty-first century, the revenues from the health and fitness industry reached about $33 billion a year, and with continued expectations for growth. Approximately 45 million Americans spend money on exercise technology and gear, club memberships, and myriad other products related to fitness. The expense and other social factors associated with exercise programs, have been cited as cause for exclusion. According to many social scientists, fitness has become a vital part of American identity, raising questions about who gets left behind from participation in it and why. The fact that there are many who cannot afford gym memberships and gear suggests a link between fitness and issues of social class.

—Trudy Mercadal, Geraldine Marrocco

References

Bennie, Jason A., et al. "Muscle Strengthening, Aerobic Exercise, and Obesity: A Pooled Analysis of 1.7 Million US Adults." *Obesity*, 11 Nov. 2019, www.onlinelibrary.wiley.com/doi/pdf/10.1002/oby.22673, 10.1002/oby.22673.

Chiu, Chih-Hui, et al. "Benefits of Different Intensity of Aerobic Exercise in Modulating Body Composition among Obese Young Adults: A Pilot Randomized Controlled Trial." *Health and Quality of Life Outcomes*, vol. 15, no. 1, 24 Aug. 2017, www.ncbi.nlm.nih.gov/pmc/articles/PMC5571495/, 10.1186/s12955-017-0743-4.

Clark, B. Ruth, et al. "Obesity and Aerobic Fitness among Urban Public School Students in Elementary, Middle, and High School." *PLOS ONE*, vol. 10, no. 9, 17 Sept. 2015, p. e0138175, 10.1371/journal.pone.0138175.

Cox, Carla E. "Role of Physical Activity for Weight Loss and Weight Maintenance." *Diabetes Spectrum*, vol. 30, no. 3, Aug. 2017, pp. 157–160, 10.2337/ds17-0013.

Donnelly, Joseph E., et al. "Aerobic Exercise Alone Results in Clinically Significant Weight Loss for Men and Women: Midwest Exercise Trial 2."

Obesity, vol. 21, no. 3, Mar. 2013, pp. E219–E228, 10.1002/oby.20145.

Jang, Sun-Hwa, et al. "Effects of Aerobic and Resistance Exercises on Circulating Apelin-12 and Apelin-36 Concentrations in Obese Middle-Aged Women: A Randomized Controlled Trial." *BMC Women's Health*, vol. 19, no. 1, 29 Jan. 2019, 10.1186/s12905-019-0722-5.

■ American Heart Association: Dietary guidelines

CATEGORY: Nutrition

The American Heart Association (AHA) is a non-profit volunteer organization with a mission statement "to build healthier lives, free of cardiovascular diseases (CVD) and stroke." Some of the contributions the AHA has made to facilitate proper care for persons with CVD and prevention of CVD in the United States include establishing standards for cardiopulmonary resuscitation (CPR) and first aid training and publishing dietary guidelines for reducing CVD risk in the general population.

The most current AHA dietary guidelines are called Diet and Lifestyle Recommendations. The recommendations are based on the findings of the AHA-appointed Dietary Committee, which reviewed hundreds of relevant research studies. Heart-healthy lifestyle patterns include regular exercise, weight maintenance, and control of cholesterol and blood pressure (BP) levels.

AHA Dietary and Lifestyle Recommendations

Balance calorie intake and physical activity to achieve or maintain a healthy body weight. Desirable body mass index (BMI) is 20–25; overweight is a BMI of 25–30 and obese is a BMI > 30. Calculate BMI using the following formulas:

- English units: (weight in pounds/[height in inches × height in inches]) × 703
- Metric units: (weight in kilograms/[height in meters × height in meters])

Education is recommended to increase awareness and understanding of information in food labels, including calorie content of food items and appropriate portion control.

Performing physical activity for 30–60 minutes is recommended for most days of the week.

Consume a diet that is rich in vegetables and fruits. The importance of eating a variety of deeply-colored fruits and vegetables (e.g., spinach, carrots, berries) should be emphasized. Drinking fruit juice should not be encouraged because it does not provide as much fiber as eating whole fruit and has a higher calorie content per serving.

Choose whole grain foods that are high in fiber. Research results show that high dietary fiber intake is associated with a lower risk for CVD and all-cause mortality, although the inverse relationship with all-cause mortality decreases with age. At least half of all grains consumed should be whole grains.

Consume fish, especially oily fish, at least twice a week. Fish is a great source of omega-3, an unsaturated fat that has many health benefits,

---

AHA GOALS FOR CVD PREVENTION

Consume an overall healthy diet.

Aim for a healthy body weight by balancing caloric intake with caloric expenditure.

Aim to meet recommended levels of low-density lipoprotein (LDL) and high density lipoprotein (HDL) cholesterol; recommended levels are LDL < 100 mg/dL and HDL > 60 mg/dL.

Aim to meet the recommended triglyceride level of < 150 mg/dL.

Aim to maintain a normal blood pressure of < 120/80 mm/Hg for adults.

Aim to maintain normal blood glucose levels of < 100 mg/dL.

Participate in regular physical activity.

Avoid the use of and exposure to tobacco products.

including reduced risk for CVD. Certain sources of fish and seafood (e.g., shark, swordfish, king mackerel, tilefish) contain high levels of mercury; although evidence suggests that there is no apparent risk of prenatal mercury exposure from ocean fish consumption alone, high levels of mercury can be harmful to fetal development, infants, younger children, and women of child-bearing age.

Limit intake of saturated fat, trans fat, and cholesterol. Choose lean meats and vegetable alternatives. Choose dairy products that are fat-free (skim), 1% fat, and low-fat. Limit consumption of partially hydrogenated fats. It is currently recommended that dietary fat and cholesterol intake should be limited as follows:

- Total dietary fat < 35% of total caloric intake but not less than 20%.
- Saturated fat < 7% of total caloric intake.
- Trans fat < 1% of total caloric intake.
- Cholesterol < 300 mg/day.

Minimize intake of beverages and foods that contain added sugar.

Choose and prepare foods with little or no salt. Sodium intake should not exceed 2,300 mg/day.

Persons who consume alcohol should do so in moderation. It is recommended that men limit alcohol intake to 2 drinks/day and women limit intake to 1 drink/day, preferably consumed with meals. 1 drink is defined as 12 oz of beer, 4 oz of wine, or 1½ oz of 80-proof liquor.

Continue to follow the AHA dietary and lifestyle recommendations when eating food that is prepared outside of the home (e.g., in restaurants, schools, or grocery stores).

Research Findings
The American Academy of Nutrition and Dietetics recommends presenting educational information regarding the AHA dietary and lifestyle recommendations as a total diet approach that focuses on consuming foods based on a variety of colors and textures, appropriate portions, and moderation rather than on focusing on details of nutrients that can be confusing.

Following the AHA dietary and lifestyle recommendations may benefit bone health according to data retrieved from a cross-sectional

study of 933 Puerto Rican adults who were 47–79 years of age.

Although it is important to limit intake of saturated fat and cholesterol, it is also important to avoid replacing saturated fat and cholesterol with food choices that are high in simple carbohydrates. Diets that are high in simple carbohydrates are associated with the development of dyslipidemia and diabetes. It is important to emphasize that prevention of CVD should focus on diet modification to increase consumption of unsaturated fats, lean proteins, complex carbohydrates, fruits, and vegetables.

Persons who consume a high-fiber diet tend to practice healthier lifestyle habits overall. They are frequently more physically active, eat a diet that is lower in fat and higher in fruits and vegetables, abstain from smoking, and consume less alcohol and caffeine.

Necessary weight loss in persons who are overweight or obese increases insulin activity, improving insulin resistance and reducing the need for medication to control diabetes in patients who have diabetes. Similarly, necessary weight loss improves hypertension and frequently alleviates the need for blood pressure medications in patients diagnosed with hypertension.

Summary
Individuals should become knowledgeable about the current AHA dietary guidelines, called Diet and Lifestyle. These guidelines include eating a well-balanced diet, regular exercise, weight maintenance, and control of cholesterol and blood pressure levels. Dietary compliance with AHA recommendations includes choosing appropriate dietary fat options, balanced with lean protein, complex carbohydrate choices, adequate fruit, vegetable and fiber intake. Research suggests that following the AHA guidelines will reduce risk factors for obesity, hypertension, diabetes, CHD, and cancer.

—Cherie Marcel

References
American Heart Association. "Diet and Lifestyle Recommendations." *American Heart Association*, 15 Aug. 2017, www.heart.org/en/healthy-living/healthy-eating/eat-smart/nutrition-basics/aha-diet-and-lifestyle-recommendations.

Beairsto, Rachael. "AHA Recommends a Focus on Healthy Dietary Choices Over Cholesterol Cut-offs." *Endocrinology Advisor*, 16 Dec. 2019, www.endocrinologyadvisor.com/home/topics/cardiovascular-and-metabolic-disorders/american-heart-association-issues-science-advisory-on-dietary-cholesterol/.

"Dietary Guidelines for Americans 2015–2020." *U.S. Department of Health and Human Services*, Office of Disease Prevention and Health Promotion, Dec. 2015, health.gov/our-work/food-nutrition/2015-2020-dietary-guidelines/guidelines/.

Pallazola, Vincent A., et al. "A Clinician's Guide to Healthy Eating for Cardiovascular Disease Prevention." *Mayo Clinic Proceedings: Innovations, Quality & Outcomes*, vol. 3, no. 3, 2019, pp. 251–267., doi:10.1016/j.mayocpiqo.2019.05.001

Sandoiu, Ana. "Cardiovascular Disease: Dietary Cholesterol May Not Raise Risk." *Medical News Today*, 20 Dec. 2019, www.medicalnewstoday.com/articles/327329.

Tapsell, Linda C, et al. "Foods, Nutrients, and Dietary Patterns: Interconnections and Implications for Dietary Guidelines." *Advances in Nutrition*, vol. 7, no. 3, 1 May 2016, pp. 445–454., doi:10.3945/an.115.011718.

■ Bariatric surgery

CATEGORY: Procedure

ALSO KNOWN AS: Gastric bypass, stomach stapling, weight loss surgery

Indications and Procedures

Candidates for bariatric surgery are the severely obese, with a body mass index (BMI) of 40 or more, or a BMI of 35 to 39 with serious medical conditions, such as diabetes mellitus, heart disease, hypertension, and sleep apnea. Typically, to qualify for surgery patients must first have tried other methods of weight loss (dietary modification, exercise, and/or drug therapy) and must be seriously impaired in their ability to perform routine activities. In addition, patients should undergo extensive psychiatric evaluation to ensure that they understand the risks of the procedure and are motivated enough to cope with its dramatic effects and permanent lifestyle changes.

There are two types of procedures. Restrictive surgery-including vertical banded gastroplasty, gastric banding, or laparoscopic gastric banding (lap band)-uses bands or staples near the top of the stomach to create a small pouch that restricts food intake to no more than one-half to one cup. The stoma, a tiny gap in the pouch that opens into the lower stomach, slows the emptying of the pouch to prolong fullness, thus reducing hunger.

Malabsorptive surgery involves surgical rearrangement of the digestive system to bypass parts of the stomach and small intestine, where most nutrients are absorbed. Rouxen-Y gastric bypass is the most commonly performed operation, derived from a procedure developed in 1966 by Edward E. Mason and named after the Y-shaped connection it creates. Roux-en-Y combines restriction with malabsorption, bypassing the lower stomach and the duodenum to connect the stomach pouch directly to the jejunum, or (less frequently) the ileum. In biliopancreatic diversion, sometimes performed on patients with a BMI of 50 or more, a portion of the stomach is actually removed, with the remaining section attached directly to the ileum, thus shortening the small intestine drastically to produce greater weight loss.

Uses and Complications

To lose weight and keep it off, surgery alone is not enough; strict diet and exercise regimens must be maintained. On average, bypass patients lose 66 percent of their excess weight after two years but gain some back as a result of stretching of the pouch over time. At five years, the loss of excess weight typically stabilizes at 33 to 50 percent. Restrictive procedures tend to result in comparatively less weight loss because there is no malabsorption. Diabetes, hypertension, and high cholesterol may improve significantly after surgery, often before marked weight loss occurs. Arthritis, sleep apnea, and other obesity-related conditions may gradually improve as weight is lost. In addition, patients often experience improved mobility and stamina and may report enhanced self-esteem and social acceptance.

Patients with very severe obesity, heart disease, diabetes, or sleep apnea and those who have inexperienced surgeons are at greater risk of developing complications. Gastric bypass patients face a 0.5 to 1.0 percent fatality rate; restrictive surgery

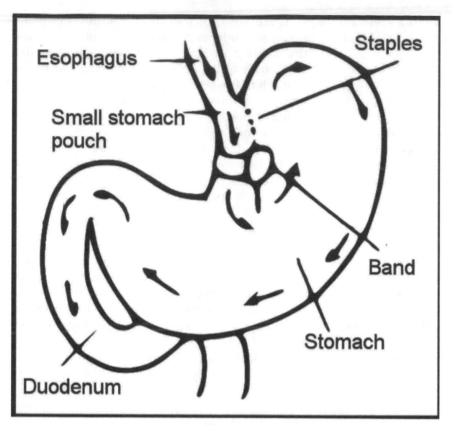

In the vertical banded gastroplasty, also called the Mason procedure or stomach stapling, a part of the stomach is permanently stapled to create a smaller pre-stomach pouch, which serves as the new stomach. (National Institute of Diabetes and Digestive and Kidney Disease)

malabsorptive procedures by definition will suffer from nutritional deficiencies, including anemia and metabolic bone disease resulting in osteoporosis, unless supplements are taken daily; regular vitamin B_{12} shots are necessary for some patients. Many patients will require further cosmetic surgery to remove large, sagging folds of skin.

All patients may experience vomiting from eating too much or too quickly. Pain behind the breastbone can result from insufficient chewing, causing large food particles to lodge in the stoma. About 70 percent of gastric bypass patients will develop dumping syndrome, a condition caused by eating too much fat or sugar, which can result in severe dizziness or weakness, abdominal cramps, nausea, vomiting, and diarrhea. Biliopancreatic bypass is further associated with chronic diarrhea and other long-term complications such as liver disease.

patients fare better at 0.1 percent. Follow-up operations are required in 10 to 20 percent of patients. Most lap band patients experience at least one side effect, including abdominal pain, heartburn, nausea, vomiting, and band slippage to the extent that up to 25 percent may have the bands removed. If staples are used, then the risk of developing a leak or rupture is around 1.5 percent, leading to serious infection and often requiring further surgeries; laparoscopic patients appear to be at higher risk. Because 30 percent of patients develop gallstones after surgery as a result of rapid weight loss, the gallbladder is often removed as well. In 2 percent of cases, the spleen may be injured, necessitating its removal.

Other complications include blood clots, gaseous distention, infection, bowel or esophageal perforation, bowel strangulation, hernias, strictures, ulcers, late staple breakdown, menstrual irregularities, and hair loss. Patients undergoing

Perspective and Prospects

Surgical treatment for obesity began in the early 1950s with dangerous intestinal bypass procedures. As techniques have improved, the number of surgeries performed has mushroomed. The American Society for Bariatric Surgery reports that its member surgeons performed 28,800 operations in 1999 and 63,100 in 2002. During the same period, however, many more of the lucrative surgeries were performed by nonmembers. As of 2007, no regulatory body oversaw bariatric surgical practices, and board certification was voluntary. Evolving surgical practices and long-term outcomes remain difficult to evaluate as clinical trial data are lacking, and proof of overall improvements in health and longevity is scanty. According to the American Medical Association (AMA), the long-term consequences of weight loss surgery remain uncertain. To establish the overall safety and efficacy of such surgery, more research and stringent clinical trials are needed.

—*Sue Tarjan*

References

Bencsath, Kalman, et al. "Outcomes of Bariatric Surgery in Morbidly Obese Patients with Multiple Sclerosis." *Journal of Obesity*, vol. 2017, 2017, pp. 1–5, 10.1155/2017/1935204.

Kang, Jenny H., and Quang A. Lc. "Effectiveness of Bariatric Surgical Procedures." *Medicine*, vol. 96, no. 46, Nov. 2017, p. e8632, journals.lww.com/md-journal/Fulltext/2017/11170/Effectiveness_of_bariatric_surgical_procedures__A.48.aspx, 10.1097/md.0000000000008632.

Khattab, Ahmed, and Mark A. Sperling. "Obesity in Adolescents and Youth: The Case for and against Bariatric Surgery." *The Journal of Pediatrics*, vol. 207, Apr. 2019, pp. 18–22, 10.1016/j.jpeds.2018.11.058.

Kizy, Scott, et al. "Bariatric Surgery: A Perspective for Primary Care." *Diabetes Spectrum*, vol. 30, no. 4, Nov. 2017, pp. 265–276, 10.2337/ds17-0034.

Maciejewski, Matthew L., et al. "Bariatric Surgery and Long-Term Durability of Weight Loss." *JAMA Surgery*, vol. 151, no. 11, 1 Nov. 2016, p. 1046, 10.1001/jamasurg.2016.2317.

Wolfe, Bruce M., et al. "Treatment of Obesity." *Circulation Research*, vol. 118, no. 11, 27 May 2016, pp. 1844–1855, 10.1161/circresaha.116.307591.

■ Breakfast consumption

CATEGORY: Nutrition

As the name implies, breakfast is the meal that breaks the fast that occurs during nighttime sleep. Research shows that breakfast plays a significant role in overall nutrient consumption, energy balance, and weight management. More than half of all adults in the United States are classified as overweight or obese, which increases risk for many chronic and potentially life-threatening diseases (e.g., diabetes mellitus type-2 [DM2], cardiovascular disease [CVD], and cancer). One simple strategy for achieving and maintaining a healthy bodyweight is to consume breakfast as part of the daily meal plan. Researchers consistently report that individuals who regularly consume breakfast are less likely to be overweight or obese, tend to have a lower body mass index (BMI; i.e., a measure of body weight in relation to height), and are more likely to consume a balanced diet and have a higher daily nutrient intake compared with persons who do not eat breakfast.

Recommendations for Breakfast Consumption

Choose nutrient-dense foods such as whole grains, fresh fruits, nuts, and low-fat dairy products.

Consume between 400–500 calories at the breakfast meal. Typical breakfasts that are served in diners and other breakfast restaurants can be in excess of 1000 calories.

Avoid foods that have the highest content of carbohydrates and simple-sugars (e.g., potatoes, sweet breads, pancakes), which can result in a sharp increase in the level of blood sugar and increased hunger. High-fiber options (e.g., whole grains, fresh fruit) slow digestion and the release of sugar into the bloodstream and increase the sensation of satiety (i.e., feeling full after eating).

Including lean sources of protein (e.g., egg whites, yogurt, quinoa) at the breakfast meal helps to increase satiety and prevents sharp increases in blood sugar levels. Although egg yolks are a significant source of cholesterol, research results indicate that eating 1–2 eggs/day does not significantly affect the blood lipid profile (i.e., level of cholesterol and triglycerides in the blood), and does not appear to increase the risk for CVD.

Research Findings

Results of studies show that fortified breakfast cereals make a significant contribution to the nutrient intake of people in developed countries. Researchers suggest that health promotion efforts should focus on encouraging consumption of breakfast.

Researchers report that consuming eggs for breakfast instead of bagels with equivalent caloric content results in less variation of plasma glucose and insulin as well as a reduction in daily caloric intake. Research also indicates that replacing bagels with eggs at breakfast can help to promote weight loss. These benefits were reported with no apparent detrimental impact on lipid profiles.

Isgin, K., et al. "Breakfast Skipping Linked to the Risk of Obesity in School-Aged Children." *Journal of the Academy of Nutrition and Dietetics*, vol. 117, no. 9, 2017, doi:10.1016/j.jand.2017.06.352.

Sievert, Katherine, et al. "Effect of Breakfast on Weight and Energy Intake: Systematic Review and Meta-Analysis of Randomised Controlled Trials." *BMJ*, 30 Jan. 2019, p. 142., doi:10.1136/bmj.l42.

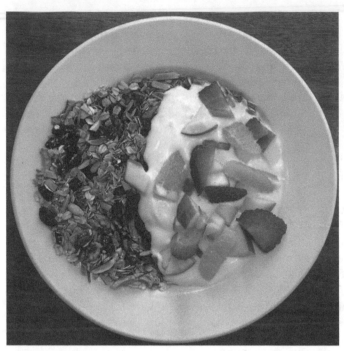

Granola, yogurt, and fruit can make a healthy breakfast. (Arnold Gatilao)

Summary

Individuals should become knowledgeable about the physiologic benefits of breakfast consumption. Research suggests that individuals who regularly consume breakfast are less likely to be overweight or obese, and are more likely to consume a balanced diet throughout the day with higher nutrient intake compared with persons who do not eat breakfast. Breakfast should consist of 400–500 calories and include a variety of foods such as, whole grains, fresh fruits, nuts, low-fat dairy products and lean protein.

—*Cherie Marcel*

References

Forkert, Elsie C. O., et al. "Skipping Breakfast Is Associated with Adiposity Markers Especially When Sleep Time Is Adequate in Adolescents." *Scientific Reports*, vol. 9, no. 1, 23 Apr. 2019, doi:10.1038/s41598-019-42859-7.

Hopkins, Laura C., et al. "Breakfast Consumption Frequency and Its Relationships to Overall Diet Quality, Using Healthy Eating Index 2010, and Body Mass Index among Adolescents in a Low-Income Urban Setting." *Ecology of Food and Nutrition*, vol. 56, no. 4, 12 Dec. 2017, pp. 297–311., doi:10.1080/03670244.2017.1327855.

■ Dance

CATEGORY: Physiology; Psychology

Overview

One of the creative arts therapies, dance movement therapy is defined by the American Dance Therapy Association (ADTA) as "the psychotherapeutic use of movement as a process that furthers the emotional, cognitive, social and physical integration of the individual." Many practitioners consider Marian Chace to be the pioneer of dance movement therapy.

Chace began teaching dance in Washington, D.C., after retiring from the Denishawn Dance Company in 1930. She had noticed that some of her students were more interested in the emotions that they felt while dancing than in learning the techniques of modern dance. Intrigued, Chace learned that they valued the catharsis of feelings they experienced while dancing. Some of these students were concurrently undergoing traditional psychotherapy with psychiatrists, who noticed that their patients felt more refreshed and unburdened after their lessons with Chace. The psychiatrists began to send other patients to Chase's classes, and they noted the positive change that dance appeared to inspire.

Chace was then invited to volunteer with those considered too disturbed to participate in therapy. The nonverbal approach of dance elicited improvement, and by the 1950s, Chace's methods were subjected to serious study.

Mechanism of Action

The principle behind dance movement therapy is that dance is the most fundamental of all the arts, requiring no external materials. It is a communication of the psyche, expressed through self-directed movement. Dance movement therapists assume that the body, mind, and spirit are interconnected, allowing for direct access to feelings, cognition, and behavior. Bodily movement simultaneously provides the means of both intervention and assessment in this mode of therapy. Participants are encouraged to choose their own music and to begin moving to it in their own ways.

The dance movement therapist begins by empathically mirroring the participant's actions, and then extends and expands them into a non-verbal statement of emotion that can release the participant from any fixed muscular patterns. Next, participants are gently coaxed into a circle and led into movement extensions with verbal narration. Once the group is a more cohesive unit, the therapist notes the styles of the participants and leads into the development of a global psychological theme for the session, with questions to shed light on individual conflicts. The session ends with communal movement from all participants to provide closure.

Uses and Applications

Chace believed that dance served as a medium for communication for the most disturbed psychiatric patients, such as schizophrenics. However, today dance movement therapists work with groups and individuals of all ages who have widely differing problems. They may work in private practice, wellness clinics, rehabilitation centers, nursing homes, and schools. The focus on positive body movement may help clients with eating disorders and body issues. The nonverbal conflict revelations and resolutions may help dysfunctional families develop communication skills, and those who have been through trauma such as abuse or violence may find a new mode of constructive coping. The physical therapy uses of dance movement therapy are self-evident, and it is often used with the frail and elderly.

Disease prevention and health promotion, a new area of specialization in dance movement therapy, is beginning to be used in programs for people with chronic medical conditions such as cardiovascular disease, chronic pain, and hypertension. Research on the effectiveness of dance movement therapy has investigated certain settings, such as prisons and homeless shelters, and specific populations, such as the mentally disabled, suicidal persons, the visually and hearing impaired, and autistic persons.

Scientific Evidence

A 1993 study suggested that dance movement therapy improved balance, rhythmic discrimination, mood, social interaction, and energy level in older persons with neurological damage. A 2010 study evaluated the influence of dance movement therapy on the perception of well-being in women with chronic fatigue syndrome. Seven persons attended a four-month program and were tested both before and after the program. Their perceptions of physical well-being improved by an average of 25.8 percent, and their perceptions of psychological well-being improved by 22.7 percent.

A 2008 dance movement therapy intervention group of persons with dementia improved in a task of visual-spatial ability and planning, whereas the control group either remained unchanged or deteriorated slightly. Dance movement therapy appears to be effective in treating cognition and self-care abilities in dementia.

A 2006 study assessed mildly depressed adolescents after twelve weeks of dance movement therapy. All self-report measurements of distress decreased significantly after the twelve weeks. In addition, both serotonin and dopamine levels increased in that group. Thus, dance movement therapy may help to decrease depression both by relieving perceptions of distress and by lowering neurotransmitter levels.

—*Eugenia M. Valentine, Ph.D.*

References

"Dance Therapy and Obesity." *Clinical Trials*, U.S. National Library of Medicine, 16 Dec. 2014, clinicaltrials.gov/ct2/show/NCT01451892. Accessed 5 Mar. 2020.

Koch, Sabine C., et al. "Effects of Dance Movement Therapy and Dance on Health-Related Psychological Outcomes. A Meta-Analysis Update." *Frontiers in Psychology*, vol. 10, 20 Aug. 2019, 10.3389/fpsyg.2019.01806.

Krishnan, Sridevi, et al. "Zumba® Dance Improves Health in Overweight/Obese or Type 2 Diabetic Women." *American Journal of Health Behavior*, vol. 39, no. 1, 1 Jan. 2015, pp. 109–120, 10.5993/ajhb.39.1.12.

Runenko, Svetlana D., et al. "Efficiency of Dance Therapy for Weight Loss and Improvement of the Psychological and Physiological State in Overweight or Obese Young Women." *Journal of Physical Education and Sport*, vol. 18, no. 2, June 2018.

■ Dietary reference intakes (DRIs)

CATEGORY: Biology

Development

The dietary reference intakes (DRIs) include four reference values that can be used in assessing and planning a healthy diet throughout the life span: estimated average requirement (EAR), recommended dietary allowance (RDA), adequate intake (AI), and tolerable upper intake limit (UL). The RDA is the amount of a nutrient needed to meet the needs of nearly all healthy individuals. In setting the RDA, an EAR is first determined. The EAR is the amount of a specific nutrient that is believed to meet the needs of half of the population. Using the assumption of a normal distribution of nutrient needs, the RDA is calculated from the EAR and the standard deviation of requirements. When data are insufficient to calculate an EAR, the available data are used to estimate an AI. The AI is similar to the RDA but acknowledges that additional research concerning nutrient requirements is needed in that area. The UL represents the highest daily intake of a nutrient that is known to pose no health risks.

The EAR, RDA, and AI cannot be used to address the needs of those with chronic or acute disease. It can be assumed that intakes below the EAR probably need to be improved, since at this level 50 percent of the population would have inadequate intake. Intakes between the EAR for a specific nutrient and the RDA also may be improved. Intakes at or above the RDA probably are adequate, although many days of intake should be evaluated because of day-to-day variation. It is more difficult to be certain of the adequacy of intake when using AIs. However, in general, intakes below the AIs should probably be improved. Intakes at or above the UL should be lowered.

Nutrients for which EARs and RDAs have been established include phosphorus, magnesium, thiamine, riboflavin, niacin, vitamin B_6, folate, vitamin B_{12}, vitamin C, vitamin E, and selenium for adults and children over one year of age. Those for which an AI has been set include calcium, vitamin D, fluoride, pantothenic acid, biotin, and choline.

Perspective and Prospects

Although these reference values could be used for labeling and fortification guidelines, they are not yet being implemented as such. The current daily value (DV percent) on the nutrition facts labels rely on the 1968 version of the nutrient reference values. The major difficulty in applying the newer reference values for labeling purposes rests on how to choose a "reference" age group or gender. Currently the DV reflect needs for a male adult.

The first nutrient-based guidelines for healthy intake were released in 1941 in the United States, with similar guidelines released in Canada in 1938. Much research has occurred since that time concerning recording and assessing nutrient intake and in determining human requirements. However, the use of these guidelines has always been to assist in planning meals for individuals and groups, including federal assistance programs.

—*Karen Chapman-Novakofski*

References

Aranceta, Javier, and Carmen Pérez-Rodrigo. "Recommended Dietary Reference Intakes, Nutritional Goals and Dietary Guidelines for Fat and Fatty Acids: a Systematic Review." *British Journal of Nutrition*, vol. 107, no. S2, 2012, doi:10.1017/s0007114512001444.

Insel, Paul M. *Discovering Nutrition*. 4th ed. Jones & Bartlett Learning, 2013.

Poli, Vanessa Fadanelli Schoenardie, et al. "The Excessive Caloric Intake and Micronutrient Deficiencies Related to Obesity after a Long-Term Interdisciplinary Therapy." *Nutrition*, vol. 38, 2017, pp. 113–119., doi:10.1016/j.nut.2017.01.012.

Ross, A. Catharine, et al., eds. *Dietary Reference Intakes for Calcium and Vitamin D*. National Academies Press, 2011.

U.S. Department of Health and Human Services and U.S. Department of Agriculture. *2015 – 2020 Dietary Guidelines for Americans*. 8th ed. USDA and HHS, 2015. https://health.gov/our-work/food-and-nutrition/2015-2020-dietary-guidelines/.

Yetley, Elizabeth A, et al. "Options for Basing Dietary Reference Intakes (DRIs) on Chronic Disease Endpoints: Report from a Joint US-/Canadian-Sponsored Working Group." *The American Journal of Clinical Nutrition*, vol. 105, no. 1, 7 Dec. 2016, doi:10.3945/ajcn.116.139097.

Substance	Amount (males)	Amount (females)	Top Sources in Common Measures
Water[i]	3.7 L/day	2.7 L/day	water, watermelon, iceberg lettuce
Carbohydrates	45-65% of calories[ii]		milk, grains, fruits, vegetables
	130 g/day	130 g/day	
Protein[iii]	10-35% of calories[iv]		meats, fish, legumes (pulses and lentils), nuts, milk, cheeses, eggs
	56 g/day	46 g/day	
Fiber	38 g/day	25 g/day	barley, bulgur, rolled oats, legumes, nuts, beans, apples
Fat	20–35% of calories		oils, butter, lard, nuts, seeds, fatty meat cuts, egg yolk, cheeses
Linoleic acid, an omega-6 fatty acid (polyunsaturated)	17 g/day	12 g/day	sunflower seeds and oil, safflower oil
alpha-Linolenic acid, an omega-3 fatty acid (polyunsaturated)	1.6 g/day	1.1 g/day	Linseed oil (flax seed), chia seed, hemp seed, walnut, soybeans
Cholesterol	300 milligrams(mg)		chicken giblets, turkey giblets, beef liver, egg yolk
Trans fatty acids	As low as possible		partially hydrogenated oils, margarine
Saturated fatty acids	As low as possible while consuming a nutritionally adequate diet		coconut meat, coconut oil, lard, cheeses, butter, chocolate, egg yolk
Added sugar	No more than 25% of calories		non-natural sweet foods: sweets, cookies, cakes, jams, energy and soda drinks, many processed foods

i Includes water from food, beverages, and drinking water.
ii Acceptable Macronutrient Distribution Range (AMDR).
iii Based on 0.8 g/kg of body weight.
iv Acceptable Macronutrient Distribution Range (AMDR).

■ Exercise

CATEGORY: Physiology

Science and Profession

The primary aim of research in the field of exercise physiology is to gain a better understanding of the quantity and type of exercise needed for health maintenance and rehabilitation. A major goal of professionals in exercise physiology is to find ways to incorporate appropriate levels of physical activity into the lifestyles of all individuals.

Physiology is the science of the physical and chemical factors and processes involved in the function of living organisms. The study of exercise physiology examines these factors and processes as they relate to physical exertion. The physical responses that occur are specific to the intensity, duration, and type of exercise performed.

Exercise of low or moderate intensity relies on oxygen to release energy for work. This process is often referred to as aerobic exercise. In the muscles, carbohydrates and fats are broken down to produce adenosine triphosphate (ATP), the basic molecule used for energy. Aerobic exercise can be sustained for several minutes to several hours.

Higher-intensity exercise is predominantly fueled anaerobically (in the absence of oxygen) and can be sustained for up to two minutes only. Muscle glycogen is broken down without oxygen to produce ATP. Anaerobic metabolism is much less efficient at producing ATP than is aerobic metabolism.

During anaerobic metabolism, a by-product called lactic acid begins to accumulate in the blood as blood lactate. The point at which this accumulation begins is called the anaerobic threshold (AT), or the onset of blood lactate accumulation (OBLA). Blood lactate can cause muscle soreness and stiffness, but it also can be used as fuel during aerobic metabolism.

A third and less often used energy system is the creatine phosphate (ATP-CP) system. Using the very limited supply of ATP that is stored in the muscles, phosphate molecules are exchanged between ATP and CP to provide energy. This system provides only enough fuel for a few seconds of maximum effort.

The type of muscle fiber recruited to perform a specific type of exercise is also dependent on exercise intensity. Skeletal muscle is composed of "slow-twitch" and two types of "fast-twitch" muscle fibers. Slow-twitch fibers are more suited to using oxygen than are fast-twitch fibers, and they are recruited primarily for aerobic exercise. One type of fast-twitch fiber also functions during aerobic activity. The second type of fast-twitch fiber serves to facilitate anaerobic, or high-intensity, exercise.

Exercise mode is also a factor in people's physiological responses to exercise. Dynamic exercise (alternating muscular contraction and relaxation through a range of motion) using many large muscles requires more oxygen than does activity using smaller and fewer muscles. The greater the oxygen requirement of the physical activity, the greater the cardiorespiratory benefits.

Many bodily adaptations occur over a training period of six to eight weeks, and other benefits are gradually manifested over several months. The positive adaptations include reduced resting and working heart rates. As the heart becomes stronger, there is a subsequent increase in stroke volume (the volume of blood the heart pumps with each beat), which allows the heart to beat less frequently while maintaining the same cardiac output (the volume of the blood pumped from the heart each minute). Another beneficial adaptation is increased metabolic efficiency. This is partially facilitated by an increase in the number of mitochondria (the organelles responsible for ATP production) in the muscle cells.

One of the most recognized representations of aerobic fitness is the maximum volume of oxygen (VO_{2max}) an individual can use during exercise. VO_{2max} is improved through habitual, relatively high-intensity aerobic activity. After three to six months of regular training, levels of high-density lipoproteins (HDLs) in the blood increase. HDL molecules remove cholesterol (a fatty substance) from the tissues to aid in protecting the heart from atherosclerosis.

Various internal and external factors influence the metabolic processes that take place during and after exercise. Internally, nutrition, degree of hydration, body composition, flexibility, sex, and age are some of the variables that play a role in the physiological responses. Other internal variables include medical conditions such as heart disease, diabetes, and hypertension (high blood pressure). Externally, environmental conditions such as temperature, humidity, and altitude alter how the exercising body functions.

Various modes of exercise testing and data collection are used to study the physiological responses of the body to exercise. Treadmills and cycle ergometers (instruments that measure work and power output) are among the most common methods of evaluating maximum oxygen consumption. During these tests, special equipment and computers analyze expired air, heart rate is monitored with an electrocardiograph (ECG), and blood pressure is taken using a sphygmomanometer. Blood and muscle-fiber samples can also be extracted to aid in identifying the fuel system and type of muscle fibers being used. Other data sometimes collected, such as skin temperature and body-core temperature, can provide pertinent information.

Metabolic equivalent units, or METs, are often used to translate a person's capability into workloads on various pieces of exercise equipment or into everyday tasks. For every 3.5 milliliters of oxygen consumed per kilogram of body weight per minute, the subject is said to be performing at a workload of one MET. One MET is approximately equivalent to 1.5 kilocalories per minute, or the amount of energy expended per kilogram of body weight in one minute when a person is at rest.

Another factor greatly affecting the physical response to exercise is body composition. The three major structural components of the body are muscle, bone, and fat. Body composition can be evaluated using a combination of anthropometric measurements. These measurements include body weight, standard height, measurements of circumferences at various locations using a tape measure, measurements of skeletal diameters using a sliding metric stick, and measurements of skinfold thicknesses using calipers.

Body fat can be estimated using several methods, the most accurate of which is based on a calculation of body density. This method, called hydrostatic weighing, involves weighing the subject under water while taking into account the residual volume of air in the lungs. The principle underlying this measurement of body density is based on the fact that fat is less dense than water and thus will float, whereas bone and muscle, which are denser than water, will sink. One biochemical technique often used to determine levels of body fat is based on the relatively constant level

of potassium-40 naturally existing in lean body mass. Another method uses ultrasound waves to measure the thickness of fat layers. X-rays and computed tomography (CT) scanning can be used to provide images from which fat and bone can be measured. Bioelectrical impedance (BIA) is a method of estimating body composition based on the resistance imposed on a low-voltage electrical current sent through the body. The most widely used and easily assessable method, however, involves measurement of skinfolds at various sites on the body using calipers. In all cases, mathematical formulas have been devised to interpret the collected data and provide the best estimate of an individual's body composition.

Other tests have been developed to determine muscular strength, muscular endurance, and flexibility. Muscular strength is often measured by performance of one maximal effort produced by a selected muscle group. Muscular endurance of a muscle or muscle group is often demonstrated by the length of time or number of repetitions a particular submaximal workload or skill can be performed.

Two major types of flexibility have been identified. One type consists of the ability to move a muscle group or joint through its full range of motion at low speeds or hold a part of the body still at the extent of its range of motion. This is called static flexibility, and it can be measured using a metric stick or a protractor-type instrument called a goniometer. Dynamic flexibility, the other major identified type of flexibility, is the flexibility through the full range of motion of a muscle group or joint at normal or high speeds. Measuring dynamic flexibility is much more difficult.

Overlapping the science of exercise physiology are the studies of biomechanics or kinesiology (sciences dealing with human movement) and nutrition. Only through an understanding of efficient body mechanics and proper nutrition can the physiological responses of the body to exercise be identified correctly.

Diagnostic and Treatment Techniques

Exercise prescription is the primary focus in the application of exercise physiology. General health maintenance, cardiac rehabilitation, and competitive athletics are three major areas of exercise prescription.

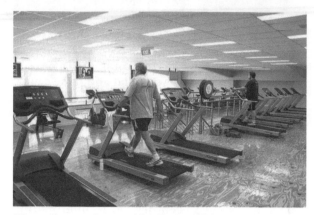

The cardio area of a gym. (Credit: LocalFitness.com.au)

Before making recommendations for an exercise program, an exercise physiologist must evaluate the physical limitations of the exerciser. In a normal health-maintenance setting, often called a "wellness" program, a health-related questionnaire can reveal relevant information. Such a questionnaire should include questions about family medical history and the subject's history of heart trouble or chest pain, bone or joint problems, and high blood pressure. The presence of any of these problems suggests the need for a physician's consent prior to exercising. After the individual has been deemed eligible to participate, an assessment of the level of physical fitness should be performed. Determining or estimating VO_{2max}, muscular strength, muscular endurance, flexibility, and body composition is usually part of this assessment. It is then possible to design a program best suited to the needs of the individual.

For the healthy adult participant, the American College of Sports Medicine (ACSM), a widely recognized authoritative body on exercise prescription, recommends three to five sessions of aerobic exercise weekly. Each session should include a five- to ten-minute warm-up period, twenty to sixty minutes of aerobic exercise at a predetermined exercise intensity, and a five- to ten-minute cool-down period.

To recommend an appropriate aerobic exercise intensity, the exercise physiologist must determine an individual's maximum heart rate. The best way to obtain this maximum heart rate is to administer a maximal exercise test. Such a test can be supervised by an exercise physiologist or an exercise-test technician; it is advisable, especially for the older

participant, that a cardiologist also be in attendance. An ECG is monitored for irregularities as the subject walks, runs, cycles, or performs some dynamic exercise to exhaustion or until the onset of irregular symptoms or discomfort.

Exercise prescription using heart rate as a measure can be achieved by various methods. A direct correlation exists between exercise intensity, in terms of oxygen consumption, and heart rate. From data collected during a maximal exercise test, a target heart-rate range of 40 to 85 percent of functional capacity can be calculated. Another method used to determine an appropriate heart-rate range is based on the difference between an individual's resting heart rate and maximum heart rate, called the heart-rate reserve (HRR). Values representing 60 percent and 80 percent of the HRR are calculated and added to the resting heart rate, yielding the individual's target heart-rate range. A third method involves calculating 70 percent and 85 percent of the maximum heart rate. Although this method is less accurate than the other two methods, it is the simplest way to estimate a target heart-rate range.

Intensity of exercise can also be prescribed using METs. This method relies on the predetermined metabolic equivalents required to perform activities at various intensities. Activity levels reflecting 40 to 85 percent of functional capacity can be calculated.

The rating of perceived exertion (RPE) is another method of prescribing exercise intensity. Verbal responses by the participant describing how an exercise feels at various intensities are assigned to a numerical scale, which is then correlated to heart rate. Through practice, the participant learns to associate heart rate with the RPE, reducing the necessity of frequent pulse monitoring in the healthy individual.

Adequate physical fitness can be defined as the ability to perform daily tasks with enough reserve for emergency situations. All aspects of health-related fitness direct attention toward this goal. Aerobic exercise often provides some conditioning for muscular endurance, but muscular strength and flexibility need to be addressed separately.

The ACSM recommends resistance training using the "overload principle," which involves placing habitual stress on a system, causing it to adapt and respond. For this training, it is suggested that eight to twelve repetitions of eight to ten strengthening exercises of the major muscle groups be performed a minimum of two days per week.

Flexibility of connective tissue and muscle tissue is essential to maximize physical performance and limit musculoskeletal injuries. At least one stretching exercise for each major muscle group should be executed three to four times per week while the muscles are warm. Three methods of stretching that have been designed to improve flexibility are ballistic stretching, static stretching, and proprioceptive neuromuscular facilitation (PNF). Ballistic stretching incorporates a bouncing motion and is generally prescribed only in sports that replicate this type of movement. During a static stretch, the muscles and connective tissue are passively stretched to their maximum lengths. PNF involves a contract-relax sequence of the muscle.

In addition to exercise prescription for cardio-respiratory fitness, muscular fitness, and flexibility, it is appropriate for the exercise physiologist to make recommendations concerning body composition. Exercise is an effective tool in fat loss. Dietary caloric restriction without exercise results in a greater loss of muscle mass along with fat than if exercise is part of a weight loss program.

For persons with special health concerns, such as diabetes mellitus or high blood pressure, the exercise physiologist works with the participant's physician. The physician prescribes necessary medications and often decides which modes of exercise are contraindicated (that is, should be avoided).

A second application, cardiac rehabilitation, takes exercise prescription a step further. Participation of a heart patient in cardiac rehabilitation is more individualized than in wellness programs. The conditions of the circulatory system, pulmonary system, and joints are only a few of the special concerns. Secondary conditions such as obesity, diabetes, and hypertension must also be considered. The responsibilities of cardiac-rehabilitation specialists include monitoring blood sugar in diabetic patients and blood pressure in all patients, especially those with hypertension. Many drugs affect heart rate or blood pressure, and most of these participants are taking more than one type of medication. Patients with heart damage caused by a heart attack may display atypical heart rhythms, which can be seen on an ECG monitor. Furthermore, the stage of recovery of the postsurgical patient is a major factor in recommending the type, frequency, intensity, and duration of exercise.

Patient education is also important. Lifestyle is usually the main factor in the development of heart disease. Cardiac patients often have never participated in a regular exercise program. They may smoke, be overweight, or have poor eating habits. Helping them to identify and correct destructive health-related behaviors is the focus of education for the heart patient.

A third application of the study of exercise physiology involves dealing with the competitive athlete. In this case, findings from the most recent research are constantly applied to yield the best athletic performance possible. A delicate balance of aerobic training, anaerobic training, strength training, endurance training, and flexibility exercises are combined with the optimum percentage of body fat, proper nutrition, and adequate sleep. The program that is designed must enhance the athletic qualities that are most beneficial to the sport in which the athlete participates.

The competitive athlete usually pushes beyond the boundaries of general exercise prescription in terms of intensity, duration, and frequency of exercise performance. As a result, the athlete risks suffering more injuries than the individual who exercises for health benefits. If the athlete sustains an injury, the exercise physiologist may work in conjunction with an athletic trainer or sports physician to return the athlete to competition as soon as possible.

Perspective and Prospects

The modern study of exercise physiology developed out of an interest in physical fitness. In the United States, the concern for development and maintenance of physical fitness was well established by the end of the twentieth century. As early as 1819, Stanford and Harvard Universities offered professional physical-education programs. At least one textbook on the physiology of exercise was published by that time.

Much of the pioneer work in this field, however, was done in Europe. Nobel Prize-winning European research on muscular exercise, oxygen utilization as it relates to the upper limits of physical performance, and production of lactic acid during glucose metabolism dates back to the 1920s.

In the early 1950s, poor performance by children in the United States on a minimal muscular fitness test helped lead to the formation of what became known as the President's Council on Physical Fitness and Sport. Concurrently, a significant number of deaths of middle-aged American males were found to be caused by poor health habits associated with coronary artery disease. A need for more research in the areas of health and physical activity was recognized by the mid-1960s. The subsequent research was facilitated by the existence of fifty-eight exercise physiology research laboratories in colleges and universities throughout the country. Organizations such as the American Physiological Society (APS), the American Alliance of Health, Physical Education, Recreation and Dance (AAH-PERD), and the American College of Sports Medicine (ACSM) were established by the mid-1950s. In an effort to ensure that well-trained professionals were involved in cardiac-rehabilitation programs, the ACSM developed a certification program in 1975. Certifications for fitness personnel were added later.

Increasingly sophisticated testing equipment should lead to a better understanding of fundamental physiological mechanisms, allowing practitioners to be more effective in measuring physical fitness and prescribing exercise programs. Health maintenance has become a priority as the number of adults over the age of fifty continues to increase. Advances in medical techniques also increase the survival rate of victims of heart attacks, creating a need for more cardiac-rehabilitation programs and practitioners. Health-care professionals and the general population need to be made more aware of the benefits of exercise for the maintenance of good health and the rehabilitation of individuals with medical problems.

—*Kathleen O'Boyle, Bradley R. A. Wilson*

References

Bray, George A, et al. "The Science of Obesity Management: An Endocrine Society Scientific Statement." *Endocrine Reviews*, vol. 39, no. 2, 6 Mar. 2018, pp. 79–132, academic.oup.com/edrv/article/39/2/79/4922247.

Koolhaas, Chantal M, et al. "Impact of Physical Activity on the Association of Overweight and Obesity with Cardiovascular Disease: The Rotterdam Study." *European Journal of Preventive Cardiology*, vol. 24, no. 9, 28 Feb. 2017, pp. 934–941, 10.1177/2047487317693952.

Richardson, Laura A., et al. "Effect of an Exercise and Weight Control Curriculum: Views of Obesity among Exercise Science Students." *Advances in Physiology Education*, vol. 39, no. 2, June 2015, pp. 43–48, 10.1152/advan.00154.2014.

Said, Mohamed Ahmed, et al. "Multidisciplinary Approach to Obesity: Aerobic or Resistance Physical Exercise?" *Journal of Exercise Science & Fitness*, vol. 16, no. 3, Dec. 2018, pp. 118–123, 10.1016/j.jesf.2018.11.001.

Wiklund, Petri. "The Role of Physical Activity and Exercise in Obesity and Weight Management: Time for Critical Appraisal." *Journal of Sport and Health Science*, vol. 5, no. 2, June 2016, pp. 151–154, www.sciencedirect.com/science/article/pii/S2095254616300060.

■ Exercise for older adults

CATEGORY: Physiology

The physiological deterioration commonly associated with aging is not entirely caused by the aging process; it is also caused by the physical inactivity that often accompanies aging. According to the 2018 National Health Survey the percent of Americans who are meeting physical activity guidelines for both aerobic and muscle strengthening activities has gradually increased since 2012 but leveled off in 2018. The numbers peak for the 18 to 24 year-old-age group and drop dramatically with age. Increased physical activity is an often suggested mechanism for reducing the rising health-care costs that accompany cardiovascular disease and deterioration of the musculoskeletal system. Even so, only 18.3 percent of men and 14.7 percent of women age sixty-five to seventy-four are participating in enough regular exercise to have a sufficient impact on their health.

Four general components collectively represent physical fitness and health: cardiorespiratory endurance (aerobic capacity), anaerobic power, muscular strength and endurance, and body composition. All these components are susceptible to decline with aging; however, the magnitude of this decline is dependent upon the extent of physical inactivity and other health factors.

Aerobic Capacity

Aerobic capacity refers to the body's ability to maximally transport and utilize oxygen to the cells (maximal volume of oxygen consumed or VO_{2max}). The body requires a higher volume of oxygen (VO_2) to sustain increased magnitudes of exercise. Aerobic capacity declines with aging because of a cumulative effect of age-related functional changes in the heart as well as muscle mass loss caused by disuse or disease. The higher the VO_2max value (measured in milliliters of oxygen used per kilogram of body weight per minute or ml/kg min), the greater the person's aerobic capacity or aerobic fitness. A higher aerobic capacity will allow an individual to exercise more comfortably and will also permit the older individual to complete activities of daily living without fatigue. Thus, functional ability is improved when aerobic fitness is improved.

Up to age thirty, VO_2max declines about 1 percent per year. Once adults reach middle age, the loss of VO_2max is accelerated unless regular aerobic exercise is undertaken. Between forty-five and fifty-five years of age, VO_2max will be lost at a rate of 9 to 15 percent. Other accelerated losses occur between the ages of sixty-five to seventy-five and from seventy-five to eighty-five years of age. However, regular participation in aerobic exercise can slow or even reverse this decline. When middle-aged or older individuals participate regularly in aerobic exercise, they can expect a 10 to 25 percent improvement in VO_2max. This can mean the difference between being functionally impaired, on one hand, and gaining back independent living skills and sports participation, on the other. Research reports on sixty-year-old endurance athletes have shown their VO_2max values to be above the values for some twenty-year-olds. For men over fifty years of age, "good" VO_2max values would be above 35 ml/kg/min; good VO_2max values for women over fifty would be above 29 ml/kg min. VO_2max values below 20

ml/kg min for either gender would indicate severe functional impairment.

Individuals can have their aerobic capacities determined with an exercise stress test administered by a team of medical professionals, including a cardiologist, a nurse, and an exercise physiologist. An aerobic exercise training program that elicits 50 to 70 percent of one's VO_2max would be sufficient to improve an older individual's aerobic capacity. Examples of aerobic exercise are walking, swimming, cycling, skiing, and dancing. Exercise of moderate intensity—enough to cause an increase in breathing and heart rate but not so much that it prevents one from being able to carry on a conversation—is sufficient for most people to gain health benefits. The experience of pain is a cue to stop exercise and reevaluate the exercise intensity level.

The Cardiovascular and Respiratory Systems

The primary purpose of the cardiovascular and respiratory or pulmonary systems (also referred to collectively as the cardiopulmonary or cardiorespiratory system) is to deliver oxygen and nutrients to the tissues while removing carbon dioxide and waste products from the tissues.

With aging, lung tissue loses elasticity, the chest wall becomes more rigid, and respiratory muscle strength is lost. This causes a loss of ventilatory (breathing) efficiency, making the mechanics of breathing harder for the aged. With exercise, the demand for more oxygen requires more frequent and deeper breaths. As the aged pulmonary system is compromised, pulmonary ventilation is decreased during maximal exercise as well as during recovery after exercise. Even with aging limitations, in the absence of pulmonary disease, the resting tissues still have an adequate oxygen supply to carry out daily functional and recreational activities. The oxygen deficit and higher respiratory work is not noticed until vigorous exercise puts a demand on the system for more oxygen, challenging the ventilatory capacity of the lungs. Although the total amount of blood flow increases as aerobic capacity increases, this does not result in an improvement in gaseous diffusion in the aged. In fact, gas exchange of oxygen and carbon dioxide in the tissues decreases with aging, and exercise training appears to have little impact on

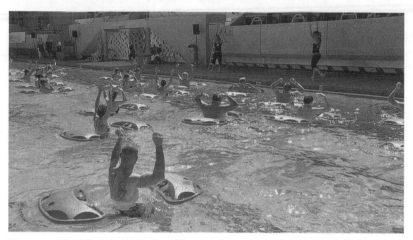

Water aerobics is beneficial for older adults as it takes strain off the bones. (Benoit Couzi)

this function. On the other hand, forced vital capacity (FVC), the maximum amount of air that can be expelled after a maximal inhalation, is one of the few pulmonary volumes influenced by both aging and exercise training. With aging, FVC declines approximately 4 to 5 percent per decade in the average individual. However, research studies that tracked aerobically trained individuals over twenty or more years found that their FVCs at age forty-five were the same as their FVCs at age twenty. This maintenance may be because of the mechanical stressing of the respiratory muscles afforded by regular aerobic exercise.

As with the pulmonary system, resting cardiovascular function experiences only moderate changes, whereas the cardiovascular response during exercise declines substantially with aging. The major reason that maximal aerobic capacity declines with aging is because of the decrease in maximal heart rate. Maximal heart rate (the highest heart rate attainable) declines approximately 6 percent per decade. Using the mathematical formula to estimate maximal heart rate (220 minus age equals heart rate in beats per minute), it can be seen that the estimated maximal heart rate of a seventy-year-old (150 beats per minute) is significantly less than that of a twenty-year-old (200 beats per minute). Heart rate is under the control of both the parasympathetic and sympathetic nervous systems. The parasympathetic nervous system is responsible for keeping the heart rate lower at rest.

The sympathetic nervous system takes over during exercise so that heart rate can be increased to meet the increased oxygen demand. The decline in maximal heart rate is caused by the aging heart becoming less sensitive to sympathetic nervous system stimulation, thereby decreasing the heart's maximal contractile capabilities. This results in the inability of the heart to attain the higher maximal values that were possible during youth. No amount of exercise training can alter this. Submaximal exercise is also more strenuous for an older adult. Exercise sessions that were once easy during youth cause higher heart rates and longer recovery times when one is older. This reflects the heightened need of the aging heart to work harder to meet the increased oxygen demands of the exercising tissues.

Regular exercise participation lowers resting heart rate (the number of times the heart beats per minute) and improves stroke volume (the volume of blood ejected with each beat of the heart) in both the young and the old. Even though cardiac contractility and total blood volume in older individuals is less and the ventricular walls are less compliant, regular aerobic exercise training increases total blood volume and tone of the peripheral vessels, thereby reducing vascular resistance and increasing the volume of blood flow back to the heart. This enables the heart to eject more blood with each beat. In aerobically trained individuals, stroke volume is improved not only during exercise but also at rest. The lower resting heart rates commonly seen in trained individuals is partially caused by the improved stroke volume. As the heart is able to deliver more blood with each beat of the heart, the heart does not need to work as hard to deliver oxygen. In addition, regular aerobic exercise enhances the heart's parasympathetic activity. Therefore, the combined effect of improved parasympathetic activity and improved stroke volume explains the bradycardia (a heart rate below 60 beats per minute) commonly observed in healthy, aerobically trained individuals.

Even though the cardiovascular parameters that determine aerobic fitness all decline with the aging process, participation in regular aerobic exercise has been shown to improve maximal stroke volume and cardiac output (the volume of blood pumped by the heart each minute, equal to heart rate minus stroke volume) by as much as 25 percent. Maximal cardiac output is increased because of the increase in stroke volume, since maximal heart rate does not increase. The types of exercise training employed, as well as the person's initial level of fitness, influences the magnitudes of these increases. Aerobic exercise, not strength training, is the type of exercise required to improve cardiovascular function. Those who are more severely deconditioned will be able to accomplish greater gains simply because they have more room for improvement.

Anaerobic Power

Converse to aerobic capacity, anaerobic power is not dependent upon the replenishment of oxygen to the cells. The fuel source used to power anaerobic movement is retrieved from energy stores located within the cell. Quick, explosive movements characterize anaerobic activities. In most athletic events, the ability to generate anaerobic power will have a direct effect upon athletic success. It is also important in daily living when one encounters an emergency situation demanding a quick, powerful response. A few examples of anaerobic activities include sprinting, throwing the discus, and lifting heavy objects.

The sports-related "anaerobic response" includes a sharp rise in lactic acid accumulation in the muscles and blood, a sharp increase in pulmonary ventilation, and a drop in the blood pH, giving rise to a more acidic state. Lactic acid accumulates with high-intensity or maximal exercise because of a combination of an increased production rate and a reduced rate of removal. The recruitment of fast-twitch muscle fibers (those fibers responsible for performing quick, explosive movements) also triggers the production of lactic acid. In addition, the need for more oxygen at maximal exercise stimulates the metabolic pathways to speed up. This results in an increase in glycolysis. Glycolysis is the energy pathway responsible for the initial breakdown of blood glucose (blood sugar) so that energy (adenosine triphosphate or ATP) can be created to perform work. At the end of glycolysis, if enough oxygen is not available, excess lactic acid will be formed. An abundance of lactic acid quickly causes muscle fatigue, and exercise soon stops.

Data on aging suggest that anaerobic power, mechanical power, and mechanical capacity peak by age forty, then decline thereafter. Several factors may explain this decline. First, older adults

EXERCISE GUIDELINES FOR OLDER ADULTS	
Aerobic Training	**Strength Training**
Duration: Minimum of 5 days a week 30 to 60 minutes per session	*Duration:* Minimum of 2 times a week, with 24 to 48 hours of rest between sessions
Intensity: Moderate intensity (one should be able to talk at same time)	*Intensity:* Exercise all the muscle groups at 40 percent to 50 percent of maximum ability; gradually increase the weight intensity
Adapt the program to individual needs (if vigorous intensity is desired and can be tolerated the guidelines change to a minimum of 3 days a week for 20 to 30 minutes per session)	*Reps:* Complete 8 to 12 repetitions for each muscle group targeted
Perform weight-bearing activities, if possible	Never hold the breath

have reduced blood glucose stores (glycogen) in the muscle tissue, which results in a decrease in glycolysis. A decrease in glycolysis will decrease energy production. Second, with aging, fewer fast-twitch muscle fibers are available because of atrophy (shrinkage from disuse). Third, the enzyme lactate dehydrogenase (LDH), which is responsible for lactic acid production when fast-twitch muscle fibers are activated, decreases with aging. Even though the anaerobic processes decline with aging, participation in anaerobic-type activities is still possible as long as the health and fitness status of the older adult is carefully considered.

The Nervous and Musculoskeletal Systems

With aging, the nervous system is unable to receive, process, and transmit messages as quickly as it did in youth. The clinical outcome is slower reaction and movement times. This is an important issue, as many aspects of functional independence require an individual to be able to react quickly in certain situations to prevent potential injury, such as when driving a car or regaining one's balance to prevent a fall. Older individuals who exercise regularly have demonstrated better reaction times, balance, and coordination in comparison to their sedentary peers. Research investigating older adults who play tennis regularly has demonstrated that active older adults can maintain and perhaps improve their motor skills with continued use. Blood flow to the brain also increases during exercise. Short-term, immediate improvements in performance of memory tasks have been demonstrated immediately following aerobic exercise. Whether there is a long-term increase in cerebral blood flow because of regular exercise participation is a question subject to continued research.

Beginning in middle age, muscular strength declines because of a combination of factors, such as muscle mass loss, decreased motor unit activation, and a decreased ability of the muscles to contract forcefully. This decline is selective as well, with some muscle groups losing substantially more strength than others. For instance, leg and trunk muscle strength appears to decline at a faster rate than arm strength. The decline in muscle mass occurs in phases. From twenty-five to fifty years of age, only about 10 percent of muscle mass is lost.

However, by age eighty, almost 40 percent of muscle mass is lost because of atrophy. This "wasting away" of muscle tissue commonly seen in the elderly is known as sarcopenia.

Weakened respiratory muscles will result in limited aerobic capabilities. Weakened lower-extremity muscles give rise to balance problems and increased risk for falls. Insufficient strength to carry out activities of daily living or functional tasks results in a loss of independent living. Although the age-related loss of muscle mass and strength cannot be totally eliminated, it can be reduced. Aging does not impair the ability of skeletal muscles to respond to exercise training. Progressive strength training programs have demonstrated that older adults can achieve gains in muscle mass (hypertrophy) and muscle strength similar to what has been observed in young individuals.

Exercise has been shown to be beneficial in reducing bone mass loss (osteoporosis). Both weight-bearing aerobic training and strength training have been found to be beneficial in improving bone mass. However, the modest improvements shown to occur with bone mass because of exercise conditioning is not great enough to prevent a fracture caused by a fall. Rather, exercise training will help to reduce the risk of falls by strengthening the ambulatory musculature. Research studies indicate that aerobic training and strength training improve neuromuscular functioning, gait, and balance, all of which are important variables in the risk profile for falls.

Psychosocial Benefits of Exercise

Psychological well-being includes components such as self-esteem, self-efficacy, depression, and anxiety. The majority of research studies investigating these factors in older individuals agree that participation in regular exercise is associated with improved psychological well-being. The benefits are greater and more consistent if the individual participates in an exercise program for at least ten weeks. Either aerobic training or strength training will work well, but very light or very vigorous exercise is not as effective as moderate-intensity exercise.

It is often cited that older individuals benefit from group activities—group interactions alleviate feelings of loneliness often encountered with aging. Although this may be true for some, home-based exercise may be preferable to the class setting for certain groups of older adults. Many older adults remain very active and are unable to fit a regularly scheduled exercise class into their own tight schedule. Others are unable to get to the exercise site because of transportation problems or physical disabilities but are still capable of performing some type of exercise or physical activity at home. A safe, moderately paced home program would better meet their needs.

Medications and the Perception of Exercise Intensity

Older adults often take several different types of medications to treat a variety of health problems. Of all the medications, beta-blockers are among the most widely prescribed. Beta-blockers are used to treat hypertension, anxiety, and heart disease. As the name suggests, these drugs block beta-receptors in the sympathetic nervous system. Among other functions, beta receptors stimulate the heart to contract and directly influence heart rate. If this action is blocked, the heart rate response will be lowered, an action necessary to reduce the workload of a diseased heart. Beta-blockers can also cause vasodilation of blood vessels, an action important for controlling hypertension. However, if an individual is going to exercise and needs to maintain his or her exercise level in the "moderate" range, heart rate will not be able to be used as an intensity index because the heart rate response will be altered by the drug. Therefore, a person will need to regulate exercise intensity based upon his or her perception of how hard the exercise feels. Perceived exertion has been shown to closely reflect the workload of the heart. The simplest advice that can be given to individuals for keeping track of exercise intensity level is the instruction to be able to "walk and talk at the same time." This eliminates the need to take heart rate measurements during exercise.

Exercise Benefits, Risks, and Guidelines

There are many exercise options available for the older adult, depending on specific goals and health status. Even though exercise is associated with a variety of health benefits, it is also associated with such health risks as worsening existing medical problems, muscle and joint injuries, and, in some cases, heart attack. Therefore, exercise programs should be designed to maximize the benefits and minimize the potential risks.

Older adults often take several different types of medications to treat a variety of health problems. Of all the medications, beta-blockers are among the most widely prescribed. Beta-blockers are used to treat hypertension, anxiety, and heart disease. As the name suggests, these drugs block beta-receptors in the sympathetic nervous system. Among other functions, beta receptors stimulate the heart to contract and directly influence heart rate. If this action is blocked, the heart rate response will be lowered, an action necessary to reduce the workload of a diseased heart. Beta-blockers can also cause vasodilation of blood vessels, an action important for controlling hypertension. However, if an individual is going to exercise and needs to maintain his or her exercise level in the "moderate" range, heart rate will not be able to be used as an intensity index because the heart rate response will be altered by the drug. Therefore, a person will need to regulate exercise intensity based upon his or her perception of how hard the exercise feels. Perceived exertion has been shown to closely reflect the workload of the heart. The simplest advice that can be given to individuals for keeping track of exercise intensity level is the instruction to be able to "walk and talk at the same time." This eliminates the need to take heart rate measurements during exercise.

Regardless of age, the Report of the Surgeon General recommends that everyone should participate in moderate exercise for at least thirty minutes on all or most days of the week for optimal health and fitness. This should be accomplished gradually. If one's goal is to improve aerobic fitness, blood pressure, cholesterol level, mood, or glucose tolerance or to reduce body fat, moderate aerobic exercise should be done at least five times per week. This requires activities that are rhythmic in nature, involve the use of larger muscle groups, and can be sustained for at least thirty to sixty continuous minutes. If the goal is to increase muscle mass, muscular endurance, or strength, then a well-rounded strength-training program should be done twice per week, with each session followed by at least one day of rest. If the goal is to maintain or improve bone mass, either weight-bearing aerobic exercise or resistance training could be used. The ideal exercise program includes both aerobic training and strength training.

—Bonita L. Marks

References

American College of Sports Medicine. *ACSM's Complete Guide to Fitness and Health*. Edited by Barbara Bushman. 2nd ed. Human Kinetics, 2017.

Owen, James P. *Just Move! A New Approach to Fitness after Fifty*. National Geographic, 2017.

Rosenbloom, Christine, and Bob Murray. *Food and Fitness after 50: Eat Well, Move Well, Be Well*. Academy of Nutrition and Dietetics, 2018.

U.S. Department of Health and Human Services. *Physical Activity Guidelines for Americans*. 2nd ed. US Department of Health and Human Services, 2018.

Westcott, Wayne L., and Thomas R. Baechle. *Strength Training Past Fifty*. 2nd ed. Human Kinetics, 2015.

■ Food labels

CATEGORY: Nutrition

Food labels by manufacturers are an important part of the marketing process. What a consumer sees on the label draws attention to the product and is a factor in determining if the consumer purchases it. Therefore, manufacturers spend considerable time and money developing labels that will help sell the products.

Another important consideration of the manufacturer is the taste of the product. Many of the ingredients that make food taste good unfortunately make the product less healthy. In particular the addition of sugars and fats can improve the taste but they also add calories. Furthermore diets high in fat and sugar increase the risk of many chronic diseases such as cardiovascular disease, diabetes and cancer. The addition of salt (which contains sodium) also enhances the flavor of food but may contribute to high blood pressure in some individuals.

Health advocates have tried for years to get food manufacturers to disclose the ingredients in the product as well as the nutritional facts. Food manufacturers have often resisted these disclosures to protect the recipes of their products and to conceal some of the unhealthy ingredients. Therefore there have been many disputes between the food manufacturers and health advocates about what data should be printed on the labels. Over time the US government has required more information to be revealed on food labels.

Nutritional Facts on Food Labels

In order to help consumers make informed decisions about their food purchases the U.S. government requires certain information to be provided on the label in a uniform format. This information is found on the label under the heading: *Nutrition Facts*. Although this information is helpful the consumer must have some basic nutrition knowledge to make healthy choices.

At the top of the *Nutrition Facts* on the label is the serving size and number of servings per container. Since all of the nutritional information that follows is based on this serving size it is important to understand what the amount is. Some products may appear to be a single serving size but actually may be two or more servings. Therefore if the product is consumed in its entirety the nutrition information must be multiplied by the number of servings.

The area beneath the serving size is the calories per serving. (The actual unit of measurement is kilocalories but on food labels it is listed as calories. This is the unit of measurement that the general public understands.) The other value listed in this section is the calories from fat. At the current time this section does not include the percent of calories from fat. Since the dietary guidelines recommend less than 30% of the calories come from fat each day this would be a helpful quantity to have printed. Because this number is not provided consumers can do a quick calculation by multiplying the calories from fat by three and if that number is less than the total calories from fat the product is in the healthier range for the overall quantity of fat.

The following section lists the quantity and percent of daily value based on a 2000 calorie diet for fat, cholesterol and sodium. Fat is recorded in grams and broken out into saturated fat and trans fat. These two are less healthy forms of fat and along with cholesterol will increase the risk of cardiovascular disease and some cancers more than polyunsaturated or monounsaturated fats. Saturated fats should be limited to less than 20 grams per day for a 2000 calorie diet (or 1 gram per 100 calories consumed). Trans fats are a processed fat and should be avoided if possible. Cholesterol is expressed in milligrams. It is recommended that cholesterol consumption be limited to 300mg per day despite

Sample label for
Macaroni & Cheese

① Start Here ➡

② **Check Calories**

③ Limit these
Nutrients

④ **Get Enough
of these
Nutrients**

⑤ **Footnote**

Nutrition Facts
Serving Size 1 cup (228g)
Servings Per Container 2

Amount Per Serving
Calories 250   Calories from Fat 110

	% Daily Value*
Total Fat 12g	18%
Saturated Fat 3g	15%
Trans Fat 3g	
Cholesterol 30mg	10%
Sodium 470mg	20%
Total Carbohydrate 31g	10%
Dietary Fiber 0g	0%
Sugars 5g	
Protein 5g	

Vitamin A	4%
Vitamin C	2%
Calcium	20%
Iron	4%

* Percent Daily Values are based on a 2,000 calorie diet.
Your Daily Values may be higher or lower depending on
your calorie needs.

	Calories	2,000	2,500
Total Fat	Less than	65g	80g
Sat Fat	Less than	20g	25g
Cholesterol	Less than	300mg	300mg
Sodium	Less than	2,400mg	2,400mg
Total Carbohydrate		300g	375g
Dietary Fiber		25g	30g

⑥ **Quick Guide
to % DV**

—————

• **5% or less
is Low**

• **20% or more
is High**

How to understand and use the US Nutritional Fact Label. (Trounce via Wikimedia Commons)

the number of calories consumed. Sodium consumption is measured in milligrams and associated with high blood pressure in some individuals. It is recommended that all people limit their sodium consumption to 2400 mg per day.

Carbohydrates which include sugars and fiber are included in the next section and are measured in grams. Total carbohydrates also have the percent daily value which should be 15 grams per 100

calories consumed or about 60% of total calories. However, these should come primarily from complex carbohydrates such as fiber and starches and not sugars. Therefore the total carbohydrates are broken down into sugars and fiber. A recent requirement is to also include the grams of sugar that was added during processing listed as *Added Sugar.* This will help consumers determine the amounts of sugar that are natural from those that were added.

The last caloric nutrient listed is protein. There is not a recommended daily value based on caloric intake for protein. Recommended intakes are based on body size and therefore cannot easily be enumerated on a label. The protein content per serving is listed simply in grams unless the food is intended for children under 4 years or if the food claims to be high in protein.

Four vitamins and minerals are commonly included on the label and are listed as a percent of the daily value. These were chosen from the many vitamins and minerals because they are the ones most Americans do not obtain in adequate amounts in the diet. Vitamins A and C are important antioxidants. Calcium is needed to build strong bones and teeth. Iron is required by the blood to carry oxygen.

At the bottom of the *Nutrition Facts* labeling is a footnote that provides general nutrition information related to the Percent Daily Value. Specific numbers are listed for a 2000 and a 2500 calorie diet to help consumers better understand the overall health-related ingredients of the food.

Ingredients on Food Labels

Also required for food labels is a list of the ingredients in the product beginning with highest quantity to the lowest quantity. The actual amounts are not required. This is helpful to identify chemical additives such as preservatives, dyes for color, artificial sweeteners and caffeine. The ingredient list is also helpful for those with allergies to avoid products that may cause reactions.

Future Directions

Over the years more labeling requirements have been added for food products. It is likely that the government will continue adding requirements to better help consumers make healthy purchasing decisions. However, there is a limit to the amount of information that can be placed on labels. Nutrition and health are very broad disciplines and putting information on labels that is understandable to the general population continues to be a challenge.

In order to simplify nutritional information on labels some non-government organizations have begun to add a seal indicating that the product is healthy or to provide summary information. Some examples include *Great for You* by Wal-Mart and *Facts Up Front* by the Grocery Manufacturer's

Association. However these programs are controversial, not universal and the nutrition facts stated are still debatable. Possibly the government one day will develop a program that would provide a universal seal for food products that would be easily understood by the general public.

—*Bradley R. A. Wilson*

References

Lafrenière, Jacynthe, et al. "The Effects of Food Labelling on Postexercise Energy Intake in Sedentary Women." *Journal of Obesity*, vol. 2017, 2017, pp. 1–10, 10.1155/2017/1048973.

Reichel, Chloe. "Journalist's Resource." *Journalist's Resource*, 4 Apr. 2018, journalistsresource.org/studies/environment/food-agriculture/food-labels-junk-nafta-obesity/.

Roberto, C A, and N Khandpur. "Improving the Design of Nutrition Labels to Promote Healthier Food Choices and Reasonable Portion Sizes." *International Journal of Obesity*, vol. 38, no. S1, July 2014, pp. S25–S33, 10.1038/ijo.2014.86.

Viola, Gaia Claudia Viviana, et al. "Are Food Labels Effective as a Means of Health Prevention?" *Journal of Public Health Research*, vol. 5, no. 3, 21 Dec. 2016, www.ncbi.nlm.nih.gov/pmc/articles/PMC5206777/, 10.4081/jphr.2016.768.

■ Hypocaloric diet

CATEGORY: Nutrition

More than half of adults in the United States are classified as overweight or obese, which increases risk for many chronic and potentially life-threatening diseases (e.g., diabetes mellitus, type2 [DM2], cardiovascular disease [CVD], cancer). Each year, approximately 280,000 individuals in the U.S. die as a result of complications related to excess body weight. Excess body weight is associated with psychological complications and can affect social relationships and status. For these reasons, weight loss/management is a major medical and societal concern. Of the treatments currently available, exercise and hypocaloric diets are the preferred methods for losing weight. A hypocaloric diet is a diet in which the daily caloric intake is less than the total daily calories burned.

Hypocaloric diets are frequently initiated for weight loss, but they are also effective for lowering blood pressure, improving blood lipid profiles (e.g., cholesterol, triglycerides), and stabilizing blood glucose levels in overweight and obese individuals. Necessary weight loss increases insulin activity, improving insulin resistance and reducing the need for medication to control DM2. Weight loss improves hypertension and frequently alleviates the need for blood pressure medication.

Hypocaloric diets are not appropriate for persons of normal weight or those who are underweight, and should be carefully considered before initiating in immunocompromised patients who frequently have increased calorie needs.

Action of a Hypocaloric Diet

Weight loss or gain is a result of energy imbalance that occurs when the number of calories consumed does not equal those used for energy. For example, a positive energy balance occurs if an individual consumes 2,500 calories/day and burns 2,000 calories/day for energy; the remaining 500 calories will be stored in the body, and the person will gain about 1 pound/week if a positive energy balance of the same amount continues. The source (e.g., protein, fat, carbohydrate) of excess calories is irrelevant, and all excess calories are stored as fat.

The reverse occurs when there is a negative energy balance. If an individual consumes a hypocaloric diet of 500 fewer calories than he/she burns in a day, the body will burn fat reserves and, if necessary, protein stores from organ and muscle mass in order to meet the required energy needs. Consumption that consistently results in the same amount of negative energy balance will result in the loss of about 1 pound/week. This equation of 500 calories to 1 pound of loss or gain is referred to as the 500 rule.

Recommendations for Implementing a Hypocaloric Diet

The Academy of Nutrition and Dietetics recommends that weight loss be limited to 1–2 pounds/week, because doing so provides for weight loss that is primarily body fat. Weight loss in excess of 2 pounds/week is usually a result of water loss or the breakdown of lean muscle tissue. The exception to this weight loss limitation is the therapeutic initiation of a very low calorie diet (VLCD) for the

treatment of extreme obesity; a VLCD should only be attempted with close medical supervision.

A hypocaloric diet should provide adequate nutrients to support overall health. It is important to choose nutrient-dense foods such as whole grains, fruits, vegetables, beans, lean proteins (e.g., fish, chicken breast), and low-fat dairy products.

A hypocaloric diet should exclude alcohol and foods that are high in fat and/or added sugar (e.g., butter, cream, desserts, pastries, soda, fast foods, prepackaged snack foods, and highly processed foods) because of their high calorie content. It is currently recommended that dietary fat intake be limited as follows:

- Total dietary fat should be < 30% of total caloric intake but not less than 20%
- Saturated fat should be < 10% of total caloric intake
- Trans fat should be < 1 % of total caloric intake

It is important to consume enough calories to support overall health. The recommended minimum calorie intake per day is 1,500 calories for men and 1,200 calories for women. Eating a diet that is too low in calories can result in inadequate nutrient intake. Manifestations of inadequate nutrition include menstrual irregularities, hormonal imbalances, loss of bone density and muscle mass, anemia, listless or apathetic demeanor, depression and irritability. fatigue and dizziness, organ malfunction due to malnutrition, brittle, spoon-shaped fingernails, dry, brittle hair, constipation and/or diarrhea, headaches, night blindness, and poor reflexes.

Research Findings

Researchers report that the inclusion of nuts and legumes in a hypocaloric diet can provide additional health benefits compared with hypocaloric diets that do not include nuts and legumes. Study subjects who consumed a hypocaloric diet enriched with almonds showed greater improvement in lipid profiles than those who consumed a nut-free hypocaloric diet, although similar results in weight loss were reported. Additionally, individuals who consumed a legume-enriched hypocaloric diet supplemented with L-arginine and selenium showed reductions in abdominal obesity, insulin resistance, hypertension, triglycerides, and pro-inflammatory markers (e.g., C-reactive protein [CRP]).

Water consumption of 500 ml prior to meals was shown to increase the weight loss achieved with hypocaloric diet intervention. Researchers believe this is due to decrease in calorie intake during the meals following water ingestion.

What We Can Do

Individuals should become knowledgeable about the physiologic effects of consuming a hypocaloric diet, in which daily caloric intake is less than the total daily calories burned. A hypocaloric diet is only recommended to help overweight and obese individuals achieve weight loss and decrease risk factors for obesity, hypertension, DM2, CVD and cancer. In order to prevent inadequate nutrient intake it is recommended to consume a well-balanced diet with a minimum daily calorie intake of 1,500 calories for men and 1,200 calories for women. Research suggests the inclusion of nuts and legumes in the diet, as well as 500 mL water consumption prior to meals may improve weight loss results while following a hypocaloric diet.

—*Cherie Marcel*

References

Benton, David, and Hayley A. Young. "Reducing Calorie Intake May Not Help You Lose Body Weight." *Perspectives on Psychological Science*, vol. 12, no. 5, 28 June 2017, pp. 703–714., doi:10.1177/1745691617690878.

Greco, Marta, et al. "Early Effects of a Hypocaloric, Mediterranean Diet on Laboratory Parameters in Obese Individuals." *Mediators of Inflammation*, 4 Mar. 2014, pp. 1–8., doi:10.1155/2014/750860.

Haywood, Cilla J, et al. "Very Low Calorie Diets for Weight Loss in Obese Older Adults—A Randomized Trial." *The Journals of Gerontology: Series A*, vol. 73, no. 1, 20 Feb. 2017, pp. 59–65., doi:10.1093/gerona/glx012.

Muscogiuri, Giovanna, et al. "The Management of Very Low-Calorie Ketogenic Diet in Obesity Outpatient Clinic: a Practical Guide." *Journal of Translational Medicine*, vol. 17, no. 1, 29 Oct. 2019, doi:10.1186/s12967-019-2104-z.

Ricci, Natalie L., and Melanie Jay. "Fast and Furious: Rapid Weight Loss Via a Very Low Calorie Diet May Lead to Better Long-Term Outcomes Than a Gradual Weight Loss Program." *Journal of Clinical Outcomes Management*, vol. 22, no. 8, Aug. 2015, pp. 346–350.

■ Ketogenic diet

CATEGORY: Nutrition

The ketogenic diet (KD) refers to a diet that is high in fat, low in carbohydrates, and adequate in protein that is initiated to control seizure activity. Eating a KD replaces glucose-based energy sources with fat-based energy sources, resulting in a physiologic state of ketosis. Ketosis is evidenced by the build-up of ketone bodies, or ketones, in the blood and urine. Ketones are water-soluble compounds that are produced as byproducts when fat-based energy sources are utilized. Although the process is not entirely understood, the increase in ketones is correlated with improved control of seizures.

The KD is structured and mathematically calculated, and should be initiated only with close medical supervision. It is a challenging diet for patients to learn and follow, and is not usually suggested by a clinician until at least 2 attempts of pharmacotherapy have failed. Although the KD is predominantly prescribed as a therapy for children with epilepsy or other seizure disorders, it has been used with good results in treatment of adults to control seizure activity. Most individuals tolerate the KD better than pharmacotherapy, but potential adverse effects include elevated low-density lipoprotein (LDL) cholesterol levels, constipation, kidney stones, and acidosis.

Action of the KD

The exact mechanism that causes the KD to be effective in reducing seizures is not fully understood. Some theories include the following:

Ketones, namely acetone, acetoacetate, and beta-hydroxybutyrate, cross the blood/brain barrier (i.e., filtering system that carries blood to the brain) and affect the onset, propagation, and/or cessation of seizures.

Ketones may be indicators of the presence of certain other substances or metabolic changes that have not been identified.

The switch from glucose-burning to fat-burning may affect physiologic use and production of insulin in such a way that improves seizure control.

Recommendations for the KD and Medication Interaction

Traditionally, the KD is initiated over a period of 3 days after a 48-hour fast, although the necessity of fasting has been questioned in results of recent research.

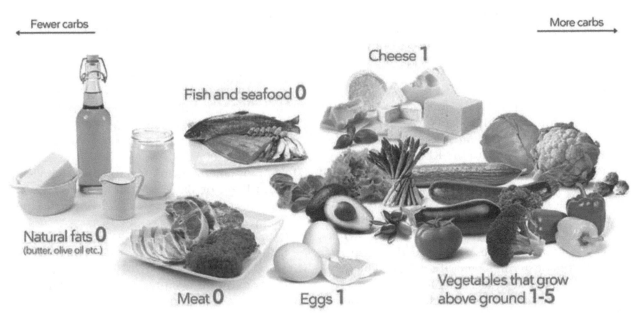

Here are typical foods to enjoy on a ketogenic diet. The numbers are net carbs, i.e. digestible carbs, per 100 grams.13 To remain in ketosis, lower is generally better. (Diet Doctor)

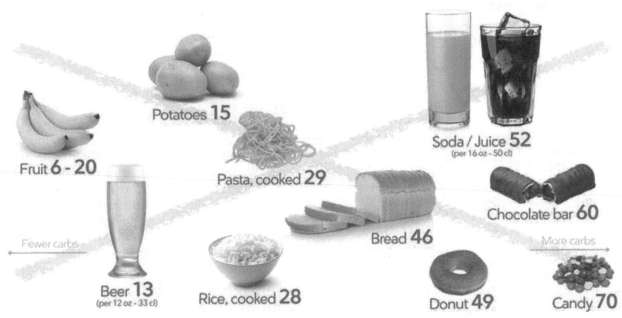

Here's what you should avoid on a keto diet – foods containing a lot of carbs, both the sugary and the starchy kind. This includes starchy foods like bread, pasta, rice, and potatoes. These foods are very high in carbs. The numbers are grams of net carbs per 100 grams, unless otherwise noted. (Diet Doctor)

The KD requires commitment, education from a physician and/or dietitian, and the ability to learn about calculating meal plans, weighing food, and initiating strategies for eating away from home. Completing these requirements takes time, and achieving and maintaining good adherence to the KD is a process that occurs over time.

The carbohydrate content of all medications should be included in the meal plan calculations in order to maintain appropriate carbohydrate intake.

Research Findings

Research results show that when adults adhere strictly to the KD they achieve significant improvement in seizure control, although establishing good adherence to the KD is challenging for adults. It can be very difficult to follow such a rigid diet after years of established dietary patterns and traditions. Another concern for recommending the KD to adults is the high likelihood that its use will result in elevated LDL levels. Results of studies show the therapeutic potential of consuming a modified Atkins diet or a low glycemic index diet to achieve better long-term adherence and fewer adverse effects among adults.

Authors of a retrospective case review of 10 cases of critically ill adult patients with super-refractory status epilepticus (SRSE) reported that treatment with the KD resulted in resolution of status epilepticus in 90% of the patients.

Summary

Individuals should become knowledgeable about the physiologic effects of the ketogenic diet (KD). The KD, which is high in fat and low in carbohydrates, is prescribed to help control seizure disorders. Patients and their family members should follow strict adherence to the prescribed KD with continued medical surveillance to monitor health status. Research suggests the KD may result in elevated LDL levels and less strict carbohydrate-controlled diets may be a good alternative.

—*Cherie Marcel*

References

Campos, Marcelo. "Ketogenic Diet: Is the Ultimate Low-Carb Diet Good for You?" *Harvard Health Blog*, Harvard Medical School, 30 July 2019.

Joshi, Shivam, et al. "The Ketogenic Diet for Obesity and Diabetes—Enthusiasm Outpaces Evidence." *JAMA Internal Medicine*, vol. 179, no. 9, 15 July 2019, p. 1163., doi:10.1001/jamainternmed.2019.2633.

Kirkpatrick, Carol F., et al. "Review of Current Evidence and Clinical Recommendations on the Effects of Low-Carbohydrate and Very-Low-Carbohydrate (Including Ketogenic) Diets for the Management of Body Weight and Other Cardiometabolic Risk Factors: A Scientific Statement from the National Lipid Association Nutrition and Lifestyle Task Force." *Journal of Clinical Lipidology*, vol. 13, no. 5, 2019, doi:10.1016/j.jacl.2019.08.003.

Mohan, Viswanathan, and Joshi Shilpa. "Ketogenic Diets: Boon or Bane?" *Indian Journal of Medical Research*, vol. 148, no. 3, 2018, p. 251., doi:10.4103/ijmr.ijmr_1666_18.

O'Connor, Anahad. "The Keto Diet Is Popular, but Is It Good for You?" *The New York Times*, 20 Aug. 2019, www.nytimes.com/2019/08/20/well/eat/the-keto-diet-is-popular-but-is-it-good-for-you.html.

■ Liposuction

CATEGORY: Procedure

Indications and Procedures

The fat contained in adipose tissue makes up 15 to 20 percent of the body weights of most healthy individuals. Much adipose tissue is found inside the abdominal cavity, but significant amounts are located under the skin of the abdomen, arms, breasts, hips, knees, legs, and throat. The quantity of this subcutaneous fat at any such site is based on individual heredity, age, and eating habits. When excessive eating greatly elevates body fat, a patient becomes obese, a condition that can be life-threatening. Until recently, the sole means for decreasing fat content resulting from obesity was time-consuming dieting, which requires much patience and will power. In addition, the positive consequences of long diets can be easily obliterated if dieters begin to overeat again. Recurrent overeating is common and often followed by the rapid regaining of the fat.

Persons who have undesired, unattractive fat deposits as a result of age, heredity, or obesity may undergo cosmetic surgery, such as so-called tummy tucks, to remove them. Such major procedures, however, often remove muscle along with fat and

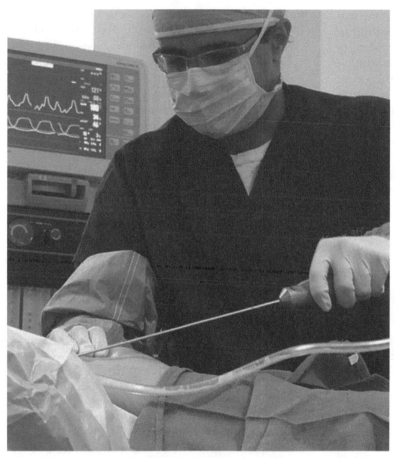

Liposuction surgery being performed by plastic surgeon with heart monitor in background. (© Photographer - James C. Mutter / Plastic Surgeon Vishal Kapoor, MD)

is made in a fold of the treated body region, so that the scar will not be noticeable after healing. At this time, a sterile cannula is introduced under the skin of the treatment area. Next, the surgeon uses suction through the cannula to remove the fat deposits. Liposuction produces temporary tunnels in adipose tissue. Upon completion of the procedure, the incision is closed and the surgical area is wrapped with tight bandages or covered with support garments. This final stage of recontouring helps the tissue to collapse back into the desired shape during healing. In most patients, the skin around the area soon shrinks into the new contours. When this does not happen easily, because of old age or other factors, liposuction is accompanied by surgical skin removal.

Uses and Complications

Liposuction can be used for body recontouring only when undesired contours are attributable to fat deposits; those attributable to anatomical features such as bone structure cannot be treated in this manner.

A major principle on which liposuction is based is the supposition that the body contains a fixed number of fat cells and that, as people become fatter, the cells fill with droplets of fat and expand. The removal of fat cells by liposuction is deemed to decrease the future ability of the treated body part to become fat because fewer cells are available to be filled. Dieting and exercise are less successful than liposuction because they do not diminish the number of fat cells in adipose tissue, only decreasing fat cell size. Hence, when dieters return to eating excess food again or exercise stops, the fat cells expand again.

Another aspect of liposuction which is becoming popular is the ability to remove undesired fat from some body sites and insert it where the fat is wanted for recontouring. Most often, this transfer involves enlarging women's breasts or correcting cases in which the two breasts are of markedly different size. Liposuction also can be used to repair asymmetry in other body parts as a result of accidents.

cause considerable scarring. Liposuction is a relatively easy way to lose unattractive body fat; it also is seen as a fast way to reverse obesity and is touted as more permanent than dieting. A cannula connected to a suction pump is inserted under the skin in the desired area. Then a chosen amount of fat is sucked out, the cannula is withdrawn, and the incision is closed. The result is a recontouring of the body part. Hence, liposuction has become a very popular cosmetic surgery procedure for the abdomen, arms, breasts, hips, knees, legs, and throat; many pounds can be removed from large areas such as the abdomen.

Liposuction begins with the administration of antibiotics and the anesthesia of the area to be recontoured. Local anesthesia is safer, but general anesthesia is used when necessary. The process usually begins after a 1.3-centimeter (0.5-inch) incision

Liposuction, as with any other surgery, has associated risks and complications. According to reputable practitioners, however, they are temporary and relatively minor, such as black-and-blue marks and the accumulation of blood and serum under the skin of treated areas. These complications are minimized by fluid removal during surgery and by the application of tight bandages or garments after the operation. Another related complication is that subcutaneous fat removal leads to fluid loss from the body. When large amounts of fat are removed, shock occurs if the fluid is not replaced quickly. Therefore, another component of successful liposuction is timely fluid replacement.

The more extensive and complex the liposuction procedure attempted, the more likely it is to cause complications. Particularly prone to problems are liposuction procedures in which major skin removal is required. Hence, surgeons who perform liposuction suggest that potential patients be realistic about the goals of the surgery. It is also recommended that patients choose reputable practitioners.

Perspective and Prospects

Liposuction, currently viewed as relatively safe cosmetic surgery, originated in Europe in the late 1960s. In 1982, it reached the United States. Since that time, its use has burgeoned, and about a half million liposuction surgeries are carried out yearly. Although its first use was as a purely cosmetic procedure, liposuction is now done for noncosmetic reasons, including repairing injuries sustained in accidents. Women were once the sole liposuction patients. Men make up about 15 percent of treated individuals; liposuction is the most popular form of cosmetic surgery among men.

In the United States, liposuction is not presently accepted by insurance companies or considered tax deductible. This situation may change because several studies have found that obese people have a greater chance of developing cardiovascular disease and cancer. It must be noted, however, that liposuction offers only temporary relief from body fat. Although it does decrease fat deposition in a treated region, lack of proper calorie intake and exercise will deposit fat elsewhere in the body.

—*Sanford S. Singer*

References

Batac, Joseph, et al. "Abdominoplasty in the Obese Patient." *Plastic and Reconstructive Surgery*, vol. 143, no. 4, Apr. 2019, pp. 721e-726e, 10.1097/prs.0000000000005413.

Geliebter, Allan. "Physiological and Psychological Changes Following Liposuction of Large Volumes of Fat in Overweight and Obese Women." *Journal of Diabetes and Obesity*, vol. 2, no. 4, 2015, pp. 1–7, 10.15436/2376-0494.15.032.

Wittgrove, Alan. "Dear Doctor, Why Doesn't Liposuction Cure Obesity?" *Obesity Action Coalition*, 2014, www.obesityaction.org/community/article-library/dear-doctor-why-doesnt-liposuction-cure-obesity/.

Wolters Kluwer Health. "No Increase in Complications with 'tummy Tuck' in Obese Patients." *ScienceDaily*, 22 Apr. 2019, www.sciencedaily.com/releases/2019/04/190422151038.htm.

■ Low glycemic index diet

CATEGORY: Nutrition

Glycemic Index

The glycemic index (GI) is a measurement of the effect of carbohydrate-containing foods on blood glucose levels (i.e., how rapidly and how high blood glucose levels rise). Using white bread, which has a GI of 100, and glucose, which has a GI of 138, as the reference foods, foods are given a numeric value according to their comparative potential to raise blood glucose levels. High GI foods (e.g., bread, potatoes, desserts) have a more dramatic effect on blood sugar levels than low GI foods (e.g., legumes, vegetables, fruits). Low GI foods promote satiety (i.e. feeling of fullness after eating) and appear to result in a spontaneous decrease in overall food consumption.

Following a low GI diet minimizes spikes in blood glucose levels, which is especially beneficial to individuals at risk for or diagnosed with diabetes mellitus, type 2 (DM2). A low GI diet is associated with weight loss and a reduction in triglycerides, low-density lipoprotein (LDL) cholesterol (called the "bad" cholesterol), and high-sensitivity C-reactive protein (hsCRP) level, which is a marker for low-grade inflammation. A low GI diet can

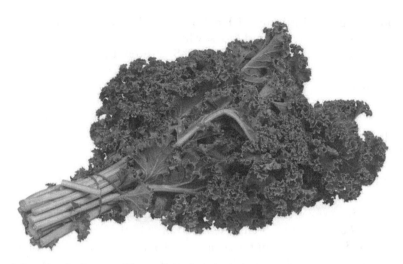

Like other leafy vegetables, curly kale is a food that is low in carbohydrates. (Evan-Amos)

potentially reduce the risk of inflammation-related comorbidities (e.g., cardiovascular disease) in overweight and obese individuals.

Low GI Recommendations

Determining the exact GI of a particular food can be difficult because there are many factors that affect GI scores, including the time of day the food is eaten, the rate of consumption, the other components in the food (e.g., protein, fat, fiber), how the food is prepared or processed (e.g., fried, pickled, blended), physiologic variations (e.g., pre-gastric hydrolysis, gastric emptying rate, hormone response) of the individual consuming the food, and the level of physical activity and stress and overall health status of the individual consuming the food.

Remembering the GI for foods when following a low GI diet can be difficult. Basic information recommended to make it easier to follow a low GI diet:

Choose fresh fruits and vegetables whenever possible.

Choose high-fiber food options, which slow digestion and the release of sugar into the bloodstream. Diets that are high in dietary fiber reduce LDL cholesterol and reduce risk of hypertension, DM2, cancer, and cardiovascular disease. Dietary sources of fiber include oat bran, barley, nuts, seeds, beans, lentils, peas, fruits, and vegetables. The recommended intake of total dietary fiber is 30 g/day; most Americans consume about half of the recommended daily intake.

Avoid foods with the highest content of carbohydrates and simple sugars (e.g., potatoes, breads, cereals, desserts, sweet foods).

Choose foods that are minimally processed. The more finely ground the carbohydrate is, the faster it affects blood glucose levels. Frying contributes a high amount of fat to the food.

It is recommended that individuals participate in physical activity for 30 minutes, 5 times a week when appropriate. Persons who are physically fit have better control of blood glucose levels than those who are sedentary.

Research Findings

Studies comparing the health benefits of a low GI diet with a generally healthy diet have produced conflicting results. The low GI diet does appear to be a useful tool for the management of blood glucose levels in persons at risk for or diagnosed with DM2, but the usefulness of the low GI diet compared with a generally healthy diet for weight loss is not conclusively known. Researchers have reported that consuming a low GI diet over time appears to increase satiety, but it is not as clearly linked to weight loss. Results of studies show strong benefits (e.g., improved insulin control and lipid profiles, weight loss) associated with a low GI diet when combined with regular exercise, but there is some question as to whether the low GI diet plays a significant role or if the exercise is the primary beneficial factor. Regardless, it is clear that diets high in simple carbohydrates are associated with dyslipidemia and DM2. Diet and lifestyle modification for the prevention of overweight and obesity, DM2, and cardiovascular disease should include choosing fresh fruits and vegetables, high-fiber complex carbohydrates, lean proteins, and unsaturated fats and engaging in regular physical exercise.

Summary

Individuals should become knowledgeable about a low GI diet and assess their own health and diet history for the quantity and type of carbohydrate intake. Eating a balanced diet that includes foods that are high in fiber and low in simple-sugar carbohydrates may reduce the risk for obesity, DM2, and cardiovascular disease. There are conflicting research results regarding the effectiveness of following a low GI diet versus an overall healthy lifestyle for weight loss and diabetes control.

—*Cherie Marcel*

References

Kohn, Jill Balla. "What Do I Tell My Clients Who Want to Follow a Low Glycemic Index Diet?" *Journal of the Academy of Nutrition and Dietetics*, vol. 117, no. 1, 2017, p. 164., doi:10.1016/j.jand.2016.10.019.

Kong, A. P. S., et al. "Role of Low-Glycemic Index Diet in Management of Childhood Obesity." *Obesity Reviews*, vol. 12, no. 7, 2010, pp. 492–498., doi:10.1111/j.1467-789x.2010.00768.x.

Pereira, Elisângela Vitoriano, et al. "Effect of Glycemic Index on Obesity Control." *Archives of Endocrinology and Metabolism*, vol. 59, no. 3, 2015, pp. 245–251., doi:10.1590/2359-3997000000045.

Rouhani, Mohammad Hossein, et al. "The Effect of Low Glycemic Index Diet on Body Weight Status and Blood Pressure in Overweight Adolescent Girls: a Randomized Clinical Trial." *Nutrition Research and Practice*, vol. 7, no. 5, 2013, p. 385., doi:10.4162/nrp.2013.7.5.385.

Schwingshackl, Lukas, et al. "Effects of Low Glycaemic Index/Low Glycaemic Load vs. High Glycaemic Index/ High Glycaemic Load Diets on Overweight/Obesity and Associated Risk Factors in Children and Adolescents: a Systematic Review and Meta-Analysis." *Nutrition Journal*, vol. 14, no. 1, 25 Aug. 2015, doi:10.1186/s12937-015-0077-1.

■ Managing Overweight/Obesity for Veterans Everywhere (MOVE!)

CATEGORY: Nutrition; Physiology

The prevalence of obesity in veterans is well documented. As a result of the increased prevalence of obesity in veterans, the Veterans Health Administration (VHA) established the MOVE! (Managing Overweight/Obesity for Veterans Everywhere) Weight Management Program for Veterans in 2006. MOVE! is an evidenced based program that provides nutrition, physical, and behavior modification counseling. The program is based on the National

Institutes of Health (NIH) Identification of Overweight and Obesity in Adults Evidence Report, suggestions from the U.S. Preventative services Task Force, the Department of Veterans Affairs/Department of Defense Clinical Practice Guideline for Screening and Management of Overweight and Obesity, and the Diabetes Prevention Program tools.

Action of the MOVE! Program

The VHA MOVE! program is the largest lifestyle change program in the U.S. Patients are eligible to participate in MOVE! if they are overweight as classified by a BMI of ≥ 25 kg/m^2 with a co-morbidity or if they are obese based on a BMI of ≥ 30 kg/m^2.

Upon entering the program, veterans complete a 23-item baseline assessment known as the MOVE!23 which collects information about medical history, weight and weight management history, motivation, barriers to changing physical activity, diet, and readiness to alter behaviors. The MOVE! program is a multidisciplinary program that consists of nutrition, physical activity, and behavioral counseling and is designed to be a part of a veteran's ongoing care from a primary care physician.

The program was implemented without designated funding and staff and the extent of implementation of the program varies across VHA institutions. For example, some institutions provided individual sessions, group sessions, or a combination of both. Institutions also may offer TeleMOVE! which consists of telephone/telehealth services and MOVE!Coach, a mobile application.

Research Findings

Research has been conducted on MOVE! programs to determine what program characteristics are associated with successful implementation and weight loss. Contextual factors that have been associated with successful program implementation included management support, establishment of a receptive implementation climate emphasizing the importance of weight management. in the control of obesity-related co-morbidities, high-functioning multidisciplinary teams, and a local champion.

Program characteristics associated with a 5% weight reduction for veterans participating in a VA program included program type (group or self-managed), and the number and type of provider contacts.

In a qualitative comparative analysis of 17 VHA institutions to determine what conditions related to a larger 6-month weight loss outcome for participants, researchers found that success of the program was enhanced by use of a standard curriculum and a group delivery format. Other conditions included the combination of high-program complexity and high staff involvement; group delivery format and low accountability to facility leadership; an active physician champion with low accountability to facility leadership; and use of a quality improvement plan without use of a waiting list.

In a study of 10 VHA institutions to explore organizational factors that supported or inhibited the implementation of MOVE!, researchers found that organizational readiness and the presence of a champion were the two factors that aligned with successful implementation. Factors that seemed to inhibit success included management support and resource availability.

Studies examining the program's effectiveness for participants have been conducted and have shown positive results for veterans engaged in the program but not for veterans with serious mental health issues. In a study of 377 veterans to investigate the effectiveness of the MOVE! program in achieving weight loss for veterans in the VA Greater Los Angeles Healthcare System, results showed that before engaging in the program a weight gain of 1.4 kg per year occurred but one year after participation in the MOVE! program participants lost and average of 2.2 kg.

In a sample of 862 veterans at the Miami VHA, investigators found that veterans gained an average of 2.0 kg/year before enrolling in MOVE! and participating in a supportive group session. An average of 1.6 kg/year was lost after participating in the program.

In a randomized controlled trial of 53 veterans with serious mental health illness from the VA Maryland and District of Columbia, researchers found that only seven participants achieved a weight loss of 5% of their baseline and there was no effect on group assignment on weight loss.

In a study of 19,367 veterans to explore whether participation in MOVE! correlated with a reduction in diabetes, investigators found that, compared with those that did not participate, the incidence of diabetes was reduced as a result of intense and sustained participation.

Studies have been conducted to explore how program factors related to participation retention and utilization rates of the MOVE! Program. In a qualitative study using semi-structured interviews with 12 MOVE! program coordinators, researchers sought to examine how program characteristics related to veteran participant retention in the program. Characteristics related to retention included: provider knowledge and referral to the program, reputation of the program within the facility, the MOVE! meeting schedule, the inclusion of physical activity in group sessions, and the involvement of a physician champion.

In a retrospective cohort study of all 140 VA institutions using the MOVE! program in 2010, investigators assessed patient and facility factors that correlated with MOVE! utilization. Investigators found that 4.39% of all eligible overweight and obese patients using VA health services used the MOVE! program at least once in fiscal year 2010. Utilization rates ranged from .05% to 16% and veterans were more likely to have had at least one MOVE! visit if they had a higher BMI, were female, not married, younger, minority or had psychiatric or obese-related comorbidities.

—*Lori Porter*

References

Batch, Bryan C., et al. "Outcome by Gender in the Veterans Health Administration Motivating Overweight/Obese Veterans Everywhere Weight Management Program." *Journal of Women's Health*, vol. 27, no. 1, Jan. 2018, pp. 32–39, 10.1089/jwh.2016.6212.

Garvin, Jane T., et al. "Characteristics Influencing Weight Reduction Among Veterans in the MOVE!® Program." *Western Journal of Nursing Research*, vol. 37, no. 1, 18 May 2014, pp. 50–65, 10.1177/0193945914534323.

Rogers, Tony B. "MOVE! Weight Management Program Home." *MOVE!*, U.S. Department of Veterans Affairs, 2020, www.move.va.gov/.

Shiroma, Paulo R, et al. "Antidepressant Effect of the VA Weight Management Program (MOVE) Among Veterans With Severe Obesity." *Military Medicine*, 20 Feb. 2020, 10.1093/milmed/usz475.

■ MyPlate nutritional model

The "2015-2020 Dietary Guidelines for Americans" that was released in December 2015 is detailed in the MyPlate nutritional model, which was launched by the United States Department of Agriculture (USDA) on June 2, 2011, as an initiative to assist healthcare professionals in providing nutrition education. MyPlate replaces MyPyramid as a practical, user friendly guide for making healthy food choices.

In MyPlate, the five food groups are presented in a simple illustration of a plate divided into four sections and a cup. The sections on the plate represent fruits, vegetables, grains, and proteins. The sections for vegetables and grains are slightly larger than those for fruits and proteins, indicating that vegetables and grains should be consumed in greater quantities. To the side of the plate illustration is a cup that represents the dairy food group. Unlike the MyPyramid model, MyPlate does not include oils and solid fats as a food choice category.

Recommendations of the "2015-2020 Dietary Guidelines for Americans" are summarized as follows:

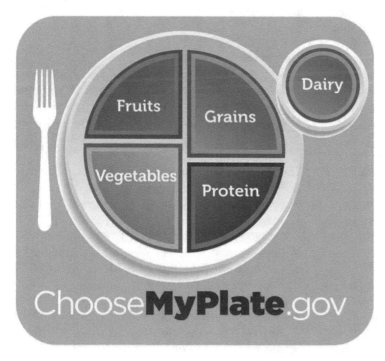

USDA MyPlate nutritional guide icon. (United States Department of Agriculture)

- Maintain calorie balance over time to achieve and sustain a healthy weight.
- Focus on consuming nutrient-dense foods and beverages.

Benefits of the MyPlate model as a replacement for the MyPyramid model

The MyPlate model is easy to understand by both adults and children. There is no need to count servings or measure portion sizes; food choices are simply placed on the plate according to the proportions in the MyPlate guidelines.

Fruits and vegetables make up half of the plate, and vegetables represent the largest section.

The former MyPyramid category of meats and beans is now referred to as the protein category. This allows for the inclusion of seafood and vegetarian protein options (e.g., eggs, fish, nuts, peas, soy).

Although the category of solid fats and oils is not represented on the plate as a separate food choice, small portions of healthy (e.g., polyunsaturated fatty acids, high-density lipoprotein cholesterols) solid fats and oils provide essential nutrients (e.g., omega-3 fatty acids, vitamins A, D, E, and K) and are considered to be included in the other sections of healthy food choices (e.g., fish, nuts, avocados, and milk, as found in the protein, vegetable, and dairy sections).

MyPlate presents a positive message regarding the inclusion of food choices instead of the former emphasis on avoidance.

Research Findings

Research evaluating the effectiveness of MyPlate in behavior modification programs is limited. Recommendations for future assessment of the MyPlate initiative include determining the degree of association between the message of MyPlate and positive behavioral changes and establishing strategies for increasing the effectiveness of the MyPlate initiative in populations that are poorly reached.

Initiatives such as MyPlate Kids' Place and MyPlate On Campus have been instituted to increase understanding and utilization of the MyPlate model among children and young adults. Social media (e.g., Twitter, Pinterest, Facebook) is also being used to increase awareness of MyPlate.

Summary

Individuals should become knowledgeable about the MyPlate model and assess their own health and diet history in relation to the MyPlate recommendations. MyPlate replaced MyPyramid in 2011 as a more practical, user friendly guide for making healthy food choices. The MyPlate model emphasizes eating a balanced diet that is high in nutritional value based on current recommendations for optimal health.

—*Cherie Marcel*

References

Chang, Sarah, and Kristin Koegel. "Back to Basics: All About MyPlate Food Groups." *Journal of the Academy of Nutrition and Dietetics*, vol. 117, no. 9, 2017, pp. 1351–1353., doi:10.1016/j.jand.2017.06.376.

"Dietary Guidelines for Americans 2015–2020." *U.S. Department of Health and Human Services*, Office of Disease Prevention and Health Promotion, Dec. 2015, health.gov/our-work/food-nutrition/2015-2020-dietary-guidelines/guidelines/.

Mulik, Kranti, and Lindsey Haynes-Maslow. "The Affordability of MyPlate: An Analysis of SNAP Benefits and the Actual Cost of Eating According to the Dietary Guidelines." *Journal of Nutrition Education and Behavior*, vol. 49, no. 8, 2017, doi:10.1016/j.jneb.2017.06.005.

"Start Simple with MyPlate." *ChooseMyPlate*, U.S. Department of Agriculture, 2020, www.choosemyplate.gov/eathealthy/start-simple-myplate.

■ Natural and alternative treatments

CATEGORY: Treatment

Losing weight can be a lifelong challenge. Researchers who study obesity consider it a chronic health condition that must be managed much like high blood pressure or high cholesterol. This means that there is no easy cure.

Losing just 5 to 10 percent of one's total weight can lower blood pressure, improve cholesterol profile, prevent diabetes, improve blood sugar control if one already has diabetes, and reduce the risk of developing osteoarthritis of the knee. A combination of improved diet and regular exercise might be the best way to lose weight and keep it off.

Although early weight-loss drugs, such as amphetamines and Fen-Phen (fenfluramine and phentermine), have had a poor safety record, sibutramine (Meridia) appears to be safe and modestly effective for weight loss. Newer drugs will likely offer greater benefits.

It is commonly stated that the high-fructose corn syrup that is added to many foods is a major cause of obesity. However, while there is little doubt that, in general, excess intake of calories promotes obesity, the specific relationship of this substance to weight gain remains questionable.

Chromium

Chromium is a mineral the body needs in only small amounts, but it is important to human nutrition. Although it has principally been studied for improving blood sugar control in people with diabetes, chromium has also been tried for reducing total weight and body fat percentage, with some success. Both of these potential benefits involve chromium's effects on insulin.

Based on this push-pull effect, to lose weight, one should keep insulin levels low. Dieting is the most obvious method of reducing insulin. When a person does not take in enough calories to supply the body's daily needs, insulin levels fall and the body breaks down fat cells. Exercising is another method to reduce insulin; by increasing the body's energy requirements, exercise causes insulin levels to fall and fat cells to break down.

It is difficult to consistently use more energy than one takes in. Hunger takes over, and a person wants to eat. If there were some way to trigger fat breakdown without going hungry, it would make weight loss much easier.

There is another important connection between insulin and weight to consider. Persons who weigh too much often develop insulin resistance. In this condition, certain cells of the body become less sensitive to insulin. The body senses this and, thus, increases insulin production until it overcomes the resistance. It is possible that fat cells respond to these increased levels of insulin by storing even more fat.

Chromium is thought to improve the body's responsiveness to insulin. Combining this belief with the insulin-weight connections, some researchers have proposed that chromium may assist in decreasing weight or improving body composition (the ratio of fatty tissue to lean tissue).

The main argument is the following: Chromium increases insulin sensitivity. This causes levels of insulin to fall. With reduced amounts of insulin in the blood, fat cells are less inclined to store fat, so weight loss may become easier. In addition, there is some evidence that chromium partially blocks insulin's effects on fat cells, interfering with its fat-building effect. This could also promote weight loss. Another small study suggests that chromium may work by influencing the brain and its role in appetite and food cravings.

There are several flaws in these arguments, though. For example, even very small amounts of insulin in the blood effectively suppress fat breakdown. Another problem is that during insulin resistance, fat cells also appear to become resistant to insulin. Insulin resistance, in other words, might be a natural method of regulating weight gain. Chromium supplements might have the undesired effect of increasing the ability of fat cells to respond to insulin, helping them to better store fat.

However, theory takes one only so far. It is more important to review the results of studies in which people were given chromium supplements to reduce their weight.

About ten well-designed, double-blind, placebo-controlled trials have evaluated chromium's potential benefit for weight loss. In the largest study, 219 people were given either placebo, 200 micrograms (mcg) of chromium picolinate daily, or 400 mcg of chromium picolinate daily. Participants were not advised to follow any particular diet. For seventy-two days, people taking chromium experienced significantly greater weight loss (more than 2.5 pounds versus about 0.25 pound) than those not taking chromium. Persons taking chromium actually gained lean body mass, so the difference in loss of fatty tissue was greater: more than 4 pounds versus less than 0.50 pound. However, a high dropout rate makes the results of this study somewhat unreliable.

In a smaller double-blind study by the same researcher, 130 moderately overweight persons attempting to lose weight were given either placebo or 400 mcg of chromium daily. Although hints of benefit were seen, they were too slight to be statistically significant. Several other small, double-blind, placebo-controlled studies also failed to find evidence of the benefit of chromium picolinate as an aid to weight loss. One study failed to find benefit with a combination of chromium and conjugated linoleic acid.

When larger studies find positive results and smaller studies do not, it often indicates that the treatment under study is only weakly effective. This may be the case with chromium as a weight-loss treatment.

Foods that are good sources of chromium include broccoli, potatoes, beef, poultry, milk, apples, bananas, and whole-grain products.

Pyruvate

Pyruvate supplies the body with pyruvic acid, a natural compound that plays important roles in the manufacture and use of energy. Theoretically, taking pyruvate might increase the body's metabolism, particularly of fat.

Several small studies enrolling about 150 people have found evidence that pyruvate or DHAP (a combination of pyruvate and the related substance dihydroxyacetone) can aid weight loss or improve body composition, or both. For example, in a six-week, double-blind, placebo-controlled trial, fifty-one people were given either pyruvate (6 grams [g] daily), placebo, or no treatment. All participated in an exercise program. In the treated group, significant decreases in fat mass (2.1 kilograms [kg]) and percentage body fat (2.6 percent) were seen, along with a significant increase in muscle mass (1.5 kg). No significant changes were seen in the placebo or nontreatment groups.

Another placebo-controlled study (blinding not stated) used a much higher dose of pyruvate (22 to 44 g daily, depending on total calorie intake). In this trial, thirty-four slightly overweight people were put on a mildly weight-reducing diet for four weeks. Subsequently, one-half were given a liquid dietary supplement containing pyruvate. In six weeks, people in the pyruvate group lost a small amount of weight (about 1.5 pounds), while those in the placebo group did not lose weight. Most of the weight loss came from fat.

Another placebo-controlled study evaluated the effects of DHAP when people who had previously lost weight increased their calorie intake. Seventeen severely overweight women were put on a restricted diet as inpatients for three weeks, during which time they lost approximately 17 pounds. They were then given a high-calorie diet. Approximately one-half of the women also received 15 g of pyruvate and 75 g of dihydroxyacetone daily. The results found that after three weeks of this weight-gaining diet, persons receiving the supplements gained only about 4 pounds, compared to about 6 pounds in the placebo group. Close evaluation showed that pyruvate specifically blocked the regain of fat weight. Larger studies (one hundred participants or more) are needed, however, to establish the benefits of pyruvate for weight loss.

Foods that contain pyruvate include apples, beer, and red wine.

Hydroxycitric Acid

Hydroxycitric acid (HCA), a derivative of citric acid, is found primarily in a small, sweet, purple fruit called *Garcinia cambogia*, the Malabar tamarind. Although animal and test-tube studies and one human trial suggest that HCA might encourage weight loss, other studies have found no benefit. In an eight-week, double-blind, placebo-controlled trial of sixty overweight people, the use of HCA at a dose of 440 mg three times daily produced significant weight loss compared with placebo.

In contrast, a twelve-week, double-blind, placebo-controlled trial of 135 overweight persons, who were given either placebo or 500 mg of HCA three times daily, found no effect on body weight or fat mass. However, this study has been criticized for using a high-fiber diet, which is thought to impair HCA absorption.

Other small placebo-controlled studies found HCA had no effect on metabolism, appetite, or weight. It is not clear whether *G. cambogia* is an effective treatment for weight loss.

Caffeine and Ephedrine

Caffeine and ephedrine (found in ephedra, an herb also known as ma huang) are central nervous system stimulants. Considerable evidence suggests ephedrine-caffeine combinations can modestly assist in weight loss.

For example, in a double-blind, placebo-controlled trial, 180 overweight people were placed on a weight-loss diet and given either ephedrine-caffeine (20 mg/200 mg), ephedrine alone (20 mg), caffeine alone (200 mg), or placebo three times daily for twenty-four weeks. The results showed that the ephedrine-caffeine treatment significantly enhanced weight loss, resulting in a loss of more than 36 pounds compared to only 29 pounds in the placebo group. Neither ephedrine nor caffeine alone produced any benefit. Contrary to some reports, participants did not develop tolerance to the treatment. For the entire six months of the trial, the treatment group maintained the same relative weight loss advantage over the placebo group. While this study found benefit only with caffeine-ephedrine and not with ephedrine alone, other studies have found that ephedrine alone also offers some weight-loss benefits.

It is not known how ephedrine-caffeine works. However, caffeine has actions that cause fat breakdown and enhance metabolism. Ephedrine suppresses appetite and increases energy expenditure. The combination appears to produce synergistic effects, with appetite suppression probably the most important overall factor.

Ephedrine presents serious medical risks and should be used only under physician supervision. In the United States, the sale of ephedrine-containing products is banned.

Medium-chain Triglycerides

Some evidence suggests that consumption of medium-chain triglycerides (MCTs) might enhance the body's tendency to burn fat. This has led to investigations of MCTs as a weight-loss aid. However, the results of clinical trials have been fairly unimpressive.

In a four-week, double-blind, placebo-controlled trial, sixty-six women were put on a diet very low in carbohydrates to induce a state called ketosis. One-half of the women received a liquid supplement containing ordinary fats; the other one-half received a similar supplement in which the ordinary fats were replaced by MCTs.

The results indicated that the MCT supplement significantly increased the rate of "fat burning" during the first two weeks of the trial and also reduced the loss of muscle mass. However, these benefits declined during the last two weeks of the trial, which suggests that the effects of MCTs are temporary. Studies that involved substituting MCTs for ordinary fats in a low- calorie diet have shown minimal relative benefits at best.

A related supplement called structured medium- and long-chain triacylglycerols (SMLCT) has been created to provide the same potential benefits as MCTs, but in a form that can be used as cooking oil. In a preliminary double-blind trial, SMLCT showed some promise as a "fat burner."

—*EBSCO CAM Review Board*

References

Bjarnadottir, Adda. "How Garcinia Cambogia Can Help You Lose Weight and Belly Fat." *Healthline*, 6 Dec. 2018, www.healthline.com/nutrition/garcinia-cambogia-weight-loss.

Maki, Kevin C, et al. "Consumption of Diacylglycerol Oil as Part of a Reduced-Energy Diet Enhances Loss of Body Weight and Fat in Comparison with Consumption of a Triacylglycerol Control Oil." *The American Journal of Clinical Nutrition*, vol. 76, no. 6, 1 Dec. 2002, pp. 1230–1236, 10.1093/ajcn/76.6.1230.

Menayang, Adi. "New Report Supports Chromium Picolinate's Weight Management Benefits." *NutraIngredients-USA*, 2 Jan. 2019, www.nutraingredients-usa.com/Article/2019/01/02/New-report-supports-chromium-picolinate-s-weight-management-benefits.

Office of Dietary Supplements. "Chromium." *National Institutes of Health*, U.S. Department of Health and Human Services, 27 Feb. 2020, ods.od.nih.gov/factsheets/Chromium-HealthProfessional/.

Onakpoya, Igho, et al. "Pyruvate Supplementation for Weight Loss: A Systematic Review and Meta-Analysis of Randomized Clinical Trials." *Critical Reviews in Food Science and Nutrition*, vol. 54, no. 1, 4 Nov. 2013, pp. 17–23, 10.1080/10408398.2011.565890.

——. "The Use of Garcinia Extract (Hydroxycitric Acid) as a Weight Loss Supplement: A Systematic Review and Meta-Analysis of Randomised Clinical Trials." *Journal of Obesity*, vol. 2011, 2011, pp. 1–9, www.hindawi.com/journals/jobe/2011/509038/, 10.1155/2011/509038.

Rumsey, Alissa. "Should You Add MCT Oil to Your Diet?" *US News & World Report*, 2019, health.usnews.com/health-news/blogs/eat-run/articles/should-you-add-mct-oil-to-your-diet.

■ Nutrition through the lifespan

CATEGORY: Nutrition

Pregnancy and Infancy

Infancy encompasses the first year of a human life. A healthy, full-term infant is born after successful development during a gestational period of 37–42 weeks. Prior to birth, fetal nutrition is provided directly from the mother's diet. A woman's diet during and preceding pregnancy can have a profound effect on the growth and development of her fetus. Unique nutritional requirements during pregnancy include the increased need for iron, folic acid, calcium, and zinc. Calorie (kcal) needs increase during pregnancy by about 300 kcal/day. Weight gain or loss throughout pregnancy is considered a good indicator of nutritional status. Research results show that when dietary and lifestyle counseling is provided, pregnant women are more likely to consume a healthy diet and gain an amount of weight that is within the recommended gestational weight gain guidelines established by the American College of Obstetricians and Gynecologists (ACOG) and the Institute of Medicine (IOM).

After birth, normal growth and development in infancy depend on the diet provided. Breast milk is considered to be excellent nutrition for infants and nutritionally superior to any available alternative. The recommendation of the American Academy of Pediatrics (AAP) is that infants should be exclusively breastfed for the first 6 months of life, and that breastfeeding should continue during the introduction of food during the first year. In cases where breastfeeding is contraindicated or is not possible (e.g., the mother is receiving therapy for cancer; the infant has an inborn error of metabolism; in cases of adoption), many types of infant formula are available to provide nutrition that is necessary for the infant to thrive.

At about 6 months of age, infants are usually ready to be introduced to solid foods. This should be done gradually, starting with small servings of simple, soft foods such as rice cereal combined with breast milk or infant formula. Foods should be introduced one at a time at intervals of 2–3 days to assess for food sensitivities or allergies. Small, cut-up pieces of soft food can be offered as the infant becomes more comfortable with solid food, which usually occurs at 8–9 months of age. The introduction of solid foods at 6–12 months of age is primarily educational for

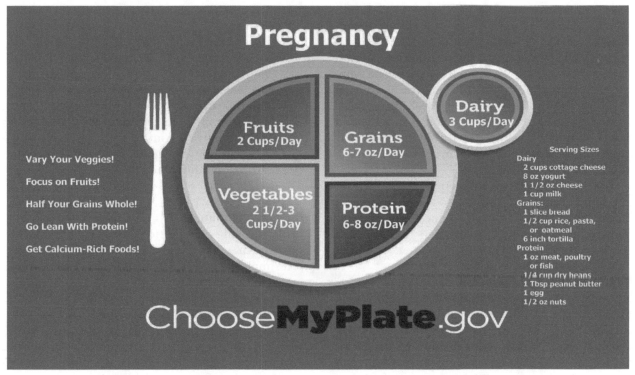

MyPlate recommendations for a pregnancy diet. (U.S. Department of Agriculture Center for Nutrition Policy and Promotion)

infants—allowing them to become familiar with the textures and flavors of food—because during this period their primary nutrition continues to be provided in breast milk or formula.

Dietary Recommendations for Pregnant Women

Eating a well-rounded diet with adequate protein (e.g., about 70 g/day) and a variety of fruits and vegetables is vital for normal fetal development. Calorie requirements increase by about 300 kcal/day, making the average intake goal 2,200–2,900 kcal/day for most pregnant women.

Prenatal supplements that include iron and folic acid are important for pregnant women to take because doing so prevents neural tube defects.

Avoidance of alcohol, tobacco, drugs, and large amounts of caffeine (e.g., > 300 mg/day) is imperative to good fetal health.

Fish and seafood provide the essential nutrient docosahexaenoic acid (DHA), which is important in fetal development. Certain types of fish (e.g., shark, swordfish, king mackerel, tilefish) should be avoided because they contain high levels of mercury, which can be harmful to fetal development.

Dietary Recommendations for Infants

Infants require only breast milk or formula for the first 6 months of life. In the first weeks of life, breastfed infants should nurse 8–12 times daily, averaging 15 minutes for each breast. Breastfed infants usually do not require supplementation with formula, although formula can be used when breast milk is unavailable (e.g., if the mother is at work or ill). In some cases, breastfed infants require vitamin D supplementation because breast milk can be deficient in vitamin D, depending on the mother's dietary intake and metabolism.

Formula-fed infants tend to consume what they require if allowed to feed on demand. Typically, feeding is required every 2–3 hours. Iron-fortified formula is recommended for infants who are fed formula because these infants tend to have inadequate iron reserves and are at risk for iron-deficiency anemia. Neither breastfed nor formula-fed infants require supplemental water because their fluid needs are met by consuming breast milk or formula.

Although breast milk or formula should be the major source of nutrition at 6–12 months of age, solid foods can be gradually introduced. When infants are able to sit independently and reach out for objects, they are ready to start eating solid food. Offering solid food should begin with simple cereal, such as rice cereal combined with warm breast milk or formula. Initial servings should be small (e.g., 1–2 spoonfuls). Infant oatmeal, mashed vegetables, and mashed fruits should be added separately over 2–3-day intervals to allow for assessment of food sensitivities or allergies.

By 8–9 months of age, infants are usually ready to try finger foods (i.e., solid foods cut into small bites). Foods that are hard to chew (e.g., raisins, nuts, popcorn) should be avoided because such foods increase risk of choking.

Common Types of Formulas

About 80% of commercial formulas are cow's milk that is treated to improve digestibility and make it as similar as possible to breast milk. Hydrolyzed formulas contain milk proteins that are broken down into very small particles to improve digestion in infants who have protein intolerance. Soy-based formulas contain soy protein and are given to infants who are lactose intolerant.

Breastfeeding

Breast milk contains antibodies and cell-mediated immunologic factors that boost the infant's immune system, providing protection against respiratory syncytial virus (RSV); pneumonia; urinary tract infection; bacterial meningitis; gastroenteritis; lymphoma; Crohn's disease; celiac disease; diabetes mellitus, types 1 and 2; and childhood obesity.

Breastfed infants show a lower incidence of certain allergies and allergic manifestations (e.g., atopic dermatitis) compared with formula-fed infants. Breastfed infants have a lower risk of sudden infant death syndrome (SIDS). Evidence suggests that breast milk enhances cognitive development.

Breastfeeding is not recommended in the following situations:

- Mother is receiving treatment for cancer
- Mother has active tuberculosis, HIV infection, or human T-cellleukemia virus type 1 (HTLV-1) infection

- Mother has a herpes simplex lesion on her breast
- Infant has galactosemia, a rare genetic disorder characterized by inability to metabolize any form of animal- or human-derived milk
- Mother is receiving certain medication (e.g., immunosuppressive or antineoplastic drugs; amphetamines) that is excreted in breast milk and can harm the infant
- Mother abuses substances (e.g., cocaine, alcohol, methamphetamines)

Research Findings

Probiotic and prebiotic formulas have been devised to encourage the growth of desirable intestinal flora (i.e., bacteria) in formula-fed infants that is similar to that in breastfed babies. These formulas prevent gastrointestinal infection, diarrhea, and onset of allergies. It has also been suggested that the improved gastrointestinal environment that is supported by probiotic and prebiotic formulas aids in the absorption of magnesium, calcium, and iron. In a recent randomized controlled trial, infants who were fed formula containing probiotics and prebiotics tolerated the formula well.

Inadequate gestational weight gain is associated with an increased rate of preterm birth and low birth weight. Excessive gestational weight gain is associated with increased rates of gestational diabetes and pre-eclampsia, which can lead to preterm birth. Results of studies show that pregnant women are more likely to gain within the recommended weight range when provided with dietary counseling. Obese women who receive dietary counseling during pregnancy are less prone to high levels of fasting insulin, leptin, and glucose. Counseling is especially effective when it focuses on beliefs regarding body shape and expected gestational weight gain.

Research conducted on mice revealed that a gluten-free diet during fetal life (via the maternal diet) and early infancy reduces the incidence of diabetes and inflammation later in life.

Summary

New parents should become knowledgeable about nutrition for healthy infants. Pregnant women may be at risk for inadequate and excessive gestational weight gain and preterm delivery, requiring dietary counseling and education on guidelines for gestational weight gain. Strict adherence to the prescribed dietary regimen and continued medical surveillance to monitor weight gain will ensure healthy progression of the pregnancy. It is recommended that infants receive breast milk or formula for the first 6 months of life, with the introduction of solid food at 6–12 months. Research suggests that pre and probiotic formulas may help increase infant tolerance.

—*Cherie Marcel*

References

Lau, Erica Y., et al. "Maternal Weight Gain in Pregnancy and Risk of Obesity among Offspring: A Systematic Review." *Journal of Obesity*, vol. 2014, 2014, pp. 1–16, 10.1155/2014/524939.

Moreno, Megan. "Early Infant Feeding and Obesity Risk." *JAMA Pediatrics*, vol. 168, no. 11, 1 Nov. 2014, p. 1084, 10.1001/jamapediatrics.2013.3379.

Robinson, S. M. "Infant Nutrition and Lifelong Health: Current Perspectives and Future Challenges." *Journal of Developmental Origins of Health and Disease*, vol. 6, no. 5, 19 June 2015, pp. 384–389, 10.1017/s2040174415001257.

Stang, Jamie, and Laurel G. Huffman. "Position of the Academy of Nutrition and Dietetics: Obesity, Reproduction, and Pregnancy Outcomes." *Journal of the Academy of Nutrition and Dietetics*, vol. 116, no. 4, Apr. 2016, pp. 677–691, 10.1016/j.jand.2016.01.008.

Symon, B, et al. "Does the Early Introduction of Solids Promote Obesity?" *Singapore Medical Journal*, vol. 58, no. 11, Nov. 2017, pp. 626–631, 10.11622/smedj.2017024.

Toddlers

Toddlerhood refers to the second and third years of a human life. It is a time of exploration in which the dramatic growth in the first year of life slows, but the motor activity increases. Toddlers are still learning self-feeding skills, such as learning to grasp finger foods, using a spoon and fork, and sipping from a cup. Eating behavior is unpredictable as the toddler experiments with flavors and textures of foods, often choosing to eat only a single type of food for a period of time and subsequently rejecting the chosen food. Although toddlers need to eat 5–7 small meals a

day, their appetite naturally decreases (i.e., a processes referred to as physiologic anorexia) after the first year of life. Toddlers frequently become distracted by the surrounding environment while eating and leaving food in inappropriate places because they run off to explore. This can be distressing for the parents/caregivers, who worry that the toddler is not consuming enough food or does not have a healthy diet. Although most toddlers naturally consume enough nutrients for normal growth, monitoring growth helps to determine if they are consuming adequate calories and reduces fears of the caregivers.

Dietary Recommendations for Toddlers Aged 1–3 Years

Toddlers should eat 5–7 small meals a day. Because lifetime eating habits are established in early childhood, it is vital that caregivers offer a variety of fruits, vegetables, whole grains, and proteins throughout the day, keeping in mind that many of the foods will be rejected several times before the toddler decides to sample them.

While eating fruit is recommended, it is best to limit fruit juice intake to 4–6 oz/day of 100% fruit juice from a cup; bottles should only be used for milk or formula. Excessive consumption of juice and other sweetened beverages is linked to dental caries, chronic diarrhea, and imbalanced diets in which fruit juice replaces necessary nutrient intake from other foods. Soda, punch, and other sugary drinks are not recommended under any circumstances.

Milk is a vital source of nutrients, including calcium and vitamin D, during toddlerhood and milk intake should average 2–3 servings (24–30 oz) per day. Drinking whole milk is important until 2 years of age because it provides the fat and cholesterol necessary for brain development. Low-fat milk can be offered after 2 years of age for moderate dietary fat intake of up to 30% of daily calories. It is not necessary or appropriate to restrict fat in the toddler's diet other than saturated and trans fats that are found in processed foods (e.g., chips, French fries).

Daily intake of 500 mg per day of calcium is recommended for toddlers. 400 international units (IU) per day of vitamin D is recommended. Iron-rich foods are recommended to prevent

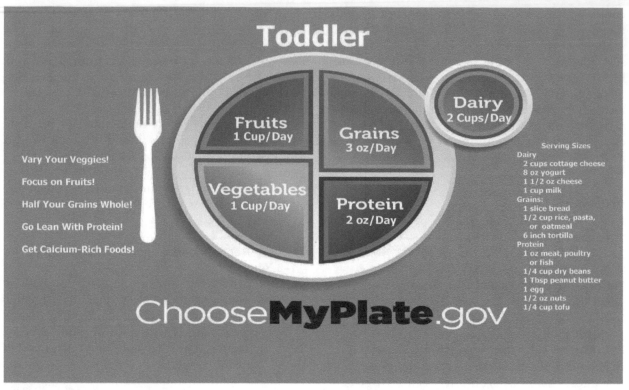

MyPlate recommendations for atoddler's diet. (U.S. Department of Agriculture Center for Nutrition Policy and Promotion)

iron-deficiency anemia, which is a common risk for young children.

Although introducing a variety of food textures can help toddlers adapt to eating a wider variety of foods, it is important to avoid foods that pose a choking hazard, including foods that are difficult to chew, do not dissolve in saliva, or are hard and round. Common foods that cause choking are whole nuts, hard candy, hotdogs, popcorn, whole grapes, raw fruits and vegetables, and globs of peanut butter. Chewing and mastication skills become more precise throughout toddlerhood, and most children are capable of self-feeding a wide range of foods by the age of 3 years.

Caregivers are encouraged to create a positive eating environment for toddlers, including the following:

- Allow ample time for the toddler to eat. Eating is a new skill to toddlers and they need time to smell, taste, and touch the food. Encouraging

them to eat rapidly increases stress during mealtimes.
- Be patient when spills and accidents occur because these are part of the toddler's learning process.
- Provide utensils toddlers can hold and put into their mouths easily and use break-resistant dinnerware.
- Create a mealtime environment that is an opportunity for family interaction so toddlers can witness positive eating habits modeled by their caregivers. Toddlers are more likely to try a new food if they see their caregivers and older siblings eating it.

Growth charts are available to monitor toddler weight gain, height, and head circumference in relation to expected norms by age. Although the goal is for the measurements to fall between the 5th and 95th percentile on the growth charts, consistent growth patterns are the best indication of nutritional adequacy in toddlers.

Research Findings

Prebiotics are food components that are not digested in the upper gastrointestinal tract, allowing them to be fermented by intestinal microflora (i.e., bacteria) into probiotic elements, which encourage the growth and activity of more desirable intestinal microflora. Studies indicate that prebiotic foods and supplements prevent the onset of allergies, gastrointestinal infection, and diarrhea and reduce the rate of overall infections in infants and toddlers up to 24 months of age.

Results of many studies show the direct impact of the dietary habits and beliefs of caregivers on the dietary habits and beliefs of their children. Researchers have documented that children tend to make food choices similar to those of both their father and their mother. Evidence suggests that even grandmothers in the toddler's home environment have a strong influence over the dietary behaviors of their grandchildren. Researchers have documented that the physical activity the family participates in has a direct influence on the activity and dietary choices of the children in the household, which indicates that health promotion interventions need to be family-based in order to be successful.

It is common for children to reject vegetables and favor fruits or cereals. In such situations, researchers suggest that using a little creativity can improve toddler intake of vegetables. Results of a recent study indicate that blending pureed vegetables into other food favorites increased vegetable intake in toddlers.

Researchers report that the results of preliminary controlled trials indicate that multi-micronutrient supplementation in children can positively impact certain aspects of cognition and behavior.

Summary

Parents and caregivers should become knowledgeable about physiologic and dietary needs during toddlerhood. Toddlers should eat 5–7 small meals a day, including a variety of fruits, vegetables, whole grains, and proteins, while keeping in mind that many of the foods will be rejected several times before the toddler decides to sample them. Toddlers should be assessed for risk of inadequate and excessive weight gain and growth, and dietary counseling to caregivers may be beneficial. It is important for caregivers to adhere to the prescribed dietary regimen of providing healthy food choices and continue medical surveillance to monitor the toddler's growth and nutritional status. Research suggests that toddlers are influenced by the dietary habits of family members.

—*Cherie Marcel*

References

Ohio State University Center for Clinical and Translational Science. "Childhood Obesity Influenced by How Kids Are Fed, Not Just What They Eat." *ScienceDaily*, 13 May 2015, w w w . s c i e n c e d a i l y . c o m / releases/2015/05/150513093358.htm.

"Tips for Parents–Ideas to Help Children Maintain a Healthy Weight." *Centers for Disease Control and Prevention*, 18 July 2018, www.cdc.gov/healthy-weight/children/index.html.

Tran, Bach Xuan, et al. "Global Evolution of Obesity Research in Children and Youths: Setting Priorities for Interventions and Policies." *Obesity Facts*, vol. 12, no. 2, 2019, pp. 137–149, 10.1159/000497121.

Wen, Li Ming, et al. "The Effect of Early Life Factors and Early Interventions on Childhood Overweight and Obesity 2016." *Journal of Obesity*, vol. 2017, 2017, pp. 1–3, 10.1155/2017/3642818.

Xu, Furong, et al. "A Community-Based Nutrition and Physical Activity Intervention for Children Who Are Overweight or Obese and Their Caregivers." *Journal of Obesity*, vol. 2017, 2017, pp. 1–9, www.ncbi.nlm.nih.gov/pmc/articles/ PMC5651117/, 10.1155/2017/2746595.

Preschool-Aged Children

Preschool-aged children (i.e., 3–5 years of age) have mastered the skill of self-feeding and are capable of eating a wide variety of foods. The preschool period is a time of activity, exploration, and learning; typically preschool-aged children show signs of independence and rebellion by around 4 years of age. The period of independence and rebellion is frequently accompanied by finicky eating that is similar to the erratic eating choices and behaviors of toddlers. Fluctuations in the preschooler's food.

References can cause parents/caregivers to become concerned about whether the child is consuming enough food or has a diet that is healthy enough. There is evidence, however, that children self-regulate their dietary intake to meet their energy needs. If they pick at one meal and do not eat well, they tend to eat more at another. By the age of 5 years, the phase of rebellion passes and most children are willing to try new foods. Monitoring the preschooler's growth patterns on a growth chart can help to determine if he/she is consuming adequate calories.

Parents/caregivers are encouraged to create a positive eating environment for children, including the following:

- Keep mealtime pleasant and avoid arguments, which can cause preschool children to attach negative feelings to eating. Children are less likely to try new foods that are introduced in a negative environment.
- Allow ample time for eating. Children need time to smell, taste, and touch their food. Rushing them can add stress during meal times.
- Be patient with spills and accidents because they are part of the preschooler's learning process.
- Provide utensils that can be held and put into the mouth easily and use break-resistant dishes and glasses.
- Create a mealtime environment that offers an opportunity for family interaction so preschoolers can witness positive eating habits modeled by their parents/caregivers. Children are more likely to try a new food if they see their parents/caregivers and older siblings eating it.

Research Findings

Results of many studies show the direct effect of parent/caregiver dietary habits and beliefs on the dietary habits and beliefs of children. Researchers have documented that children tend to make food choices similar to those of both their father and mother. Evidence suggests that even grandmothers in the home environment have a strong influence over the dietary behaviors of their grandchildren. Researchers have documented that the physical activity the family participates in has a direct effect on the activity and dietary choices of the children in the household, which indicates that health promotion interventions should be family- and community-based to be successful, supporting families where they live and work.

Researchers in a recent study investigated the association between family meals, viewing television during meals, and food choices made by children. Results were that children who ate breakfast, lunch, or dinner with their family at least 4 days/week ate more fruits and vegetables than those who did not participate in family meals 4 days/week. Children who rarely or never watched television during family meals were less likely to eat soda and chips.

Researchers report that introducing nutrition and physical activity interventions through child care (or daycare) centers reduces dietary risk factors, such as obesity, for preschool children and their families.

It is common for children to reject vegetable food choices and favor fruits and cereals. In such situations, researchers suggest that using a little creativity can improve vegetable intake during

---

RECOMMENDATIONS FOR CHILDREN 3–5 YEARS OF AGE

Calories: 1,000–1,400 kcal/day

Protein: 13–19 g/day

Carbohydrates: 50–60% of total calories consumed/day, with no more than 10% from simple sugars (e.g., white bread, candy, chips)

Fiber: 8–11 g/day

Fat: Total fat intake averaged over 2–3 days should be 20–30% of total caloric intake, with saturated fat consumption comprising less than 10% of total caloric intake. Trans fats, such as those found in many processed foods, should be avoided.

Cholesterol: should not exceed 300 mg/day.

Milk : 2–3 servings (24–30 oz) per day

Calcium: 500 mg for children 1–3 years of age, 800 mg/day for children 4–8 years of age.

Vitamin D: 400 international units (IU) per day

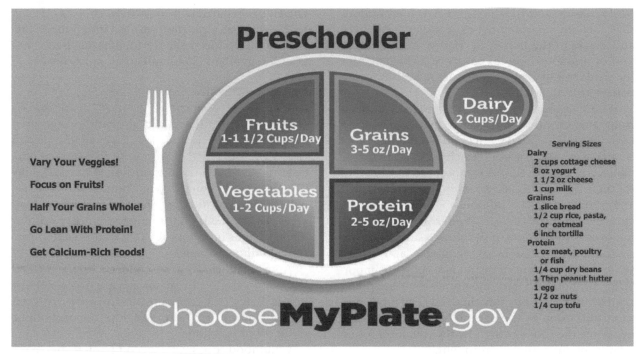

MyPlate recommendations for a preschooler's diet. (U.S. Department of Agriculture Center for Nutrition Policy and Promotion)

childhood. Results of a recent study found that blending pureed vegetables into other food favorites increased vegetable intake in children.

Summary

Parents and caregivers should become knowledgeable about nutrition for healthy preschool children. Preschool children should consume a variety of fruits, vegetables, whole grains, and lean proteins throughout the day. Family dietary counseling may be necessary if children are experiencing inadequate or excessive weight gain and growth. The prescribed dietary regimen should emphasize the importance of healthy food choices and continued medical surveillance to monitor the preschooler's growth and nutritional status. Research suggests that minimizing television watching results in better dietary choices, and healthy food choices during childhood reduces the risk of obesity.

—*Cherie Marcel*

References

Khalsa, Amrik Singh, et al. "Attainment of '5-2-1-0' Obesity Recommendations in Preschool-Aged Children." *Preventive Medicine Reports*, vol. 8, Dec. 2017, pp. 79–87, 10.1016/j.pmedr.2017.08.003.

Towner, Elizabeth K., et al. "Treating Obesity in Preschoolers." *Pediatric Clinics of North America*, vol. 63, no. 3, June 2016, pp. 481–510, 10.1016/j.pcl.2016.02.005.

Volger, Sheri, et al. "Early Childhood Obesity Prevention Efforts through a Life Course Health Development Perspective: A Scoping Review." *PLOS ONE*, vol. 13, no. 12, 28 Dec. 2018, p. e0209787, www.ncbi.nlm.nih.gov/pmc/articles/PMC6310279/, 10.1371/journal.pone.0209787.

School-Age Children

School-age children (i.e., 6–12 years of age) are in the stage of development referred to as the latent time of growth. During this period, growth rate slows and developmental changes are gradual as the physiologic foundation is established for the wide-ranging and rapid transformation that occurs in adolescence.

Although school-age children have established habits for food choices and eating meals in their home environment, the introduction of school and other outside activities presents new food options that include school lunches, vending machines, and snacks in the homes of friends. The presentation of new food options can pose a challenge for the parents/caregivers to encourage healthy eating behaviors in their children.

With many children receiving their noon meals from school lunch programs, parent/caregiver knowledge of the food choices offered by the school is important. If the school lunch options are inadequate, parents/caregivers can prepare sack lunches for their children to take to school.

Parent/caregiver influence over children's choices at breakfast and dinner becomes more important. Results of studies show a strong positive association between breakfast intake and school performance. Research results also show the importance of family-shared mealtimes in developing positive dietary choices in children. The foods provided and eaten by the parents/caregivers strongly influence the foods chosen by their children when away from the home environment.

Because lifetime eating habits are established in early childhood, it is vital that caregivers begin to encourage healthy eating habits in their children at a young age. Encouraging healthy eating habits involves offering a variety of fruits, vegetables, whole grains, and lean proteins at mealtimes and providing healthy food choices for snacks that are appealing and easy to carry.

The U.S. Department of Agriculture (USDA) produced the *MyPlate for Kids*, which provides age-appropriate materials and information designed to help children 6–11 years of age increase their knowledge regarding healthy food choices. *MyPlate for Kids* depicts a pyramid divided into 5 food categories that children should include in their diets: grains, vegetables, fruits, milk, and meat/beans.

Childhood Obesity

In developed countries, coronary heart disease (CHD) is the leading cause of death in both men and women, with death from cancer a close second cause. Diets that are high in saturated fat and cholesterol have been definitively linked to CHD, obesity, and certain cancers (e.g., cancer of the breast, colon, endometrium, gallbladder, esophagus, pancreas, and kidney). Continuing to reinforce positive dietary habits in school-age children is vital to prevent childhood obesity.

Approximately 35% of children in the United States who are 6–19 years of age are overweight or obese. Rates of overweight and obesity are even higher among minority and low socioeconomic status subpopulations.

Childhood obesity is accompanied by many comorbid conditions, including cardiovascular and endocrine dysfunction (e.g., type 2 diabetes mellitus [DM2], dyslipidemia), obstructive sleep apnea (OSA), asthma, and orthopedic impairments. The likelihood that obesity will persist into adulthood increases from 20% in obese 4-year-olds to 80% in obese adolescents.

Research Findings

Results of many studies show that the dietary habits and beliefs of parents/caregivers have a direct effect on the dietary habits and beliefs of their

---

RECOMMENDATIONS FOR SCHOOL-AGE CHILDREN

Calories: 1,500–3,000 kcal/day

Protein: 34 g/day

Carbohydrates: 50–60% of total calories consumed daily with no more than 10% from simple sugars (e.g., white bread, candy, chips).

Fiber: 11–17 g/day

Fat: Total fat intake averaged over 2–3 days should be 20–30% of total caloric intake, and saturated fat consumption should be less than 10% of total caloric intake. Trans fats, such as those found in many processed foods, should be avoided.

Cholesterol: should not exceed 300 mg/day.

Milk: 2–3servings (24–30 oz) per day

Calcium: 800 mg/day for children 4–8 years of age; 1,300 mg/day for children 9–13years of age.

Vitamin D: 400 international units (IU) per day

children. Researchers have documented that children tend to make food choices similar to those of their fathers and mothers. Evidence suggests that even grandmothers have a strong influence over dietary behaviors in their grandchildren's homes. Researchers have documented that the physical activity the family participates in has a direct effect on the activity and dietary choices of the children in the household, indicating that health promotion interventions should be family- and community-based to be successful, supporting families where they live and work.

A study investigating the association between family meals, viewing television during meals, and food choices made by the children in the family showed that children who ate breakfast, lunch, or dinner with their families at least 4 days/week ate more fruits and vegetables than those who did not participate in family meals 4 days/week. Children who rarely or never watched television during family meals were less likely to consume soda and chips.

Childhood obesity is a major public health concern in the U.S. and other developed countries. Behavior modification strategies focused on eating a healthy diet and increasing physical activity have produced the best short- and long-term results for weight loss in children. However, there are few treatment programs available to obese children and families who are economically disadvantaged. This is a significant concern considering that rates of overweight and obesity are higher in economically disadvantaged populations. Researchers have suggested that group-based behavioral interventions for the family would lower the expense of treatment and make treatment resources more accessible. Another important focus for intervention is the quality of nutrition standards for foods in schools. Studies have shown that increasing the availability of fruits, vegetables, whole grains, and low-fat dairy products in the school setting can positively affect the food choices of children. Unfortunately, many schools are also equipped with vending machines that provide unhealthy food options, which undermines the effectiveness of the school nutrition programs.

Researchers in a study of children aged 6–13 years living in the inner-city reported that the biggest perceived barrier to physical activity was lack of correct information and that insufficient access to healthy foods acted as a barrier to consuming a healthy diet.

Upon review of a comprehensive obesity prevention program implemented in an underserved Hispanic community, researchers found that, after 2 years, the nutrition-related knowledge, attitudes, and behaviors of school staff and students improved significantly. Evidence also suggests that learning activities focused on promoting healthy energy balance and reducing the risk for DM2 in middle school children were most effective if they required peer interaction.

Summary

Parents and caregivers should become knowledgeable about nutrition in healthy school-age children. Children should be encouraged to consume a variety of fruits, vegetables, whole grains, and lean proteins, including snacks that are appealing and easy to carry. School-age children may be at risk of inadequate and excessive weight gain and growth, requiring dietary counseling. The prescribed dietary regimen should emphasize the importance of healthy food choices and continued medical surveillance to monitor the growth and nutritional status. Research suggests a positive association between breakfast intake and school performance. Study results also show the importance of family-shared mealtimes in developing positive dietary choices in children.

—*Cherie Marcel*

References

Arteaga, S. Sonia, et al. "Childhood Obesity Research at the NIH: Efforts, Gaps, and Opportunities." *Translational Behavioral Medicine*, vol. 8, no. 6, 21 Nov. 2018, pp. 962–967, academic.oup.com/tbm/article/8/6/962/5134051, 10.1093/tbm/iby090.

Kim, Hee Soon, et al. "What Are the Barriers at Home and School to Healthy Eating?" *Journal of Nursing Research*, vol. 27, no. 5, Apr. 2019, p. 1, 10.1097/jnr.0000000000000321.

Pandita, Aaakash, et al. "Childhood Obesity: Prevention Is Better than Cure." *Diabetes, Metabolic Syndrome and Obesity: Targets and Therapy*, vol. 9, Mar. 2016, p. 83, www.ncbi.nlm.nih.gov/pmc/articles/PMC4801195/, 10.2147/dmso.s90783.

Yale University. "School-Based Nutritional Programs Reduce Student Obesity." *ScienceDaily*, 17 Dec. 2018, www.sciencedaily.com/releases/2018/12/181217101814.htm.

Adolescents

Adolescence marks the onset of puberty, which is the final growth spurt of childhood. This phase of development is a time of accelerated and significant physical changes. The adolescent body is maturing and developing sexual characteristics due to the release of estrogen and testosterone. The characteristic changes vary widely in timing and manifestation among adolescents. Girls tend to develop earlier and more rapidly than boys, but weight and height in boys eventually surpass that of girls.

Adolescence can be a distressing stage of life due to the physical transformation of the body. In some cases, girls become insecure about their degree of developing breasts and hips and boys feel inadequate and impatient if their height and weight are less optimal than their peers. Psychosocial development during adolescence is significant, and a sense of growing independence leads adolescents to begin looking to their friends rather than family members for affirmation. The pressure to be accepted by peers is strong and affects the adolescent's perceptions of style, social norms, physical activity, and dietary habits.

Although the influence of the adolescent's parents/caregivers largely shifts to a focus on peer influence, the role of family support during this growth period should not be underestimated. Most adolescents eat their initial meal of the day at home. Results of studies show a strong positive association between breakfast intake and school performance. Many adolescents eat the majority of their dinners at home even though their evening activities outside the home have increased. Research results show the importance of family-shared, television-free mealtimes in developing positive dietary choices in adolescents. Foods provided and eaten by the family remain a strong influence on the adolescent's choice of foods outside of the home.

Dietary Challenges for Adolescents

Eating Disorders. Because of the rapid growth and changes that occur during adolescence, the body's demand for energy, protein, vitamins, and minerals increases. The heightened hunger that adolescents experience can result in consuming unhealthy snacks (e.g., chips, sodas, candy bars) that have poor nutritional value and are readily available in vending machines, fast-food restaurants, and certain friends' homes. Many girls begin to gain weight during adolescence, which can cause them to feel insecure even if the weight gain and fat deposits are simply due to normal maturation. Social pressure to be thin frequently drives affected girls to self-impose a poorly planned diet for weight loss. For many, this is the beginning of an eating disorder such as anorexia nervosa and bulimia nervosa. The harmful effects of severe dieting and eating disorders during adolescence can extend into adulthood and cause infertility, metabolism dysfunctions, and difficulty with weight control. Treatment for eating disorders involves psychological and nutritional counseling, either individually or in group settings, and hospitalization is necessary in some cases to manage fluid imbalances, vitamin and mineral deficiencies, protein and energy malnutrition, and/or depression.

Anorexia nervosa develops when a person consumes too few calories to support normal body functions and growth. Due to an intense fear of weight gain and negative self-image, persons with anorexia nervosa will starve themselves and/or exercise excessively, losing more weight than is healthy.

Bulimia also occurs as the result of irrational fear of weight gain and/or body dysmorphia (i.e., misperception of body image). A person with bulimia may eat large amounts of food and induce vomiting or abuse laxatives in an attempt to avoid weight gain.

Obesity. In developed countries, coronary heart disease (CHD) is the leading cause of death in both men and women, with death from cancer a close second. It has been speculated that 10–70% of cancer-related deaths are preventable by alterations in diet. Diets that are high in saturated fat and cholesterol are definitely linked to CHD, obesity, and certain cancers (e.g., cancer of the breast, colon, endometrium, gallbladder, esophagus, pancreas, and kidney). Continuing to reinforce positive dietary habits in children is vital to prevent childhood obesity. Current statistics show that about 35% of children in the United States who are 6–19 years of age are overweight or obese. Rates of overweight and obesity are even higher among minority and low socioeconomic status subpopulations. Childhood obesity is accompanied by many

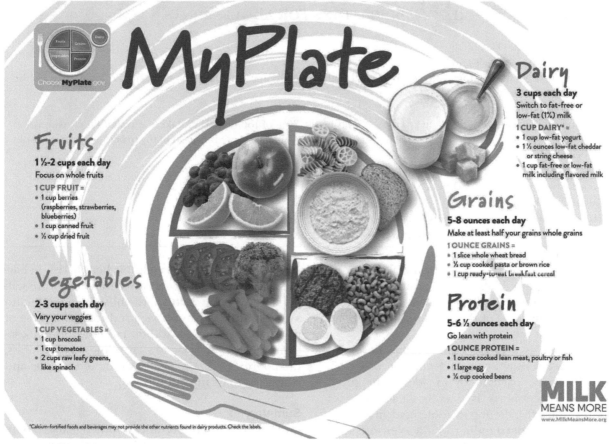

MyPlate recommendations for a preschooler's diet. (U.S. Department of Agriculture Center for Nutrition Policy and Promotion)

comorbid conditions, including cardiovascular and endocrine dysfunction (e.g., diabetes mellitus, type 2 [DM2], dyslipidemia), obstructive sleep apnea, asthma, and orthopedic impairments. The likelihood of obesity persisting into adulthood increases from 20% in obese 4-year-olds to 80% in obese adolescents.

Research Findings

Results of a study investigating the association between family meals, viewing television during meals, and food choices made by the children in the family showed that children who ate breakfast, lunch, or dinner with their family at least 4 days/week ate more fruits and vegetables than those who did not participate in family meals 4 days/week. Children who rarely or never watched television during family meals were less likely to consume soda and chips.

Obesity is a major public health concern in the U.S. and other developed countries. Behavior modification strategies that focus on eating a healthy diet and increasing physical activity have produced the best short- and long-term results for weight loss in children and adolescents. However, there are few treatment programs available to obese children and their families who are economically disadvantaged. This is a significant concern because rates of overweight and obesity are higher in this subpopulation. Researchers suggest that behavioral interventions that are group-based would lower the expense of treatment and make treatment resources more accessible for families with limited funds. Another important focus for intervention is the quality of nutrition standards for food in schools. Results of studies show that increasing the availability of fruits, vegetables, whole grains, and low-fat dairy products in the school setting can positively

RECOMMENDATIONS FOR ADOLESCENTS

Calories: 1,500–3,000 kcal/day

Protein: 46 g/day for girls and 52 g/day for boys

Carbohydrates: 50–60% of total calories consumed each day, with no more than 10% from simple sugars (e.g., white bread, candy, chips)

Fiber: 36–38 g/day

Fat: Total fat intake averaged over 2–3 days should be 20–30% of total caloric intake; saturated fat consumption should be less than 10% of total caloric intake. Trans fats, such as those found in many processed foods, should be avoided

Cholesterol: should not exceed 300 mg/day

Milk: 2–3 servings (24–30 oz) per day.

Calcium: 1,300 mg/day

Vitamin D: 400 international units (IU) per day

Activity: 30 minutes of moderate-intensity physical activity 5 times a week.

affect the food choices that children make. Unfortunately, many schools also have vending machines that provide unhealthy food options that undermine the effectiveness of the school nutrition programs.

Adolescence is a phase of childhood development that is strongly associated with the onset of eating disorders, particularly in adolescent girls. Early onset of puberty is a well-established risk factor for restrictive dieting in adolescent girls. This reinforces the understanding that adolescents are profoundly influenced by the acceptance of their peers. As a girl's body changes, she becomes aware of the other girls in her age group. Early maturation can lead to feelings of conspicuousness and insecurity about the body. Study results show that girls who develop an eating disorder in adolescence have a high likelihood of continuing to have an eating disorder in adulthood. Evidence also indicates that eating disorders and unhealthy dieting can result in difficulty with metabolism and weight control, including obesity, later in life. Researchers suggest that intervention strategies should target the peer groups of adolescent girls rather than focusing exclusively on the affected individual because motivation to change eating habits frequently stems from peer influence. Identifying the eating habits of the peer group can help formulate strategies to assist the affected individual in overcoming the eating disorder, potentially preventing future complications.

Research confirms that adolescents who embrace healthy dietary practices and participate in physical activity are less likely to exhibit health risk behaviors (e.g., substance use), have a more accurate self-perceived health status, are more optimistic and satisfied with life, and have a reduced incidence of depressive symptoms. Additionally, the more obesogenic lifestyle risk factors an adolescent exhibits, the poorer his or her quality of life tends to be and continues to be into adulthood.

Summary

Individuals should become knowledgeable about nutrition in adolescents. Adolescents should consume a variety of vegetables, fruits, whole grains, low-fat dairy products, lean proteins, and healthy fats, while minimizing simple sugars and highly processed foods. Adolescents may be at risk for inadequate and excessive weight gain and growth; possibly requiring dietary counseling. A prescribed dietary regimen may be necessary to emphasize the importance of healthy food choices. Research suggests that adolescents who embrace healthy dietary practices are less likely to struggle with obesity later in life.

—*Cherie Marcel*

References

Ajie, Whitney N., and Karen M. Chapman-Novakofski. "Impact of Computer-Mediated, Obesity-Related Nutrition Education Interventions for Adolescents: A Systematic Review." *Journal of Adolescent Health*, vol. 54, no. 6, June 2014, pp. 631–645, www.sciencedirect.com/science/article/pii/S1054139X13008422, 10.1016/j.jadohealth.2013.12.019.

Golden, N. H., et al. "Preventing Obesity and Eating Disorders in Adolescents." *PEDIATRICS*, vol. 138, no. 3, 22 Aug. 2016, pp. e20161649–e20161649, 10.1542/peds.2016-1649.

Hilger-Kolb, Jennifer, et al. "Associations between Dietary Factors and Obesity-Related Biomarkers in Healthy Children and Adolescents - a Systematic Review." *Nutrition Journal*, vol. 16, no. 1, Dec. 2017, 10.1186/s12937-017-0300-3.

Øen, Gudbjørg, et al. "Adolescents' Perspectives on Everyday Life with Obesity: A Qualitative Study." *International Journal of Qualitative Studies on Health and Well-Being*, vol. 13, no. 1, Jan. 2018, p. 1479581, 10.1080/17482631.2018.1479581.

Todd, Alwyn, et al. "Overweight and Obese Adolescent Girls: The Importance of Promoting Sensible Eating and Activity Behaviors from the Start of the Adolescent Period." *International Journal of Environmental Research and Public Health*, vol. 12, no. 2, 17 Feb. 2015, pp. 2306–2329, www.ncbi.nlm.nih.gov/pmc/articles/PMC4344727/, 10.3390/ijerph120202306.

Zalewska, Magdalena, and El bieta Maciorkowska. "Selected Nutritional Habits of Teenagers Associated with Overweight and Obesity." *PeerJ*, vol. 5, 22 Sept. 2017, p. e3681, 10.7717/peerj.3681.

Adults and Older Adults

Over the past century, life expectancy has increased. Since 1870, the number of persons over the age of 65 has increased from 1 million to 32 million, and is expected to reach 71 million by the year 2030. Ten percent of older adults are 85 years of age and older, making this the fastest growing age group among the aging population.

As the human body ages, physiologic changes occur that can affect nutritional status. For example, muscle mass and bone density diminishes; changes occur in the perception of flavor, taste, and odor; hearing and vision become less acute; cognitive capacity diminishes; and circadian rhythms shift, which affects sleep/wake patterns and overall energy. Organ function declines, and the gastrointestinal (GI) system slows, which affects the body's ability to digest, metabolize, and absorb nutrients, and inhibits efficient elimination of waste.

Although age-related changes occur gradually, they tend to accelerate after 55 years of age. The incidence of chronic diseases such as cardiovascular disease (CVD), type 2 diabetes mellitus (DM2), and osteoporosis increases in older adults. Researchers consistently report that these chronic conditions are directly correlated to dietary habits, exercise, and stress management. Initiating and maintaining healthy dietary and other lifestyle behaviors can prevent or postpone the onset of a chronic disease, or slow its progress.

Signs and Symptoms of Dementia

In the United States, dementia affects approximately 14% of persons over 71 years of age, and is the leading cause of dependence among older adults. Individuals with dementia experience variable changes in appetite, nutritional patterns, and the ability to perform basic activities of daily living (ADLs), such as shopping for and preparing food.

Signs and symptoms of dementia include the following:

- Memory loss and disorientation, which often manifests by pacing and wandering
- Communication impairment
- Inability to recognize persons or things that were once familiar
- Inability to learn, comprehend, or reason
- Significant weight changes
- Mood swings, personality and behavioral changes (e.g., aggression, suspicion, agitation), and insomnia
- Hallucinations and delusions
- Loss of independence due to inability to perform ADLs

Dietary and Lifestyle Recommendations that Promote Healthy Aging

It is important to consume enough calories to support general health. The recommended minimum calorie intake per day is 1,500 calories for men and 1,200 calories for women.

In order to provide adequate nutrients to support overall health, it is important to choose nutrient-dense foods such as whole grains, fresh fruits, vegetables, beans, nuts, lean proteins (e.g., fish, chicken breast), and low-fat dairy products.

RECOMMENDATIONS FOR ADULTS

Calories: 2,000 calories a day for women and 2,500 for men

Protein: 56 g/day for men; 46 g/day for women

Carbohydrates: 45-65% of total calories consumed daily with no more than 10% from simple sugars (e.g., white bread, candy, chips).

Fiber: 25-30 g/day

Fat: Total fat intake averaged over 2–3 days should be 20–35% of total caloric intake, and saturated fat consumption should be less than 10% of total caloric intake. Trans fats, such as those found in many processed foods, should be avoided.

Cholesterol: should not exceed 300 mg/day.

Milk: 3 cups or 732 mL/d per day

Calcium: 1,000 mg/day

Vitamin D: 400 international units (IU) per day

The American Heart Association (AHA) has outlined dietary guidelines:

Consume a diet that is rich in vegetables and fruits. Eating a variety of deeply-colored fruits and vegetables (e.g., spinach, carrots, berries) should be emphasized. Drinking fruit juice should not be encouraged because it does not provide the fiber of whole fruit and has a higher calorie content per serving.

Choose whole-grain, high-fiber foods. Research results have shown that a high intake of dietary fiber is associated with lower risk for CVD and lower all-cause mortality, although the inverse relationship with all-cause mortality decreases with age. At least half of the grains consumed should be whole grains.

Consume fish, especially oily fish, at least twice a week. Fish is a great source of the unsaturated fat omega-3, which has many health benefits, including reduced risk for CVD.

Limit intake of saturated fat, trans fat, and cholesterol. Choose lean meats. Choose dairy products that are fat-free (i.e., skim), 1% fat, or low-fat. Limit consumption of partially hydrogenated fats. It is currently recommended that dietary fat and cholesterol intake should be limited as follows:

- Total dietary fat < 35% of total caloric intake but not less than 20%
- Saturated fat < 7% of total caloric intake
- Trans fat < 1 % of total caloric intake
- Cholesterol < 300 mg/day

Minimize intake of beverages and foods that contain added sugar.

Choose and prepare foods with little or no salt. Sodium intake should not exceed 2,300 mg/day.

For those who consume alcohol, moderate consumption is recommended. It is recommended that men limit alcohol intake to

DEMENTIA AND NUTRITION

Provide familiar foods that the person has previously liked.

Provide small, frequent meals.

Enable self-feeding for as long as possible by providing finger foods and utensils that are easily held (e.g., a fork with a large handle), and/or assisting with eating.

Fortify foods with whole milk or protein supplements, and provide high-calorie snacks if calorie consumption is inadequate.

Serve food at a comfortable temperature (e.g., not excessively hot or cold).

Provide a dining area that is familiar and quiet, with adequate lighting.

Follow a consistent meal schedule.

Encourage physical activity, if possible, to stimulate appetite and circulation.

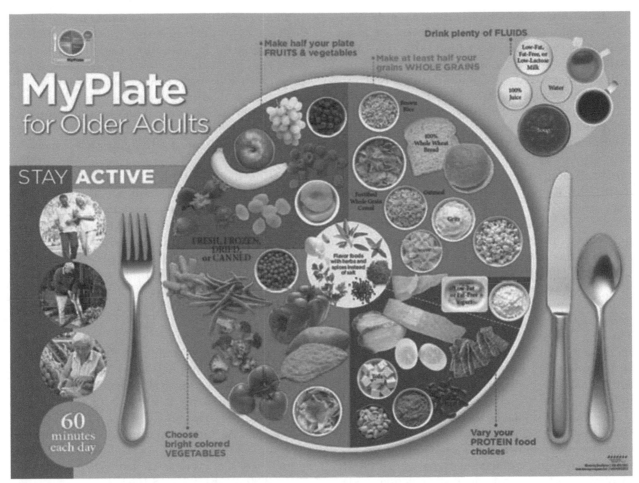

MyPlate recommendations for an older adult's diet. (U.S. Department of Agriculture Center for Nutrition Policy and Promotion)

2 drinks/day and women limit alcohol intake to 1 drink/day, preferably consumed with meals. 1 drink = 12 oz of beer , 4 oz of wine, or 1 and a half oz of 80 proof liquor.

Older women are at an increased risk for developing osteoporosis due to the drop in estrogen that occurs with menopause. Additionally, many older persons do not consume or absorb (i.e., from the sun) enough vitamin D each day. Among its many functions, vitamin D is vital for the absorption of calcium. Consuming adequate calcium and vitamin D can help to maintain healthy bones in aging persons.

The recommended daily intake of calcium is at least 1,200 mg/day. Sources of calcium include dairy products, fish with bones, broccoli, and legumes.

It is recommended that adults aged 51–70 years should take 400 international units (IU) of vitamin D/day, and adults over age 70 should take 600 IU/day. Most vitamin D is absorbed through the skin from exposure to sunlight. Food sources of vitamin D include salmon, egg yolks, cheese, and dairy products that have been fortified with vitamin D.

Regular physical activity for 30–60 minutes at least 5 times a week is recommended to maintain muscle mass and bone density, and to promote cardiovascular health.

Research Findings
The Mediterranean diet, originally based on the dietary patterns of persons living in the Mediterranean basin during the 1960s, replaces saturated

fats with unsaturated fats (predominantly olive oil); encourages consuming a variety of fresh fruits and vegetables, and foods that are minimally processed; and limits consumption of dairy products, eggs, and red meat. Emphasis is placed on using seasonally fresh and locally grown foods. Potential benefits to following the Mediterranean diet include weight loss, reduced pain and swelling for individuals with rheumatoid arthritis, and lower risk for cardiovascular events and cancer. Along with the physical benefits of following the Mediterranean diet, there is evidence that psychological well-being is enhanced. Researchers have reported that the Mediterranean diet exhibits potential for protection against age-related cognitive decline.

Evidence has shown that daily intake of the recommended amount of vitamin D and calcium can result in improvement in bone mineral density in the skeletal system of postmenopausal women. The U.S. Food and Drug Administration (FDA) states that the combination of adequate calcium and vitamin D, along with increased physical activity, can decrease the risk for osteoporosis later in life.

The linolenic metabolites eicosapentaenoic acid (EPA) and docosahexaenoic acid (DHA), which can be found in fatty fish (e.g., salmon, mackerel), walnuts, soybeans, and flax seeds, have been shown to play a protective role against dementia, CVD, inflammatory bowel disease, cancer, and rheumatoid arthritis, which may be due to their anti-inflammatory activity.

According to researchers, consuming egg yolks can increase macular pigment concentration in older adults who are taking cholesterol-lowering statins. Results of other studies show that eggs contain highly bioavailable lutein, which is a carotenoid that is believed to prevent age-related macular degeneration and cataracts. Although egg yolks are a significant source of cholesterol, research indicates that eating 1–2 eggs/day does not significantly affect the blood lipid profile and does not appear to increase the risk for CVD.

Summary

Individuals should become knowledgeable about diet and aging. Older adults are at risk for CVD, DM2, osteoporosis, dementia, and malnutrition. In order to receive adequate nutrients to support overall health, it is important for older adults to choose nutrient-dense foods such as whole grains, fresh fruits, vegetables, beans, nuts, lean proteins, and low-fat dairy products. A prescribed dietary regimen emphasizing the importance of adherence to the plan of care and continued medical surveillance to monitor nutritional and overall health status may help reduce risk factors associated with aging. It is especially important for family and caregivers to understand the signs and symptoms of dementia and make sure these individuals are receiving adequate nutrition. Research suggests that following the Mediterranean diet, receiving adequate vitamin D and calcium, EPA and DHA fatty acids intake, and eating 1–2 eggs per day may be dietary factors that contribute to healthy aging in older adults.

—*Cherie Marcel*

References

Bales, Connie W, and Kathryn N Porter Starr. "Obesity Interventions for Older Adults: Diet as a Determinant of Physical Function." *Advances in Nutrition*, vol. 9, no. 2, 1 Mar. 2018, pp. 151–159, 10.1093/advances/nmx016.

Batsis, John A. "Obesity in the Older Adult: Special Issue." *Journal of Nutrition in Gerontology and Geriatrics*, vol. 38, no. 1, 2 Jan. 2019, pp. 1–5, 10.1080/21551197.2018.1564197.

Batsis, John A., and Alexandra B. Zagaria. "Addressing Obesity in Aging Patients." *The Medical Clinics of North America*, vol. 102, no. 1, 1 Jan. 2018, pp. 65–85, www.ncbi.nlm.nih.gov/pmc/articles/PMC5724972/, 10.1016/j.mcna.2017.08.007.

Hruby, Adela, and Frank B. Hu. "The Epidemiology of Obesity: A Big Picture." *PharmacoEconomics*, vol. 33, no. 7, 4 Dec. 2014, pp. 673–689, www.ncbi.nlm.nih.gov/pmc/articles/PMC4859313/, 10.1007/s40273-014-0243-x.

Qi, Lu. "Personalized Nutrition and Obesity." *Annals of Medicine*, vol. 46, no. 5, 10 Apr. 2014, pp. 247–252, www.ncbi.nlm.nih.gov/pmc/articles/PMC5330214/, 10.3109/07853890.2014.891802.

Zhou, Lin, et al. "The Impact of Changes in Dietary Knowledge on Adult Overweight and Obesity in China." *PLOS ONE*, vol. 12, no. 6, 23 June 2017, p. e0179551, 10.1371/journal.pone.0179551.

■ Overeaters Anonymous

CATEGORY: Treatment

Overeaters Anonymous (OA) is a twelve-step recovery program based on the methods and philosophy of Alcoholics Anonymous. OA members profess that they are "powerless over food" and that their "lives have become unmanageable." The purpose of the group is not to promote weight loss and dieting but to support inner changes and daily actions that remove the feeling that one must consume excess and addictive foods.

Background

Overeaters Anonymous (OA) was founded by Rozanne S., Jo S., and Bernice S. in 1960 after Rozanne had attended a Gamblers Anonymous (GA) meeting to support a friend. Rozanne discovered that the members' stories of compulsive gambling mirrored her own story of compulsive overeating. She recognized that the twelve steps and twelve traditions of recovery that were the foundation of Alcoholics Anonymous (AA) and adopted by GA could be applied to recovery from compulsive overeating.

The OA program is based on twelve steps, twelve traditions, and eight tools of recovery. The twelve steps are almost identical to those of AA. In AA literature, the word alcohol can be replaced with trigger food and the word drinking can be replaced with compulsive overeating to make the principles applicable to OA members. However, an important distinction between the two groups is that although AA members can abstain from all alcohol, OA members cannot abstain from all food.

Persons who wish to disengage from compulsive overeating must identify and refrain from ingesting specific food ingredients that trigger the compulsion. The most common trigger foods are wheat and sugar. In addition, compulsive overeating may be triggered by compulsive food behaviors, such as the need to empty a package of food or the need to finish food on a plate rather than leaving a portion or discarding food. In 2009, OA defined abstinence as "the action of refraining from compulsive eating and compulsive food behaviors."

The twelve traditions, nearly identical to those of AA, are guidelines for conducting meetings and sustaining the principles of the organization. Each of the twelve traditions has a related

spiritual principle: unity, trust, identity, autonomy, purpose, solidarity, responsibility, fellowship, structure, neutrality, anonymity, and spirituality.

By using the eight tools of recovery, members are better able to achieve and maintain abstinence from compulsive overeating. The first tool is a plan of eating. (OA does not promote a specific dietary plan but encourages members to develop a personal eating plan after consulting a physician or dietitian and identifying trigger foods to avoid.) The second tool is sponsorship. A sponsor is an experienced OA member who helps a new member understand and work the twelve steps. The third tool is the OA meeting, which provides regular support from other OA members and helps members to overcome the isolation and shame that impede recovery.

The fourth tool of recovery is the telephone. Members are encouraged to ask for help from one another, especially when emotions are overwhelming. The fifth tool is writing as a way of examining one's reactions to difficult situations and discovering alternative coping mechanisms. The sixth tool is literature, particularly the publications of OA and the *Big Book* of AA. Such reading material provides insight into the nature and consequences of compulsive overeating and provides hope for recovery.

The seventh tool is anonymity, which protects members from gossip as they express their pain and struggles and also asserts equality among members. The eighth tool is service. Members are asked to sustain the organization with acts such as welcoming new members, setting up and cleaning up meeting rooms, and sharing news of upcoming OA events.

OA is a nonprofit organization. All funding comes from the sale of OA literature and voluntary contributions collected at meetings. The program has not changed over time. The demographics of its members have changed only as a reflection of trends in the general population. More participants today have college degrees, more work full-time, and more are divorced.

Mission and Goals

The official literature of OA states that "Our primary purpose is to abstain from compulsive overeating and to carry this message of recovery to those who still suffer." OA has an estimated fifty-four thousand members in more than seventy-five countries, with sixty-five hundred groups meeting each week. Most members are white females who have been in the program an average of 5.7 years. They began the program with moderate obesity.

Although OA does not focus on diet and calorie counting, members of OA experience an average weight loss of 21.8 pounds as a result of working the program. Like other twelve-step programs, OA seeks to improve the physical, mental, and spiritual facets of the lives of its members. A 2002 survey found that 90 percent of OA members reported improvements in these areas.

Specific OA practices have a demonstrated significant relationship with the maintenance of abstinence from foods that trigger compulsive overeating: weighing and measuring foods on a deliberate food plan; regular communication with other OA members, specifically a sponsor; spending time in introspection; writing as a form of personal expression and investigation; attending OA meetings regularly; reading OA literature for inspiration; and working the steps, particularly the fourth and ninth steps. Abstinence and spirituality were strongly correlated with self-reported success.

—*Bethany Thivierge*

References

McKenna, Rebecca A, et al. "Food Addiction Support: Website Content Analysis." *JMIR Cardio*, vol. 2, no. 1, 24 Apr. 2018, p. e10, 10.2196/cardio.8718.

Redif, Zibe. "Overeaters Anonymous Saved My Life — But Here's Why I Quit." *Healthline*, 30 July 2019, www.healthline.com/health/mental-health/leaving-overeaters-anonymous#1.

Rodríguez-Martín, Boris C., and Belén Gallego-Arjiz. "Overeaters Anonymous: A Mutual-Help Fellowship for Food Addiction Recovery." *Frontiers in Psychology*, vol. 9, 20 Aug. 2018, 10.3389/fpsyg.2018.01491.

Russell-Mayhew, Shelly, et al. "How Does Overeaters Anonymous Help Its Members? A Qualitative Analysis." *European Eating Disorders Review*, vol. 18, no. 1, Jan. 2010, pp. 33–42, 10.1002/erv.966.

■ Sleep

CATEGORY: Physiology

Sleep is a physical and mental state of deep rest in which a person is not conscious of their surroundings. In addition to a balanced diet and regular exercise, adequate sleep is a vital component of a healthy life. The amount of sleep considered adequate varies depending on age, health, and activity level. Most adults require 7–8 hours/day of sleep, and children require 10–15 hours/day. Although the exact mechanisms of sleep are not fully understood, results of studies show that sleep is necessary for the brain to function properly and for the body to restore itself. Sleep deprivation is associated with increased risk for hypertension, diabetes mellitus, type 2 (DM2), obesity, depression, heart attack, and stroke.

Structure and Functions

All multicellular animals cycle through daily fluctuations in biological activity known as circadian rhythms, with the alternation of sleep and wakefulness being the most obvious example. In humans, a polycyclic sleep/wake cycle-several periods of sleep and arousal during a twenty-four-hour period-becomes evident in the fetus during the latter stages of pregnancy. As children progress from infancy through childhood, they gradually settle into a mainly diurnal pattern, with one long period of sleep during the day. A complex interaction of several external and internal events determines the timing and duration of sleep.

The key exogenous factor that influences sleep is light. In the absence of the alternation of day and night, people will usually develop a sleep/wake cycle that is a little longer (from a few minutes to an hour) than a twenty-four-hour day. Two neurological structures detect light and synchronize the body's sleep/wake cycle with the presence or absence of light. The pineal gland is a photosensitive endocrine gland centrally located in the brain that secretes the hormone melatonin, which causes drowsiness. When darkness increases, the pineal gland steps up production of melatonin; levels of melatonin decline as light increases. Melatonin levels also affect the structure of the brain that plays the key role in regulating circadian rhythms, the suprachiasmatic nucleus of the hypothalamus (SCN). The SCN serves as the body's primary

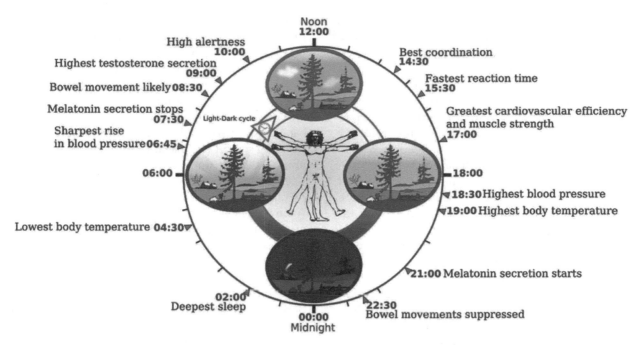

The human biological clock. (Yassine Mrabe)

biological clock, containing cells that will pulse in rhythmic activity in the absence of light. The activity of these cells, however, is influenced by output from the pineal gland and also from the eye's retinal cells, providing two avenues by which light can affect the SCN. Light causes the SCN to alter levels of Tim, a protein which, when it interacts with two other proteins known as Per and Clock, will induce sleepiness at high levels. Levels of Tim, in turn, will increase activity in certain cells of the SCN. Thus, light serves as the *zeitgeber* (time-giver) for the sleep/wake cycle by changing the activity of the pineal gland and SCN, thereby altering levels of sleep-inducing chemicals.

Although damage to the pineal gland and SCN will significantly disrupt the quality and quantity of sleep, periods of sleep will still occur. That observation, in addition to the fact that animals will develop sleep/wake cycles in the absence of light changes, points to other, internal mechanisms that control sleep and arousal. One of these mechanisms is body temperature. Body temperature fluctuates from approximately 98 degrees Fahrenheit (36.7 degrees Celsius) to 99 degrees Fahrenheit (37.2 degrees Celsius) during the day. Rising body temperature is associated with arousal; declining body temperature is correlated with drowsiness. Vigorously

rubbing the hands together can increase blood flow to the hands, dropping the blood supply to the brain, thereby decreasing the temperature of the brain and making it easier to fall asleep. While blood flow has an impact on the level of alertness, it is the flow of several neurotransmitters-chemicals that bridge the synaptic gap between one neuron (nerve cell) and another-that play the crucial role in regulating sleep and arousal.

Neurotransmitters generally have excitatory or inhibitory effects on arousal, but their impact on sleep is dependent on the neurological structures that they affect. Overall, more neurotransmitters appear to facilitate arousal rather than sleepiness. Acetylcholine and glutamate are the primary neurotransmitters for learning, so it is not surprising that they mediate the brain's alertness to external stimuli. The pontomesencephalon portion of the reticular formation-the brain's major arousal system-releases these two neurotransmitters, which activate regions of the brain from top (the cortex) to bottom (the medulla). Acetylcholine is also released by excitatory basal forebrain cells that have direct connections with the thalamus, the brain's center for the integration and processing of sensory information. Close to the bottom of the brain in the pons is the locus coeruleus, which promotes wakefulness and helps to consolidate memories. Norepineph-rine, the neurotransmitter that is involved in the display of active emotions such as fear or anger, is released from this structure and arouses many areas of the brain. Between the locus coeruleus and the basal forebrain is the hypothalamus, which influences many aspects of motivation and emotion, particularly through its regulation of the pituitary gland, the master gland of the endocrine system. Anterior cells of the hypothalamus release histamine, which, like acetylcholine, has widespread arousing effects on the brain. Taking antihistamine drugs to subdue the symptoms of allergies and colds will militate against those arousing effects. Lateral cells of the hypothalamus produce orexin, a neurotransmitter that is necessary for staying awake, especially as the day transpires.

Three neurotransmitters promote the induction and maintenance of sleep; two of them exert their effects via the basal forebrain. Gamma-aminobutyric acid (GABA), the brain's primary inhibitory neurotransmitter, is released by inhibitory cells in the basal forebrain and dampens arousal in the cortex and thalamus. Adenosine decreases activity in the acetylcholine-producing cells of the basal forebrain, thereby inhibiting arousal. Caffeine derives its stimulating effects by blocking adenosine receptors. Moderate levels of serotonin have a calming effect and can facilitate the induction of sleep. However, serotonin (and norepinephrine) can decrease the quantity of REM sleep. Other chemicals, such as prostaglandins, work in conjunction with these three neurotransmitters to promote the induction and maintenance of sleep.

The interplay of various levels of neurotransmitters and hormones effect changes in the electrical activity of the brain. Recordings of the electrical potentials of brain cells made with an electroencephalograph (EEG) have resulted in the identification of four succeeding distinct patterns of brain wave activity that occur in approximately ninety-minute cycles. Prior to falling asleep, a person manifests mostly alpha EEG readings-high amplitude (top-to-bottom distance), medium wavelength (peak-to-peak distance) brain wave activity-characteristic of an alert, relaxed state. When a person slips into the first stage of sleep, a theta EEG pattern-low amplitude, short wavelengths-predominates. As sleep progresses, brief periods of very short wavelengths (sleep spindles) and bursts of high amplitude waves (K-complexes) punctuate the theta EEG pattern, marking the appearance of stage 2 sleep. Eventually, high amplitude and long wavelength brain activity-a delta EEG record-becomes more prevalent and stage 3 sleep is evident. Finally, delta EEG waves predominate as the person settles into stage 4 sleep. The individual will then cycle back through the third and second stages before reaching stage 1 sleep again, completing the ninety-minute biorhythm. The second period of stage 1 sleep is usually accompanied by the first appearance of rapid eye movement (REM) sleep in humans (many species lack the eye movements), a phenomenon in which brain activity is high but many signs of physiological arousal, such as muscle tension, are low. The time spent in each stage varies, depending on how long the person has been sleeping: stages 3 and 4 predominate during the first half of a sleep period, while stages 1 and 2 predominate (stage 4 sleep is often absent) during the second half.

Differences in sleep stage characteristics and their associated phenomena have led some researchers to distinguish between two basic types of sleep: S-sleep (more neural synchrony, similar activity in diverse brain regions), which combines stages 3 and 4, and D-sleep (more neural desynchrony, diverse brain regions active at different times), which combines stages 1 and 2. S-sleep is characterized by many signs of a deeper physical rest: lower body temperature, generally lower autonomic arousal, difficult arousal. Moreover, sleep loss and physical injuries or deprivations tend to increase the percentage of S-sleep over D-sleep. In contrast, more signs of psychological restoration are associated with D-sleep: increased cortical blood flow and more vivid and prevalent dreams, especially during REM sleep. Additionally, deprivation of REM sleep tends to impair memory and increase irritability more so than deprivation of S-sleep. Because the distinctions between S-sleep and D-sleep are not always clear-cut-for example, S-sleep is essential for some types of memory formation-some researchers prefer to distinguish between REM sleep and non-REM (NREM) sleep.

Sleep and Diet

More research is needed to understand the complex interrelationship between sleep and diet. There is evidence that individuals who sleep less have a tendency to consume foods that are higher in fats and simple sugars, eat fewer fruits and vegetables, snack more often, and have more irregular meal patterns than individuals who sleep more. Further study is necessary to discern the effect of dietary choices on sleep patterns, and the influence of sleep patterns on dietary choices.

Caffeine induces wakefulness. The primary action of caffeine is antagonism of the adenosine receptor. Adenosine dilates blood vessels and facilitates sleep. By binding with the adenosine receptor, caffeine interferes with the ability of adenosine to slow the body, which results in increased neural activity. Caffeine is readily absorbed and its effects last 4–6 hours, although the effects of caffeine can last up to 20 hours in older persons with slower metabolism. Individuals with insomnia are advised to avoid drinking coffee during the afternoon and evening. Dietary sources of caffeine include coffee and tea, certain soft drinks, cocoa beans/chocolate, kola nuts, and certain medications (e.g., pain relievers, cold medications, diet pills).

Carbohydrates (e.g., bread, pasta, white rice, potatoes, cake and desserts) are rapidly absorbed and induce sleepiness. Eating a carbohydrate-rich meal results in a rapid increase of insulin. Insulin stimulates the uptake of large neutral amino acids (LNAAs) into muscle tissue, but insulin has no effect on the amino acid tryptophan, which results in an increased ratio of tryptophan to LNAAs, and elevated levels of tryptophan in the brain. Tryptophan contributes to the synthesis of serotonin, which is a neurotransmitter that causes calmness and fatigue.

Eating a larger meal is more likely to result in sleepiness than eating a smaller meal. Solid foods cause tiredness more often than liquid foods. One or 2 glasses of alcohol can induce sleepiness, but excessive alcohol intake can cause awakening, and disrupt the quality of sleep.

Research Findings

Sleep disorders are common among children with attention deficit hyperactivity disorder (ADHD). Study results show that improvement in sleep patterns can reduce the symptoms of ADHD. There is also evidence that eating a diet high in sugar contributes to ADHD symptomology. Because of the interrelationship between diet and sleep, and the knowledge that both sleep and diet contribute to the symptoms of ADHD, researchers are investigating the potential of holistic therapies for ADHD that focus on dietary changes and improvement in sleep patterns.

Researchers report that insufficient sleep appears to impede weight loss by slowing the loss of body fat, increasing the loss of lean body mass, and increasing the sensation of hunger. Diet quality is also reduced with insufficient sleep. Results of a recent study revealed that women who sleep fewer than 6 hours/day are more likely to be overweight and obese, and tend to consume more calories, more carbohydrates, and less fiber than women who sleep 6 hours/day or longer. The women who slept for longer periods consumed higher amounts of key nutrients, including vitamin C, niacin, vitamin B12, and calcium.

PROMOTING ADEQUATE SLEEP

- Avoid consuming rapidly absorbing carbohydrates at the midday meal to prevent afternoon fatigue. Eating a small evening meal that is rich in complex carbohydrates (e.g., quinoa, wild rice, legumes) can be conducive to falling asleep.
- Include foods rich in B-complex vitamins (e.g., leafy greens, meat), vitamin C (e.g., orange and red fruits and vegetables), magnesium (e.g., beans, leafy greens), and protein (e.g., lean meat, beans, nuts) that contribute to the synthesis of tryptophan and are quickly depleted during times of stress and sleep deprivation.
- Avoid ingesting caffeine (e.g., coffee, certain soft drinks, tea) in the evening.
- Limit alcohol consumption to 1–2 drinks/day to avoid disruption of normal sleep patterns.
- Keep healthier snack choices (e.g., unsalted nuts, fresh fruit, dried fruit) on hand to prevent impulse snacking on junk foods.
- Engage in daily physical activity. Exercise reduces stress hormones, boosts a sense of well-being, and improves sleep and overall health.

Summary

Individuals should become knowledgeable about the relationship between diet and sleep. Sleep is necessary for the brain to function properly and for the body to restore itself. Sleep deprivation is associated with increased risk for hypertension, DM2, obesity, depression, heart attack, and stroke. A balanced diet that includes appropriate options for dietary fat, lean proteins, complex carbohydrates, and a variety of fruits and vegetables may help improve sleep patterns. Research suggests that sleep deprived individuals often make unhealthy food choices and may experience difficulty with weight loss efforts.

—*Paul J. Chara Jr., Cherie Marcel*

References

Bonanno, Lilla, et al. "Assessment of Sleep and Obesity in Adults and Children." *Medicine*, vol. 98, no. 46, Nov. 2019, p. e17642, 10.1097/md.0000000000017642.

Cooper, Christopher B, et al. "Sleep Deprivation and Obesity in Adults: A Brief Narrative Review." *BMJ Open Sport & Exercise Medicine*, vol. 4, no. 1, Oct. 2018, p. e000392, 10.1136/bmjsem-2018-000392.

Gohil, Anisha, and Tamara S. Hannon. "Poor Sleep and Obesity: Concurrent Epidemics in Adolescent Youth." *Frontiers in Endocrinology*, vol. 9, 10 July 2018, 10.3389/fendo.2018.00364.

Ogilvie, Rachel P., and Sanjay R. Patel. "The Epidemiology of Sleep and Obesity." *Sleep Health*, vol. 3, no. 5, 1 Oct. 2017, pp. 383–388, www.sciencedirect.com/science/article/abs/pii/S2352721817301481?via%3Dihub, 10.1016/j.sleh.2017.07.013.

■ Sports

CATEGORY: Physiology

Introduction

In the U.S. organized sports for boys were initiated in the early 1920s. Business leaders realized that young boys needed to develop character and skills, and sports were a good way to accomplish it. Over time this lead to business funding and support for sports leagues such as Pop Warner Football, Little League Baseball and the American Youth Soccer Association. By the 1970s the Women's Movement began to address the gender inequities and advocated for similar sports programs for girls. Title IX legislation expanded the sport opportunities for females.

Currently girls and boys have many opportunities to play competitive sports at many different levels, from recreation to elite programs. Whatever level is chosen athletes can develop many skills that will benefit them later in life, whether in their career, family or community. In addition to physical well-being the potential benefits are many and include social, behavioral, and intellectual growth. Not everyone has to play at the highest levels. For example, an athlete playing at a high level may not have the opportunity to develop as many leadership skills when spending more time on the bench compared to playing at a lower level and spending more time on the field. All types of sport participation can help youth to begin developing important life skills.

Health Benefits

Since there is physical activity involved in most sports, playing can have health benefits. Training or working the body to perform well causes many physiological changes over time that can benefit health. Muscles, heart, lungs and bones become stronger which can have lifelong benefits when reinforced with continued regular exercise. Serious athletes tend to eat healthier diets to help improve training and performance. Fewer athletes are overweight compared with non-athletes.

Other health benefits include the ability to handle stress. Although competition can be very stressful for some, athletes actually have less stress and depression than non-athletes. One reason is regular exercise helps to reduce stress and depression. Athletes also have better mood states. These noted benefits may be in part due to the fact that athletes sleep better. The recovery provided by sleep is instrumental in managing stress.

Developing the healthy habits of exercise, good nutrition and stress management will help athletes get a better start toward a lifetime of healthy living. It is easier to develop healthy habits during the younger years than to change bad habits later in life.

Social Benefits

Participation in sports, particularly team sports, helps to develop the social skills needed later in life.

Most young people will eventually have to work in an organization with other workers. Some will become involved in community and civic programs. Others may become coaches. In all of these situations people must work together toward a common goal. Whether a sports team or a work organization the members must have the social skills for the group as a whole to be successful.

Teamwork is one of the fundamental skills developed in sport participation. Several people, each with specific responsibilities, must do their part for the whole to be successful. In sports success is generally winning. In work success may be completing a project and getting a contract. Either way the skills required for success are the same, and those learned as a child playing sports also benefit the worker later in life. An important part of the teamwork is accepting individual responsibilities, being accountable for them, and doing one's best to complete them effectively and unselfishly.

Sports and life are competitive and participants must be humble in success and accepting in defeat. There should be respect for the rules, authority and others involved on both sides. No one is successful all of the time and learning to handle failure is an important lesson in life.

One common desire in sports and life is to have fun. Most athletes play sports because they have fun playing them. Not all parts of sports training is fun but athletes learn to work through the hard times because they enjoy the competition. This is often called delayed gratification. Just like later in life people must work hard at responsibilities they do not enjoy to experience the successes that the hard work produces.

Behavioral Benefits

Being an effective team member requires many individual skills. Communication is the transfer of information among the team members. Playing sports help members learn, through action, how to effectively disseminate information to team members and listen to accurately interpret the information from others. Developing communication skills will help young athletes in future interactions at work, in the family and in the community.

Discipline, motivation, dedication and sacrifice are needed when playing sports. Regularly attending organized practices and training sessions help athletes develop discipline. Having training rules and following them consistently teaches athletes to meet expectations of others now and in the future. To be disciplined requires motivation or the desire to do well in the sport and make continual improvements. This develops dedication, or a commitment to the sport. However, these traits are not developed without sacrifice. Discipline, motivation and dedication require athletes to give up time that could be spent doing something else fun. However, sacrifice for a sport can result in the development of behavioral skills that will prepare them for future challenges in work, family and life. It helps to form a positive work ethic.

Playing sports also provides the opportunity to develop leadership skills. Although some athletes will develop better leadership skills than others, those that do will benefit from the sport experience in the future. There are many types of leaders. Not all are formal, obvious leaders. Even learning subtle leadership skills can be beneficial later in life.

A major benefit of playing sports is the development of self-esteem, or having a positive impression of one's self. Certainly sports can have a very negative effect on self-esteem if the athlete is unsuccessful and does not meet individual expectations of performance. Those who have realistic goals and see consistent development in sport skills and performance can benefit from improvements in self-esteem. This will help build confidence to meet other challenges in life.

Intellectual Benefits

Although playing sports is a very physical activity, successful athletes also have to understand how to play the game. Therefore playing sports can also develop cognitive skills. All sports have different strategies that must be understood to win. Athletes must learn to analyze the competitive situation and make good strategic decisions quickly. This requires focus, concentration and confidence. These are also skills needed to be successful in life. Sport participation can also improve math skills as athletes calculate in their minds how far the team is ahead or behind and then use that information to make appropriate adjustments in strategy.

—*Bradley R. A. Wilson*

207

References

Cvetkovi, N., et al. "Exercise Training in Overweight and Obese Children: Recreational Football and High-Intensity Interval Training Provide Similar Benefits to Physical Fitness." *Scandinavian Journal of Medicine & Science in Sports*, vol. 28, 6 July 2018, pp. 18–32, onlinelibrary.wiley.com/doi/full/10.1111/sms.13241, 10.1111/sms.13241.

Learmonth, Yvonne C., et al. "Physical Education and Leisure-Time Sport Reduce Overweight and Obesity: A Number Needed to Treat Analysis." *International Journal of Obesity*, vol. 43, no. 10, 8 Jan. 2019, pp. 2076–2084, 10.1038/s41366-018-0300-1.

Turner, Robert W., et al. "Reported Sports Participation, Race, Sex, Ethnicity, and Obesity in US Adolescents From NHANES Physical Activity (PAQ_D)." *Global Pediatric Health*, vol. 2, 6 Apr. 2015, p. 2333794X1557794, www.ncbi.nlm.nih.gov/pmc/articles/PMC4784630/, 10.1177/2333794x15577944.

Vincent, Heather K. "Advising the Obese Patient on Starting a Running Program." *Current Sports Medicine Reports*, vol. 14, no. 4, 2015, p. 278, 10.1249/jsr.0000000000000171.

Wiklund, Petri. "The Role of Physical Activity and Exercise in Obesity and Weight Management: Time for Critical Appraisal." *Journal of Sport and Health Science*, vol. 5, no. 2, June 2016, pp. 151–154, www.sciencedirect.com/science/article/pii/S2095254616300060, 10.1016/j.jshs.2016.04.001.

■ Stress reduction

CATEGORY: Physiology; Psychology

Indications and Procedures

Stress can exacerbate difficulties in daily functioning, slow recovery from mental or physical problems, and impede immunological functioning. Stress reduction techniques represent a cluster of procedures that share the goal of reducing bodily and emotional tension: drug and physical therapies, exercise, biofeedback training, meditation, hypnosis, psychotherapy, relaxation training, and stress inoculation therapy.

The drugs used in stress reduction are designed to provide overall bodily relaxation, to induce rest, or to decrease the anxious thinking that exacerbates stressful experiences. Sedatives, tranquilizers, benzodiazepines, antihistamines, beta-blockers, and barbiturates are examples of such drugs. Similarly, physical therapies and exercise are recommended for these purposes. Baths (hydrotherapy), massages, and moderate exercise can also be part of a stress reduction program.

Psychotherapy is a common treatment for stress implemented by psychiatrists, psychologists, social workers, psychiatric nurses, and counselors. Not only does it help individuals to sort out their problems mentally but it is also an effective stress management strategy. When individuals analyze their lifestyles and life events, stress-inducing behaviors and life patterns can be explored and targeted for modification.

Biofeedback training, meditation, hypnosis, and relaxation training all focus on inducing relaxation or altered consciousness by shifting a person's attention. Biofeedback uses monitoring devices attached to the body to provide visual or aural feedback to the trainee. Such devices include the electromyograph (EMG), which measures muscle tension, and the psychogalvanometer, which measures galvanic skin response (GSR). An EMG involves placing sensors on various muscle groups to record muscular electrical potentials. GSR also relies on sensors, but these sensors record bodily responses caused by sweat gland activity and emotional arousal. The feedback from such devices allows a trainee to learn to control certain bodily processes (for example, muscle tension, brain waves, heart rate, temperature, and blood pressure). Biofeedback training is used to treat headaches, temporomandibular joint (TMJ) syndrome, high blood pressure, and tics, and it can also facilitate neuromuscular responses in stroke patients.

Meditation is a focused thinking exercise involving a quiet setting and the repetition of a word or phrase called a mantra. By blocking distracting thoughts and refocusing attention, meditation reduces anxious thinking. It is useful for mild anxiety, minor concentration difficulties, and daily relaxation.

Hypnosis involves the use of suggestion, concentrated attention, and/or drugs to induce a sleeplike state, or trance. Hypnosis can be induced

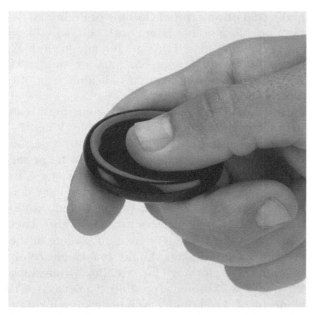

Some people use "worry stones" to cope with stress. (Wikimedia Commons)

by a hypnotist or via self-hypnosis. Hypnotic states are characterized by increased suggestibility, ability to recall forgotten events, decreased pain sensitivity, and increased vasomotor control. The ability to be hypnotized varies from person to person based on susceptibility to suggestion and psychological needs. Hypnosis is used as a brief therapy targeting such problems as insomnia, pain, panic, and sexual dysfunction. In addition, hypnosis is sometimes used when drugs are contraindicated for anesthetic use, particularly for dental procedures.

Relaxation training involves three primary methods: autogenic training, which involves such techniques as head, heart, and abdominal exercises; progressive relaxation, which involves becoming aware of tension in the various muscle groups by relaxing one group at a time in a specific order; and breathing exercises. Relaxation training is best learned when a therapist trains an individual in person and then the exercises are practiced independently. Relaxation can be practiced several times daily, as well as in response to stressful events. High blood pressure, ulcers, insomnia, asthma, drug and alcohol problems, spastic colitis, tachycardia (rapid heartbeat), pain management, and moderate-to-severe anxiety disorders are treated with relaxation training.

Stress inoculation therapy is a specific type of psychotherapy involving techniques that alter patterns of thinking and acting. It comprises three steps: education about stress and fear reactions, rehearsal of coping behaviors, and application of coping behaviors in stress-provoking situations. It is useful for treating anxiety disorders related to stress.

Uses and Complications

Individuals should not apply stress reduction procedures without proper consultation; medical conditions that might be causing symptoms should be assessed or ruled out first. Biofeedback training for headaches, for example, would be unwarranted until other, more serious causes of headaches had been eliminated from consideration. Similarly, exercise, drug, and physical therapies could actually worsen conditions such as high blood pressure, alcohol and drug problems, and chronic pain if applied incorrectly. For example, where stress or pain is chronic, drug therapies might encourage the development of drug dependence.

Instead, skilled providers should administer these procedures. Training via self-help materials alone or by an unskilled provider may provide no benefit or create difficulties. Poor training could result in frustration, hypervigilance, heightened anxiety, depression, or pain caused by overattention to symptoms or conflicts. In fact, some individuals are prone to these effects even with good training. Therefore, ongoing assessment is necessary. Finally, interpretation of any memories provoked by hypnosis should be done with caution because of the suggestibility that is characteristic of hypnotic states.

—*Nancy A. Piotrowski*

References

Daubenmier, Jennifer, et al. "Mindfulness Intervention for Stress Eating to Reduce Cortisol and Abdominal Fat among Overweight and Obese Women: An Exploratory Randomized Controlled Study." *Journal of Obesity*, vol. 2011, 2011, pp. 1–13, www.ncbi.nlm.nih.gov/pmc/articles/PMC3184496/, 10.1155/2011/651936.

Dutheil, Frédéric, et al. "Stress Management in Obesity during a Thermal Spa Residential Programme (ObesiStress): Protocol for a Randomised Controlled Trial Study." *BMJ Open,* vol. 9, no. 12, Dec. 2019, p. e027058, 10.1136/bmjopen-2018-027058.

Jääskeläinen, Anne, et al. "Stress-Related Eating, Obesity and Associated Behavioural Traits in Adolescents: A Prospective Population-Based Cohort Study." *BMC Public Health*, vol. 14, no. 1, 7 Apr. 2014, bmcpublichealth.biomedcentral.com/articles/10.1186/1471-2458-14-321, 10.1186/1471-2458-14-321.

Scott, Karen A., et al. "Effects of Chronic Social Stress on Obesity." *Current Obesity Reports*, vol. 1, no. 1, 11 Jan. 2012, pp. 16–25, www.ncbi.nlm.nih.gov/pmc/articles/PMC3428710/, 10.1007/s13679-011-0006-3.

Xenaki, Niovi, et al. "Impact of a Stress Management Program on Weight Loss, Mental Health and Lifestyle in Adults with Obesity: A Randomized Controlled Trial." *Journal of Molecular Biochemistry*, vol. 7, no. 2, 3 Oct. 2018, pp. 78–84.

◼ Walking

CATEGORY: Physiology

Walking is a physical activity that helps to strengthen the heart. Walking is a readily accessible physical activity that most people can participate in for health reasons. Physical activity has many benefits. It strengthens the heart, muscles, and bones; helps a person manage his or her weight; prevents disease; and improves mood. Walking programs can be tailored for individuals of all fitness levels.

Getting Started

Walking is an easy way to add physical activity to a person's life. Regular walks can ward off weight gain and prevent some conditions and diseases. It does not have costs involved since a person can just get up and walk just about anywhere. People do not only have to walk outdoors, which can be inconvenient at times, such as during inclement weather. They can choose to walk indoors at a mall or on a treadmill.

Walking does not require any special equipment—other than a proper pair of sneakers. Sneakers should have arch support and be flexible to absorb shock. Clothing should be comfortable and weather appropriate (hats, gloves, and scarves in the cold or waterproof clothing or umbrellas for the rain). Removable layers work best, so walkers can remove clothing if they get hot or add clothing if they get cold. Sunscreen, hats, or sunglasses should be worn to protect an individual from the ultraviolet rays of the sun.

Adding a friend to chat with or some music can help make the activity more enjoyable. When listening to music during physical activity, a person should keep the volume low enough so he or she still can be aware of surroundings, for example, by hearing car horns or sirens from emergency personnel. For safety reasons, people should avoid walking on uneven surfaces to avoid injury. They also should walk in well-lit areas (if walking in the evening). Night walkers should wear bright colors or reflective clothing for visibility. Individuals should not walk alone, if possible. If a person walks alone, he or she should let someone know the time and route of the walk. Walkers should keep a cell phone and identification with them in case of emergencies.

Walking can take on meditative state of mind or enhance reflections on recent or past events, which have been called Medicine Walks. Medicine Walks involve 3 phases, including preparation, solo time, and returning to community. Preparation involves thinking about what you many want to learn or understand during the walk. Reflections on natural surroundings while walking and taking note of personal thoughts or feelings are parts of the solo time phase. Sharing what was learned or experiences during the walk with friends or family are part of the Medicine Walk community experience.

Before individuals begin any type of physical activity such as walking, they should visit their health care provider to make sure they are healthy enough to be participating in exercise. A health care provider can assess a person's overall health to determine if there will be any risks associated with exercise. The following are some health concerns to address with the provider:

- Do conditions such as heart trouble, diabetes, or asthma exist?
- Does physical activity cause chest pain or pain in the neck, shoulder, or arm?
- Are faintness or dizzy spells present?
- Does physical activity cause shortness of breath?

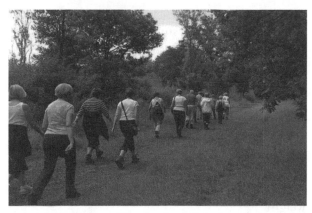

A group of walkers are following the walk leader, who is wearing a yellow jacket. (Walking for Health, Paul Glendell)

- Is walking difficult because of bone or joint problems, such as arthritis?
- Will a walking regimen impact any existing health problems?

Developing a Walking Program

Once individuals have determined that they are healthy enough to begin a walking program, then they are ready to develop a plan. The plan should include the route or location of the walk (inside versus outside); times they will walk, including how often (thirty minutes for five days a week); and with whom they will walk.

Before beginning the walk, a person should gently warm the muscles by walking slowly for five to ten minutes to prepare the body for exercise. The person should increase the pace and try to maintain or exceed this pace during the entirety of the walk. When walking, people should consider their technique or form to avoid injury. The following are some tips a person should remember while walking:

- Look forward.
- Keep the chin up.
- Keep the shoulders slightly back.
- Keep the neck and back straight and relaxed, not stiff.
- Keep the abdominal muscles tight.
- Make sure the foot rolls from heel to toe.
- Walk with toes pointed forward.

- Swing arms naturally with a slight bend at the elbows (some people prefer to pump the arms).

Individuals should cool down their muscles toward the end of the walk. This can be done by walking at a slower pace for five to ten minutes. In addition, stretching is an important part of all physical activity. A person should stretch his or her muscles after warming up or after cooling down to prevent injury.

Seeing Benefits and Staying on Track

Walking can lower the risk of a person developing conditions such as high blood pressure, heart disease, and diabetes. It strengthens the heart, bones, and muscles. It burns calories, helping a person to maintain or lose weight—especially when paired with a healthy diet plan. Walking can help improve balance and coordination. It also helps to improve a person's mood. The more a person participates in physical activity, the more benefits he or she will see. Pairing a healthy diet with a walking plan can further improve a person's overall health.

Individuals should plan to walk for at least thirty minutes most days of the week. As a person becomes comfortable with a walking regimen, he or she can gradually increase goals. These can include walking longer distances, for greater amounts of time, or on more challenging terrain, such as hills.

Also, individuals can track their progress by recording the time spent walking, how many steps they take, and the distance they walk each day. These details can be recorded in a journal, on a spreadsheet, or in a physical fitness app on a smartphone or mobile device. Pedometers or other electronic devices can keep track of a person's steps and distance walked to help mark progress of the walking program.

—Angela Harmon, Richard P. Capriccioso

References

Baker, E.H., et al. "A Pilot Study to Promote Walking among Obese and Overweight Individuals: Walking Buses for Adults." *Public Health*, vol. 129, no. 6, June 2015, pp. 822–824, 10.1016/j. puhe.2015.03.021.

Correia de Faria Santarém, G, et al. "Correlation between Body Composition and Walking Capacity in Severe Obesity." *PLOS ONE*, vol. 10, no. 6, 22 June 2015, p. e0130268, 10.1371/journal.pone.0130268.

Forjuoh, Samuel N., et al. "Determinants of Walking among Middle-Aged and Older Overweight and Obese Adults: Sociodemographic, Health, and Built Environmental Factors." *Journal of Obesity*, vol. 2017, 2017, pp. 1–11, 10.1155/2017/9565430.

Son, Sungmin, et al. "Effects of a Walking Exercise Program for Obese Individuals with Intellectual Disability Staying in a Residential Care Facility." *Journal of Physical Therapy Science*, vol. 28, no. 3, 2016, pp. 788–793, 10.1589/jpts.28.788.

University of Cambridge. "Children Who Walk to School Less Likely to Be Overweight or Obese." *ScienceDaily*, 21 May 2019, www.sciencedaily.com/releases/2019/05/190521101344.htm.

"Walking: Trim Your Waistline, Improve Your Health." Mayo Clinic. Mayo Foundation for Medical Education and Research. 18 Apr. 2013, http://www.mayoclinic.org/healthy-lifestyle/fitness/in-depth/walking/art-20046261

■ Weight loss medications

CATEGORY: Pharmacology

Indications and Procedures

By the mid-1990s, several drugs had come onto the market showing promise in helping people achieve weight loss. The most widely sought and prescribed of these were Fen-Phen (combining serotonergic fenfluramine and amphetamine-like phentermine) and Redux (dexfenfluramine, with similar properties and actions to fenfluramine). Fen-Phen inhibited the brain's utilization of the neurochemical serotonin, which acts on the brain's appetite control center in the hypothalamus, and suppressed appetite directly, much as traditional over-the-counter diet pills do. Other drugs, less widely used, included phentermine, mazindol, and fluoxetine.

The hope and early evidence were that these medications would produce improved cardiac function, cholesterol and triglyceride profiles, blood sugar concentrations, and blood pressure; assist in the treatment of bulimia; and reduce weight in the obese and prevent weight gain in those at high risk for it, such as individuals who recently have quit smoking. The drugs were intended to assist those with morbid obesity, obese persons with serious medical conditions, and obese persons who had failed to manage their weight using more conservative nutritional and behavioral methods. At no point did researchers intend the medications as quick fixes for those unwilling to exercise or unwilling to change their eating habits. Nevertheless, many physicians prescribed them to patients who were not significantly obese or who were merely overweight.

Uses and Complications

Multiple studies across many different populations have tended to show the same results: Measurable weight loss in those taking the drugs was between 5 and 15 percent, with weight regained one year after patients had stopped taking the drug. The medications had few initial side effects-dry mouth, constipation, and drowsiness being the most common-and were unlikely to become physically addicting.

Health providers across all disciplines were particularly concerned, however, that some patients were coming to rely on these medications as alternatives to the sustained, hard work of developing lifestyle habits of healthy, proportional eating and exercise. In addition, concerns grew over the drugs' potential to cause neurotoxicity and primary pulmonary hypertension. Fen-Phen, in particular, was responsible for numerous reports of valvular heart disease and pulmonary hypertension.

Perspective and Prospects

In 1997, the Food and Drug Administration (FDA) withdrew approval of Fen-Phen and Redux for treating obesity, and their marketing and distribution were discontinued. Class-action lawsuits were filed-former Fen-Phen users alone have filed approximately fifty thousand lawsuits against the makers of the drug-and large settlements were reached for those who had used Fen-Phen and other such drugs.

The government then set its sights on dietary products containing ephedra. Manufacturers claimed that ephedra, a botanical source of ephedrine, is a "fat-burning" supplement that could

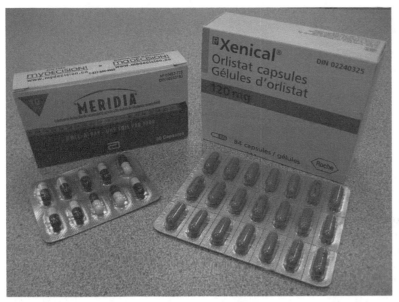

Orlistat (Xenical), the most commonly used medication to treat obesity and sibutramine (Meridia), a medication that was recently withdrawn due to cardiovascular side effects. (James Heilman, MD)

boost energy and enhance athletic performance, but reports began to surface about seizures, strokes, heart attacks, and even deaths in otherwise healthy users. In 2003, the FDA banned the use of ephedra.

—*Paul Moglia, LeAnna DeAngelo*

References

"Are Weight-Loss Drugs Worth Trying? - Harvard Health." *Harvard Health Publishing*, Harvard Medical School, 22 May 2018, www.health.harvard.edu/staying-healthy/are-weight-loss-drugs-worth-trying.

Khera, Rohan, et al. "Association of Pharmacological Treatments for Obesity With Weight Loss and Adverse Events: A Systematic Review and Meta-Analysis." *JAMA*, vol. 315, no. 22, 2016, pp. 2424–34, www.ncbi.nlm.nih.gov/pubmed/27299618, 10.1001/jama.2016.7602.

Van Gaal, Luc, and Eveline Dirinck. "Pharmacological Approaches in the Treatment and Maintenance of Weight Loss." *Diabetes Care*, vol. 39, no. Supplement 2, 19 July 2016, pp. S260–S267, 10.2337/dcs15-3016.

Yanovski, Susan Z., and Jack A. Yanovski. "Long-Term Drug Treatment for Obesity." *JAMA*, vol. 311, no. 1, 1 Jan. 2014, p. 74, 10.1001/jama.2013.281361.

■ Yoga

CATEGORY: Physiology

Introduction

The word "yoga" comes from the Sanskrit word *Yuj*, meaning to "yoke," "join," or "unite." The word implies joining or integrating all aspects of the body with the mind to achieve a healthy and balanced life. The true purpose of the ancient practices of yoga is to bring a proper balance between the physical and mental aspects of a person and to awaken what yoga practitioners understand to be subtle energies of the body. Yoga cultivates muscular strength, endurance, and flexibility and enhances the practitioner's mental acuity. Meditative breathing calms a person's nerves and sharpens a person's focus. With regular yoga practice, individuals are known to gain physical health, mental relaxation, and inner tranquility.

Yoga has been practiced in India, in one form or another, for more than four thousand years. More than two thousand years ago, the Indian scholar Patanjali codified the various yoga practices into a written collection called the *YogaSutras*. According to Patanjali, there are three critical components of yoga: physical postures (*asanas*), breath control (*pranayama*), and meditation (*samyana*). The main purpose of *asanas* and *pranayam* is to cleanse the body, increase energy, and raise the level of consciousness. Yoga styles have come to include a strong component of meditation to enhance the union of mind, body, and soul. Patanjali showed how, through the practice of yoga, one could gain mastery over mind and emotion. Advanced yoga practitioners are known to have incredible control over several autonomic functions such as respiration, heart rate, and blood flow.

While the ancient practice of yoga focused more on access to a higher level of consciousness and spirituality, modern yoga focuses more on the physical and mental health benefits of the practice. Yoga has enjoyed rising popularity in recent years in the U.S., particularly among younger, college-educated females.

FINDING THE RIGHT TYPE OF YOGA AND THE RIGHT TEACHER

The word "yoga" as used in the United States refers to a broad range of different kinds of mental, physical, and spiritual practices. Persons who have a desire to learn should take some time to get acquainted with the different schools and styles to appreciate what various teachers have to offer. Yoga is a most personal kind of exercise, and the benefits accrue slowly and subtly over time.

Many different schools and styles of yoga are taught in the United States. Some teachers have been certified in particular traditions, others offer a synthesis based on their own practice with yoga masters. The various major traditions include the following:

Astanga yoga. This form of yoga, developed by K. Pattabhi Jois, is a demanding form of the practice. This yoga uses a concept of "flow" that has participants moving continuously and jumping from one posture to another, building strength, flexibility, and stamina. Astanga yoga is an intense workout and is not recommended for persons looking for leisurely stretching exercises.

Integral yoga. This form of yoga was developed by Swami Satchidananda. It relies on breathing exercises (*pranayama*) and meditation as much as on postures for the practice.

Iyengar yoga. Iyengar yoga is a style of yoga developed by B. K. S. Iyengar, who systemized his training and certified teachers who have completed an extensive two-to-five-year training program. Iyengar practitioners use props such as blocks and belts to aid them in performing many of the more difficult postures, and great attention is paid to a precise alignment of postures.

Kripalu yoga. This form of yoga places emphasis on "honoring the wisdom of the body" and allowing each student to develop an awareness of mind, body, emotion, and spirit. The practice is delineated into three stages: learning the postures and exploring the body's abilities, holding the postures for an extended time and developing an inner awareness, and moving from one posture to another in a spontaneous movement.

Kundalini yoga. This form of yoga involves postures, meditation, and the coordination of breath. The practice is said to create a controlled release of kundalini energy, a creative force thought to be at the base of the spine.

Viniyoga. Viniyoga was developed by Krishnamacharya, a teacher whose disciples have created numerous other yoga forms. Viniyoga is a gentle form of flow yoga (continuous movement) that focuses on a student's ability rather than on idealized form.

Bikram yoga. Bikram yoga, founded by Bikram Choudhury, utilizes yoga postures practiced in a heated environment.

Sivananda yoga. This form of yoga involves a set structure that includes relaxation, pranayama (breathing), and classic asana postures.

Many excellent yoga books explain the postures and feature beautiful photographs and illustrations. Teachers, however, can impart an understanding of the poses and the practice of yoga in ways that books cannot. A teacher can also help one develop correct alignment in the various poses so that one gets the greatest benefit and so that internal stretching and healing begin.

While there is still an emphasis on yoga as a physical exercise, many teachers now address the more spiritual aspects of practice too. Other teachers take a holistic or even therapeutic approach with their students, reading their yoga practice as an open book on their personality and behavior.

The kind of relationship one develops with his or her yoga teacher depends on the teacher's philosophy and on what kind of response the student wants. However, certain basic rules should be followed in assessing a yoga teacher's capabilities.

Upon seeing a new student in class, most teachers will acknowledge that the student is new to class and will have a short chat with the student. Teachers also might ask the student if he or she has any injuries so they can recommend alternative poses if they think some routines are too difficult. Good yoga teachers will carefully watch the new student, make adjustments to postures, and push the student beyond perceived limits.

—Reviewed by Brian Randall, M.D.

Health Benefits

Research, mostly performed in India, suggests a wide variety of positive health effects from the daily practice of yoga, including, but not limited to, pain reduction in arthritis and carpal tunnel syndrome, reduction of coronary artery disease, and relief from asthma and other respiratory ailments. Situated in Bangalore, India, the Swami Vivekananda Yoga Anusandhana Samsthana (SVYASA) University treats people with such

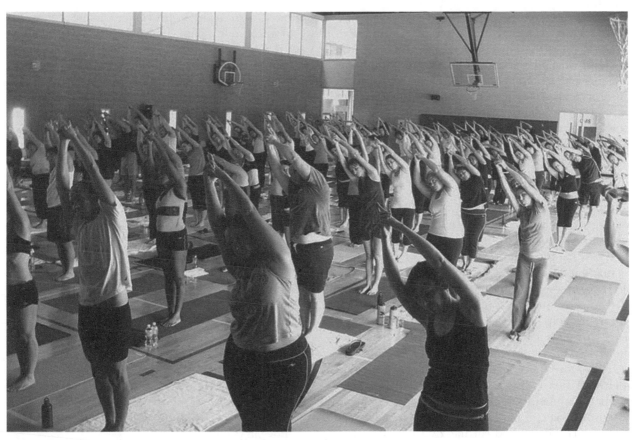

A yoga class in Cresent Moon pose. (Jessmcintyre via Wikimedia Commons)

ailments as asthma, arthritis, heart disease, high blood pressure, psychiatric ailments, and eating disorders. The center uses an integrated approach of yoga therapies that includes *asanas*, chanting, *kriya* (yoga cleansing techniques), meditation, *pranayam*, and lectures on yoga philosophy. The system, according to their research, has been shown to benefit people with asthma, intellectual disabilities, rheumatoid arthritis, and type 1 diabetes mellitus. It is believed to improve visual perception, manual dexterity, and spatial memory. However, the quality of the research in Indian institutes must be taken into consideration, since a Cochrane Airways Group review of literature found that "no reliable conclusions could be drawn concerning the use of breathing exercises for asthma in clinical practice. This was a result of methodological differences among the included studies and poor reporting of methodological aspects in most of the included studies."

With support from other organizations, SVYASA has been engaged in a vast variety of research, including studies regarding the use of yoga to treat obsessive-compulsive disorder; the effects of yoga on people with multiple sclerosis; and the use of yoga for assessing alertness, ability to focus, flexibility, balance, quality of life, and fatigue in healthy elderly people. *Pranayam* has been shown to lower blood pressure in people with hypertension, to alleviate discomfort from gastritis, and to reduce stress and anxiety. One difficulty with the work in India, however, has been a lack of rigor in research design and protocol. For example, the yoga practices are traditionally combined with chanting, discourse, and other activities, and it is difficult to determine the effects of such extra variables when comparing the results of one study with another.

Studies suggest that yoga can have benefits on several parameters including physical and mental health, quality of life, and pain relief, though no association has been shown with decreased mortality. Benefits in cardiovascular fitness have been shown primarily among older adults. Evidence suggests that yoga is associated with improved flexibility, balance and pain relief, particularly for patients with low back pain and rheumatologic conditions. There may also be benefits for pregnant patients, particularly with regards to decreased pelvic pain and improved perinatal outcomes. Evidence from randomized trials also indicate improvements in sleep quality and fatigue in cancer survivors.

Perspective and Prospects

With growing interest in alternative therapies, several individuals and institutions have initiated extensive studies on the effects of yoga. For example, researchers at Ball State University found that fifteen weeks of yoga training brought a 10-percent improvement in lung capacity. Yoga has been found to help fight cardiovascular disease when used in conjunction with other lifestyle changes, such as a low-fat diet; however, the *European Journal of Preventative Cardiology* reviewed the literature on yoga and heart disease and concluded that only "weak recommendations can be made for the ancillary use of yoga for patients with coronary heart disease, heart failure, and cardiac dysrhythmia." The National Institutes of Health (NIH) is supporting research on yoga, including its use for treating insomnia and chronic lower back pain.

In a study at the University of Iowa, some patients with chronic fatigue syndrome were shown to benefit from yoga. Yoga prevailed among numerous conventional and alternative therapies as an effective fatigue fighter. At the end of the two-year study, yoga was the only therapy linked to a statistically significant positive outcome by linear regression analysis.

Marian Garfinkel, a yoga teacher turned researcher, has demonstrated that practicing certain yoga postures can relieve the symptoms of carpal tunnel syndrome, the common ailment resulting from repetitive hand activities such as typing. Patients practicing prescribed yoga postures showed significant improvement in grip strength and suffered less pain. There was also improvement on a nerve test used to measure the severity of carpal tunnel syndrome. Studies are in progress to observe the effect of yoga on osteoarthritis of the knee and on repetitive strain injuries. However, later work reviewing the effects of yoga on carpal tunnel syndrome has come to more modest conclusions.

Because each patient is unique in their different abilities and weaknesses, a yoga approach should be tailored to specific problems as well as specific potentials. It is also important to look at the studies in which yoga did not prove effective and to determine which variables led to these failures.

—*Tulsi B. Saral, Ananya Anand*

References

Cramer, Holger, et al. "A Systematic Review of Yoga for Heart Disease." *European Journal of Preventive Cardiology*, vol. 22, no. 3, 3 Feb. 2014, pp. 284–295, 10.1177/2047487314523132.

Rathi, SunanadaSurendra, et al. "Development and Validation of Integrated Yoga Module for Obesity in Adolescents." *International Journal of Yoga*, vol. 11, no. 3, 2018, p. 231, 10.4103/ijoy.ijoy_38_17.

Ross, A., et al. "A Different Weight Loss Experience: A Qualitative Study Exploring the Behavioral, Physical, and Psychosocial Changes Associated with Yoga That Promote Weight Loss." *Evidence-Based Complementary and Alternative Medicine*, vol. 2016, 2016, pp. 1–11, www.ncbi.nlm.nih.gov/pmc/articles/PMC4995338/, 10.1155/2016/2914745.

Rshikesan, P. B. "Yoga Practice for Reducing the Male Obesity and Weight Related Psychological Difficulties-A Randomized Controlled Trial." *Journal of Clinical and Diagnostic Research*, vol. 10, no. 11, 2016, 10.7860/jcdr/2016/22720.8940.

Telles, Shirley, et al. "Twelve Weeks of Yoga or Nutritional Advice for Centrally Obese Adult Females." *Frontiers in Endocrinology*, vol. 9, 17 Aug. 2018, 10.3389/fendo.2018.00466.

Conditions In Depth

■ Conditions In Depth: Coronary Artery Disease (CAD)

Coronary Artery Disease (CAD)

The coronary arteries supply blood to the heart muscle. CAD is damage or disease of these arteries. These changes slow or stop the flow of blood.

Regular blood flow is needed to bring oxygen and nutrients to the heart muscle. Without this supply the heart muscle cannot work well. A lack of oxygen can also lead to damage or death of heart muscle. Blood flow changes can lead to:

- Ischemia—damage to heart tissue.
- Angina—Chest pain caused by slowed blood flow to the heart. For some this may feel like a pressure or even shortness of breath.
- Myocardial infarction—blood flow is completely cut off. Also called heart attack.

CAD is the most common life-threatening disease in the US.

CAD Causes

A narrowing of the blood vessels called atherosclerosis is the most common cause of CAD. This is a buildup of plaque on the walls of the blood vessels. The plaque begins because of:

- Injury to the blood vessel walls
- Substances in the blood that stick to walls

After an injury tissue collects or is deposited at the site. This helps the blood vessel heal. However, it can also make it easier for substances in the blood to stick to the area. Substances may include LDL "bad" cholesterol and cells linked to inflammation. They can remain even after the injury has healed. Over time, more substances can get trapped. Together they form plaque. The plaque irritates the blood vessel walls. This causes more injury and creates a new cycle that develops more plaque.

The blood vessel opening gets more narrow with each layer of plaque.

Damage to blood vessels can occur from multiple factors such as:

- High blood pressure—causes rough blood flow that can injure the walls of blood vessels
- High cholesterol—"bad" cholesterol can stick to and irritate the walls of the blood vessels
- Diabetes—excess glucose in the blood can add to plaque build up in blood vessels
- Smoking—chemicals from cigarette smoke can irritate blood vessel walls and make deposits in the walls of blood vessels
- Radiation therapy

—*Michael J. Fucci, DO, FACC*

References

"Angina (Chest Pain)." *American Heart Association*, 14 Dec. 2017, www.heart.org/en/health-topics/heart-attack/angina-chest-pain#.Wp1fXGrwZQI.

"Coronary Artery Disease (CAD)." *DynaMed*, EBSCO Information Services, 28 Feb. 2018, www.dynamed.com/topics/dmp~AN~T116156/Coronary-artery-disease-CAD.

"Coronary Heart Disease." *National Heart, Lung, and Blood Institute*, U.S. Department of Health & Human Services, www.nhlbi.nih.gov/health-topics/coronary-heart-disease. Accessed 6 Mar. 2020.

■ Risk factors for Coronary Artery Disease (CAD)

A risk factor is something that increases your likelihood of getting a disease or condition.

It is possible to develop CAD with or without the risk factors listed below. However, the more risk factors you have, the greater your likelihood of developing CAD. Some risk factors can't be changed, but many can. Talk to your doctor about how you can reduce the number of risk factors you have.

Lifestyle Factors

Certain lifestyle factors may increase your risk of atherosclerosis, which can lead to CAD. These include:

- Physical inactivity—Contributes to an increase in weight, high cholesterol, high blood pressure, and other heart-related risk factors.
- Smoking—Includes cigarettes, cigars, and second hand smoke. Smoking narrows blood vessels and irritates blood vessel walls, which both contribute to atherosclerosis.
- A diet high in saturated fat, trans fat, cholesterol, and/or calories. Increased fats in the diet are directly associated arterial plaque build-up.
- Excess alcohol intake—Contributes to high triglycerides in the blood, increasing your risk of arterial plaque build-up.

Health Conditions

Having certain health conditions put you are at greater risk of developing CAD. These may include:

- High blood pressure—Can lead to turbulent blood flow that can damage blood vessel walls.
- Lipid disorders—High cholesterol and/or triglycerides in the blood contribute to plaque build up in the arteries.
- Diabetes/glucose intolerance—High levels of glucose in the blood contribute to the risk of atherosclerosis and blood vessel damage.
- Obesity and overweight—Excess weight puts you at higher risk for high blood pressure, high cholesterol, and diabetes.
- Metabolic syndrome—A condition marked by elevated blood pressure, cholesterol, blood glucose, and body weight. Excess weight centered around the midsection is of particular concern.
- Chronic stress—Contributes to high blood pressure, depression, and may contribute to making poor decisions that affect your health, such as smoking.
- Psychological disorders, such as depression or anxiety—It is not known how depression, anxiety, and CAD are linked, but psychological

problems do affect overall mental and physical well being. Fatigue, stress, or disinterest can lead you to make poor decisions about your health, such as ignoring treatment plans that reduce your risk of CAD.

Genetic Factors

Genetics are believed to play a role in risk factors that lead to CAD. A family history of CAD or heart disease can increase your risk of CAD. The risk increases when combined with other unhealthy lifestyle choices.

Sex

Men tend to develop atherosclerosis earlier than women. However, a woman's risk increases to that of men with the onset of menopause. Heart disease is the leading cause of death in both men and women.

Certain Blood Test Results

Recent research has found that higher levels of homocysteine and C-reactive proteins in the blood may increase the risk of developing CAD. However, it is not clear the exact relationship and what levels are desirable.

Talk to your doctor to see if these blood tests will benefit you. They may be done if you are considered to be a high-risk candidate for CAD.

Advancing Age

Your risk of CAD increases as you get older. Men older than 45 and women older than 55 (younger in cases of premature menopause) are at greater risk of heart disease.

Race and Ethnicity

African Americans have a higher incidence of high blood pressure than Caucasians and, therefore, a higher risk of developing CAD. Heart disease risk is also higher among Mexican Americans, American Indians, native Hawaiians, and some Asian Americans.

—*Michael J. Fucci, DO, FACC*

References

"Cardiovascular Disease Major Risk Factors." *DynaMed*, EBSCO Information Systems, 12 June 2017, www.dynamed.com/condition/cardiovascular-disease-major-risk-factors.

"Cardiovascular Disease Possible Risk Factors." *DynaMed*, EBSCO Information Services, 26 Feb. 2018, www.dynamed.com/prevention/cardiovascular-disease-possible-risk-factors.

"Coronary Artery Disease - Coronary Heart Disease." *American Heart Association*, 26 Apr. 2017, www.heart.org/en/health-topics/consumer-healthcare/what-is-cardiovascular-disease/coronary-artery-disease#.Wp14QmrwbIV.

"Coronary Heart Disease." *National Heart, Lung, and Blood Institute*, U.S. Department of Health & Human Services, www.nhlbi.nih.gov/health-topics/coronary-heart-disease. Accessed 6 Mar. 2020.

"C-Reactive Protein (CRP) and Other Biomarkers as Cardiac Risk Factors." *DynaMed*, EBSCO Information Services, 25 Feb. 2016, www.dynamed.com/evaluation/c-reactive-protein-crp-and-other-biomarkers-as-cardiac-risk-factors.

Emdin, Connor A., et al. "Meta-Analysis of Anxiety as a Risk Factor for Cardiovascular Disease." *The American Journal of Cardiology*, vol. 118, no. 4, Aug. 2016, pp. 511–519, 10.1016/j.amjcard.2016.05.041.

Fung, Teresa T., et al. "Sweetened Beverage Consumption and Risk of Coronary Heart Disease in Women." *The American Journal of Clinical Nutrition*, vol. 89, no. 4, 1 Apr. 2009, pp. 1037–1042, www.ncbi.nlm.nih.gov/pubmed/19211821/, 10.3945/ajcn.2008.27140.

"Homocysteine and Cardiovascular Disease." *DynaMed*, EBSCO Information Services, 23 Aug. 2016, www.dynamed.com/evaluation/homocysteine-and-cardiovascular-disease.

Kodama, Satoru. "Cardiorespiratory Fitness as a Quantitative Predictor of All-Cause Mortality and Cardiovascular Events in Healthy Men and Women." *JAMA*, vol. 301, no. 19, 20 May 2009, p. 2024, 10.1001/jama.2009.681.

Park, Chan Seok, et al. "Relation Between C-Reactive Protein, Homocysteine Levels, Fibrinogen, and Lipoprotein Levels and Leukocyte and Platelet Counts, and 10-Year Risk for Cardiovascular Disease Among Healthy Adults in the USA." *The American Journal of Cardiology*, vol. 105, no. 9, May 2010, pp. 1284–1288, 10.1016/j.amjcard.2009.12.045.

Ridker, Paul M., et al. "Comparison of C-Reactive Protein and Low-Density Lipoprotein Cholesterol Levels in the Prediction of First Cardiovascular Events." *New England Journal of Medicine*, vol. 347, no. 20, 14 Nov. 2002, pp. 1557–1565, 10.1056/nejmoa021993.

■ Reducing your risk of Coronary Artery Disease (CAD)

There are a variety of issues that can contribute to CAD and fortunately many of the risk factors can be managed or avoided. The more factors you control, the more you reduce your risk of CAD.

Aim for a Healthy Weight

If you are overweight or obese, adopt a sensible eating plan. Exercise regularly to lose weight gradually, and maintain your weight at the desired level. Consider consulting with a dietitian who can help you with meal planning and portion sizing.

Quit Smoking

Chemicals in tobacco smoke contribute to the build-up of plaque in the arteries, increasing your risk of atherosclerosis. It also irritates the lining of the blood vessels which can cause further damage.

Quitting smoking is the best way to put yourself on the right track. Talk with your doctor about tools and programs to help you quit. Secondhand smoke can be damaging as well.

Drink Alcohol in Moderation

Excess alcohol intake is also associated with an increased risk of CAD. If you drink alcohol, aim for moderation. Moderate alcohol intake means 2 drinks or less a day for men, and 1 drink a day or less for women. Some studies have suggested that moderate alcohol consumption may help increase the beneficial high-density lipoprotein (HDL) cholesterol, which may help reduce plaque build-up.

Eat a Healthful Diet

Your diet can have a significant impact on your "bad" and "good" cholesterol levels. Managing your cholesterol levels with a well-balanced diet can reduce your risk for CAD by reducing the amount of plaque build-up.

A well-balanced diet includes plenty of whole grains, fruits and vegetables, and nuts. Also consider substituting bad fats for good fats. This means eating more mono- or polyunsaturated fats like olive and canola oils, and less saturated and trans fats which can raise the levels of bad cholesterol.

Foods to consider limiting or avoiding include:

- High-fat processed meats such as bologna, sausage, hot dogs
- Solid fats such as shortening, stick butter, or lard
- Whole milk, cream, ice cream, and cheese
- Baked goods that contain egg yolks and butter
- Fried foods such as fried chicken, french fries, and potato chips
- Fatty red meats or organ meats such as liver
- Saturated oils like coconut oil, palm oil, and palm kernel oil

Control Blood Glucose Levels If You have Diabetes

High blood glucose levels can cause damage to smaller blood vessels and contribute to atherosclerosis. Managing blood glucose levels can reduce the risk or delay onset of CAD for people with diabetes. If you have diabetes, work with your doctor to develop a plan to manage your blood glucose levels.

Maintain Normal Blood Pressure

High blood pressure is a major cause of CAD. Dietary changes, regular exercise, and medications can help you control your blood pressure. If you are being treated for high blood pressure, adhere to the treatment plan outlined by your doctor. Stay in contact with your medical team and have your blood pressure tested regularly.

Too much sodium has also been linked to high blood pressure. Aim for sodium levels less than 2,300 mg per day. Read food labels to find the hidden sodium in your diet in addition to limiting use of table salt.

The DASH diet is a plan designed to help reduce blood pressure.

Exercise Regularly

Regular aerobic exercise, such as brisk walking, using a stationary bike, or treadmill, can help reduce the risk of heart disease including CAD. In general, it is recommended that you exercise at least 30 minutes per day on most days of the week.

If you have a sedentary job, it may be beneficial to aim for 60 minutes of exercise a day. Overall, exercise will help strengthen the heart muscle, decrease the heart's workload, and lower blood pressure.

Talk to your doctor before starting any exercise program.

Michael J. Fucci, DO, FACC

References

"Cardiovascular Disease Prevention Overview." *DynaMed*, EBSCO Information Services, 22 Feb. 2018, www.dynamed.com/prevention/cardiovascular-disease-prevention-overview.

"Coronary Heart Disease." *National Heart, Lung, and Blood Institute*, U.S. Department of Health & Human Services, www.nhlbi.nih.gov/health-topics/coronary-heart-disease. Accessed 6 Mar. 2020.

Ebbing, Marta. "Cancer Incidence and Mortality After Treatment With Folic Acid and Vitamin B$_{12}$." *JAMA*, vol. 302, no. 19, 18 Nov. 2009, p. 2119, 10.1001/jama.2009.1622.

Ekelund, Ulf, et al. "Does Physical Activity Attenuate, or Even Eliminate, the Detrimental Association of Sitting Time with Mortality? A Harmonised Meta-Analysis of Data from More than 1 Million Men and Women." *The Lancet*, vol. 388, no. 10051, Sept. 2016, pp. 1302–1310, www.thelancet.com/journals/lancet/article/PIIS0140-6736(16)30370-1/fulltext, 10.1016/s0140-6736(16)30370-1.

"Homocysteine and Cardiovascular Disease." *DynaMed*, EBSCO Information Services, 23 Aug. 2016, www.dynamed.com/evaluation/homocysteine-and-cardiovascular-disease.

Thavendiranathan, Paaladinesh, et al. "Primary Prevention of Cardiovascular Diseases With Statin Therapy." *Archives of Internal Medicine*, vol. 166, no. 21, 27 Nov. 2006, p. 2307, 10.1001/archinte.166.21.2307.

■ Symptoms of Coronary Artery Disease (CAD)

CAD gets worse over time. Symptoms may not appear in early stages. It is possible to not know you have CAD until complications appear. Over time, CAD may lead to:

Angina

Angina is the most common symptom of CAD. It is chest pain or discomfort with a squeezing or pressure-like quality. It is most often felt behind the

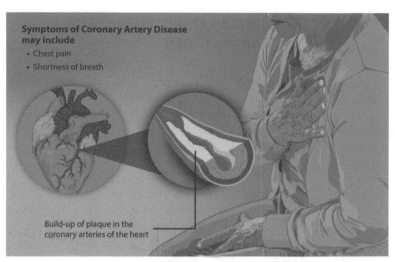

Depiction of a person suffering from Coronary Artery Disease. The build-up of plaque in a coronary artery has been shown as well. (MyUpchar)

breastbone. It may sometimes be felt in the shoulders, arms, neck, jaws, or back. Angina is a sign that your heart tissue is not getting all the oxygen it needs. People who have angina are at an increased risk of having a heart attack.

Types of angina include:

- Stable angina or angina pectoris—attacks can be predicted. The triggers are known. This type of angina does not occur when you are at rest or relaxed. It often disappears after a few minutes of rest.
- Unstable angina—less predictable. Chest pain may occur while at rest. The discomfort may last longer and be more intense.
- Variant or Prinzmetal angina—usually caused by the spasm of a coronary vessel. It occurs when you are at rest. Often happens in the middle of the night. It can be quite severe. In some cases, it may be linked to arrhythmias.
- Microvascular angina—caused by spasms in the smallest arterial vessels of the heart. Spasms cause a decrease in the heart's blood supply.

Complications
CAD can eventually lead to severe complications such as:

- Heart attack—blockage of blood flow to the heart. Can cause severe damage to the heart or death.

- Heart arrhythmias—irregular heartbeats. They can cause symptoms like fatigue or shortness of breath. They can also lead to sudden cardiac arrest
- Heart failure—heart cannot pump enough blood to meet the needs of the body. Can cause shortness of breath and swelling of ankles, feet, or abdomen. Heart failure can lead to early death as well.

Differences Between Angina and a Heart Attack
Note of Caution: An angina attack can be frightening. People may mistake it for having a heart attack or just think it is heartburn. A stable pattern of angina does not definitely mean a heart attack is about to occur. Some differences include:

Duration of pain
- Anginal pain often lasts for only a few minutes. It is relieved by rest or medicine called nitroglycerin.
- Heart attack pain may last longer. It may also fade and return. A heart attack may also change the pattern of angina you are used to.

External factors
- Anginal pain is often brought on certain factors. The symptoms will stop once the trigger is stopped or removed.
- Heart attack pain will usually not subside with rest. Other symptoms like shortness of breath, nausea, or sweating may also be present.

If you have chest pain that is new, worsening, or persistent, call for emergency medical services right away.

- Do not try to determine the cause of chest pain for yourself.
- Do not drive yourself to the hospital.

Heart attacks can cause severe, permanent damage to the heart, or death. Quick medical care may stop some of the damage and increase survival. Ideally care should be given within the first hour after symptoms begin. Emergency medical service can give these treatments on the way to the hospital.

NOTE: Women, the elderly, or people with diabetes may have less typical symptoms. Some people may have silent ischemia and experience no symptoms at all.

Associated Conditions

Build up of plaque and damage to blood vessels rarely occurs in the heart's blood vessels alone. Blood vessel damage in other areas of the body may lead to other conditions such as:

- Erectile dysfunction (ED)—ED is often caused by a blood flow problem in the penis. It may be an early sign of blood vessel problems in the body.
- Peripheral artery disease (PAD)—Narrowing and blockage of arteries outside of the heart and brain.
- Chronic kidney disease—May often be caused by blood vessel damage.
- Stroke —Blood flow to the brain is completely blocked in one or more arteries in the brain.

—Michael J. Fucci, DO, FACC</item>

References

"Coronary Artery Disease (CAD)." *DynaMed*, EBSCO Information Services, 28 Feb. 2018, www.dynamed.com/condition/coronary-artery-disease-cad.

"Coronary Heart Disease." *National Heart, Lung, and Blood Institute*, U.S. Department of Health & Human Services, www.nhlbi.nih.gov/health-topics/coronary-heart-disease. Accessed 6 Mar. 2020.

Nascimento, E. R., et al. "Sexual Dysfunction and Cardiovascular Diseases: A Systematic Review of Prevalence." *Clinics*, vol. 68, no. 11, 1 Nov. 2013, pp. 1462–1468, 10.6061/clinics/2013(11)13.

"Warning Signs of a Heart Attack." *American Heart Association*, 2016, www.heart.org/en/health-topics/heart-attack/warning-signs-of-a-heart-attack.

■ Screening for Coronary Artery Disease (CAD)

The purpose of screening is to find a disease in early stages. Some tests are given to people that do not yet have symptoms. Other tests may only be given to those at high risk. Early diagnosis of CAD may slow or prevent future damage to the heart.

Screening Guidelines and Tests

CAD screening is often done as part of regular exams. The following are regular screening tests that help to identify risk factors for developing CAD:

Blood Tests

Blood tests can identify factors that can lead to CAD. These include:

- High cholesterol. Your total cholesterol should be checked every 5 years once you reach the age of 20. More frequent testing may be recommended if you have had:
    ◦ High LDL cholesterol or triglycerides
    ◦ Low HDL cholesterol
    ◦ Other factors that increase your risk of heart disease
- Blood glucose. Screens for diabetes or pre-diabetes.nShould be checked every 3 years after age 45 years

Body Weight

Your body weight should be checked at each exam once you reach the age of 20. Your doctor will assess:

- Body mass index (BMI)
- Waist circumference

Excess weight is a risk factor for CAD.

Screening Tests for High Risk Populations

If you are at high risk of developing CAD, you doctor may recommend screening tests such as:

Blood Tests

Elevated C-reactive is a protein marker found in the blood. This marker appears when there is an inflammatory response in the body. An increased level is linked with a higher risk for CAD.

ECG

An ECG records the electrical activity of your heart. It is done with electrodes that are placed on the skin. An ECG may be able to s how changes in your heart's rhythm. It can also show if the heart has been damaged. However, a normal ECG does not mean you are free of CAD. Most early changes are not seen on this test.

Chest X-ray

Your doctor may order chest x-rays. It will show your heart's size. Your doctor will also be able to see any signs of congestion in the lungs.

Cardiac CT Scan

This CT scan is also known as coronary artery calcium scoring. It is an advanced x-ray that can show calcium levels in the arteries of the heart. The results are shown as a calcium score. Calcium build-up is a marker of CAD.

Ankle-brachial Indices

Peripheral arterial disease (PAD), the hardening of the arteries outside of the heart. It is also a marker for increased risk of artery disease in the heart. An ankle-brachial index measurement is done to screen for and diagnose PAD. Blood pressure is measured at your ankle and at your arm. If blood pressure is lower in your ankle, it indicates a blockage between your heart and your leg.

Atherosclerosis is a systemic disease. If it is present in one area of the body it is likely present in other areas.

Carotid Intima-media Thickness (IMT)

Measuring the thickness of the two innermost layers of the arterial wall. It may detect the presence of atherosclerosis. However, research has not determined if the relationship to CAD is clinically significant enough. It is not clear whether IMT is a good screening tool for CAD.

—*Michael J. Fucci, DO, FACC*

References

Buttitta, Flavio, et al. "Usefulness of Carotid Intima-Media Thickness Measurement and Peripheral B-Mode Ultrasound Scan in the Clinical Screening of Patients with Coronary Artery Disease." *Angiology,* vol. 51, no. 4, Apr. 2000, pp. 269–279, 10.1177/000331970005100401.

"Cardiac CT for Calcium Scoring." *Radiologyinfo. Org,* Radiological Society of North America, 28 Jan. 2020, www.radiologyinfo.org/en/info.cfm?pg=ct%5Fcalscoring.

"Coronary Artery Disease (CAD)." *DynaMed,* EBSCO Information Services, 28 Feb. 2018, www.dynamed.com/condition/coronary-artery-disease-cad.

"C-Reactive Protein (CRP) and Other Biomarkers as Cardiac Risk Factors." *DynaMed,* EBSCO Information Services, 25 Feb. 2016, www.dynamed.com/evaluation/c-reactive-protein-crp-and-other-biomarkers-as-cardiac-risk-factors.

"Heart-Health Screenings." *American Heart Association,* 22 Mar. 2019, www.heart.org/en/health-topics/consumer-healthcare/what-is-cardiovascular-disease/heart-health-screenings#.Wp2AzmrwbIU.

Zebrack, James S, et al. "C-Reactive Protein and Angiographic Coronary Artery Disease: Independent and Additive Predictors of Risk in Subjects with Angina." *Journal of the American College of Cardiology,* vol. 39, no. 4, Feb. 2002, pp. 632–637, 10.1016/s0735-1097(01)01804-6.

■ Medications for Coronary Artery Disease (CAD)

The information provided here is meant to give you a general idea about each of the medications listed below. Only the most general side effects are included, so ask your doctor if you need to take any special precautions. Use each of these medications as recommended by your doctor, or according to the instructions provided. If you have further questions about usage or side effects, contact your doctor.

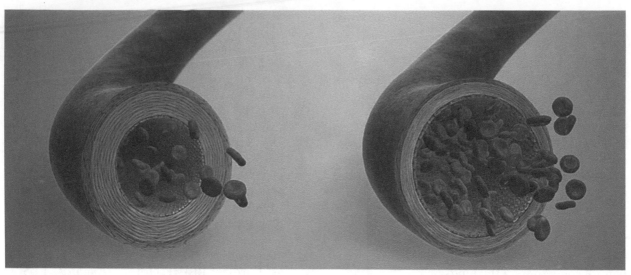

Normal blood vessel (left) vs. vasodilation (right). (Scientific Animations)

Prescription Medications

Vasodilators

Vasodilators help dilate or widen blood vessels. People with CAD have blood vessels that are narrowed, which reduces the amount of blood that can be delivered to the heart muscle. Nitrates or nitroglycerin may be used to immediately relieve an attack of angina that is occurring, or prevent or reduce future attacks. Nitrates come in many preparations, including tablets, sprays for use under the tongue, ointments, or patches for placement on the skin. The tablets or sprays are used at times of anginal episodes, while the ointment or patch is used on a daily basis for prevention of attacks.

Common names include:	Possible side effects include:
Nitroglycerin	Headache
	Lightheadedness or faintness from low blood pressure
	Rapid heart rate—tachycardia
	Flushing of face and neck
	Nausea or vomiting
	Restlessness

Beta-Blockers

These medications help slow the heart rate and reduce blood pressure, especially during exercise. They are intended to prevent anginal attacks or heart attacks. Beta-blockers are also prescribed when recovering from a heart attack in order to lessen the likelihood of recurrence.

Common names include:	Possible side effects include:
Metoprolol	Decreased sexual ability
Atenolol	Lightheadedness or faintness from low blood pressure
Nadolol	Trouble sleeping/nightmares
Propranolol	Unusual tiredness or weakness
Carvedilol	Breathing difficulty or asthma
Bisoprolol	
Pindolol	
Timolol	
Acebutolol	
Labetalol	
Betaxolol	
Carteolol	
Penbutolol	
Esmolol	

Statins

Statins are drugs that help to lower cholesterol levels and decrease inflammation. They are often prescribed to people diagnosed with CAD. These medications may reduce the risk of stroke and heart attack.

Common names include:	Possible side effects include:
Atorvastatin	Headache
Pravastatin	Stomach ache
Lovastatin	Diarrhea
Simvastatin	Muscle weakness
Fluvastatin	Rarely, liver damage
Rosuvastatin	

Calcium Channel Blockers

These medications affect the movement of calcium into the cells of the heart and blood vessels. As a result, blood vessels dilate. The supply of blood and oxygen to the heart is increased, while the heart's workload is decreased. This helps to prevent anginal attacks, as well as lessen the possibility of heart attacks.

Common names include:	Possible side effects include
Nifedipine	Constipation
Verapamil	Swollen legs
Diltiazem	Unusual tiredness or weakness
Amlodipine	Headache
Felodipine	Palpitations
Isradipine	
Nisoldipine:	

Antiplatelet Agents

Antiplatelet agents prevent the formation of blood clots by keeping platelets from clumping and sticking together.

Common names include:	Possible side effects include:
Aspirin	Nausea and vomiting
Clopidogrel	Diarrhea
Ticlopidine	Skin rash
Dipyridamole	Ringing in the ears— tinnitus
	Skin bruising
	Irritation of the stomach lining
	Bleeding from the digestive system and other internal organs
	Allergic reaction

Anticoagulants

Anticoagulants are given to "thin" the blood, in an effort to prevent the formation of blood clots. The most serious side effect is bleeding.

Common names include:	Possible side effects include:
Warfarin	Bloody or tarry black stools
	Nosebleeds
	Heavy menstrual periods
	Easy bruising
	Allergic reaction

Nicorandil

This medication, which contains a nitrate, dilates blood vessels by affecting the potassium flow in the heart cells and blood vessels.

Ranolazine

Ranolazine is an anti-anginal medication that does not depend on reductions in heart rate or blood pressure. It reduces the frequency of anginal chest pain, but has not been shown to reduce heart attacks.

Common names include:	Possible side effects include:
Ranexa	Lightheadedness
	Headache
	Nausea
	Constipation
	Potential to interact with other medication—This medication should be avoided in people with liver or severe kidney disease.

Angiotensin-converting Enzyme (ACE Inhibitors)

ACE inhibitors work to dilate blood vessels by interfering with the action of angiotensin, a chemical that contracts and narrows blood vessels.

Common names include:	Possible side effects include:
Benazepril	Cough
Captopril	Headache
Enalapril	Lightheadedness
Fosinopril	Increased levels of potassium in the blood
Lisinopril	
Moexipril	
Perindopril	
Quinapril	
Ramipril	

Over-the-Counter Medication

Aspirin

A small, daily dose of aspirin has been shown to decrease the risk of heart attack by preventing blood clots from forming. Ask your doctor before taking aspirin daily. A possible side effect of taking aspirin regularly is bleeding in the stomach and gastrointestinal tract.

Special Considerations

If you are taking medications, follow these general guidelines:
- Take the medication as directed. Do not change the amount or the schedule.

- Ask what side effects could occur. Report them to your doctor.
- Talk to your doctor before you stop taking any prescription medication.
- Do not share your prescription medication.
- Medications can be dangerous when mixed. Talk to your doctor or pharmacist if you are taking more than one medication, including over-the-counter products and supplements.
- Plan ahead for refills as needed.

—*Michael J. Fucci, DO, FACC*

References

"Antiplatelet and Anticoagulant Drugs for Coronary Artery Disease." *DynaMed*, EBSCO Information Services, 26 Jan. 2018, www.dynamed.com/topics/dmp~AN~T114649/Antiplatelet-and-anticoagulant-drugs-for-coronary-artery-disease.

"Coronary Heart Disease." *National Heart, Lung, and Blood Institute*, U.S. Department of Health & Human Services, www.nhlbi.nih.gov/health-topics/coronary-heart-disease.

"Hypertension Medication Selection and Management." *DynaMed*, EBSCO Information Services, 8 Feb. 2018, www.dynamed.com/management/hypertension-medication-selection-and-management.

LaRosa, John C., et al. "Comparison of 80 versus 10 Mg of Atorvastatin on Occurrence of Cardiovascular Events After the First Event (from the Treating to New Targets [TNT] Trial)." *The American Journal of Cardiology*, vol. 105, no. 3, Feb. 2010, pp. 283–287, 10.1016/j.amjcard.2009.09.025.

"Management of Stable Angina." *DynaMed*, EBSCO Information Services, 15 Nov. 2017, www.dynamed.com/management/management-of-stable-angina.

"Statins for Primary and Secondary Prevention of Cardiovascular Disease." *DynaMed*, EBSCO Information Services, 22 Feb. 2018, dynamed.com/prevention/statins-for-primary-and-secondary-prevention-of-cardiovascular-disease.

■ Lifestyle changes to manage Coronary Artery Disease (CAD)

The goal of lifestyle changes is to prevent further build up of plaque and decrease damage to your blood vessels. Some steps may even help reduce the amount of plaque in your blood vessels. These changes will also reduce your risk of heart attack and stroke.

Dietary Changes

If you are not on a special diet to manage other conditions, your doctor may recommend dietary changes.

Diets that are high in saturated fat and cholesterol increase your risk of CAD. Saturated fat and cholesterol are found in animal products, full-fat dairy products, lard, and palm and coconut oils, among other foods. These foods contribute to build up of plaque.

A dietitian can help you reduce saturated fats and cholesterol in your diet and teach you how to make healthier substitutions. Good dietary choices include fresh fruits and vegetables, as well as lean meats and fish—particularly fish rich in omega-3 fatty acids such as salmon.

Decreasing low-density lipoprotein (LDL) cholesterol intake while increasing high-density lipoprotein (HDL) cholesterol intake may improve blood flow to the heart by reducing the amount of plaque in your arteries. Limiting fat and cholesterol in your diet can also help you lose weight.

Exercise Regularly

Note—Do not begin any exercise program without consulting your doctor.

Regular aerobic training can help increase your physical abilities and quality of life. You should aim to exercise for at least 30 minutes per day on most days of the week. Begin slowly and work your way to this goal. Depending on the symptoms and severity of your condition, your doctor may have you do an exercise test before starting a program.

Quit Smoking

Smoking damages your blood vessels and lung tissue, reduces the amount of oxygen in your blood, and forces your heart to beat faster. Talk to your doctor about the best way to quit smoking.

Remember that secondhand smoke is also harmful. Make sure you are not exposed to cigarette smoke if at all possible. Not smoking improves blood flow by relaxing constricted blood vessels.

Reduce or Avoid Excess Weight

Excess weight strains the heart muscle and is associated with increased risk of atherosclerosis. If you are overweight, talk with a dietitian who can help

you with portion control and meal planning. To achieve your goal weight, you should also participate in regular exercise most days of the week.

If you are struggling to lose weight, talk to your doctor about your options and what your ideal weight range may be.

Decrease or Discontinue Alcohol Consumption

Excess alcohol increases triglyceride levels in the blood, which contribute to atherosclerosis and heart arrhythmias. Alcohol also may react with certain medications.

Reduction or elimination of alcohol can help improve symptoms associated with angina. Moderate drinking is considered2 or less drinks a day for men and 1 drink or less a day for women. Small amounts of alcohol in this range may have beneficial effects such as raising your HDL cholesterol.

Manage Chronic Conditions

It is just as important to follow any treatment plans for other chronic conditions you may have. Managing chronic conditions will help with your treatment of CAD.

Control Blood Glucose Levels

People who have diabetes may reduce their risk of heart attack or other cardiac events if they maintain their blood glucose near normal levels. There are many other proven health benefits to maintaining tight control of blood glucose. If you have diabetes, talk to your doctor about ways to keep your blood glucose in a healthy range.

Maintain Normal Blood Pressure

High blood pressure is one of the most critical risk factors CAD. High blood pressure causes the heart muscle to work harder to pump blood through narrowed blood vessels. The increased strain on the heart can also lead to heart failure. Maintaining a healthy blood pressure involves weight management, salt reduction, regular exercise, and stress management. If none of these methods work, talk to your doctor about blood pressure medications and home monitoring.

Take Prescribed Medications

Take any medications your doctor has prescribed, such as statins for high cholesterol. Use medications as recommended by your doctor, or according to the instructions provided. Talk with your doctor if you have questions about usage or side effects.

Communication

Maintain regular communication with your healthcare team, adhere to your treatment plan, and go to any recommended appointments. Your needs may change over time. Regular contact with your healthcare team will help you stay on top of any changes.

Identifying and Managing Depression

People with depression are less likely to adhere to their treatment plans for other chronic conditions. This contributes to an increased risk of complications associated with CAD.

Other Management

- Sexual activity—It is normal for you or your partner to feel concerned about whether it is safe for you to resume sexual activity. In general, people who have CAD that is stable and properly treated can engage in sexual activity. To find out what is safe for you, make an appointment to discuss this issue with your doctor.
- Counseling—Depression is common with many cardiovascular disorders. If you are feeling depressed or are having trouble managing your CAD, ask your doctor about counseling. Counselors can help you navigate challenges of living with a chronic condition. It also may be beneficial to join a support group so you can interact with others who have CAD. They offer an environment of encouragement and support that will help you adjust and adhere to your treatment.
- Cardiac rehabilitation—Provides supervised education and counseling to increase exercise, manage symptoms, and reduce the risk of further heart-related conditions.

Be an active participant in your care. Talk to your team about symptoms or treatments that you are having difficulty with. Other treatments options may be available to help you better manage your CAD.

When to Contact Your Doctor

- Contact your doctor if you notice changes in any of these symptoms:
- Chest pain

- Usual patterns of angina
- Shortness of breath, especially when out of proportion to exercise or exertion
- Fatigue

—Michael J. Fucci, DO, FACC

References

"Coronary Artery Disease (CAD)." *DynaMed*, EBSCO Information Services, 28 Feb. 2018, www.dynamed.com/condition/coronary-artery-disease-cad.

"Coronary Heart Disease." *National Heart, Lung, and Blood Institute*, U.S. Department of Health & Human Services, www.nhlbi.nih.gov/health-topics/coronary-heart-disease.

"Management of Stable Angina." *DynaMed*, EBSCO Information Services, 15 Nov. 2017, www.dynamed.com/management/management-of-stable-angina.

Martí-Carvajal, Arturo J, et al. "Homocysteine-Lowering Interventions for Preventing Cardiovascular Events." *Cochrane Database of Systematic Reviews*, vol. 8, 17 Aug. 2017, 10.1002/14651858.cd006612.pub5.

■ Surgical and other procedures for Coronary Artery Disease (CAD)

Surgery may be needed to treat severe CAD. It may also treat CAD that is causing angina despite treatment.

Surgical Procedures

Coronary Artery Bypass Graft (CABG)

CABG is also known as open heart or bypass surgery. It is the most common type of heart surgery in the US.

A healthy blood vessel is removed from another area of the body. (A vein if it is from the leg, an artery if it is taken from the chest.) The healthy blood vessel is connected to the damaged artery. It is placed just above and just below the blocked area. This allows some blood to pass around the damaged area through the new pathway. If more than one area is blocked, a bypass can be done for each area. Two areas are called a double bypass, three is called triple bypass and so on.

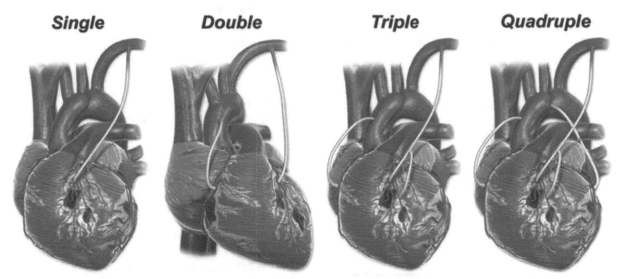

Coronary Artery Bypass Graft (CABG)

Illustration depicting single, double, triple, and quadruple bypass. (BruceBlaus)

Types of CABG include:

- Traditional CABG
  - The heart is stopped for surgery.
  - A heart-lung machine takes over the job of the heart until surgery is done.

- Off-pump CABG
  - No heart-lung machine is needed.
  - The surgeon works on the heart while it is still beating.

- Minimally invasive direct CABG
  - Small incisions are made along the left side of the chest.
  - May not be an option for everyone or widely available.

Talk to your doctor about which option is better for you. Although CABG may relieve symptoms, it does not cure heart disease. You still must maintain a healthy lifestyle. That includes reaching a healthy weight, heart healthy diet, not smoking, and taking medicine

Other Procedures

Other procedures are used to open blocked arteries include:

- Coronary angioplasty—also called a percutaneous coronary intervention (PCI). A tube is inserted into the artery in your groin. It is passed up to blockage in the heart. There a balloon is quickly inflated and deflated. This opens the artery and improves blood flow. The balloon and catheter are then removed.
- Stent—A mesh stent may be placed in the artery during angioplasty. This will help to keep it open. The stent may be coated with a medicine. It will help to prevent blockage from coming back.
- Atherectomy—A tube is passed through blood vessels to the heart. Once the blockage is reached, a tool is used to slice the plaque away.

—*Michael J. Fucci, DO, FACC</item>*

References

"Cardiac Procedures and Surgeries." *American Heart Association*, 31 Mar. 2017, www.heart.org/en/health-topics/heart-attack/treatment-of-a-heart-attack/cardiac-procedures-and-surgeries#.Wp2C22rwbIU.

"Coronary Artery Bypass Graft (CABG) Surgery." *DynaMed*, EBSCO Information Services, 28 Dec. 2017, www.dynamed.com/procedure/coronary-artery-bypass-graft-cabg-surgery.

"Coronary Artery Bypass Grafting." *National Heart, Lung, and Blood Institute*, U.S. Department of Health & Human Services, 18 Nov. 2014, www.nhlbi.nih.gov/health-topics/coronary-artery-bypass-grafting.

"Percutaneous Coronary Intervention (PCI) Procedure." *DynaMed*, EBSCO Information Services, 26 July 2017, www.dynamed.com/procedure/percutaneous-coronary-intervention-pci-procedure.

"Revascularization for Coronary Artery Disease (CAD)." *DynaMed*, EBSCO Information Services, 1 Feb. 2018, www.dynamed.com/management/revascularization-for-coronary-artery-disease-cad.

■ Talking to your doctor about Coronary Artery Disease (CAD)

You have a unique medical history. Therefore, it is essential to talk with your doctor about your personal risk factors and/or experience with CAD. By talking openly and regularly with your doctor, you can take an active role in your care.

General Tips for Gathering Information

Here are some tips that will make it easier for you to talk to your doctor:

- Bring someone else with you. It helps to have another person hear what is said and think of questions to ask.
- Write out your questions ahead of time, so you don't forget them.
- Write down the answers you get, and make sure you understand what you are hearing. Ask for clarification, if necessary.
- Don't be afraid to ask your questions or ask where you can find more information about what you are discussing. You have a right to know.

Specific Questions to Ask Your Doctor

About CAD
- Do I have CAD?
- How much blockage do I have in my arteries?

About Your Risk of Developing CAD
- Based on my medical history, lifestyle, and family background, am I at risk for CAD?
- How can I prevent CAD?

About Treatment Options
- What are all my treatment options?
- Do I have to take medications or will I need surgery?
- If I have surgery, will I be cured?

About Medication
- What kind of medication do I have to take?
- What is the medication supposed to do?
- Will I always have to take medication?
- What are the possible side effects? What should be done if they occur?
- Where can I get more information about the medication?
- If the side effects are bad, can I take something else that works as well?

About Lifestyle Changes
- Are there certain activities or sports that I should avoid? Is it safe to have sex?
- How can I find help to quit smoking?
- Can you refer me to a registered dietitian to help me with my diet?
- What exercises are best and how much do I need?
- Should I need to stop drinking alcohol?
- If I change my lifestyle habits, will I still need to take medication?

About Outlook
- What will happen over the next few weeks, months, and years?
- Will my condition get worse?
- What are the most important things I can do to manage this condition?

—*Michael J. Fucci, DO, FACC*

References

"Getting the Most Out of Your Doctor Appointment." *FamilyDoctor.Org*, American Academy of Family Physicians, 19 Jan. 2018, familydoctor.org/tips-for-talking-to-your-doctor/.

"Heart-to-Heart: Talking to Your Doctor." *American Heart Association*, 26 Oct. 2015, www.heart.org/en/health-topics/consumer-healthcare/doctor-appointments-questions-to-ask-your-doctor/heart-to-heart-talking-to-your-doctor#.Wp2GUmrwbIU.

"Preparing for Medical Visits." *American Heart Association*, 8 Jan. 2018, www.heart.org/en/health-topics/cardiac-rehab/communicating-with-professionals/preparing-for-medical-visits#.Wp2Ga2rwbIU.

"Talking to Your Doctor." *National Institutes of Health*, U.S. Department of Health & Human Services, 8 May 2015, www.nih.gov/institutes-nih/nih-office-director/office-communications-public-liaison/clear-communication/talking-your-doctor.

■ Resource guide for Coronary Artery Disease (CAD)

American Heart Association
7272 Greenville Avenue
Dallas, TX 75231
1-800-AHA-USA-1
http://www.heart.org

On this site, you will find general information about heart disease, including educational information, news, research, health programs, and dietary information.

Centers for Disease Control
1600 Clifton Rd.
Atlanta, GA 30333
1-800-CDC-INFO
http://www.cdc.gov

This site provides educational and statistical information about heart disease, as well as information about several other conditions.

National Heart, Lung, and Blood Institute (NHLBI)
NHLBI Health Information Center
PO Box 30105
Bethesda, MD 20824
(301) 592-8573
http://www.nhlbi.nih.gov

The NHLBI is a part of the National Institutes of Health. The site provides information about cholesterol, heart disease risk factors, and various heart conditions. The institute conducts and supports research related to the causes, prevention, diagnosis, and treatment of heart, blood vessel, lung, and blood diseases as well as sleep disorders.

—*Michael J. Fucci, DO, FACC*

■ Conditions In Depth: Gout

Gout is a form of arthritis caused by a build up of crystals in a joint. It most often affects the joint of the big toe, but can but it can affect other joints as well. Gout may occur in a single attack or become a recurrent problem. During acute attacks, gout can cause pain, swelling, and redness in the affected joint. Periods between acute attacks are usually symptom-free.

Gout can also create a collection of crystals under the skin called tophi. The tophi are visible lumps under the skin that can show up anywhere in the body and become tender during acute attacks.

Over time, gout can cause permanent damage to the affected joints and the kidneys. Fortunately, these long term factors are less likely to occur with proper treatment. The earlier gout is detected and treated, the better it can be managed.

Types of Gout

Asymptomatic hyperuricemia:
- Elevated levels of uric acid in the blood (hyperuricemia), but no other symptoms.
- Present before the first gout attack.

Acute gout (gout attack)
- Chronically increased uric acid levels result in the deposit of uric acid crystals in the joint spaces.
- Symptoms develop quickly, usually overnight and after some stimulus or trigger.
- Will usually resolve within 3 to 14 days, even without treatment.

Interval gout:
- A symptom-free time between attacks.
- Crystals usually present in the joint.
- Low-level inflammation may damage the joints.

Chronic tophaceous gout:
- Occurs in people with gout and uric acid levels that remain high for a long time.
- Attacks become more frequent and the pain may not resolve completely between episodes.
- Joints may become damaged and be persistently stiff and swollen.
- Crystal may build up in the skin (tophi) or around the joints as subcutaneous nodules.
- The kidneys may be damaged.

Causes of Gout

Gout is caused by the build-up of uric acid crystals in and around a joint. Crystals often form because of high levels of uric acid in the blood.

Uric acid is created in the liver and released into the blood during the breakdown of a substance in food called purines. The uric acid is then filtered out of the blood through the kidneys and passes out of the body through urine. Higher than normal levels of uric acid in the blood may be caused by:

Increased production of uric acid from:

- Excess consumption of foods high in purines like steak, seafood, and organ meats
- Certain medications, such as cytotoxic agent (chemotherapy) or vitamin B12

Decreased excretion of uric acid from:

- Impaired ability to clear the uric acid in the kidneys, which may occur with kidney damage or disease
- Consumption of foods such as alcohol or sugary drinks
- Certain medications, such as diuretics, salicylate containing medications (like aspirin), niacin, or levodopa

Medical conditions, such as high blood pressure, obesity, hypothyroidism, Kelley-Seegmiller syndrome or Lesch-Nyhan syndrome

—*Michael Woods, MD, FAAP*

References

Bolster, Marcy. "Gout." *American College of Rheumatology*, Mar. 2019, www.rheumatology.org/I-Am-A/Patient-Caregiver/Diseases-Conditions/Gout.

"Gout." *DynaMed*, EBSCO Information Services, 2 Sept. 2016, www.dynamed.com/condition/gout.

——. *National Institute of Arthritis and Musculoskeletal and Skin Diseases*, National Institutes of Health, 12 Apr. 2017, www.niams.nih.gov/health-topics/gout.

——. *Arthritis Foundation*, arthritis.org/diseases/gout. Accessed 13 Mar. 2020.

■ Risk factors for gout

A risk factor is something that increases your likelihood of getting a disease or condition. It is possible to develop gout with or without the risk factors listed below. However, the more risk factors you have, the greater your likelihood of developing gout. If you have a number of risk factors, ask your doctor what you can do to reduce your risk.

High levels of uric acid in the blood is the main risk factor for gout. Gout is more common in men over 30 years old, and usually doesn't usually affect women until after menopause. The risk for gout is increased if other family members have gout.

Other factors that may increase your chance of gout include:

Lifestyle Factors

Lifestyle factors that increase the risk of gout include:

- Obesity—the extra tissue increases the production of uric acid, which affects blood levels
- Eating a diet high in foods with purines, such as seafood, shellfish, or red meat
- Excess intake of alcohol
- Drinking high-fructose beverages, such as sugar-sweetened sodas and orange juice

Medical Conditions

Serious illness, such as a heart attack or stroke , can trigger a gout attack. Other illnesses that may increase the risk for developing gout include:

- High blood pressure
- Vascular diseases that affect blood vessels

- Diabetes
- Hyperlipidemia
- Kidney disease
- Thyroid disorders
- Organ transplantation

Medical Treatments

Medications and vitamins that may increase the risk of gout include:

- Diuretics—often used to treat high blood pressure
- Salicylates and medications made from salicylic acid, such as aspirin
- Levodopa—used in the treatment of Parkinson's disease
- Cyclosporine—used to help control rejection of transplanted organs
- Niacin

—*Michael Woods, MD, FAAP*

References

Bolster, Marcy. "Gout." *American College of Rheumatology*, Mar. 2019, www.rheumatology.org/I-Am-A/Patient-Caregiver/Diseases-Conditions/Gout.

"Gout." *DynaMed*, EBSCO Information Services, 2 Sept. 2016, www.dynamed.com/condition/gout.

——. *National Institute of Arthritis and Musculoskeletal and Skin Diseases*, National Institutes of Health, 12 Apr. 2017, www.niams.nih.gov/health-topics/gout.

——. *Arthritis Foundation*, arthritis.org/diseases/gout. Accessed 13 Mar. 2020.

■ Reducing your risk of gout

There are no specific guidelines to help prevent gout, but there are ways to reduce the risk of acute attacks and maintain joint health. Managing certain risk factors may help. Steps include:

- Maintain a healthy weight—Obesity is linked to increased uric acid levels. Eat more vegetables, low- or non-fat dairy, and mono- and polyunsaturated fats.

- Exercise regularly—Moderate exercise helps with weight control and overall well-being. Talk to your doctor about which exercises will benefit you the most. Avoid intense exercises that strain muscles and joints.
- Drink alcohol in moderation—Excess alcohol consumption is associated with gout. Moderate alcohol intake means 2 drinks or less per day for men, and 1 drink or less per day for women. Choosing not to drink alcohol is also acceptable.
- Avoid foods that contain high amounts of purines. These include red meats, seafood, and foods high in salt or fructose.

Talk to your doctor about adding bing sweet cherries and/or vitamin C supplements to your diet. These may help reduce uric acid levels. Keep in mind that supplements and herbal medications may interact with medications you currently take. Talk to your doctor or pharmacist about medications and supplements you may be taking to learn about possible problems.

—*Michael Woods, MD, FAAP*

References

Bolster, Marcy. "Gout." *American College of Rheumatology*, Mar. 2019, www.rheumatology.org/I-Am-A/Patient-Caregiver/Diseases-Conditions/Gout.

"Gout." *DynaMed*, EBSCO Information Services, 2 Sept. 2016, www.dynamed.com/condition/gout.

——. *National Institute of Arthritis and Musculoskeletal and Skin Diseases*, National Institutes of Health, 12 Apr. 2017, www.niams.nih.gov/health-topics/gout.

——. *Arthritis Foundation*, arthritis.org/diseases/gout. Accessed 13 Mar. 2020.

"Gout Management - Prevention of Recurrent Attacks." *DynaMed*, EBSCO Information Services, 4 Nov. 2016, www.dynamed.com/management/gout-management-prevention-of-recurrent-attacks.

"What Are Purines and How Are They Related to Food and Health?" *World's Healthiest Foods*, The George Mateljan Foundation, www.whfoods.org/genpage.php?tname=george&dbid=51.

■ Symptoms of Gout

Gout attack symptoms often develop rapidly over-night and worsen over the next 24-48 hours. They can happen one time, several times, or chronically. They can be triggered by many things including:

- Joint injury or other trauma
- Surgery or sudden, severe illness
- Psoriasis flares
- Infection
- Certain medications, such as chemotherapy, diuretics, or intravenous contrast media
- Crash diets and fasting
- Drinking too much alcohol
- Eating large portions of certain foods high in purines
- Dehydration (not getting enough fluids)
- Fructose sweetened drinks

A single gout attack usually only affects only one joint, but recurrent attacks may affect more than one joint. The big toe is the most common site of gout. Other sites include the ankle, heel, foot instep, wrist, elbow, or fingers.

Common symptoms in the joint include:

- Severe pain and sensitivity of the joint
- Extreme tenderness
- Swelling<
- Redness
- Warmth
- Fever and flu-like symptoms may also be present.

Recurrent attacks can lead to permanent joint damage, especially if gout remains untreated. Uric acids can build up and create deposits called tophi. They can lead to:

- Hard lumps under the skin near or around joints
- Hard lumps at the rim of the ear, fingertips, cornea of eye, aorta, spine, or around the brain
- High levels of uric acid in the body can also lead to complications in other areas of the body, such as the kidney stones or chronic renal failure.

—Michael Woods, MD, FAAP

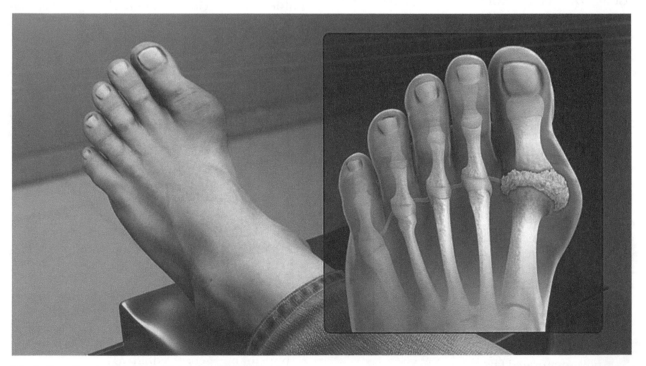

Illustration of gout affected foot. (Scientific Animations)

References

Bolster, Marcy. "Gout." *American College of Rheumatology*, Mar. 2019, www.rheumatology.org/I-Am-A/Patient-Caregiver/Diseases-Conditions/Gout.

"Gout." *DynaMed*, EBSCO Information Services, 2 Sept. 2016, www.dynamed.com/condition/gout.

——. *National Institute of Arthritis and Musculoskeletal and Skin Diseases*, National Institutes of Health, 12 Apr. 2017, www.niams.nih.gov/health-topics/gout.

——. *Arthritis Foundation*, arthritis.org/diseases/gout. Accessed 13 Mar. 2020.

■ Medications for Gout

The information provided here is meant to give you a general idea about each of the medications listed below. Only the most general side effects are included. Ask your doctor if you need to take any special precautions. Use each of these medications only as recommended by your doctor, and according to the instructions provided. If you have further questions about usage or side effects, contact your doctor. Medications can be used to treat the symptoms of acute attacks and help prevent future recurrent attacks.

In general medications for acute treatment will reduce inflammation and pain. Medications include colchicine, corticosteroids, and nonsteroidal anti-inflammatory drugs. Allopurinol may also be used during a severe acute episode to reduce uric acid production.

Some medications for prevention may treat chronic inflammation, but most of them are given to reduce uric acid. They will be considered if you have 2 or more attacks per year, skin lesions (tophi or subcutaneous nodules), a uric acid kidney stone,

or reduced kidney function. Medications include colchicine, nonsteroidal anti-inflammatory drugs, xanthine oxidase inhibitors, uricosuric medications, and pegloticase.

The choice and duration of medication will depend on many things, including your age, severity of disease and the number of joints affected, previous responses to treatment, overall health, and ability to tolerate the medication. Medications for acute attacks work best if taken within 24 hours of symptom onset. They may only be needed for a short time. Preventive medications will have to be taken on a regular basis.

Prescription Medications

Colchicine
Colchicine is given during a gout attack to relieve the pain, swelling, and inflammation. It works by decreasing the acidity of joint tissue and preventing deposits of uric acid crystals in joints. This medication may also be taken in smaller doses to help prevent recurrent gout attacks when people are started on urate-lowering medications. Consult your doctor before taking colchicine if you have liver or kidney disease.

Possible side effects include:
Diarrhea
Nausea
Vomiting
Abdominal pain
Muscle pain

Corticosteroids
Corticosteroids can control the pain, swelling, and inflammation of joints caused by gout. The medication can be given as a tablet or in liquid

Common names include:	*Possible side effects include:*	*Long term use may cause:*
Prednisone Prednisolone	Indigestion, nausea, or vomiting	Glaucoma Cataracts
Betametasone (for joint injection) Triamcinalone (for joint injection)	Thrush Diarrhea	Diabetes Thinning of the skin
Methylprednisolone (given IV, usually for severe cases)	Headache Psychiatric disturbances Weight gain	Weak, fragile bones High blood pressure

form or by injection into a joint—or in severe cases, as an IV. If taken orally, corticosteroids are best taken at the same time(s) each day and should be taken with liquid or food to lessen stomach upset.

Xanthine Oxidase Inhibitors

Xanthine oxidase inhibitors are sometimes given to people who suffer repeated gout attacks. This medication slows the development of uric acid by inhibiting the activity of certain enzymes. It's given in tablet form and should be taken at the same time(s) each day. Allopurinol should be taken with food or liquid to help avoid stomach upset. Febuxostat may be given if you cannot tolerate allopurinol or have kidney disease.

Common names include:	Possible side effects include:
Allopurinol	Rash
Febuxostat	Nausea
	Liver problems
	Joint pain (febuxostat)

Uricosuric Medications

These medications are sometimes given to those who suffer repeated gout attacks (especially when tophi deposits develop). This medication forces the kidneys to excrete additional uric acid. It's given in tablet form and should be taken at the same time each day with food or liquid to help avoid stomach upset. People with uric acid kidney stones or with certain blood disorders should not take these medications.

Common names include:	Possible side effects include:
Probenecid	Headache
Sulfinpyrazone	Appetite loss
Benzbromarone	Nausea
	Vomiting
	Kidney stones
	Lightheadedness (sulfinpyrazone)
	Severe rash from allergic reaction

	Ringing or buzzing in the ear—tinnitus (sulfinpyrazone)
	Flare-up of peptic ulcer (sulfinpyrazone)

Pegloticase

Pegloticase has been approved by the US Food and Drug Administration (FDA) to treat adults who have severe gout that has not been relieved by other treatments. This medication is an enzyme that works by turning uric acid into a chemical that does not cause gout symptoms. This chemical leaves the body through the urine. Pegloticase is given by injection every 2 weeks. Since severe allergic reactions are common with this medication, a corticosteroid and an antihistamine are given before the injection of pegloticase.

Other possible side effects include:
Flare-up of gout
Nausea and vomiting
Constipation
Bruise at the injection site
Nasal irritation
Chest pain
Runny nose

Prescription and Over-the-Counter Medications

Nonsteroidal Anti-inflammatory Drugs (NSAIDs)

Some can be purchased over the counter or your doctor may prescribe a higher dosage. They work by decreasing prostaglandins, hormones that produce inflammation and pain. The medication may also be taken in smaller doses to help prevent attacks in those with recurrent gout attacks who are started on urate-lowering medications. NSAIDs are given by mouth. They should be taken at the same time (or times) each day and should be taken with food or liquid to help avoid stomach upset. NSAIDs are given to treat the pain, inflammation, and swelling caused by gout attacks.

Common names include:	Possible side effects include:
Ibuprofen—OTC or prescription Indomethacin—prescription only	Stomach problems, such as stomach upset, ulcers, and bleeding
Naproxen—OTC or prescription Diclofenac—prescription only	Worsening of chronic conditions, such as high blood pressure, heart failure, or kidney disease
	Kidney damage
	Severe allergic reaction, such as hives, difficulty breathing, or swelling around the eyes
	Increased risk of bleeding—always inform your doctor that you are taking an NSAID before having any medical or dental procedures or surgeries

NSAIDs may cause an increased risk of serious cardiovascular problems, like heart attack and stroke. This risk is especially important for those with cardiovascular disease or who are have risk factors for cardiovascular disease.

Special Considerations

If you are taking medications, follow these general guidelines:

- Take the medication as directed. Do not change the amount or the schedule.
- Ask what side effects could occur. Report them to your doctor.
- Talk to your doctor before you stop taking any prescription medication.
- Do not share your prescription medication.
- Medications can be dangerous when mixed. Talk to your doctor or pharmacist if you are taking more than one medication, including over-the-counter products and supplements.
- Plan ahead for refills as needed.

—*Michael Woods, MD, FAAP*

References

"Allopurinol." *DynaMed*, EBSCO Information Services, 6 Feb. 2017, www.dynamed.com/drug-monograph/allopurinol.

Bolster, Marcy. "Gout." *American College of Rheumatology*, Mar. 2019, www.rheumatology.org/I-Am-A/Patient-Caregiver/Diseases-Conditions/Gout.

"Colchicine." *DynaMed*, EBSCO Information Services, 6 Feb. 2017, www.dynamed.com/drug-monograph/colchicine.

"Febuxostat." *DynaMed*, EBSCO Information Services, 27 Sept. 2016, www.dynamed.com/drug-monograph/febuxostat.

"Gout." *DynaMed*, EBSCO Information Services, 2 Sept. 2016, www.dynamed.com/condition/gout.

——. *Arthritis Foundation*, arthritis.org/diseases/gout. Accessed 13 Mar. 2020.

"Gout Management - Prevention of Recurrent Attacks." *DynaMed*, EBSCO Information Services, 4 Nov. 2016, www.dynamed.com/management/gout-management-prevention-of-recurrent-attacks.

"Gout Management - Treatment of Acute Attack." *DynaMed*, EBSCO Information Services, 13 Oct. 2014, www.dynamed.com/management/gout-management-treatment-of-acute-attack.

"Pegloticase." *DynaMed*, EBSCO Information Services, 6 Feb. 2017, www.dynamed.com/drug-monograph/pegloticase.

"Probenecid." *DynaMed*, EBSCO Information Services, 6 Feb. 2017, www.dynamed.com/drug-monograph/probenecid.

■ Lifestyle changes to manage gout

Lifestyle changes cannot cure gout, but they can help control uric acid levels in the blood, which lead to gout attacks. Lifestyle recommendations include:

Avoid Certain Foods and Beverages

Uric acid is created by the breakdown of purines found in certain foods. Avoid or limit foods and beverages that are high in purines such as:

- Organ meats, such as liver, kidney, and sweetbreads
- Seafood and shellfish, such as lobster, crab, or sardines
- Red meat, such as beef or lamb
- Some vegetables, such as asparagus, cauliflower, and mushrooms
- Salty foods, sauces, and gravies

Blood uric acid levels can also be influenced by some foods and beverages that aren't high in purines such as:

- Alcoholic beverages, especially beer, during an acute attack—people with recurrent gout should always avoid alcohol
- High-fructose drinks, which include sugar-sweetened soda and sweetened juice

Diet

A well-rounded, healthful diet is important for overall well-being and maintaining a healthy weight. Be sure to get adequate amounts of calories, protein, and calcium. In general, eat less saturated and more mono- and polyunsaturated fats. Increase intake of fruits, vegetables, and whole grains. Excess weight can put extra stress on your joints. If you are overweight, talk to your doctor or a dietitian about dietary options.

It's important to drink plenty of fluids throughout the day. Fluids help flush uric acid from the body and help prevent recurrent gout attacks.

Talk to your doctor about adding bing sweetcherries and/or vitamin C supplements to your diet. These may help reduce uric acid levels and gout symptoms.

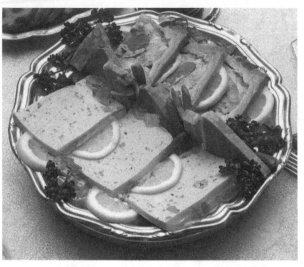

A variety of pâtés (containing liver) on a platter. Organ meats like liver are high in purines and can cause gout. (David Monniaux)

Be an active participant in your care. Talk to your healthcare team about symptoms or treatments that you are having difficulty with. Other treatments options may be available to help you better manage your health.

—*Michael Woods, MD, FAAP*

References

Bolster, Marcy. "Gout." *American College of Rheumatology*, Mar. 2019, www.rheumatology.org/I-Am-A/Patient-Caregiver/Diseases-Conditions/Gout.

"Gout." *DynaMed*, EBSCO Information Services, 2 Sept. 2016, www.dynamed.com/condition/gout.

——. *National Institute of Arthritis and Musculoskeletal and Skin Diseases*, National Institutes of Health, 12 Apr. 2017, www.niams.nih.gov/health-topics/gout.

——. *Arthritis Foundation*, arthritis.org/diseases/gout. Accessed 13 Mar. 2020.

"Gout Management - Prevention of Recurrent Attacks." *DynaMed*, EBSCO Information Services, 4 Nov. 2016, www.dynamed.com/management/gout-management-prevention-of-recurrent-attacks.

"Gout Management - Treatment of Acute Attack." *DynaMed*, EBSCO Information Services, 13 Oct. 2014, www.dynamed.com/management/gout-management-treatment-of-acute-attack.

"What Are Purines and How Are They Related to Food and Health?" *World's Healthiest Foods*, The George Mateljan Foundation, www.whfoods.org/genpage.php?tname=george&dbid=51.

■ Talking to your doctor about gout

You have a unique medical history. Therefore, it is essential to talk with your doctor about your personal risk factors and/or experience with gout. By talking openly and regularly with your doctor, you can take an active role in your care.

General Tips for Gathering Information

Here are some tips that will make it easier for you to talk to your doctor:

- Bring someone else with you. It helps to have another person hear what is said and think of questions to ask.
- Write out your questions ahead of time, so you don't forget them.
- Write down the answers you get, and make sure you understand what you are hearing. Ask for clarification, if necessary.
- Don't be afraid to ask your questions or ask where you can find more information about what you are discussing. You have a right to know.

Specific Questions to Ask Your Doctor

About Gout

- Do my symptoms suggest that I have gout?
- Could these symptoms be caused by any other joint diseases?
- What kinds of tests will I need to have a firm diagnosis?
- I've had one gout attack:
  ◦ What are the chances of my having another?
  ◦ What can I do to avoid having another?

About Treatment Options

- When can I expect to feel improvement from the treatment?
- Will I have to take medications to control my gout for the rest of my life?
- What side effects can occur from taking medications for gout?
- Will these medications interfere with any other medications, supplements, or over the counter drugs I am already taking?
- Are there any complementary or alternative therapies I should consider?

About Lifestyle Changes

- What lifestyle changes will help control my gout?
- How does my diet affect my gout?
- Do I have to avoid all foods containing purines?
- If my gout is under control, can I drink alcohol at all?

About Outlook

- What possible long-term complications may occur from gout?
- If I keep my gout under good control, what are the chances that I can avoid long-term complications from the disorder?
- Do I have to keep taking medications if lifestyle changes work for me?

—Michael Woods, MD, FAAP

References

Bolster, Marcy. "Gout." *American College of Rheumatology*, Mar. 2019, www.rheumatology.org/I-Am-A/Patient-Caregiver/Diseases-Conditions/Gout.

"Getting the Most Out of Your Doctor Appointment." *FamilyDoctor.Org*, American Academy of Family Physicians, 19 Jan. 2018, familydoctor.org/tips-for-talking-to-your-doctor/.

"Gout." *DynaMed*, EBSCO Information Services, 2 Sept. 2016, www.dynamed.com/condition/gout.

——. *National Institute of Arthritis and Musculoskeletal and Skin Diseases*, National Institutes of Health, 12 Apr. 2017, www.niams.nih.gov/health-topics/gout.

——. *Arthritis Foundation*, arthritis.org/diseases/gout. Accessed 13 Mar. 2020.

■ Resource guide for Gout

Arthritis Foundation

1355 Peachtree Street NE, Suite 600
Atlanta, GA 30309
800-283-7800
https://www.arthritis.org

The Arthritis Foundation provides information and resources about gout, a type of inflammatory arthritis. Their goal is to chart a winning course and make each day another stride towards a cure.

Foot Health Facts—American College of Foot and Ankle Surgeons
8725 West Higgins Road, Suite 555
Chicago, IL 60631
800-421-2237
https://www.foothealthfacts.org

Gout most often affects the joint of the big toe. The Foot Health Facts website contains information about the cause of gout and how to treat it. It is the official consumer website of the American College of Foot and Ankle Surgeons.

—*Michael Woods, MD, FAAP*

■ Conditions In Depth: Heart Attack

A heart attack is caused by a sudden loss of blood flow to the heart muscle. The loss of blood will make it hard or impossible for the heart to pump blood out to the body. Heart tissue can also die if blood flow is stopped long enough. This leads to permanent damage. Heart attacks can range from minor to severe and fatal. The outcome is based on how much heart tissue was affected and what care was given. Immediate medical care can make a drastic difference in the outcome of most heart attacks.

Causes of Heart Attack
All cells in the body need oxygen. Working muscles like the heart need a regular supply of oxygen. Blood vessels called coronary arteries carry oxygen to heart muscle. A blockage in these arteries causes immediate problems. Heart cells will die within a few minutes when they do not get the oxygen they need. A blockage in a large artery will affect a larger area of the heart. This will lead to a more severe heart attack. A blockage in a smaller blood vessel will affect a smaller area. It will cause a minor heart attack. The amount of damage will also depend on the degree of blockage. The artery may be completely blocked, others may only be

blocked when the blood vessel squeezes down. Blood flow through the coronary arteries can be slowed or blocked by:

Atherosclerosis and Coronary Artery Disease
Atherosclerosis is the buildup of plaque in the arteries. It builds up over many years. Items in your blood, such as fat and cholesterol, stick to blood vessel walls and slowly build up a hardened plaque. This causes tears in the wall of the artery. Blood clots help the wall heal but also adds to the bulk of the plaque. The plaque narrows the artery as it grows. This makes it easier for new blood clots or plaque build up to completely block the artery and stop blood flow.

Coronary artery disease (CAD) is reduced blood flow to the heart because of plaque buildup. It is the leading killer of men and women in the US. A heart attack can be the first sign of CAD.

Coronary Artery Spasm
The muscular walls of blood vessels tighten or loosen to help blood flow. It is controlled by the nervous system to help manage blood flow and blood pressure. Illnesses, injuries, or medicine and supplements can cause these muscles to spasm and tighten. It will slow the flow of blood to the heart. In a blood vessel with plaque buildup this could easily lead to a complete blockage of blood flow.

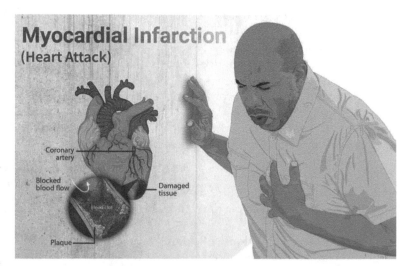

Depiction of a person suffering from a heart attack (Myocardial Infarction). Blood clot in the artery leading to the artery, along with chest pain - the primary symptom - has been shown. (MyUpchar)

Blood Clot

Blood clots collect around an injury site or where blood has pooled. Blood clots that form in blood vessels can break off and travel in the blood stream. It can travel through the body until it becomes stuck in smaller blood vessels. There it will block blood flow until the body can clear the clot. A heart attack happens when the clot sticks in one of the coronary arteries.

—Michael J. Fucci, DO, FACC

References

"About Heart Attacks." *American Heart Association*, 31 July 2016, www.heart.org/en/health-topics/heart-attack/about-heart-attacks.

"Acute Coronary Syndromes." *DynaMed*, EBSCO Information Services, 15 Mar. 2019, www.dynamed.com/condition/acute-coronary-syndromes.

"ST-Elevation Myocardial Infarction (STEMI)." *DynaMed*, EBSCO Information Services, 10 July 2018, www.dynamed.com/condition/st-elevation-myocardial-infarction-stemi.

Sweis, Ranya N. "Acute Myocardial Infarction (MI)." *Merck Manuals Professional Edition*, Merck Manuals, 2018, www.merckmanuals.com/professional/cardiovascular-disorders/coronary-artery-disease/acute-myocardial-infarction-mi.

■ Risk factors for Heart Attack

A risk factor is something that raises your chances of getting a health problem. You can have a heart attack with or without the factors listed below. The more risks you have, the greater your chances of having a heart attack. Ask your doctor what you can to do lower your risk.

Factors That Can Be Changed

Smoking

Smoking harms blood vessels. It causes plaque buildup and narrowing which makes the heart work harder. Heart attack risk for smokers is 2 times higher than those who do not smoke. They are also more likely to die from a heart attack. Smokers who have a heart attack and do not quit have a much higher risk of having more heart attacks and sudden cardiac arrest.

Lack of Exercise

Exercise keeps the heart and blood vessels healthy. Not getting enough makes the risk of a heart attack or stroke up to 2 times higher. Talk to your doctor before starting a program. Even small amounts of exercise have can make a big difference in risk.

Alcohol Use

Drinking too much alcohol raises blood pressure and triglycerides. Triglycerides are a type of fat in the blood linked to plaque buildup. Alcohol is also linked to abnormal heart rhythms. Drink in moderation. This is 1 drink or less a day for women and 2 drinks or less a day for men.

Certain Medicines

Nonsteroidal anti-inflammatory drugs (NSAIDs) ease pain, swelling, or fever. Risk of a heart attack is higher within the first week of regular NSAID use. Talk to your doctor about other medicine you can take.

Illegal drugs

Drugs, such as cocaine, damage the heart. This can lead to heart attacks or sudden cardiac arrest.

Testosterone

Men aged 65 years and older who are taking testosterone are more likely to have a heart attack. It is used to treat health problems like erectile dysfunction.

Health Conditions

High Blood Pressure

High blood pressure makes the heart work harder. Over time, it can lead to damaged blood vessels, which increases the risk of heart disease. People who have high blood pressure and do not keep it in a healthy range have a higher risk of having a heart attack.

High Cholesterol

Cholesterol carries out certain jobs in the body. The body makes and uses what it needs. But, cholesterol from food can make levels too high. This can lead to plaque buildup in the arteries.

Excess Weight

Obesity or excess weight is linked to heart attacks and heart disease. Excess weight makes the heart work harder. Losing a small amount of weight can make a big difference in lowering heart attack risk.

Diabetes

With diabetes, the body does not make or use insulin the way it should. in the blood lead a higher risk of a heart attack and early death. Glucose levels should be kept in a healthy range to lower the risk.

Metabolic Syndrome

Metabolic syndrome is marked by higher than normal blood pressure, cholesterol, glucose, and body weight, mainly around the middle part of the body. These, either alone or together, increase heart attack risk.

Obstructive Sleep Apnea (OSA)

OSA is a pattern of disrupted sleep. The airway is blocked many times a night during sleep. This raises blood pressure and lowers the amount of oxygen in the blood. OSA is linked to heart disease and early death.

Factors That Cannot Be Changed

Age

Aging changes how the heart works. Most times, it does not cause problems. Some changes are a larger heart, slower heart rate, and stiffer blood vessels and valves.

Gender

Men have a higher risk of heart disease overall. A women's risk increases after menopause, which may be related to a drop in the amount of estrogen. As a result, heart attacks are more likely in men over the age of 45 and in women over the age of 55.

Genetics and Background

Family members who have heart attacks increase your risk as well. In general, Blacks have a higher rate of high blood pressure than Whites: This causes a higher risk of getting heart disease and having a heart attack. Heart disease risk is also higher among Mexican Americans, Native Americans, native Hawaiians, and some Asian Americans.

—*Michael J. Fucci, DO, FACC*

References

"Alcohol and Heart Health." *American Heart Association*, 12 Jan. 2015, www.heart.org/HEARTORG/HealthyLiving/HealthyEating/Nutrition/Alcohol-and-Heart-Disease_UCM_305173_Article.jsp#.XJuGkFVKgzx.

Bally, Michèle, et al. "Risk of Acute Myocardial Infarction with NSAIDs in Real World Use: Bayesian Meta-Analysis of Individual Patient Data." *BMJ*, 9 May 2017, p. j1909, doi: 10.1136/bmj.j1909.

"Cardiovascular Disease Major Risk Factors." *DynaMed*, EBSCO Information Services, 20 Aug. 2018, www.dynamed.com/condition/cardiovascular-disease-major-risk-factors.

"Cardiovascular Disease Possible Risk Factors." *DynaMed*, EBSCO Information Services, 28 Nov. 2018, www.dynamed.com/prevention/cardiovascular-disease-possible-risk-factors.

"Illegal Drugs and Heart Disease." *American Heart Association*, 3 May 2018, www.heart.org/HEARTORG/Conditions/More/MyHeartandStrokeNews/Cocaine-Marijuana-and-Other-Drugs-and-Heart-Disease_UCM_428537_Article.jsp#.XJuGvVVKgzx.

"Secondhand Smoke (SHS) Facts." *Centers for Disease Control and Prevention*, 17 Jan. 2018, www.cdc.gov/tobacco/data_statistics/fact_sheets/secondhand_smoke/general_facts/index.htm.

"Understand Your Risks to Prevent a Heart Attack." *American Heart Association*, 30 June 2016, www.heart.org/en/health-topics/heart-attack/understand-your-risks-to-prevent-a-heart-attack.

■ Reducing your risk of Heart Attack

A risk factor is something that raises your chances of getting a health problem. Some of these, such as family history or age, cannot be changed. Luckily, many can be. These will help lower the risk of a heart attack:

Eat a Heart-Healthy Diet

Aim for a diet with plenty of whole grains, fruits and vegetables, and nuts. Learn how to swap foods that are bad for you for ones that are healthy. Start with snacks, then move onto meals. Focus on lean proteins such as fish or chicken. Aim for fish 2 times a week. It has omega-3 fatty acids, which are good for your heart.

If you are overweight or obese, your doctor can help you lose weight safely. Plan to lose weight slowly so you can learn to keep your weight in the right range. A dietitian can teach you about portion sizing and meal planning.

Quit Smoking
Smoking is linked to a buildup of plaque in the arteries. Narrowed blood vessels make it harder for oxygen to get to the heart muscle, which can result in a heart attack.

Quitting smoking is the best way to put yourself on the right track. There are many programs that can help you quit. Try to stay away from other people's smoke as much as you can.

Drink Alcohol in Moderation
Moderation is 2 drinks or less a day for men and 1 drink or less a day for women. Drinking too much alcohol is linked to abnormal heart rhythms and other heart problems. Abnormal heart rhythms increase the risk of a heart attack.

Exercise Regularly
Regular aerobic exercise, such as brisk walking, or using a stationary bike or treadmill, lowers the risk of a heart attack. It also helps with overall heart health. Exercise makes the heart stronger, eases the heart's workload, and lowers blood pressure. Aim for at least 150 minutes a week. Try to get more if you have a job where you spend most of the day sitting. Talk to your doctor before starting any exercise program.

Daily Aspirin
Some people may can take an aspirin a day to lower the risk of a heart attack. This may not work for all people and it does carry risk. Talk to your doctor before taking daily aspirin.

Control Other Health Conditions
Certain health problems, are linked with a higher risk of heart disease or heart attack. While not all risk can be eliminated, controlling these problems greatly lower the risk of heart problems.

High Blood Pressure
Keep with your treatment plan for high blood pressure. Learn how to track your blood pressure at home. Changing how you eat, adding regular exercise, and using medicine can help you control your blood pressure. The DASH diet is designed to lower blood pressure.

Diabetes
Diabetes damages small blood vessels and causes plaque buildup in their walls. Controlling glucose can delay heart problems that can lead to a heart attack. If you have diabetes, work with your care team to keep glucose levels in a healthy range.

Obstructive Sleep Apnea (OSA)
OSA is marked by repeated airway blockage during sleep. OSA lowers the amount of oxygen in the blood and is linked to high blood pressure, heart failure, diabetes, stroke, and heart attack. OSA can be treated by using continuous positive airway pressure (CPAP) machine or having surgery.

—*Michael J. Fucci, DO, FACC*</item>

References
"Cardiovascular Disease Prevention Overview." *DynaMed*, EBSCO Information Services, 22 Feb. 2018, www.dynamed.com/prevention/cardiovascular-disease-prevention-overview.

Ekelund, Ulf, et al. "Does Physical Activity Attenuate, or Even Eliminate, the Detrimental Association of Sitting Time with Mortality? A Harmonised Meta-Analysis of Data from More than 1 Million Men and Women." *The Lancet*, vol. 388, no. 10051, Sept. 2016, pp. 1302–1310, 10.1016/s0140-6736(16)30370-1.

"Fish and Omega-3 Fatty Acids." *American Heart Association*, 23 Mar. 2017, www.heart.org/en/healthy-living/healthy-eating/eat-smart/fats/fish-and-omega-3-fatty-acids.

"Hypertension Alternative Treatments." *DynaMed*, EBSCO Information Services, 17 Nov. 2017, www.dynamed.com/management/hypertension-alternative-treatments.

"ST-Elevation Myocardial Infarction (STEMI)." *DynaMed*, EBSCO Information Services, 10 July 2018, www.dynamed.com/condition/st-elevation-myocardial-infarction-stemi.

■ Symptoms of a Heart Attack

Chest pain is often thought of as the main sign of a heart attack. It can feel like squeezing or pressure in the middle of the chest. It may last a while, or go away and come back. But, not all people having a heart attack feel the same pain. Women, older people, or people with certain health problems may not feel pain or have classic symptoms.

Other common symptoms include:

- Discomfort or pain in the arms, back, jaw, neck, or stomach
- Trouble catching your breath with or without chest pain
- Cold sweat
- Nausea or vomiting
- Lightheadedness
- Anxiety
- Feelings of doom or death

Women may have other symptoms that are not as clear or obvious. They may or may not be with those listed above. These are:

- Feeling very tired—can happen days or weeks ahead of other symptoms
- Pressure or pain in the lower chest, upper belly, or upper back
- Lightheadedness—may lead to fainting

Heart attacks can cause lasting heart damage or death. Do not drive yourself or someone to the hospital. Call emergency medical services so treatment can be started on the way to the hospital. Doing so will lower the amount of heart damage and increase the chances of survival.

—*Michael J. Fucci, DO, FACC*

References

"Acute Coronary Syndromes." *DynaMed*, EBSCO Information Services, 15 Mar. 2019, www.dynamed.com/condition/acute-coronary-syndromes.

"Heart Attack Symptoms in Women." *American Heart Association*, 31 July 2015, www.heart.org/en/health-topics/heart-attack/warning-signs-of-a-heart-attack/heart-attack-symptoms-in-women.

"ST-Elevation Myocardial Infarction (STEMI)." *DynaMed*, EBSCO Information Services, 10 July 2018, www.dynamed.com/condition/st-elevation-myocardial-infarction-stemi.

Sweis, Ranya N. "Acute Myocardial Infarction (MI)." *Merck Manuals Professional Edition*, Merck Manuals, 2018, www.merckmanuals.com/professional/cardiovascular-disorders/coronary-artery-disease/acute-myocardial-infarction-mi.

"Warning Signs of a Heart Attack." *American Heart Association*, 30 June 2016, www.heart.org/en/health-topics/heart-attack/warning-signs-of-a-heart-attack.

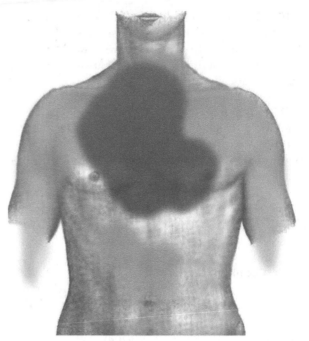

Areas where pain is experienced in myocardial infarction, showing common (darker) and less common (lighter) areas on the chest. (J. Heuser)

■ Medications for Heart Attack

Here are the basics about each of the medicines below. Only the most common reactions are listed. Ask your doctor if you need to take any special steps. Use each of these drugs as advised by your doctor or the booklet they came with. If you have any questions, call your doctor.

Treatment with medicine starts on the way to the hospital and continues after you get home. They are used to open blood vessels and prevent blood clots, and treat high blood pressure or cholesterol. The medicines used will change over time depending on your needs.

Prescription Medicine

Opioids

Opioids are used to ease pain and anxicty.

Common names include:	Possible side effects include:
Morphine	Constipation
Dilaudid	Nausea and vomiting
Fentanyl	Itching
	Lightheadedness
	Sedation

Nitrates

Nitrates ease chest pain by widening the arteries. This lets more blood to flow to the heart muscle. There are many ways to take nitrates.

Common names include:	Possible side effects include:
Nitroglycerin	Low blood pressure
	Headache

Thrombolytic Agents

These will break up blood clots in the arteries of the heart to improve blood flow.

Common names include:	Possible side effects include:
Tissue plasminogen activator (tPA)	Stroke
Streptokinase	Hemorrhage
Reteplase	
Tenecteplase	
Lanoteplase	

Antiarrhythmic Drugs

These drugs help regulate heart rhythm so the blood can get to the heart muscle.

Sodium Channel Blockers

Common names include:
Procainamide
Quinidine
Disopyramide
Lidocaine
Flecainide
Tocainide
Amiodarone
Mexiletine
Propafenone
Moricizine

Beta-blockers

Beta-blockers ease the heart's workload and lowers blood pressure. They can also be used to regulate heart rhythm.

Common names include:	Possible side effects include:
Acebutolol	Low blood pressure
Atenolol	Slow heart rate
Betaxolol	Fatigue
Metoprolol	Problems having sex
Nadolol	
Pindolol	
Propranolol	
Timolol	
Carvedilol	
Nebivolol	

Action Potential-Prolonging Agents

Common names include:
Bretylium
Sotalol
Dofetilide

Calcium Channel Blockers

These lower blood pressure and slow the heart rate. They can also be used to regulate heart rhythm.

Common names include:	Possible side effects include:
Amlodipine	Low blood pressure
Felodipine	Lightheadedness
Isradipine	Constipation
Nicardipine	
Nifedipine	
Verapamil	
Diltiazem	

ACE Inhibitors

ACE inhibitors lower blood pressure. They can also extend life in those with severe heart damage.

Common names include:	Possible side effects include:
Enalapril	Lasting dry, unproductive cough
Lisinopril	Low blood pressure
Quinapril	Headache
	Lightheadedness
	Swelling
	Skin rashes

ARBs

Common names include:	Possible side effects include:
Candesartan	Headache
Irbesartan	Lightheadedness
Losartan	Nasal congestion
Valsartan	Back and leg pain
	Diarrhea

Antiplatelet Drugs

These drugs help keep the blood from clotting. They may be given when aspirin cannot be used. They may also be given with aspirin to people who have had an angioplasty.

Common names include:	Possible side effects include:
Ticlopidine	Bleeding
Clopidogrel	Diarrhea
Prasugrel	Stomach upset

Anticoagulants

Anticoagulants help to keep the blood from clotting. It is often given to people during heart procedures or after other clot-busting drug treatment.

Common names include:	Possible side effects include:
Heparin	Internal bleeding
Warfarin	Stroke
Bivalirudin	

Statins

Statins lower cholesterol levels in the blood. Atorvastatin may reduce the risk of repeat stroke or heart attack. These drugs may be used with other methods to treat high cholesterol such as changes in how you eat.

Common names include:	Possible side effects include:
Atorvastatin	Headache
Pravastatin	Muscle pain
Lovastatin	Liver damage—rare
Simvastatin	
Fluvastatin	
Rosuvastatin	

Over-the-Counter Medications

Aspirin

Aspirin helps prevent clotting and reclosing of the artery. Aspirin may become part of long-term treatment. Possible side effects include:

- Stomach upset
- Gastrointestinal bleeding and stroke

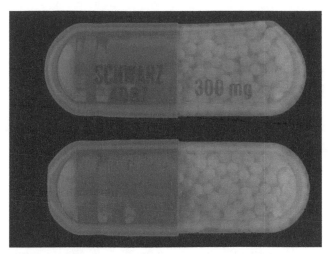

Verapamil (brand name Verelan) 300-mg extended-release capsule.
(National Library of Medicine)

Special Considerations

If you are taking medicine:

- Take medicine as directed. Do not change the amount or the schedule.
- Ask what side effects could occur. Report them to your doctor.
- Talk to your doctor before you stop taking any prescription medicine.
- Do not share your prescription medicine.
- Medicine can be dangerous when mixed. Talk to your doctor or pharmacist if you are taking more than one medicine. This includes over-the-counter products and supplements.
- Plan for refills as needed.

—Michael J. Fucci, DO, FACC

References

"Acute Coronary Syndromes." *DynaMed*, EBSCO Information Services, 15 Mar. 2019, www.dynamed.com/condition/acute-coronary-syndromes.

"Cardiac Medications." *American Heart Association*, 15 Jan. 2020, www.heart.org/en/health-topics/heart-attack/treatment-of-a-heart-attack/cardiac-medications.

"Hypertension Medication Selection and Management." *DynaMed*, EBSCO Information Services, 16 Nov. 2018, www.dynamed.com/management/hypertension-medication-selection-and-management.

"ST-Elevation Myocardial Infarction (STEMI)." *DynaMed*, EBSCO Information Services, 10 July 2018, www.dynamed.com/condition/st-elevation-myocardial-infarction-stemi.

"Statins." *DynaMed*, EBSCO Information Services, 5 Apr. 2018, www.dynamed.com/drug-review/statins.

Sweis, Ranya N. "Acute Myocardial Infarction (MI)." *Merck Manuals Professional Edition*, Merck Manuals, 2018, www.merckmanuals.com/professional/cardiovascular-disorders/coronary-artery-disease/acute-myocardial-infarction-mi.

■ Lifestyle changes to manage Heart Attack

There are many steps involved in recovering from a heart attack. Some habits will need to be changed to make the heart stronger. Focus on what you can change. Doing so will improve your quality of life. Changes are focused on:

Quit Smoking

Smoking narrows blood vessels, and makes your heart rate and blood pressure go up. People who keep smoking after a first heart attack are twice as likely to have a second one. Quitting smoking will drop the risk of a heart attack to that of a non-smoker within 3 years.

Being around smokers or in smoky places is also harmful. Try to stay away from them if you can.

Diet and Weight Loss

Eat a balanced diet with many types of foods. You may need to focus on foods with less fat and salt in them. It is hard to make changes, so start out slowly and move forward. Swap good foods for bad foods when you can such as eating an apple instead of a candy bar.

Eating foods low in saturated fat and cholesterol, and rich in whole grains, and fruits and vegetables will help lower cholesterol levels, blood pressure, and body weight. Eat less red meat and more lean proteins like chicken or fish. Add fish 2 days a week to get heart-healthy omega-3 into your diet.

Excess weight causes stress on the heart. Losing as little as 10 pounds can drastically lower the risk of having heart problems. Your doctor will help you find a way to lose excess weight safely. This makes it easier to stay in a healthy weight range. Keeping weight in a healthy range lowers the risk of high cholesterol, high blood pressure, and other heart diseases that can lead to a heart attack.

A dietitian will help you learn how to read food labels, shop for food, and plan meals.

Exercise Regularly

Cardiac rehab is a structured program to help you get into a regular exercise routine. Choose activities you like so they become a normal part of the day. This also helps with weight loss and keeping a healthy weight. Exercise can be as easy as a brisk walk. Aim for at least 150 minutes a week.

Manage Any Health Problems

Stick with your treatment for other health problems such as diabetes or high blood pressure. Taking medicine as directed lowers the risk of further heart attacks. Talk to your doctor if you need to make changes.

Drink Alcohol in Moderation

Talk to your doctor about drinking alcohol. You may need to avoid it. If it is okay, then limit drinking to moderation. This is 1 drink per day for women and 2 drinks per day for men. One drink equals 12 ounces of beer, or 4 ounces of wine, or 1 ounce of 100-proof spirits. Keep in mind that alcohol may interact with how well your medicine works.

Watch for Depression

It is common to have mood changes after a heart attack. Depression can slow healing and put you at risk for other heart problems or death. Signs of depression that last longer than 2 weeks should prompt a call to your doctor. These are feelings of sadness, hopelessness, and loss of interest in doing favorite activities. Depression is treatable.

Returning to Everyday Life

Recovery from a heart attack also involves:

- Sex—It is normal for you or your partner to feel concerned about having sex. In general,

people who have a heart attack can have sex after a short time. Feel free to talk about this with your doctor. You and your partner may also find sex therapy helpful. It will allow you both to talk about your concerns and learn how to return to having sex.

- Therapy—Support groups or one-on-one counseling can help you cope with challenges that come after having a heart attack. Support groups let you to meet others who have had a heart attack. They offer encouragement and support that will help you cope and stick with your long-term goals.

- Participate in your care—Talk to your care team about symptoms or treatments that you are having problems with. Other treatments may be available to help you better manage your health.

—*Michael J. Fucci, DO, FACC*

References

"Acute Coronary Syndromes." *DynaMed*, EBSCO Information Services, 15 Mar. 2019, www.dynamed.com/condition/acute-coronary-syndromes.

"Heart Attack Tools and Resources." *American Heart Association*, www.heart.org/en/health-topics/heart-attack/heart-attack-tools-and-resources.

"ST-Elevation Myocardial Infarction (STEMI)." *DynaMed*, EBSCO Information Services, 10 July 2018, www.dynamed.com/condition/st-elevation-myocardial-infarction-stemi.

Steinke, Elaine E., et al. "Sexual Counselling for Individuals with Cardiovascular Disease and Their Partners." *European Heart Journal*, vol. 34, no. 41, 29 July 2013, pp. 3217–3235, 10.1093/eurheartj/eht270.

"Treatment for Tobacco Use." *DynaMed*, EBSCO Information Services, 17 Oct. 2018, www.dynamed.com/management/treatment-for-tobacco-use-19.

■ Surgical and other invasive procedures for Heart Attack

Surgery can be done to restore or improve blood flow to the heart muscle. This helps the heart work better. When heart attacks are severe, surgery may be done right away.

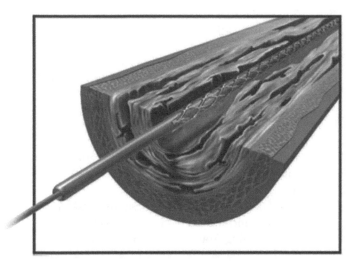

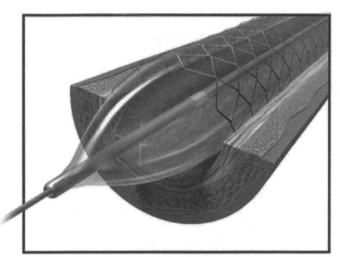

Balloon angioplasty with stent. (BruceBlaus)

Surgery to Relieve a Heart Attack

Coronary Artery Bypass Grafting (CABG)
During CABG, a healthy blood vessel is taken from somewhere in the body. The healthy blood vessel is attached to an artery in the heart just above and below the blockage. The new blood vessel lets blood move around the blockage. Bypass can be done for each blocked artery in the heart. CABG can be done as:

- On-pump—Done while the heart is stopped. A machine moves blood and oxygen around the body for the heart and lungs. Once the arteries are fixed, the heart is restarted.

- Off-pump—No machine is needed. The arteries are fixed while the heart is beating.
- Minimally invasive direct—Small cuts are made along the left side of the chest and between the ribs to get to the blood vessels. </item>

Angioplasty
A catheter is threaded through an artery in the groin and passed to the problem artery. Imaging tracks the catheter and watches blood flow.

Types of angioplasty are:

- Balloon—The catheter is placed in the near-blocked artery. A small balloon is quickly inflated and deflated. This lets theballoon press the plaque on the walls of the artery to open reopen it.The catheter is taken out when blood flow returns to normal.
- Stent—A mesh stent may be placed in the artery to keep it open. The stent may be coated with medicine to keep it from narrowing again.
- Laser—A laser beam vaporizes the plaque to open the artery.
- Atherectomy—A shaver on the tip of the guided catheter slices the plaque away.

Although these procedures may ease symptoms, it does not cure heart disease. Other steps such as keeping a healthy weight, eating right, and quitting smoking will need to be taken.

Surgery to Treat Damage from a Heart Attack
Heart attacks can cause permanent heart damage. This can change the heart's structure and how it works. Surgery is used to move blood around damaged tissue or to fix heart rhythm problems. They are not a cure, but they do improve quality of life. These are:

- Intra-aortic balloon counterpulsation (IABP)—A small balloon is threaded into the aorta, the body's largest artery. It moves with your heart rhythm, bringing the heart muscle more blood.
- Transmyocardial laser revascularization (TMR)—TMR is mainly used in people who have severe angina. A laser is placed through small cuts on the left side of the chest. These make small channels the parts of the heart that need them.

- Implantable cardioverter defibrillator (ICD)—An ICD is placed in the chest. People having a heart attack are more prone to heart rhythm problems. ICDs help keep the heart rhythm normal.
- Coronary artery radiation—Radiation is sometimes used to reopen arteries in the heartthat have narrowed after a stent was placed.

—Michael J. Fucci, DO, FACC

References

"Acute Coronary Syndromes." *DynaMed*, EBSCO Information Services, 15 Mar. 2019, www.dynamed.com/condition/acute-coronary-syndromes.

"Cardiac Procedures and Surgeries." *American Heart Association*, 31 Mar. 2017, www.heart.org/en/health-topics/heart-attack/treatment-of-a-heart-attack/cardiac-procedures-and-surgeries.

"Coronary Artery Bypass Graft (CABG) Surgery." *DynaMed*, EBSCO Information Services, 20 Feb. 2019, www.dynamed.com/procedure/coronary-artery-bypass-graft-cabg-surgery.

"Coronary Artery Bypass Grafting." *National Heart, Lung, and Blood Institute*, U.S. Department of Health & Human Services, 18 Nov. 2014, www.nhlbi.nih.gov/health-topics/coronary-artery-bypass-grafting.

"Percutaneous Coronary Intervention (PCI) Procedure." *DynaMed*, EBSCO Information Services, 18 Jan. 2019, www.dynamed.com/procedure/percutaneous-coronary-intervention-pci-procedure.

"ST-Elevation Myocardial Infarction (STEMI)." *DynaMed*, EBSCO Information Services, 10 July 2018, www.dynamed.com/condition/st-elevation-myocardial-infarction-stemi.

"Ventricular Assist Devices (VADs)." *Texas Heart Institute*, www.texasheart.org/heart-health/heart-information-center/topics/ventricular-assist-devices/.

■ Talking to your doctor about Heart Attack

General Tips for Gathering Information

You have your own health past. Talk with your doctor about your risk factors and background with heart disease. By talking openly and often with your doctor, you can make the best choices for you and your family. Here are some tips that will make it easier for you to talk to your doctor:

- Bring someone else with you. It helps to have another person hear what is said and think of questions to ask.
- Bring the list of current medicine with you.
- Write your questions ahead of time, so you don't forget them.
- Write down the answers you get and make sure you grasp what you are hearing. Ask for help, if needed.
- Don't be afraid to ask your questions or ask where you can find more information about what you are discussing. You have a right to know.

Specific Questions to Ask Your Doctor

About Your Risk of Developing Heart Disease and Heart Attack

- Based on my medical history, lifestyle, and family background, am I at risk for a heart attack?
- How do I best prevent heart disease and heart attack?
- How do I know if my blood pressure or cholesterol is high?

About Treatment Options

- What are the risks and benefits of the various methods to reopen the artery?
- What medicine is available to help me?
- What are the benefits and side effects of these medicines?
- Will these medicines interact with other medicines, over-the-counter products, or dietary or herbal supplements I am already taking?

About Lifestyle Changes

- How soon after my heart attack can I begin exercising?
- What type of exercise is best?
- How much should I be exercising?
- How do I get started with an exercise program?
- Do I have to change my diet? If so, how do I go about it?
- Should I stop drinking alcohol?
- How can I find help to quit smoking?
- Do I need to lose weight? If so, how much?

- How soon after my heart attack is it safe to have sex?

About Your Outlook

- How do I know if my cholesterol and blood pressure are staying within healthy limits?
- How often will you monitor my blood pressure and cholesterol levels?
- How likely am I to have another heart attack?
- How extensive is the damage to my heart? How will that affect my quality of life?

—Michael J. Fucci, DO, FACC

References

"Acute Coronary Syndromes." *DynaMed*, EBSCO Information Services, 15 Mar. 2019, www.dynamed.com/condition/acute-coronary-syndromes.

"Getting the Most Out of Your Doctor Appointment." *FamilyDoctor.Org*, American Academy of Family Physicians, 19 Jan. 2018, familydoctor.org/tips-for-talking-to-your-doctor/.

"Heart-to-Heart: Talking to Your Doctor." *American Heart Association*, www.heart.org/en/health-topics/consumer-healthcare/doctor-appointments-questions-to-ask-your-doctor/heart-to-heart-talking-to-your-doctor.

"Preparing for Medical Visits." *American Heart Association*, 31 Jan. 2018, www.heart.org/en/health-topics/cardiac-rehab/communicating-with-professionals/preparing-for-medical-visits.

"ST-Elevation Myocardial Infarction (STEMI)." *DynaMed*, EBSCO Information Services, 10 July 2018, www.dynamed.com/condition/st-elevation-myocardial-infarction-stemi.

■ Resource guide for Heart Attack

American Heart Association

7272 Greenville Avenue
Dallas, TX 75231
1-800-AHA-USA-1
http://www.heart.org

On this site, you will find general information about heart disease, including educational information, news, research, health programs, and dietary information.

Centers for Disease Control

1600 Clifton Rd.
Atlanta, GA 30333
1-800-CDC-INFO
http://www.cdc.gov

This site provides educational and statistical information about heart disease, as well as information about several other conditions.

National Heart, Lung, and Blood Institute (NHLBI)

NHLBI Health Information Center
Building 31, Room 5A52
31 Center Drive MSC 2486
Bethesda, MD 20892
(301) 592-8573
http://www.nhlbi.nih.gov

The NHLBI is a part of the National Institutes of Health. The site provides information about cholesterol, heart disease risk factors, and various heart conditions. The institute conducts and supports research related to the causes, prevention, diagnosis, and treatment of heart, blood vessel, lung, and blood diseases as well as sleep disorders.

—Michael J. Fucci, DO, FACC

■ Conditions In Depth: Peripheral Artery Disease (PAD)

Peripheral artery disease (PAD) is damage or disease of the arteries outside of the heart and brain. Blood carries oxygen and nutrients to organs and tissues. Problems with the arteries can affect the health of tissue in the arms, legs, and body core.

If PAD isn't treated, it can lead to problems like tissue death, infection, and amputation. Things that cause PAD can also harm blood vessels in the heart and brain. This means people with PAD are at risk for heart attack and stroke.

PAD Causes

Atherosclerosis is the most common cause of PAD. This is a build up of plaque on the walls of the vessels. Plaque is a waxy matter made of fats and other matter in the blood. It sticks to the walls. It can also be made of scar tissue or fibers used to fix damage to the walls. Overtime, plaque grows by trapping other matter in the blood, such as bad cholesterol and blood sugar. As it grows, the blood vessel gets narrow and makes it harder for blood to flow. Things that can lead to atherosclerosis are:

- Smoking—can bother vessel walls and make deposits on them
- High cholesterol—bad cholesterol can stick to and bother the walls of the vessels
- High blood pressure—causes strong blood flow that can injure the walls of vessels
- Diabetes—too much sugar in the blood can lead to plaque build up
- Radiation therapy

—*Daniel A. Ostrovsky, MD*

References

"About Peripheral Artery Disease (PAD)." *American Heart Association*, 31 Oct. 2016, www.heart.org/en/health-topics/peripheral-artery-disease/about-peripheral-artery-disease-pad.

Hills, Alexander J, et al. "Peripheral Arterial Disease." *British Journal of Hospital Medicine*, vol. 70, no. 10, Oct. 2009, pp. 560–565, 10.12968/hmed.2009.70.10.44622.

Jurado, Javier A., et al. "Radiation-Induced Peripheral Artery Disease." *Catheterization and Cardiovascular Interventions*, vol. 72, no. 4, 1 Oct. 2008, pp. 563–568, 10.1002/ccd.21681.

"Peripheral Artery Disease (PAD) of Lower Extremities." *DynaMed*, EBSCO Information Services, 23 Aug. 2018, www.dynamed.com/condition/peripheral-artery-disease-pad-of-lower-extremities.

"What Is Peripheral Artery Disease?" *National Heart, Lung, and Blood Institute*, US Department of Health & Human Services, 23 Jan. 2019, www.nhlbi.nih.gov/health-topics/peripheral-artery-disease.

■ Risk factors for Peripheral Artery Disease (PAD)

You can get PAD with or without the risks below. The more you have, the greater your chances of getting PAD. If you have many, ask your doctor what you can do to lower them.

Things You Can Change

Smoking

Smoking makes blood vessels narrow. It also builds up plaque in the arteries and raises your pulse and blood pressure. The risk of PAD is four times higher in smokers and former smokers. It can also happen up to 10 years earlier in smokers.

Inactivity

Not being active lowers the health of your vessels and heart. It also raises the chance of other PAD risks. Talk to your doctor before you start any workout program. Grow the intensity slowly over time.

Long Term Health Problems

High Cholesterol

Cholesterol is a waxy matter used by the body. The body makes it and some also comes from the foods you eat. High levels of certain cholesterol in your blood can lead to atherosclerosis. This is the main cause of PAD.

High Blood Pressure

Blood pressure is the force of blood on the walls of your arteries. It can cause too much stress and force on blood vessel walls when it is too high. Over time, this causes damage. It also raises the risk of PAD. If you have high blood pressure, talk with your doctor about how to control it.

Glucose Intolerance

Glucose intolerance and diabetes happen when the body does not make insulin or does not use it well. Insulin is a hormone that helps pull sugar out of the blood and into cells for use. High levels of it can lead to atherosclerosis and blood vessel damage. Controlling your blood sugar can help lower the risk of diseases like PAD.

Obesity and Overweight

Being obese or overweight raises your risk of PAD even if you do not have other factors. Talk to your doctor about your ideal weight range. Make a plan to help you reach your goal weight.

Metabolic Syndrome

Metabolic syndrome is high blood pressure, cholesterol, blood sugar, and body weight, mainly around

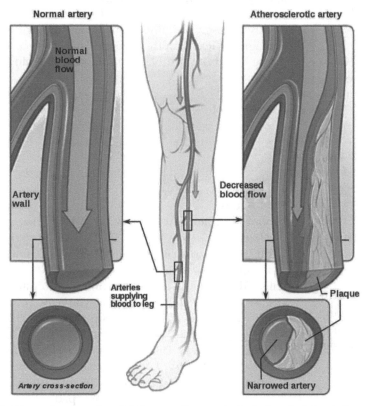

The illustration shows how P.A.D. can affect arteries in the legs. Left figure shows a normal artery with normal blood flow. The inset image shows a cross-section of the normal artery. Right figure shows an artery with plaque buildup that's partially blocking blood flow. The inset image shows a cross-section of the narrowed artery. (Jmarchn)

the midsection. People with this health problem have an greater risk of PAD because of too much stress on their heart.

HIV Infection

People with long term HIV infection may have a greater risk of PAD. The reason why is not clear.

Factors That You Can't Change

Age

PAD and atherosclerosis get worse over time. This means the older you are, the greater the buildup may be. The heart and blood vessels also have normal changes that can affect function, such as an increase in heart size, slower heart rate, and stiffer

blood vessels and valves. This decrease is often not enough to cause problems. But problems can happen when they combine with current vascular diseases, like PAD.

Gender

Men have a higher risk of heart disease, but the risk in women raises sharply after menopause. Estrogen is thought to protect blood vessels before that time. The natural drop in estrogen after menopause can lower this protection. This brings risk levels that are like those in men. As a result, men tend to get PAD earlier than women.

PAD is more likely to happen in men over the age of 40, and in women over the age of 50.

Genetics

Your genes can also play a role in your risk of PAD with or without other risks listed here. Your risk of getting PAD is higher if you have a family history of PAD, high blood pressure, or high cholesterol.

—*Daniel A. Ostrovsky, MD*

References

Beckman, Joshua A., et al. "Association of Human Immunodeficiency Virus Infection and Risk of Peripheral Artery Disease." *Circulation*, vol. 138, no. 3, 17 July 2018, pp. 255–265, 10.1161/circulationaha.117.032647.

Hills, Alexander J, et al. "Peripheral Arterial Disease." *British Journal of Hospital Medicine*, vol. 70, no. 10, Oct. 2009, pp. 560–565, 10.12968/hmed.2009.70.10.44622.

"Peripheral Artery Disease (PAD) of Lower Extremities." *DynaMed*, EBSCO Information Services, 23 Aug. 2018, www.dynamed.com/condition/peripheral-artery-disease-pad-of-lower-extremities.

"Understand Your Risk for PAD." *American Heart Association*, 31 Oct. 2016, www.heart.org/en/health-topics/peripheral-artery-disease/understand-your-risk-for-pad.

Reducing your risk of Peripheral Artery Disease (PAD)

There are a range of factors that can raise the risk of having a PAD. Many of them can be avoided or managed. The more factors you control, the more you lower your risk.

Quit Smoking

Chemicals in smoke add to the build-up of plaque in the arteries. This raises your risk of atherosclerosis. Smoking can also cause changes in blood vessels. These changes can affect blood flow.

If you smoke, talk with your doctor about tools and programs to help you quit. Secondhand smoke can also cause harm. Try to avoid it.

Reach and Maintain a Healthy Weight

If you are overweight or obese , talk to your doctor about a plan to lose weight. Adopt a healthy eating plan and make exercise part of your daily routine. Plan to lose weight slowly over time. A dietitian can help you with meal planning and portion sizing.

Eat a Healthy Diet

Your diet can affect your bad and good cholesterol levels and blood pressure. A healthy diet includes plenty of whole grains, fruits and vegetables, and nuts. Also consider eating good fats instead of bad fats. This means eating more good fats like olive and canola oil, and less bad fats that can raise your bad cholesterol levels. General guidelines include adding fish to your diet at least twice per week.

Exercise Regularly

Regular aerobic exercise, such as walking, biking, or running, can help improve blood vessel health and blood flow. It will also help strengthen the heart muscle, reduce the heart's workload, and lower blood pressure. Ask your doctor if you are healthy enough to exercise If you are, aim for at least 30 minutes of exercise per day on most days of the week.

Daily Aspirin

If you are at high risk, your doctor may suggest taking daily aspirin to help control blood clots. Blood clots may be more likely to form and cause bigger problems in people with PAD. Since aspirin therapy has risks, be sure to talk with your doctor before you start.

Manage Other Health Problems

Certain health problems are linked to a higher risk of this disease. While not all risk can be removed, managing these health problems can reduce the risk of blood flow problems. Work with your doctor to help manage:

- High cholesterol
- Diabetes
- Hypertension

—*Daniel A. Ostrovsky, MD*

References

"About Peripheral Artery Disease (PAD)." *American Heart Association*, 31 Oct. 2016, www.heart.org/en/health-topics/peripheral-artery-disease/about-peripheral-artery-disease-pad.

Hills, Alexander J, et al. "Peripheral Arterial Disease." *British Journal of Hospital Medicine*, vol. 70, no. 10, Oct. 2009, pp. 560–565, 10.12968/hmed.2009.70.10.44622.

"Peripheral Artery Disease." *National Heart, Lung, and Blood Institute*, US Department of Health & Human Services, 23 Jan. 2019, www.nhlbi.nih.gov/health/health-topics/topics/pad.

"Peripheral Artery Disease (PAD) of Lower Extremities." *DynaMed*, EBSCO Information Services, 23 Aug. 2018, www.dynamed.com/condition/peripheral-artery-disease-pad-of-lower-extremities.

"Prevention and Treatment of PAD." *American Heart Association*, 31 Oct. 2016, www.heart.org/en/health-topics/peripheral-artery-disease/prevention-and-treatment-of-pad.

Symptoms of Peripheral Artery Disease (PAD)

PAD is a disease that gets worse over time. You may not have symptoms until the disease gets much worse. Over time, PAD may lead to:

Intermittent Claudication

This is the most common symptom of PAD. Claudication is pain that occurs in the thigh, hip, calf, or foot. It may happen when you walk, use stairs, or workout.

You may have cramping or limping. You may also feel heavy, weak, or tired. Symptoms often begin after walking a certain distance, such as a block or two, and end after you rest for the same amount of time.

Other Symptoms

You may also have:

- A numb feeling in your legs or feet when you are resting
- Cold legs or feet
- Muscle pain in the thighs, calves, or feet
- Loss of hair on the lower limbs
- Poorly growing or thick toenails
- Pale or blue legs or feet
- Problems walking
- Foot wounds that heal slowly

Complications

PAD can lead to severe problems, such as:

- Critical limb ischemia—Ulcers that are slow to heal because of low or blocked blood flow. They can lead to gangrene. When the blood supply is cut off, the tissue does not get enough oxygen and begins to die. Gangrene can lead to amputation of the limb.
- Functional decline—As PAD progresses, you won't be able to walk as far.
- Erectile dysfunction

—Daniel A. Ostrovsky, MD</item>

References

Hills, Alexander J, et al. "Peripheral Arterial Disease." *British Journal of Hospital Medicine*, vol. 70, no. 10, Oct. 2009, pp. 560–565, 10.12968/hmed.2009.70.10.44622.

"Peripheral Artery Disease (PAD) of Lower Extremities." *DynaMed*, EBSCO Information Services, 23 Aug. 2018, www.dynamed.com/condition/peripheral-artery-disease-pad-of-lower-extremities.

"Symptoms and Diagnosis of PAD." *American Heart Association*, 31 Oct. 2016, www.heart.org/en/health-topics/peripheral-artery-disease/symptoms-and-diagnosis-of-pad.

■ Screening for Peripheral Artery Disease (PAD)

Screening helps find and treat diseases earlier. Tests are given to people who don't have signs, but who may be at high risk for certain health problems. There are no tests for PAD. But your doctor will screen for problems that lead to vascular disease. These tests will be done at your routine checkups:

- Blood pressure readings
- Blood tests to check your cholesterol and blood sugar
- Body weight checks, such as checking your body mass index (BMI) and waist size
- Asking about your habits, such as eating, smoking, and exercise

If you are at high risk, your doctor may want to do:

- Visual exam—Your doctor should look at the skin of all of your limbs during check-ups. Changes in skin texture and color, sores, or nonhealing wounds may be a sign of PAD.
- Pulses—Your doctor can listen and feel for pulses in your feet and groin. Unusual sounds in the arteries and weak pulses are signs of PAD.
- Ankle-brachial index (ABI)—Your doctor takes pressures in both arms and ankles using a blood pressure cuff and an ultrasound. The readings are used to find out your ABI. A value less than or equal to 0.9 is a sign of PAD.

—Daniel A. Ostrovsky, MD

References

"Peripheral Artery Disease (PAD) of Lower Extremities." *DynaMed*, EBSCO Information Services, 23 Aug. 2018, www.dynamed.com/condition/peripheral-artery-disease-pad-of-lower-extremities.

"Prevention and Treatment of PAD." *American Heart Association*, 31 Oct. 2016, www.heart.org/en/health-topics/peripheral-artery-disease/prevention-and-treatment-of-pad.

■ Medications for Peripheral Artery Disease (PAD)

Here are some facts about medicines that can help treat PAD. Only the most general side effects are listed. Ask your doctor if you need to take any special steps. Use each of these drugs the way your doctor tells you to. Or, follow the fact sheet that come with them. If you have questions, call your doctor. Medicines can help treat PAD. There are two types:

- Ones that help your blood flow through narrowed arteries
- Ones that thin the blood so that it does not clot as easily

Prescription Medications

Pentoxifylline
Pentoxifylline helps blood flow by lowering its thickness and making red blood cells move more easily.

Possible side effects include:
Stomach upset
Nausea
Lightheadedness

Antiplatelet Agents
Cilostazol is the only antiplatelet agent labeled to treat intermittent claudication. People who use it have been able to walk for longer periods of time and distance. It should not be taken if you have heart failure.

Common names include:	Possible side effects include:
Clopidogrel	Headache
Ticlopidine	Runny nose, sore throat
Dipyridamole	Bowel changes
Cilostazol	Bleeding

Clot-busting Drugs (Thrombolytic Drugs)
Given by IV, this drug is only given to people in the hospital. These drugs may be used if you get acute limb ischemia. This is a serious problem from PAD. It causes blood flow into a limb to lower quickly.

None of these drugs are FDA approved for treating peripheral vascular occlusion. These drugs break down the chemicals that hold blood clots together. Thrombolysis must be safely controlled.

Common name:	Possible side effects include:
Recombinant tissue plasminogen activator (rt-PA, Alteplase)	Bleeding, such as in sites where you have had surgery or have stomach ulcers
	Allergic reactions
	Heart and lung events

Anticoagulants
These drugs may be used if you get acute limb ischemia. This is a problem from PAD. This is a serious problem from PAD. It causes blood flow into a limb to lower quickly. If this happens, the doctor may inject you with heparin in the hospital. Once at home, an oral version, such as warfarin, may be used.

These drugs work right away to stop blood from clotting. They do not break down a clot after it has formed. If you are at high risk of a repeat clot, these drugs may be needed.

Common names include:	Possible side effects include:
Heparin	Bleeding
Warfarin	Allergic reactions
	Too few platelets

Over the Counter Medications

Aspirin
Aspirin is often used for problems with blood flow due to its safety, low cost, and the way it can reduce heart attacks and other occlusive vascular diseases. Lower doses are less likely to cause stomach problems or bleeding ulcers that are common with higher doses.

Possible side effects include:
Indigestion
Peptic ulcers
Bleeding

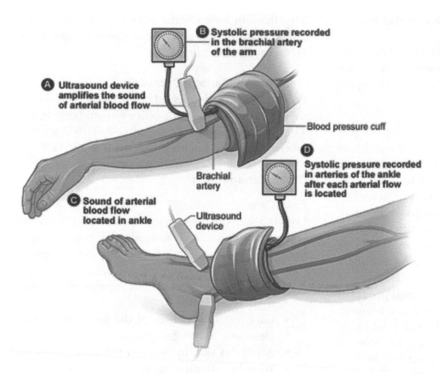

The illustration shows the ankle-brachial index test. The test compares blood pressure in the ankle to blood pressure in the arm. As the blood pressure cuff deflates, the blood pressure in the arteries is recorded. (National Heart Lung and Blood Insitute)

When to Contact Your Doctor

- New or worsening symptoms
- Drug side effects
- Foot wounds that do not heal

Special Considerations

Whenever you are taking a prescription medication, take the following precautions:

- Take your medicine as advised. Do not change the amount or schedule.
- Ask what side effects could happen. Tell them to your doctor.
- Talk to your doctor before you stop taking any prescription medicine.
- Do not share your prescription medicine.
- Medicines can be harmful when mixed. Talk to your doctor or pharmacist if you are taking more than one, including over the counter products and supplements.
- Plan ahead for refills.

—*Daniel A. Ostrovsky, MD*

References

Hills, Alexander J, et al. "Peripheral Arterial Disease." *British Journal of Hospital Medicine,* vol. 70, no. 10, Oct. 2009, pp. 560–565, 10.12968/hmed.2009.70.10.44622.

"Peripheral Artery Disease (PAD) of Lower Extremities." *DynaMed,* EBSCO Information Services, 23 Aug. 2018, www.dynamed.com/condition/peripheral-artery-disease-pad-of-lower-extremities.

"Prevention and Treatment of PAD." *American Heart Association,* 31 Oct. 2016, www.heart.org/en/health-topics/peripheral-artery-disease/prevention-and-treatment-of-pad.

Rooke, Thom W., et al. "2011 ACCF/AHA Focused Update of the Guideline for the Management of Patients With Peripheral Artery Disease (Updating the 2005 Guideline)." *Journal of the American College of Cardiology,* vol. 58, no. 19, Nov. 2011, pp. 2020–2045, 10.1016/j.jacc.2011.08.023.

Sontheimer, Daniel L. "Peripheral Vascular Disease: Diagnosis and Treatment." *American Family Physician,* vol. 73, no. 11, 1 June 2006, pp. 1971–1976.

■ Lifestyle changes to manage Peripheral Artery Disease (PAD)

Lifestyle changes can help reduce symptoms, slow disease, and improve your heart health. These changes can also lower your risk of health problems.

Quit Smoking

Quitting smoking is a critical step. Smoking can cause blood vessels to twitch. This lowers the amount of oxygen in your blood. Both of these things lower the amount of oxygen that is in your legs and feet. Chemicals in smoke can also lead to plaque buildup over time.

Talk to your doctor about ways to quit. There are many tools, such as patches, therapies, and drugs that may help. Keep in mind that breathing in smoke from other people is also harmful.

Exercise Often

Do not start any exercise program without talking to your doctor. Exercise can help new, small blood vessels grow. These blood vessels can grow in areas with poor blood flow. This can let blood flow to tissues that need it, which may reduce symptoms. Regular aerobic training can also help raise your physical skills, quality of life, and help handle other things that lead to PAD, such as high cholesterol and high blood pressure.

You may need to start with a supervised program that will help you help your ability to move around. Aim to get 30-45 minutes of exercise at least three times a week. From there, you may be able to increase your frequency and intensity of activity based on your progress.

Reduce or Avoid Excess Weight

Excess weight is linked to a greater risk of atherosclerosis. If you are struggling to lose weight, talk to your doctor about what you can do about it and what your ideal weight range may be. A dietitian can also help you with meal planning.

Manage Chronic Health Problems

Follow any plans for other health problems you may have. Stay in contact with your medical team to make sure you are on track and make any changes. Managing other health problems will help with your treatment of PAD.

Control Blood Sugar Levels

High blood sugar levels can lead to plaque buildup in the blood vessels. Over time, it can also harm smaller vessels. Although diabetes is linked to a greater risk of heart problems, that risk can be lowered if you control your blood sugar levels. Work with your health care team to learn how to do this.

Maintain Normal Blood Pressure

High blood pressure causes strong blood flow. This can damage blood vessels. Work with your medical team to monitor and manage your blood pressure.

This may include weight management, salt reduction, exercise, and stress management. For some, medicines may be needed.

Identify and Manage Depression

People who are depressed are less likely to stick to their treatment plans for other chronic conditions. They are also less likely to exercise. This leadsto an increased risk of health problems from PAD.

Other Management

Foot Care

Looking at your feet every day will help prevent serious problems that can lead to ulcers or amputation. To keep your feet healthy, take these steps:

- Look at your feet daily for injuries, ingrown toenails, or cuts.
- Care for any injuries of the feet with regular cleansing and dressings.
- Avoid dry skin by using moisturizing creams.
- Wear breathable, but close-toed, shoes.
- Get properly fitted for shoes.
- Talk to your doctor or podiatrist about any toe or toenail problems. Make sure they know you have PAD.

Be active in your care. Talk to your team about symptoms or treatments if you are having a hard time with them.

—Daniel A. Ostrovsky, MD

References

Bondke Persson, A., et al. "Therapeutic Arteriogenesis in Peripheral Arterial Disease: Combining Intervention and Passive Training." *Vasa*, vol. 40, no. 3, 1 May 2011, pp. 177–187, 10.1024/0301-1526/a000092.

Haas, Tara L., et al. "Exercise Training and Peripheral Arterial Disease." Comprehensive *Physiology*, vol. 2, no. 4, Oct. 2012, www.ncbi.nlm.nih.gov/pmc/articles/PMC3767482/, 10.1002/cphy.c110065.

Hills, Alexander J, et al. "Peripheral Arterial Disease." *British Journal of Hospital Medicine*, vol. 70, no. 10, Oct. 2009, pp. 560–565, 10.12968/hmed.2009.70.10.44622.

"Peripheral Artery Disease (PAD) of Lower Extremities." *DynaMed*, EBSCO Information

Services, 23 Aug. 2018, www.dynamed.com/condition/peripheral-artery-disease-pad-of-lower-extremities.

"Prevention and Treatment of PAD." *American Heart Association*, 31 Oct. 2016, www.heart.org/en/health-topics/peripheral-artery-disease/prevention-and-treatment-of-pad.

"What Is Peripheral Artery Disease." *National Heart, Lung, and Blood Institute*, US Department of Health & Human Services, 23 Aug. 2018, www.nhlbi.nih.gov/health/health-topics/topics/pad.

Reviews, 11 Aug. 2013, 10.1002/14651858.cd005507.pub3.

"Peripheral Artery Disease (PAD) of Lower Extremities." *DynaMed*, EBSCO Information Services, 23 Aug. 2018, www.dynamed.com/condition/peripheral-artery-disease-pad-of-lower-extremities.

"Prevention and Treatment of PAD." *American Heart Association*, 31 Oct. 2016, www.heart.org/en/health-topics/peripheral-artery-disease/prevention-and-treatment-of-pad.

■ Surgical procedures for Peripheral Artery Disease (PAD)

Surgery may be used for PAD that is causing bad health problems. It may also be used when other methods fail or there is a danger of limb loss. The main goal is to get blood to flow better.

Bypass Grafting

If blood can't flow to your limb, your doctor may want to do bypass grafting It removes a healthy blood vessel from the leg or somewhere else the body. The vessel is attached to the problem artery just above and just below the part that isn't working right. Blood will then be able to go around it by moving through the new blood vessel.

Percutaneous Angioplasty

Percutaneous angioplasty uses tubes to help view and open vessels. A thin tube is passed into larger arteries like those in your groin and passed through vessels to the blocked part. Tools can then be used to remove or break up clots, press down on plaque, or place devices that help prop vessels open. Cryoplasty is one more method. It uses nitrous oxide to cool and open the artery.

—*Daniel A. Ostrovsky, MD*

References

Hills, Alexander J, et al. "Peripheral Arterial Disease." *British Journal of Hospital Medicine*, vol. 70, no. 10, Oct. 2009, pp. 560–565, 10.12968/hmed.2009.70.10.44622.

McCaslin, James E, et al. "Cryoplasty for Peripheral Arterial Disease." *Cochrane Database of Systematic*

■ Talking to your doctor about Peripheral Artery Disease (PAD)

General Tips for Gathering Information

You have a unique medical history. Therefore, it is essential to talk with your doctor about your personal risk factors and/or experience with PAD. By talking openly and regularly with your doctor, you can take an active role in your care. Here are some tips that will make it easier for you to talk to your doctor:

- Bring someone else with you. It helps to have another person hear what is said and think of things you may have missed.
- Write out your questions ahead of time, so you don't forget them.
- Write down the answers you get, and make sure you understand what you are hearing. Ask for clarification, if necessary.
- Don't be afraid to ask questions and learn where you can find more information about what you are discussing. You have a right to know.

Specific Questions to Ask Your Doctor

About Your Risk of Developing Symptomatic Disease

- Will I develop symptoms in the future?
- How soon will that happen?

About Your Risk of Developing Severe Complications

- How likely is it that I will have complications like infection or gangrene?
- Can you help me with foot care and advice, or do I have to see a podiatrist?

About Treatment Options

- What medications do you recommend?
- What effects, both positive and negative, can I expect?
- Will they interact with anything I am already taking?
- How long will I have to take them?
- Are there alternative therapies that have been shown to help treat PAD?
- Will surgery ever be necessary?

About Lifestyle Changes

- Am I doing all I can to address the causes of this condition to help keep it from getting worse?
- Please give me the information I need to engage in a proper, safe exercise program.

About Outlook

- What can I expect in the future?
- Do I have any other conditions that affect my blood vessels?
- How and why does AD (with other conditions) affect my risk for heart attack and stroke?

—*Daniel A. Ostrovsky, MD*

References

"Getting the Most Out of Your Doctor Appointment." *FamilyDoctor.Org*, American Academy of Family Physicians, 19 Jan. 2018, familydoctor.org/tips-for-talking-to-your-doctor/.

"Heart-to-Heart: Talking to Your Doctor." *American Heart Association*, www.heart.org/en/health-topics/consumer-healthcare/doctor-appointments-questions-to-ask-your-doctor/heart-to-heart-talking-to-your-doctor.

"Peripheral Artery Disease (PAD) of Lower Extremities." *DynaMed*, EBSCO Information Services, 23 Aug. 2018, www.dynamed.com/condition/peripheral-artery-disease-pad-of-lower-extremities.

"Preparing for Medical Visits." *American Heart Association*, 31 Jan. 2018, www.heart.org/en/health-topics/cardiac-rehab/communicating-with-professionals/preparing-for-medical-visits.

"Talking to Your Doctor." *National Institutes of Health*, 8 May 2015, www.nih.gov/institutes-nih/nih-office-director/office-communications-public-liaison/clear-communication/talking-your-doctor. Accessed 10 Dec. 2018.

■ Resource guide for Peripheral Artery Disease (PAD)

American Heart Association

National Center
7272 Greenville Avenue
Dallas, TX 75231
1-800-242-8721
http://www.heart.org

On this site, you will find general information about heart disease, including educational information, news, research, health programs, and dietary information.

Society of Interventional Radiology

3975 Fair Ridge Drive
Suite 400 North
Fairfax, VA 22033
703-691-1805
https://www.sirweb.org

The Society of Interventional Radiology provides general information about PAD, screening guidelines, clinical trials, and self-testing. Their website also offers information about the "Legs for Life" PAD screening program.

Vascular Cures

274 Redwood Shores Parkway
Suite 717
Redwood City, CA 94065
650-368-6022
http://vascularcures.org

This site provides a glossary, FAQs, and a physician finder sponsored through the American Association of Vascular Surgeons.

Heart and Stroke Foundation of Canada

110-1525 Carling Avenue
Ottawa, ON K1Z 8R9
1-888-473-4636
http://www.heartandstroke.ca

The Heart and Stroke Foundation of Canada provides educational materials about heart attack, stroke, and other heart conditions. The national voluntary health agency's mission is to reduce disability and death from cardiovascular diseases and stroke.

■ Conditions In Depth: Sleep Apnea

Sleep apnea occurs when breathing stops for brief periods of time while a person is sleeping. It can last for 10-30 seconds, and may occur up to 20-30 times per hour. During one night of sleep, this can cause up to 400 episodes of interrupted breathing.

Every time you stop breathing, you interfere with the normal patterns of deep sleep. The quality of sleep that you get is greatly impaired. Your level of alertness and your ability to pay attention may be seriously affected.

If you have sleep apnea, you are also more likely to have:

- Accidents, especially car accidents
- Coronary artery disease
- Stroke
- Lung disease
- High blood pressure
- Diabetes
- Kidney disease

There are several kinds of sleep apnea. These include:

Obstructive Sleep Apnea

This is caused by a temporary airway obstruction. This blockage may be partial or complete. Obstructive sleep apnea can occur when the tissues of your throat relax too much and cave in on each other. If you are overweight, then your excess tissue might be putting too much pressure on your airway, causing it to collapse.

You may have a deviated septum, nasal polyps, large tonsils, or an elongated soft palate and uvula that obstruct your airway while you are sleeping.

For children, enlarged tonsils and adenoids are the most common reason for obstructive sleep apnea.

Central Sleep Apnea

This occurs when the lower brain stem fails to send signals to the muscles that control breathing. Conditions that cause problems with the lower brain stem include certain types of polio, encephalitis, stroke, brain tumors, and other diseases that affect the brain and central nervous system. For children, the most common reason for central sleep apnea is prematurity.

Mixed Sleep Apnea

Mixed sleep apnea includes aspects of both obstructive and central sleep apnea.

—*Marcie L. Sidman, MD*

References

Botros, Nader, et al. "Obstructive Sleep Apnea as a Risk Factor for Type 2 Diabetes." *The American Journal of Medicine*, vol. 122, no. 12, Dec. 2009, pp. 1122–1127, www.ncbi.nlm.nih.gov/pmc/articles/PMC2799991/, 10.1016/j.amjmed.2009.04.026.

Molnar, Miklos Z, et al. "Association of Incident Obstructive Sleep Apnoea with Outcomes in a Large Cohort of US Veterans." *Thorax*, vol. 70, no. 9, 2 June 2015, pp. 888–895, 10.1136/thoraxjnl-2015-206970.

"Obstructive Sleep Apnea (OSA) in Adults." *DynaMed*, EBSCO Information Services, 5 Oct. 2016, www.dynamed.com/condition/obstructive-sleep-apnea-osa-in-adults.

"Sleep Apnea." National Heart, Lung, and Blood Institute, US Department of Health & Human Services, 10 Dec. 2018, www.nhlbi.nih.gov/health-topics/sleep-apnea.

"Sleep Apnea Information." *American Sleep Apnea Association*, 5 Apr. 2019, www.sleepapnea.org/learn/sleep-apnea/.

"Sleep Apnea Information Page." *National Institute of Neurological Disorders and Stroke*, National Institutes of Health, 27 Mar. 2019, www.ninds.nih.gov/Disorders/All-Disorders/Sleep-Apnea-Information-Page.

■ Risk factors for Sleep Apnea

A risk factor is something that increases your likelihood of getting a disease or condition.

It is possible to develop sleep apnea with or without the risk factors listed below. However, the more risk factors you have, the greater your likelihood of developing sleep apnea. If you have a number of risk factors, ask your doctor what you can do to reduce your risk. Risk factors for sleep apnea include:

Smoking
People who smoke more than 2 packs per day are more likely to develop sleep apnea than non-smokers.

Alcohol
Some studies have shown that people who use alcohol regularly have an increased risk of sleep apnea.

Sedative Medications
Using sedative medications can increase your risk of sleep apnea.

Medical Conditions
The following conditions may increase your risk of obstructive sleep apnea:

- Obesity
- Pregnancy
- Diabetes
- Polycystic ovary syndrome
- High blood pressure
- Facial deformities
- Hypothyroidism
- Gastroesophageal reflux disease (GERD)
- Enlarged tonsils or adenoids
- Chronic respiratory tract conditions, such as:
  - Asthma
  - Allergies
  - Chronic bronchitis
  - Chronic obstructive pulmonary disease (COPD)

The following conditions may increase your risk of central sleep apnea:

- Bulbar poliomyelitis
- Encephalitis
- Neurodegenerative diseases
- Stroke
- Problems after cervical spine surgery
- Primary hypoventilation syndrome
- Brain tumors
- Down syndrome

Gender
Men are thought to be 2 to 4 times more likely to develop sleep apnea than women. However, some researchers have suggested that this difference may be because women are underdiagnosed with the condition.

Genetic Factors
Sleep apnea appears to run in certain families.

Ethnic Background
Sleep apnea is more common among:

- African Americans
- People of Mexican origin
- Pacific Islanders

Physical Characteristics
You have an increased risk of developing sleep apnea if you have the following physical characteristics:

- Thick neck
- Obstructed nasal passages
- Large tongue
- Narrow airway
- Receding chin
- Overbite
- Certain shapes and increased rigidity of the palate and jaw

You also have an increased risk of developing sleep apnea if you breathe through your mouth while sleeping, or if you snore.

—*Marcie L. Sidman, MD*

References
"Obstructive Sleep Apnea (OSA) in Adults." *DynaMed*, EBSCO Information Services, 5 Oct. 2016, www.dynamed.com/condition/obstructive-sleep-apnea-osa-in-adults.

"Sleep Apnea Information." *American Sleep Apnea Association*, 5 Apr. 2019, www.sleepapnea.org/learn/sleep-apnea/.

"Sleep Apnea Information Page." *National Institute of Neurological Disorders and Stroke*, National Institutes of Health, 27 Mar. 2019, www.ninds.nih.gov/Disorders/All-Disorders/Sleep-Apnea-Information-Page.

"Who Is at Risk for Sleep Apnea." *National Heart, Lung, and Blood Institute*, US Department of Health & Human Services, 10 Dec. 2018, www.nhlbi.nih.gov/health-topics/sleep-apnea.

■ Reducing your Risk of Sleep Apnea

There are a few things you can do to lower your risk of sleep apnea. These include:

Maintain an Appropriate Weight
Obesity is the main risk factor for sleep apnea. If you are overweight, you may be able to prevent sleep apnea by talking to your doctor about a weight loss program. If you're not overweight, try to maintain an appropriate weight through proper diet and exercise.

Limit Alcohol Intake
Drinking alcohol can increase the number of sleep apnea episodes you have each night. Therefore, limit your intake of alcohol.

Avoid Taking Sedative Medications
Sedative medications can worsen sleep apnea. Try to avoid using these medications.

Don't Smoke
Heavy smokers are more likely to develop sleep apnea than nonsmokers. If you smoke, talk to your doctor about how to quit.

Exercise Regularly
Regular exercise may decrease sleep apnea symptoms. Try to exercise at least 4 times a week for 30 minutes each time.
—*Marcie L. Sidman, MD*

References
"Obstructive Sleep Apnea (OSA) in Adults." *DynaMed*, EBSCO Information Services, 5 Oct. 2016, www.dynamed.com/condition/obstructive-sleep-apnea-osa-in-adults.

"Sleep Apnea Information Page." *National Institute of Neurological Disorders and Stroke*, National Institutes of Health, 27 Mar. 2019, www.ninds.nih.gov/Disorders/All-Disorders/Sleep-Apnea-Information-Page.

■ Symptoms of Sleep Apnea

The symptoms of sleep apnea when it's occurring may include:

- Very loud snoring
- Episodes of long pauses of interrupted breathing during sleep
- Possibly struggling, snorting, gasping, choking, and partially or completely awakening in an attempt to restart breathing

Symptoms that occur as a result of these episodes of sleep apnea may include:

- Disturbed rest
- Daytime sleepiness
- Problems staying alert or paying attention
- Irritability
- Poor memory
- Difficulty learning
- Decreased energy
- Headache
- Sexual problems
- Depression
- Anxiety
- Weight gain
- Hyperactivity in children
- Confusion

—*Marcie L. Sidman, MD*

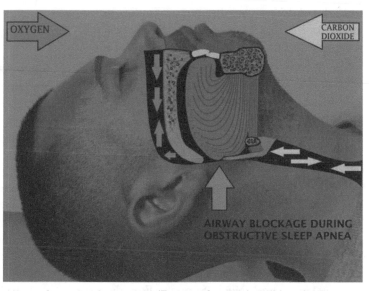

Airway obstruction during sleep. (Drcamachoent via Wikimedia Commons)

References

"Obstructive Sleep Apnea (OSA) in Adults." *DynaMed*, EBSCO Information Services, 5 Oct. 2016, www.dynamed.com/condition/obstructive-sleep-apnea-osa-in-adults.

"Pediatric Sleep-Disordered Breathing." *ENT Health*, American Academy of Otolaryngology–Head and Neck Surgery Foundation, Dec. 2018, www.enthealth.org/conditions/pediatric-sleep-disordered-breathing/. Accessed 16 Mar. 2020.

"Sleep Apnea Information Page." *National Institute of Neurological Disorders and Stroke*, National Institutes of Health, 27 Mar. 2019, www.ninds.nih.gov/Disorders/All-Disorders/Sleep-Apnea-Information-Page.

"What Are the Signs and Symptoms of Sleep Apnea." *National Heart, Lung, and Blood Institute*, US Department of Health & Human Services, 10 Dec. 2018, www.nhlbi.nih.gov/health-topics/sleep-apnea.

Screening for Sleep Apnea

The purpose of screening is early diagnosis and treatment. Screening tests are usually administered to people without current symptoms, but who may be at high risk for certain diseases or conditions.

Your doctor may give you a test, such as the Berlin Questionnaire or the Epworth Sleepiness Scale, to gain information about your symptoms. The American Academy of Pediatrics recommends that children are screened for sleep apnea by asking about snoring.

—*Marcie L. Sidman, MD*

References

"Obstructive Sleep Apnea (OSA) in Adults." *DynaMed*, EBSCO Information Services, 5 Oct. 2016, www.dynamed.com/condition/obstructive-sleep-apnea-osa-in-adults.

"Snoring, Sleeping Disorders, and Sleep Apnea." *ENT Health*, American Academy of Otolaryngology–Head and Neck Surgery Foundation, Aug. 2018, www.enthealth.org/conditions/snoring-sleeping-disorders-and-sleep-apnea/.

Lifestyle changes to manage Sleep Apnea

General Guidelines for Managing Sleep Apnea

Lose Weight

Obesity is a major risk factor for sleep apnea. If you're overweight, talk to your doctor about a reasonable weight loss goal and a safe weight loss program. As little as 10% weight loss can greatly reduce the number of sleep apnea episodes that occur each night.

Stop Using Alcohol and Sedative Medications

Alcohol and sedative medications are nervous system depressants. They affect the brain, causing it to function more slowly and less effectively. Using alcohol and/or sedatives will increase the frequency and number of sleep apnea episodes that occur each night. When you stop taking these products, your sleep apnea may improve.

Stop Smoking

If you smoke, talk to your doctor about ways to quit. Nicotine can worsen sleep apnea.

Exercise

There is evidence that exercise helps to improve sleep apnea even without weight loss. Talk to your doctor about which exercises are right for you.

Sleep on Your Side

Some people find that sleeping on one side, rather than sleeping on their backs or stomachs, greatly reduces sleep apnea. You can use a variety of pillows to comfortably prop yourself on your side.

—*Marcie L. Sidman, MD*

References

"How Is Sleep Apnea Treated." *National Heart, Lung, and Blood Institute*, US Department of Health & Human Services, 10 Dec. 2018, www.nhlbi.nih.gov/health-topics/sleep-apnea.

"Obstructive Sleep Apnea (OSA) in Adults." *DynaMed*, EBSCO Information Services, 5 Oct. 2016, www.dynamed.com/condition/obstructive-sleep-apnea-osa-in-adults.

"Sleep Apnea Information." *American Sleep Apnea Association*, 5 Apr. 2019, www.sleepapnea.org/learn/sleep-apnea/.

"Sleep Apnea Information Page." *National Institute of Neurological Disorders and Stroke*, National Institutes of Health, 27 Mar. 2019, www.ninds.nih.gov/Disorders/All-Disorders/Sleep-Apnea-Information-Page.

"Snoring, Sleeping Disorders, and Sleep Apnea." *ENT Health*, American Academy of Otolaryngology–Head and Neck Surgery Foundation, Aug. 2018, www.enthealth.org/conditions/snoring-sleeping-disorders-and-sleep-apnea/.

■ Surgical procedures for Sleep Apnea

Surgery may be considered if other treatments do not help. The goal of treatment is to remove or shift excess tissue in the airway. Surgical options include:

- Tonsillectomy for enlarged tonsils
- Removal of nasal polyps
- Surgery to straighten a deviated septum
- Correction of facial or jaw deformities
- Removal of tissue in the throat
- Palate implants

Success from the surgery can be different for person to person. Any surgery also has a chance of complications. You and your doctor will talk about risks and benefits of surgery for you. Some surgical options include:

Uvulopalatopharyngoplasty (UPPP)

UPPP will remove extra tissue from the back of the throat. This includes the tonsils and part of the soft palate.

Laser-assisted Uvulopalatoplasty (LAUP)

LAUP also removes extra tissue in the back of the throat. It is done with lasers. LAUP seems to help improve snoring. It's not clear what effect it may have on sleep apnea.

Radiofrequency Ablation

Extra tissue at the base of the tongue is removed. A tool uses radio waves to destroy tissue. It is done over a number of treatments. Snoring and decreased daytime sleepiness may decrease after ten treatments. It is more effective for snoring. It is not clear if it is effective as a treatment of sleep apnea.

Tracheostomy

Tracheostomy is a surgery that creates a new airway. An opening is made in the base of the throat. A tube will allow air to pass through this hole and into the lungs. It will bypass tissue in the back of the mouth and throat which causes the problem. This may be needed for severe apnea.

Pillar Palatal Implants

Implants can help to stiffen tissue at the back of the mouth. This may help keep tissue from falling into airway. It may be more effective for treating snoring than sleep apnea. It may help to reduce daytime sleepiness in those with sleep apnea.

—*Marcie L. Sidman, MD*

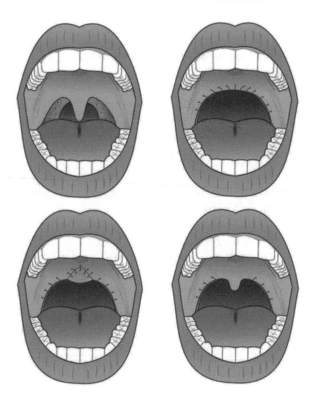

Uvulopalatopharyngoplasty. A) pre-operative, B) original UPPP, C) modified UPPP, and D) minimal UPPP. (Drcamachoent via Wikimedia Commons)

References

Costanzo, Maria Rosa, et al. "Transvenous Neuro-stimulation for Central Sleep Apnoea: A Randomised Controlled Trial." *The Lancet*, vol. 388, no. 10048, Sept. 2016, pp. 974–982, 10.1016/s0140-6736(16)30961-8.

"How Is Sleep Apnea Treated." *National Heart, Lung, and Blood Institute*, US Department of Health & Human Services, 10 Dec. 2018, www.nhlbi.nih.gov/health-topics/sleep-apnea.

"Obstructive Sleep Apnea (OSA) in Adults." *DynaMed*, EBSCO Information Services, 5 Oct. 2016, www.dynamed.com/condition/obstructive-sleep-apnea-osa-in-adults.

"Position Statement: Surgical Management of Obstructive Sleep Apnea." *American Academy of Otolaryngology-Head and Neck Surgery*, 20 Mar. 2014, www.entnet.org/content/surgical-management-obstructive-sleep-apnea.

■ Talking to your doctor about Sleep Apnea

General Tips for Gathering Information

You have a unique medical history. It is important to talk with your doctor about your personal risk factors and/or experience with sleep apnea. By talking openly and regularly with your doctor, you can take an active role in your care. Here are some tips that will make it easier for you to talk to your doctor:

- Bring someone else with you. It helps to have another person hear what is said and think of questions to ask.
- Write your questions ahead of time so you don't forget them.
- Write down the answers you get and make sure you understand what you are hearing. Ask for clarification, if necessary.

Don't be afraid to ask your questions or ask where you can find more information about what you are discussing. You have a right to know.

Specific Questions to Ask Your Doctor

About Sleep Apnea

- Could my daytime sleepiness be due to sleep apnea?

- How do I get tested for sleep apnea?
- Will I need to see a specialist?
- How can I or my sleep partner tell if I'm having apnea episodes?
- Is it safe for me to continue to drive?
- Is it safe for me to operate heavy machinery?
- Is it safe for me to continue to participate in my usual activities?
- Is sleep apnea the only reason for my symptoms?
- What else could be causing my fatigue?

About Your Risk of Developing Sleep Apnea

- Since I'm overweight, could I develop sleep apnea?
- Do I have any other risk factors for this condition?
- Are there other measures I can take to lower my risk?

About Treatment Options

- Are there any new trials of medications for sleep apnea that you would advise?
- Are there dental or orthodontic devices that might be helpful for my degree of sleep apnea?
- Is my condition severe enough that you would recommend surgery in order to avoid potential complications?
- What are the success rates of the different types of surgical interventions?

About Lifestyle Changes

- How much weight should I lose in order to reduce my risk of sleep apnea?
- Which weight loss program would you recommend?
- Are there pillow systems to help me sleep on my side?
- Should I discontinue using alcohol and sedatives?
- Can you recommend a program to help me quit smoking?

About Outlook

- What kinds of sleep apnea complications might I be at risk for?
- Does sleep apnea stay the same or worsen?

- How severe does sleep apnea have to be to produce serious complications?
- What signs of complications should I be alert for?

—*Marcie L. Sidman, MD*

References

"Getting the Most Out of Your Doctor Appointment." *FamilyDoctor.Org*, American Academy of Family Physicians, 19 Jan. 2018, familydoctor. org/tips-for-talking-to-your-doctor/.

"Obstructive Sleep Apnea (OSA) in Adults." *DynaMed*, EBSCO Information Services, 5 Oct. 2016, www.dynamed.com/condition/obstructive-sleep-apnea-osa-in-adults.

"Sleep Apnea Information Page." *National Institute of Neurological Disorders and Stroke*, National Institutes of Health, 27 Mar. 2019, www.ninds.nih. gov/Disorders/All-Disorders/Sleep-Apnea-Information-Page.

■ Resource guide for Sleep Apnea

American Sleep Apnea Association

641 S Street NW
3rd Floor
Washington, DC 20001-5196
1-888-293-3650
https://www.sleepapnea.org

This website provides a variety of materials discussing sleep apnea, including a brochure, a phone app,and many other educational materials. You can participate in the "Sleep Apnea Support Forum" and post questions about the condition and treatments.

National Heart, Lung, and Blood Institute

Building 31
31 Center Drive
Bethesda, MD 20892
301-592-8573
https://www.nhlbi.nih.gov

NHLBI provides fact sheets on sleep apnea and other sleep disorders, as well as heart, lung, and blood disorders. Look here for information on current areas of research, clinical trials seeking subjects, meetings and conferences, and a link to the organization's sister website, the National Center on Sleep Disorders Research (NCSDR).

National Sleep Foundation

https://sleepfoundation.org

Here you will find brochures, newsletters, and reports on narcolepsy and other sleep disorders; a long list of links to other websites with good information on sleep disorders; and information about sleep disorder specialists in your area.

American Academy of Otolaryngology—Head and Neck Surgery

1650 Diagonal Road
Alexandria, VA 22314
703-836-4444
http://www.entnet.org

The American Academy of Otolaryngology—Head and Neck Surgery (AAO-HNS) is the world's largest organization representing specialists who treat the ear, nose, throat, and related structures of the head and neck.

On this website, you can find newsletters, reports about obstructive sleep apnea and other sleep disorders, and a lengthy list of links to related websites.

■ Conditions In Depth: Type 2 Diabetes

Insulin is a hormone normally produced by the pancreas. Insulin helps your body convert food into energy. Without insulin, glucose (sugar) from food cannot enter cells, and glucose builds up in the blood. Your body tissues become starved for energy.

Type 2 diabetes is primarily a disorder in which the cells are not responding to the high levels of insulin circulating in the body. The body becomes increasingly resistant to insulin. As type 2 diabetes progresses, the over-worked beta cells of the pancreas start to make less insulin.

Type 2 diabetes occurs because either one or both of the following conditions exist:

- Fat, muscle, or liver cells do not respond to the high levels of insulin (called insulin resistance)
- Beta cells in the pancreas do not make enough insulin relative to the demands of the body

People older than age 45 years are at higher risk of developing this condition, but it can occur at any age—even during childhood. Excess weight and obesity is the primary cause of insulin resistance, and it increases the chance of developing type 2 diabetes.

If diabetes is left untreated, serious health complications can occur. These complications affect the eyes, heart, kidneys, blood and nerve supply, and immune system.

—*Kim Carmichael, MD*

References

"Diabetes Mellitus Type 2 in Adults." *DynaMed*, EBSCO Information Services, 29 Aug. 2016, www.dynamed.com/condition/diabetes-mellitus-type-2-in-adults.

"Type 2 Diabetes." *American Diabetes Association*, www.diabetes.org/diabetes/type-2?loc=DropDownDB-type2.

■ Risk factors for Type 2 Diabetes

It is possible to develop type 2 diabetes with or without the risk factors listed below. But, the more risk factors you have, the greater your likelihood of developing type 2 diabetes. If you have a number of risk factors, ask your doctor what you can do to reduce your risk.

Excess Weight and Obesity

Carrying excess weight, especially in the upper body and abdomen, increases your risk of type 2 diabetes. This is especially true for overweight young adults, people who have been overweight for a long time. But is it also true for middle-aged adults who gain weight.

There has been a marked increase in type 2 diabetes among overweight children. Until recently, this disease was rarely found in people under the age of 40. The development of type 2 diabetes is increasingly seen in overweight children.

Insulin is a hormone made in the body. It is needed to move glucose from the blood to body tissue. The tissues of overweight or obese people can become less sensitive to insulin. This is called insulin resistance. Insulin resistance can lead to diabetes and contribute significantly to many of its complications.

Sedentary Lifestyle and Poor Dietary Patterns

Type 2 diabetes is very common in the US. A major risk factor is the typical American or Westernized lifestyle, which is characterized by:

- Lack of physical activity
- Consumption of high-calorie, high-fat, high-carbohydrate foods and beverages, such as sugar-sweetened sodas and juices
- High intake of processed meats

Sleep Problems

Having sleep problems may put you at an increased risk for diabetes. Sleep problems include having difficulty falling asleep, having difficulty staying asleep, sleeping too long (over 9 hours), or not sleeping enough (less than 5 hours).

Conditions

Certain conditions that can increase the risk of developing type 2 diabetes include:

- Lipid disorders—low high-density lipoprotein (HDL) "good" cholesterol, high triglycerides levels
- High blood pressure
- Cardiovascular disease
- Gestational diabetes—or having had a baby weighing 9 pounds or more at birth
- Prediabetes—blood sugar level is higher than normal, but not high enough to meet the criteria for diabetes
- Nonalcoholic fatty liver disease
- Polycystic ovary syndrome or other condition associated with insulin resistance
- Drug-induced diabetes from taking certain medications

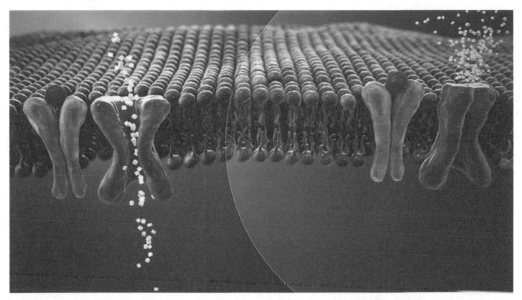

Mechanism of normal blood sugar absorption (left) vs. insulin resistance in type 2 diabetes (right). (Scientific Animations)

- Endocrine disorders—Cushing's syndrome, hyperthyroidism, or acute pancreatitis
- Genetic disorders—Down syndrome, porphyria, hemochromatosis,
- Turner syndrome,
- Klinefelter syndrome
- Depression

Age

If you are aged 45 or older, the American Diabetes Association (ADA) recommends screening. Regardless of age, though, if you are overweight and have other risk factors, then you should be screened for diabetes. Overweight children who are aged 10 or older should be screened, as well.

Ethnic Background

In the United States, people of the following ethnic groups are at greater risk of type 2 diabetes:

- African American
- Hispanic American
- Pima Indian
- Native American
- Asian American
- Pacific Islander

Many people in these groups have a lower risk of type 2 diabetes when they do not live in a Westernized culture.

Genetics

Having family members with type 2 diabetes increases your risk of developing the condition.

—*Kim Carmichael, MD*

References

American Diabetes Association. "Diagnosis and Classification of Diabetes Mellitus." *Diabetes Care,* vol. 33, no. Suppl 1, Jan. 2010, pp. S62–S69, 10.2337/dc10-s062.

"Diabetes Mellitus Type 2 in Adults." *DynaMed,* EBSCO Information Services, 29 Aug. 2016, www.dynamed.com/condition/diabetes-mellitus-type-2-in-adults.

Mantovani, Alessandro, et al. "Nonalcoholic Fatty Liver Disease and Risk of Incident Type 2 Diabetes: A Meta-Analysis." *Diabetes Care,* vol. 41, no. 2, 22 Jan. 2018, pp. 372–382, 10.2337/dc17-1902.

Shen, Hsiu-Nien, et al. "Risk of Diabetes Mellitus after First-Attack Acute Pancreatitis: A National Population-Based Study." *American Journal of Gastroenterology,* vol. 110, no. 12, Dec. 2015, pp. 1698–1706, 10.1038/ajg.2015.356.

"Statistics About Diabetes." *American Diabetes Association,* 22 Mar. 2018, www.diabetes.org/resources/statistics/statistics-about-diabetes.

■ Reducing your risk of developing Type 2 Diabetes

If you have been diagnosed with prediabetes or have risk factors for type 2 diabetes, there are steps you can take to lower your risk of developing the condition. These steps include:

Regular Exercise and Weight Loss

Insulin is a hormone produced in the body. It helps glucose move out of the blood and into body tissue for use as energy. Excess body weight makes your tissue less responsive to insulin. This can lead to high blood glucose levels. By losing weight, your body tissue will be more sensitive to insulin and will be better able to use insulin.

Regular exercise can help reduce your risk of type 2 diabetes in 2 ways:

- Exercise alone lowers blood glucose levels by making your cells more sensitive to insulin.
- Regular exercise will help you lose weight.

Heart disease is a common complication of diabetes. Regular exercise can help lower the levels of fat and cholesterol in your blood and lower your blood pressure. This will decrease your risk for heart disease.

Choose exercises that you enjoy. Make it part of your daily routine. Strive to maintain an exercise program that keeps you fit and at a healthy weight. The goal should be to exercise for at least 150 minutes/week. This should be moderate-intensity aerobic exercise, like brisk walking, riding a bicycle, playing tennis, or doing water aerobics. In addition, strength training should be done at least twice a week. Examples of strength training include using free weights, weight machines, or resistance bands.

Before you start any exercise program, talk to your doctor. It is important that you wear a diabetes identification bracelet when you exercise.

Too little sleep can contribute to weight gain. Aim for 7-8 hours of good sleep each night.

Dietary Changes

The American Diabetes Association (ADA) offers these guidelines for reducing your risk of developing diabetes:

- Eat a healthy diet that includes whole grains, fruits, vegetables, and low-fat dairy products.
- Reduce your intake of saturated fats (such as whole milk, cream, ice cream, meat).
- Eat a diet low in cholesterol.

If you want to change your eating habits, ask your doctor for a referral to a registered dietitian. A dietitian can help you create an individualized eating plan that includes all of the nutrients your body needs.

Medications

Medications commonly used to treat type 2 diabetes may also be prescribed to prevent the condition in people who are at high risk. Examples of these medications include:

- Metformin
- Pioglitazone
- Acarbose

—*Kim A. Carmichael, MD, FACP*

References

American Diabetes Association. "Executive Summary: Standards of Medical Care in Diabetes–2010." *Diabetes Care,* vol. 33, no. Suppl 1, Jan. 2010, pp. S4–S10, 10.2337/dc10-s004.

—. "Standards of Medical Care in Diabetes–2010." *Diabetes Care,* vol. 33, no. Suppl 1, Jan. 2010, pp. S11–S61, 10.2337/dc10-s011.

Carter, P., et al. "Fruit and Vegetable Intake and Incidence of Type 2 Diabetes Mellitus: Systematic Review and Meta-Analysis." *BMJ,* vol. 341, no. aug18 4, 19 Aug. 2010, pp. c4229–c4229, www.bmj.com/content/341/bmj.c4229, 10.1136/bmj.c4229.

Crandall, Jill P, et al. "Alcohol Consumption and Diabetes Risk in the Diabetes Prevention Program." *The American Journal of Clinical Nutrition,* vol. 90, no. 3, 29 July 2009, pp. 595–601, 10.3945/ajcn.2008.27382.

"Diabetes Mellitus Type 2 in Adults." *DynaMed,* EBSCO Information Services, 29 Aug. 2016, www.dynamed.com/condition/diabetes-mellitus-type-2-in-adults.

DREAM (Diabetes REduction Assessment with ramipril and rosiglitazone Medication) Trial Investigators. "Effect of Rosiglitazone on the Frequency of Diabetes in Patients with Impaired Glucose Tolerance or Impaired Fasting Glucose: A Randomised Controlled Trial." *The Lancet*, vol. 368, no. 9541, Sept. 2006, pp. 1096–1105, 10.1016/s0140-6736(06)69420-8.

"Evidence-Based Nutrition Principles and Recommendations for the Treatment and Prevention of Diabetes and Related Complications." *Diabetes Care*, vol. 25, no. Suppl1, 1 Jan. 2002, pp. S50–S60, doi: 10.2337/diacare.25.2007.s50.

Lindström, Jaana, et al. "Sustained Reduction in the Incidence of Type 2 Diabetes by Lifestyle Intervention: Follow-up of the Finnish Diabetes Prevention Study." *The Lancet*, vol. 368, no. 9548, Nov. 2006, pp. 1673–1679, 10.1016/s0140-6736(06)69701-8.

"Measuring Physical Activity Intensity." *Centers for Disease Control and Prevention*, 29 Jan. 2020, www.cdc.gov/physicalactivity/basics/measuring/index.html.

Phung, O. J., et al. "Oral Anti-Diabetic Drugs for the Prevention of Type 2 Diabetes." *Diabetic Medicine*, vol. 28, no. 8, 13 July 2011, pp. 948–964, 10.1111/j.1464-5491.2011.03303.x.

"Prediabetes." *American Diabetes Association*, 2019, www.diabetes.org/diabetes-risk/prediabetes.

Salas-Salvado, J., et al. "Reduction in the Incidence of Type 2 Diabetes With the Mediterranean Diet: Results of the PREDIMED-Reus Nutrition Intervention Randomized Trial." *Diabetes Care*, vol. 34, no. 1, 7 Oct. 2010, pp. 14–19, 10.2337/dc10-1288.

■ Symptoms of Type 2 Diabetes

You may have type 2 diabetes for years before you start to have symptoms. Symptoms may be difficult to notice if they are mild. High blood glucose levels may cause the symptoms, or they may be due to complications from diabetes. Symptoms may include:

- Weight loss
- Increased urination
- Increased thirst
- Increased hunger
- Fatigue
- Lightheadedness while standing
- Blurry vision
- Irritability
- Frequent or recurring infections
- Slow wound healing
- Foot ulcers
- Numbness or tingling in the hands or feet
- Problems with gums and teeth
- Itching

—Kim Carmichael, MD, FACP

References

"Diabetes Mellitus Type 2 in Adults." *DynaMed*, EBSCO Information Services, 29 Aug. 2016, www.dynamed.com/condition/diabetes-mellitus-type-2-in-adults.

"Type 2 Diabetes." *American Diabetes Association*, www.diabetes.org/diabetes/type-2?loc=DropDownDB-type2.

"Types of Diabetes." *National Institute of Diabetes and Digestive and Kidney Diseases*, US Department of Health & Human Services, 11 Nov. 2019, www.niddk.nih.gov/health-information/diabetes/overview/what-is-diabetes#types.

■ Screening for Type 2 Diabetes

Finding diabetes can help to decrease complications. It may also find a condition called prediabetes. This is a blood glucose level that is high but not yet diabetes. It will often move on to type 2 diabetes. Finding it early may help to prevent diabetes from starting.

Screening tests are given to people who may be at high risk.

Screening Guidelines

American Diabetes Association (ADA) recommends screening for prediabetes and type 2 diabetes in the following:

- Adults who are overweight or obese with one or more of these risk factors:
  - First-degree relative with diabetes

- High-risk group (African American, Latino, Native American, Hispanic American, Asian American, or Pacific Islander)
- History of cardiovascular disease
- High blood pressure
- Low high-density lipoprotein (HDL) (good) cholesterol level and high triglycerides levels
- Polycystic ovary syndrome
- Inactive lifestyle
- Other conditions that can cause insulin resistance such as severe obesity, acanthosis nigricans

- Women who have had gestational diabetes
- Adults aged 45 and older with or without risk factors
- Overweight children over 10 years old (or after puberty starts) with 1 or more of these risk factors:
  - High body mass index (BMI) based on child's weight and height
  - Family history of any type of diabetes, including during pregnancy
  - Signs of insulin resistance or having a condition associated with insulin resistance

At-risk ethnic background

Screening may be repeated again in 3 years.

Screening Tests

HbA1c Test

The HbA1c test is a good indicator of your average blood glucose levels over the past 2-4 months. This test usually does not require any dietary restrictions.

Fasting Plasma Glucose

With this blood test, you need to fast (not eat anything) for at least 8 hours before the test.

Two-Hour Oral Glucose Tolerance Test

After fasting overnight, the doctor tests your glucose level. You are then asked to drink 75 grams of glucose dissolved in water. Two hours later, the doctor tests your glucose level again.

—*James P. Cornell, MD*

References

American Diabetes Association. "Classification and Diagnosis of Diabetes: Standards of Medical Care in Diabetes—2019." *Diabetes Care*, vol. 42, no. Suppl 1, 17 Dec. 2018, pp. S13–S28, 10.2337/dc19-s002.

—. "Standards of Medical Care in Diabetes—2018." *Diabetes Care*, vol. 41, no. Suppl 1, Jan. 2018, pp. S1–S172.

"Diabetes Mellitus Type 2 in Adults." *DynaMed*, EBSCO Information Services, 29 Aug. 2016, www.dynamed.com/condition/diabetes-mellitus-type-2-in-adults.

"Prediabetes." *DynaMed*, EBSCO Information Services, 16 Nov. 2018, www.dynamed.com/condition/prediabetes.

■ Medications for Type 2 Diabetes

The information provided here is meant to give you a general idea about each of the medications listed below. Only the most general side effects are included. Ask your doctor if you need to take any special precautions. Use each of these medications only as recommended by your doctor, and according to the instructions provided. If you have further questions about usage or side effects, contact your doctor.

Some people are able to manage type 2 diabetes with diet and exercise alone. But, in many cases, medications are added to this treatment plan to help you control your blood glucose (sugar) levels.

Anti-diabetes medications that are taken by mouth, often referred to as oral agents, are used to treat type 2 diabetes. They lower blood glucose levels in a variety of ways. Since each class works differently, these medications may be used in combination. All of these drugs work best when they are part of a total treatment program that includes healthy eating and regular exercise.

Despite diet, exercise, and oral medications, some people with long-standing type 2 diabetes may need to take insulin or other medications to control their glucose levels.

Prescription Medications

Biguanides

Metformin

Metformin works in the liver to make it produce less glucose and make your body more sensitive to insulin. Metformin can also lower blood fat levels and possibly lead to minor weight loss, which can ultimately help with blood glucose control.

Metformin is usually taken 1-2 times a day with meals. Metformin does not cause the body to make more insulin. When it is used alone, it rarely causes hypoglycemia (low blood glucose levels). However, when combined with other diabetes drugs, it can cause hypoglycemia.

Special Considerations

Tell your doctor if you drink more than 2-4 alcoholic drinks a week, since metformin is poorly tolerated with alcohol. Also, if you are having surgery or a test that requires contrast dye for scans, make sure the doctor knows you are taking metformin. The medication will need to be stopped temporarily.

Sulfonylurea Drugs

Sulfonylurea drugs stimulate the beta cells in the pancreas to make more insulin. They also help your body's cells use insulin better.

These medications are generally taken 1-2 times per day, 30 minutes before a meal. This medication should always be taken with food. This is to reduce the risk of developing hypoglycemia.

All sulfonylureas have similar effects on your blood glucose level, but they may have different side effects. Based on the results of your blood glucose monitoring, your doctor will work with you to adjust your dosage. Talk to your doctor about which side effects you should watch for.

Common names include:
Chlorpropamide
Glipizide
Glyburide
Glimepiride
Tolazamide
Tolbutamide

Special Considerations

Sulfonylurea drugs help to control your blood glucose by stimulating the production and the release of insulin. Therefore, there is the chance that they can cause hypoglycemia. Be sure to talk with your doctor and a registered dietitian about balancing the amount of food you eat with the amount of medication you take to help reduce the risk of hypoglycemia.

Some of these drugs may cause negative effects if taken with alcohol. Chlorpropamide is the most common drug to cause these effects, which includes vomiting and flushing.

Sulfonylurea drugs can also increase the risk of heart attack and heart failure. Talk to your doctor about your individual risk factors for heart disease.

Meglitinides

Like sulfonylureas, these medications help the pancreas produce more insulin. However, it works faster than sulfonylureas, allowing for more flexible timing of doses and meals.

Also like sulfonylureas, these medications can increase the risk of hypoglycemia. So, you should talk with your doctor and/or a registered dietitian about balancing the amount of food you eat with the amount of medication you take. This will help to reduce the risk of hypoglycemia. Repaglinide is usually taken 2-4 times a day, within 15-30 minutes before each meal.

Common names include:
Repaglinide
Nateglinide

Thiazolidinediones

These medications are also called insulin sensitizers because they make the cells in your body more sensitive to or better able to use insulin. Specifically, they work in the muscle and fat cells. They may also help decrease the amount of glucose released by the liver.

These drugs do not cause the body to make more insulin. Therefore, when they are used alone, they rarely cause hypoglycemia. Pioglitazone has an added benefit of improving cholesterol levels.

When combined with other diabetes drugs, thiazolidinediones may cause hypoglycemia.

This type of medication is usually prescribed once per day. It may be taken with or without food, at about the same time each day.

Common names include:

Rosiglitazone

Pioglitazone

Special Considerations

- In rare cases, thiazolidinediones can harm your liver. Therefore, your doctor will regularly monitor your liver function with blood tests when you are taking one of these drugs.
- This group of medications can increase your risk of edema and heart failure.
- This group of medications may also increase the risk of fractures in women.
- Pioglitazone may increase your risk of bladder cancer.

Alpha-glucosidase Inhibitors

These medications are also called starch blockers because they slow down the digestion of carbohydrates (starches and sugars), which are the major food sources of glucose. This slow-down in digestion leads to a slow-down in absorption, and therefore, a slower increase in blood glucose after a meal. When used alone, alpha-glucosidase inhibitors do not cause hypoglycemia. However, when combined with other diabetes drugs, they may cause this side effect.

Alpha-glucosidase inhibitors should be taken with the first bite of each main meal. When you initially start this medication, your doctor may have you take it less frequently. You will build up the dose over time as your body adjusts to the medication.

Common names include:

Acarbose

Miglitol

Special Considerations

Table sugar (sucrose) is not effective at treating hypoglycemia when you are taking these drugs because alpha-glucosidase inhibitors slow the digestion of sucrose. If symptoms of hypoglycemia occur while you are taking one of these medications, glucose tablets should be used to treat it.

Dipeptidyl Peptidase-4 (DPP-4) Inhibitors

DPP-4 inhibitors lengthen the activity of certain proteins, which increase the release of insulin after your blood glucose level rises with a meal. The medication does this by blocking a specific enzyme (DPP-4), which is responsible for breaking down these proteins. These drugs can enhance your body's own ability to reduce the elevated blood glucose levels.

This class of medication is meant to be used together with diet and exercise to help improve the blood glucose levels. It can be used alone or added to other commonly prescribed oral antidiabetic drugs.

Common names include:

Sitagliptin

Vildagliptin

Saxagliptin

Linagliptin

Glucagon-like Peptide-1 Receptor Agonist

After eating a meal, a hormone called glucagon-like peptide-1 (GLP-1) is produced in the stomach and intestines. This hormone leads to insulin being released from the beta cells in the pancreas.

GLP-1 agonists are meant to be used in people with type 2 diabetes whose blood glucose is not controlled with oral anti-diabetes medications. There is also a concern that some of these agents may increase the risk of developing a rare type of thyroid tumor (medullary cancer) in certain people Discuss this with your doctor.

Common names include:	*Possible side effects include:*
Exenatide	Low blood glucose
Liraglutide	Headache
	Nausea, vomiting
	Diarrhea
	Irritation where the shot is given

Pramlintide

Pramlintide Amylin is a hormone produced by the same beta cells which produce insulin. Amylin is released at the same time as insulin. Moreover, amylin reduces glucagon's release and enhances the sense of fullness after eating a meal. Together with insulin, amylin helps lower the blood glucose level. Pramlintide is chemically related to amylin. And like amylin, Pramlintide reduces appetite, and its use has been associated with weight loss.

Pramlintide is used together with insulin in people who fail to achieve the desired blood glucose levels despite getting the optimal doses of insulin. This drug is given by injection immediately before a meal. The elderly should use this drug with special care.

Sodium-Glucose Co-Transporter 2 (SGLT-2) Inhibitors

SGLT-2 inhibitors are oral medications that block the reabsorption of glucose in the kidneys. This means more glucose is passed in the urine.

Possible side effects include:

High blood pressure
Kidney problems
Hypoglycemia
Increased risk of genital fungal infections
Increased low-density lipoprotein (LDL) cholesterol

Bile Acid Binders

Colesevelam is an oral medication. The medication binds to food in the intestines and blocks it from being absorbed into the body. It is used with other antidiabetes drugs, and with diet and exercise. It is not recommended in people with a history of bowel obstruction, high triglycerides, or pancreatitis caused by high triglycerides.

Common name:	Possible side effects include:
Colesevelam	Constipation
	Cold symptoms, including stuffy nose or sore throat
	Indigestion
	Hypoglycemia
	Nausea
	High blood pressure

Dopamine Agonists

Dopamine agonists reduce the amount of prolactin in the bloodstream by blocking the release of prolactin from the pituitary gland. It has also been shown to reduce blood glucose leves in people with diabetes.

It is used in the treatment of pituitary and endocrine disorders. It is not recommended in people who have uncontrolled high blood pressure, women who are breastfeeding, or those who experience fainting with migraine headaches. Talk to your doctor if you have liver or kidney problems.

Common name:	Possible side effects include:
Bromocriptine	Nausea, vomiting
	Low blood pressure, which can lead to lightheadedness and fainting
	Headaches
	Raynaud's phenomenon
	Daytime sleepiness

Insulin

In almost all patients with type 2 diabetes, the pancreas eventually no longer makes enough insulin for the body. To help control your diabetes, you may need to inject insulin. Insulin must be taken as an injection. If it were taken by mouth, it would be digested by the stomach before it reached your bloodstream where it needs to do its work.

To work properly, the amount of insulin you use must be balanced with the amount and type of food you eat, the amount of exercise you do, and the other diabetes medications you are taking.

If you change your eating habits, your exercise, or both without changing your insulin dose, your blood glucose level can drop too low or rise too

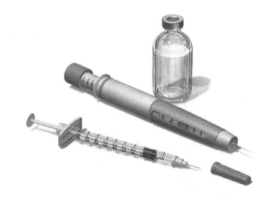

Insulin syringe and pen. (BruceBlaus)

high. Current insulin treatment regimens usually employ some combination of rapid-acting and long- or very long-acting insulin.

All About Insulin

The 3 characteristics of insulin are:

- Onset—the length of time it takes for the insulin to reach the bloodstream and begin lowering blood glucose after it is injected
- Peak time—the time during which insulin is at its maximum strength in terms of lowering blood glucose levels
- Duration—how long the insulin continues to lower blood glucose

The main types of insulin available are:

Type of insulin	Description
Rapid-acting	This type of insulin works in about 5 minutes. It reaches its peak in about 1 hour and lasts for 2-4 hours.
Regular- or Short-acting	This type of insulin works in about 30 minutes. It reaches its peak in about 2-3 hours and lasts about 3-6 hours.
Intermediate-acting	This type of insulin works in about 2-4 hours. It reaches its peak in about 4-12 hours and lasts about 12-18 hours.
Long-acting	This type of insulin works in about 6-10 hours and lasts for about 20-24 hours.

Insulin can also come in premixed forms, which combine intermediate-acting insulin with rapid- or short-acting insulin.

Methods of Insulin Delivery

There are several different ways of getting insulin into your body by injection. Some examples are:

- Syringe—The syringes you will use are small and have fine needles with special coatings that help to make injecting as easy and painless as possible. When insulin injections are done properly, most people find that they are relatively painless.

- Pen—The insulin pen looks very much like an old-fashioned cartridge pen, except that it has a needle and holds a cartridge of insulin. Pens are particularly useful for people who are often on the go or who have poor coordination. The majority of pens are disposable.
- Pump—This is a small computerized device that you wear on your belt or in your pocket. It delivers a steady, measured dose of insulin through a flexible plastic tube called a cannula. With the aid of a small needle, the cannula is inserted through the skin into the fatty tissue and is taped in place. In some products, the needle is removed and only a soft catheter remains in place. Because the pump continuously releases tiny doses of insulin, this delivery system most closely mimics the body's normal release of insulin.

Note:

- Check your insulin's expiration date. If you haven't finished it before then, throw the rest away.
- Store unopened bottles of insulin in the refrigerator. Do not store your insulin at extreme temperatures.
- Keep the bottle of insulin you are using at room temperature. Injecting cold insulin can sometimes make the injection more painful. (Most pharmacists believe that insulin kept at room temperature will last for about one month.)

When to Contact Your Doctor

Diabetes pills do not work for everyone. Also, they may become less effective after a few months or years. Until you are well accustomed to your medications, be sure to monitor your blood glucose levels regularly and record the information to tell your doctor. This will help you and your doctor recognize if your pills are not working properly and if you need a change in dosage or even treatment. Report any low blood sugars or symptoms of hypoglycemia to your doctor immediately.

When you start taking diabetes medications, they may cause some side effects. (Each drug can cause different effects, so ask your doctor what to expect from your drug regimen.) However, many of these effects go away as your body adjusts to the medication. If side effects persist, tell your doctor.

Once your diabetes is under adequate control on oral medications, it may not be necessary to continue monitoring your blood sugar levels on a regular basis. Type 2 diabetes (when not taking insulin) can be adequately managed by using another test called glycosylated hemoglobin or hemoglobin A1c (HbA1c), which is done in a doctor's office. Unlike blood sugar levels, HbA1c has the advantage of measuring average blood glucose levels over the last 3-month period, which marks the effectiveness of diabetes management over the long-term. Most people with diabetes are recommended to keep their HbA1c levels below 7% to avoid or delay diabetic complications. But individual goals may vary.

Special Considerations

If you are taking medications, follow these general guidelines:

- Take the medication as directed. Do not change the amount or the schedule.
- Ask what side effects could occur. Report them to your doctor.\Talk to your doctor before you stop taking any prescription medication.
- Plan ahead for refills if you need them.
- Do not share your prescription medication with anyone.
- Medications can be dangerous when mixed. Talk to your doctor if you are taking more than one medication, including over-the-counter products and supplements.

—*Kim A. Carmichael, MD, FACP*

References

American Diabetes Association. "Executive Summary: Standards of Medical Care in Diabetes–2010." *Diabetes Care,* vol. 33, no. Suppl 1, Jan. 2010, pp. S4–S10, 10.2337/dc10-s004.

——. "Standards of Medical Care in Diabetes–2010." *Diabetes Care,* vol. 33, no. Suppl 1, Jan. 2010, pp. S11–S61, 10.2337/dc10-s011.

Bode, B. W., et al. "Patient-Reported Outcomes Following Treatment with the Human GLP-1 Analogue Liraglutide or Glimepiride in Monotherapy: Results from a Randomized Controlled Trial in Patients with Type 2 Diabetes." *Diabetes, Obesity and Metabolism,* vol. 12, no. 7, 7 Jan. 2010, pp. 604–612, 10.1111/j.1463-1326.2010.01196.x.

Bohannon, Nancy. "Overview of the Gliptin Class (Dipeptidyl Peptidase-4 Inhibitors) in Clinical Practice." *Postgraduate Medicine,* vol. 121, no. 1, Jan. 2009, pp. 40–45, 10.3810/pgm.2009.01.1953.

"Colesevelam." *DynaMed,* EBSCO Information Services, 6 Sept. 2016, www.dynamed.com/drug-monograph/colesevelam.

"Diabetes Mellitus Type 2 in Adults." *DynaMed,* EBSCO Information Services, 29 Aug. 2016, www.dynamed.com/condition/diabetes-mellitus-type-2-in-adults.

"Exenatide." *DynaMed,* EBSCO Information Services, 6 Sept. 2016, www.dynamed.com/drug-monograph/exenatide.

Farmer, Andrew, et al. "Impact of Self Monitoring of Blood Glucose in the Management of Patients with Non-Insulin Treated Diabetes: Open Parallel Group Randomised Trial." *BMJ,* vol. 335, no. 7611, 25 June 2007, p. 132, 10.1136/bmj.39247.447431.be.

"Insulin Basics." *American Diabetes Association,* 16 July 2015, www.diabetes.org/diabetes/medication-management/insulin-other-injectables/insulin-basics.

"Insulin, Medicines, & Other Diabetes Treatments." *National Institute of Diabetes and Digestive and Kidney Diseases,* US Department of Health & Human Services, Dec. 2016, www.niddk.nih.gov/health-information/diabetes/overview/insulin-medicines-treatments?dkrd=hiscr0023.

"Invokana." *DailyMed,* US National Library of Medicine, 4 Aug. 2016, dailymed.nlm.nih.gov/dailymed/search.cfm?labeltype=all&query=Invokana.

"Liraglutide." *DynaMed,* EBSCO Information Services, 27 Sept. 2016, www.dynamed.com/drug-monograph/liraglutide.

Loke, Y. K., et al. "Long-Term Use of Thiazolidinediones and Fractures in Type 2 Diabetes: A Meta-Analysis." *Canadian Medical Association Journal,* vol. 180, no. 1, 6 Jan. 2009, pp. 32–39, 10.1503/cmaj.080486.

Nissen, Steven E., and Kathy Wolski. "Effect of Rosiglitazone on the Risk of Myocardial Infarction and Death from Cardiovascular Causes." *New*

England Journal of Medicine, vol. 356, no. 24, 14 June 2007, pp. 2457–2471, 10.1056/nejmoa072761.

"Sitagliptin." *DynaMed*, EBSCO Information Services, 27 Sept. 2016, www.dynamed.com/drug-monograph/sitagliptin.

Traina, Andrea N., and Michael P. Kane. "Primer on Pramlintide, an Amylin Analog." *The Diabetes Educator*, vol. 37, no. 3, 6 Apr. 2011, pp. 426–431, 10.1177/0145721711403011.

Tzoulaki, I., et al. "Risk of Cardiovascular Disease and All Cause Mortality among Patients with Type 2 Diabetes Prescribed Oral Antidiabetes Drugs: Retrospective Cohort Study Using UK General Practice Research Database." *BMJ*, vol. 339, no. dec03 1, 3 Dec. 2009, pp. b4731–b4731, 10.1136/bmj.b4731.

Lifestyle changes to manage Type 2 Diabetes

Losing weight and beginning a regular exercise program can help bring your blood glucose levels to within the normal range. However, this does not mean that your diabetes has been cured. Rather, you must maintain these lifestyle habits, including eating healthy foods, to keep your blood glucose in control and to minimize the chances of complications.

Diet and exercise alone may not be enough to maintain blood glucose levels within a normal range. You may need to take anti-diabetes medications, including insulin, to control glucose levels.

Weight Loss
Weight loss is the first step you can take to help lower your blood glucose level. As you lose weight, your body's cells will be more responsive to insulin. This can lead to improved blood glucose control.

The safest and most effective way to lose weight is by eating fewer calories, eating healthy food, and exercising regularly. You should strive for gradual and continual weight loss until you reach your ideal weight. If you are overweight, losing just 5%-10% of your body weight can make a difference in your blood glucose control.

Diet
The nutrition guidelines for managing diabetes can seem complicated. However, you will see that the guidelines are similar as those for general good health. A registered dietitian can help you develop healthy eating patterns that will work for you. Ask your doctor for a referral to a registered dietitian. The basic eating guidelines for people with type 2 diabetes are:

Planning Meals and Snacks
Eat 3meals per day, and do not skip meals. Each meal should be at about the same time each day and contain about the same amount of carbohydrate, protein, and fat as the same meal the day before. Your blood glucose rises and falls in response to your eating patterns. Therefore, by eating about the same amounts and types of food at the same times each day, you can more easily predict when your blood glucose level will rise.

Snacks are also important. Eat 2-3 snacks per day, and keep them with you at all times in case a meal is delayed. Just before bedtime, have a snack that contains both protein and starch. Eating at this time can help control the changes in blood glucose that may occur while you sleep.

Filling Your Plate
To make sure that you are getting the nutrients that you need, follow the US Department of Agriculture's ChooseMyPlate guidelines. MyPlate encourages you to:

- Fill half of your plate with fruits and vegetables.
- Eat whole grains, lean protein, and fat-free or low-fat dairy products.
- Watch your portion size! Avoid overeating.
- Choose low-sodium foods.
- Opt for water instead of sugary drinks.

In addition, the American Diabetes Association (ADA) offers these tips for creating a healthy plate:

- Give yourself a larger amount of non-starchy vegetables. There are many kinds to choose from like spinach, carrots, broccoli, cucumbers, mushrooms, and peppers.
- Add a small serving of starchy foods. Some examples include: whole grain bread, rice, cooked beans, peas, corn and potatoes.

- Add a small serving of meat or meat substitute (such as chicken, fish, shrimp, tofu).
- Drink a glass of fat-free milk with your meal.

Focusing on Carbohydrates

Sugar and starch are both carbohydrates. Your body reacts to any type of carbohydrate in the same way, so the total amount of carbohydrate you eat is more important for blood glucose control than the source.

A dietitian can help you determine how many grams of carbohydrate you should eat per day. This amount should be dispersed evenly throughout your meals and snacks, and you may need to avoid foods that are high in sugar. Many foods contain carbohydrates. Grain products, fruits, and milk products contain the most. Soda has a lot of sugars and should be avoided.

Keeping a Record

Keep a record of your meals, include the time you ate, what you ate, and how much you ate. Include this information with your blood glucose levels and insulin dosages. This information is very helpful when you discuss how to modify your medication and/or diet with your doctor.

Exercise

The ADA recommends exercising for at least 150 minutes a week. This should be moderate-intensity aerobic exercise, like brisk walking, riding a bicycle, playing tennis, or doing water aerobics. In addition, strength training should be done at least twice a week. Examples of strength training include using free weights, weight machines, or resistance bands.

Talk with your doctor about an exercise program that is safe for you. Since exercise usually causes your blood glucose to drop, you may need to make some modifications in your medication dose and schedule, as well as your eating plan. Also, when you exercise, remember to wear your diabetes identification bracelet.

When to Contact Your Doctor

Contact your doctor if you:

- Are having difficulty losing weight
- Have any questions about your eating plan

- Feel that your eating plan is too difficult to follow
- Want to start an exercise program or make significant changes in your present program
- Have any symptoms of hypoglycemia after exercising
  - Shakiness
  - Lightheadedness
  - Extreme sweating<
  - Hunger
  - Headache
  - Pale skin color

—Kim A. Carmichael, MD, FACP

References

Christian, James G. "Clinic-Based Support to Help Overweight Patients With Type 2 Diabetes Increase Physical Activity and Lose Weight." *Archives of Internal Medicine*, vol. 168, no. 2, 28 Jan. 2008, p. 141, 10.1001/archinternmed.2007.13.

Davies, M J, et al. "Effectiveness of the Diabetes Education and Self Management for Ongoing and Newly Diagnosed (DESMOND) Programme for People with Newly Diagnosed Type 2 Diabetes: Cluster Randomised Controlled Trial." *BMJ*, vol. 336, no. 7642, 14 Feb. 2008, pp. 491–495, 10.1136/bmj.39474.922025.be.

"Diabetes Mellitus Type 2 in Adults." *DynaMed*, EBSCO Information Services, 29 Aug. 2016, www.dynamed.com/condition/diabetes-mellitus-type-2-in-adults.

Li, Tricia Y., et al. "Regular Consumption of Nuts Is Associated with a Lower Risk of Cardiovascular Disease in Women with Type 2 Diabetes." *The Journal of Nutrition*, vol. 139, no. 7, 6 May 2009, pp. 1333–1338, 10.3945/jn.108.103622.

Loimaala, Antti, et al. "Effect of Long-Term Endurance and Strength Training on Metabolic Control and Arterial Elasticity in Patients With Type 2 Diabetes Mellitus." *The American Journal of Cardiology*, vol. 103, no. 7, Apr. 2009, pp. 972–977, 10.1016/j.amjcard.2008.12.026.

"Nutrition Overview." *American Diabetes Association*, 2019, www.diabetes.org/nutrition.

"What Is MyPlate." *Choose MyPlate*, US Department of Agriculture, 7 Jan. 2016, www.choosemyplate.gov/.

■ Talking to your doctor about Type 2 Diabetes

General Tips for Gathering Information

You have a unique medical history. Therefore, it is essential to talk with your doctor about your personal risk factors and/or experience with type 2 diabetes. By talking openly and regularly with your doctor, you can take an active role in your care. Here are some tips that will make it easier for you to talk to your doctor:

- Bring someone else with you. It helps to have another person hear what is said and think of questions to ask.
- Write out your questions ahead of time, so you do not forget them.
- Write down the answers you get, and make sure you understand what you are hearing. Ask for clarification, if necessary.
- Don't be afraid to ask your questions or ask where you can find more information about what you are discussing. You have a right to know.

You'll likely have many questions about diabetes, and it is important to discuss them with your doctor. Here are some questions to get you started.

Specific Questions to Ask Your Doctor

About Your Risk of Developing Type 2 Diabetes

- Based on my medical history, lifestyle, and family background, am I at risk for type 2 diabetes?
- Are there changes I can make to reduce my risk?
- Are other people in my family at risk, as well?

About Type 2 Diabetes

- What caused my diabetes?
- Which of the complications am I at risk for?
- What is the difference between type 1 and type 2 diabetes?
- What are realistic and healthy blood glucose and HbA1c levels for me?

About Treatment Options

- Will I need to take medication?
- What medication is best for me?
- What benefits and side effects should I watch for from this medication?
- Will I need to take insulin?
- What type of insulin will I use?
- How do I inject the insulin?
- Are insulin injections painful?
- Is an insulin pen or pump appropriate for me?
- How can I discreetly inject insulin when I am in public places or social situations?
- What about using insulin when I travel?
- How do I adjust my medications for changes in eating and exercise?
- Are there any complementary or alternative therapies I can try?

About Monitoring

- How do I use the blood glucose monitor and how often should I use it?
- What does the HbA1c level mean?
- When was the last time I had my HbA1c levels measured?
  - What were the results and what do they mean?
  - How often should I have this test?
- When was the last time I had a lipid profile done?
  - What were the results and what do they mean?
  - How often should I have this test?
- How can I reduce my risk of complications?
- How often should I be checked for complications?
- Can you refer me to specialists to help prevent and/or manage some of the complications?
- Are there any problems with my feet?
- What should I do to prevent problems with my feet?
- Are there any problems with my eyes?
- What should I do to prevent problems with my eyes?
- What is my blood pressure? How often should I have it checked?

About Lifestyle Changes
- How do I go about losing weight?
- How can I improve my health?
- Can you refer me to a registered dietitian to help me plan my meals?
- Can I still eat sweets? How do I fit them into my meal plan?
- Can I drink alcohol?
- Do I have to eat differently than the rest of my family?
- How can I eat when I go out to restaurants?
- Can you recommend some cookbooks for people with diabetes?
- Can I continue to or begin to exercise?
- What type of exercise is best for me?
- When should I not exercise?
- Are there classes or programs that can help me make these lifestyle changes?

About Your Outlook
- Can you recommend some diabetes support groups for me and for my family?
- What can I tell my husband, children, parents, and other family members and friends about my condition?
- How often will I need checkups?
- What is my expected prognosis?

—Kim Carmichael, MD, FACP

References
"Diabetes Mellitus Type 2 in Adults." *DynaMed*, EBSCO Information Services, 29 Aug. 2016, www.dynamed.com/condition/diabetes-mellitus-type-2-in-adults.

"Getting the Most Out of Your Doctor Appointment." *FamilyDoctor.Org*, American Academy of Family Physicians, 19 Jan. 2018, familydoctor.org/tips-for-talking-to-your-doctor/.

"Type 2 Diabetes." *American Diabetes Association*, www.diabetes.org/diabetes/type-2?loc=DropDownDB-type2.

■ Resource guide for Type 2 Diabetes

American Diabetes Association
2451 Crystal Drive
Suite 900
Alexandria, VA 22202
1-800-342-2383
http://www.diabetes.org

This site is a comprehensive resource for people with diabetes and healthcare professionals alike. You'll learn the details of the disease, from diagnosis to complications, as well as find links to health insurance information. You can also read issues of Diabetes Forecast, the association's consumer magazine.

Joslin Diabetes Center
One Joslin Place
Boston, MA 02215
617-309-2400
diabetes@joslin.harvard.edu
http://www.joslin.harvard.edu

Joslin's Online Diabetes Library provides a wealth of useful information explaining in detail such topics as carbohydrate counting, artificial sweeteners, blood sugar changes with exercise, and the effects of diabetes on sexuality.

National Institute of Diabetes and Digestive and Kidney Diseases
9000 Rockville Pike
Bethesda, MD 20892
301-496-3583
https://www.niddk.nih.gov

The NIDDK offers a collection of booklets on everything from glucose monitors to alternative treatments for diabetes. There are also materials in Spanish, and several designed for lower literacy levels. You can view them online or order hard copies; many are free.

—Michael Woods, MD, FAAP

APPENDICES

Bibliography

General Bibliography

Aarestrup, Julie, et al. Childhood Overweight, Tallness, and Growth Increase Risks of Ovarian Cancer. *Cancer Epidemiology Biomarkers & Prevention*, vol. 28, no. 1, Jan. 2019, pp. 183–188., doi:10.1158/1055-9965.epi-18-0024.

About Heart Attacks. *American Heart Association*, 31 July 2016, www.heart.org/en/health-topics/heart-attack/about-heart-attacks.

About Peripheral Artery Disease (PAD). *American Heart Association*, 31 Oct. 2016, www.heart.org/en/health-topics/peripheral-artery-disease/about-peripheral-artery-disease-pad.

Acute Coronary Syndromes. *DynaMed*, EBSCO Information Services, 15 Mar. 2019, www.dynamed.com/condition/acute-coronary-syndromes.

Adelizzi, Angela. Obesity and Obstructive Sleep Apnea. *Obesity Medicine Association*, 2 Aug. 2018, obesitymedicine.org/obesity-and-sleep-apnea/.

Ajie, Whitney N., and Karen M. Chapman-Novakofski. Impact of Computer-Mediated, Obesity-Related Nutrition Education Interventions for Adolescents: A Systematic Review. *Journal of Adolescent Health*, vol. 54, no. 6, June 2014, pp. 631–645, www.sciencedirect.com/science/article/pii/S1054139X13008422, 10.1016/j.jadohealth.2013.12.019.

Alberga, Angela S., et al. Weight Bias: a Call to Action. *Journal of Eating Disorders*, vol. 4, no. 1, 7 Nov. 2016, doi:10.1186/s40337-016-0112-4.

Alcohol and Heart Health. *American Heart Association*, 12 Jan. 2015, www.heart.org/HEARTORG/HealthyLiving/HealthyEating/Nutrition/Alcohol-and-Heart-Disease_UCM_305173_Article.jsp#.XJuGkFVKgzx.

Alexandre, Leo. Pathophysiological Mechanisms Linking Obesity and Esophageal Adenocarcinoma. *World Journal of Gastrointestinal Pathophysiology*, vol. 5, no. 4, 2014, p. 534., doi:10.4291/wjgp.v5.i4.534.

Algoblan, Abdullah, et al. Mechanism Linking Diabetes Mellitus and Obesity. *Diabetes, Metabolic Syndrome and Obesity: Targets and Therapy*, 2014, p. 587., doi:10.2147/dmso.s67400.

Allopurinol. *DynaMed*, EBSCO Information Services, 6 Feb. 2017, www.dynamed.com/drug-monograph/allopurinol.

Alpert, Martin A., et al. Obesity and Heart Failure: Epidemiology, Pathophysiology, Clinical Manifestations, and Management. *Translational Research*, vol. 164, no. 4, 2014, pp. 345–356., doi:10.1016/j.trsl.2014.04.010.

Al-Safi, Zain A., and Alex J. Polotsky. Obesity and Menopause. *Best Practice & Research Clinical Obstetrics & Gynaecology*, vol. 29, no. 4, 2015, pp. 548–553., doi:10.1016/j.bpobgyn.2014.12.002.

American Association for Cancer Research. Excess Body Weight before 50 Is Associated with Higher Risk of Dying from Pancreatic Cancer. *ScienceDaily*, 31 Mar. 2019, www.sciencedaily.com/releases/2019/03/190331192525.htm.

American College of Sports Medicine. *ACSM's Complete Guide to Fitness and Health.* Edited by Barbara Bushman. 2nd ed. Human Kinetics, 2017.

American Diabetes Association. Classification and Diagnosis of Diabetes: Standards of Medical Care in Diabetes—2019. *Diabetes Care*, vol. 42, no. Suppl 1, 17 Dec. 2018, pp. S13–S28, 10.2337/dc19-s002.

American Diabetes Association. Diagnosis and Classification of Diabetes Mellitus. *Diabetes Care*, vol. 33, no. Suppl 1, Jan. 2010, pp. S62–S69, 10.2337/dc10-s062.

American Diabetes Association. Executive Summary: Standards of Medical Care in Diabetes–2010. *Diabetes Care*, vol. 33, no. Suppl 1, Jan. 2010, pp. S4–S10, 10.2337/dc10-s004.

American Heart Association.Diet and Lifestyle Recommendations.*American Heart Association*, 15 Aug. 2017, www.heart.org/en/healthy-living/healthy-eating/eat-smart/nutrition-basics/aha-diet-and-lifestyle-recommendations.

Angina (Chest Pain).*American Heart Association*, 14 Dec. 2017, www.heart.org/en/health-topics/heart-attack/angina-chest-pain#. Wp1fXGrwZQI.

Annamalai, Aniyizhai, et al. Prevalence of Obesity and Diabetes in Patients with Schizophrenia. *World Journal of Diabetes*, vol. 8, no. 8, 2017, p. 390., doi:10.4239/wjd.v8.i8.390.

Anonymous. I'm a Fat Bulimic – Here's Why the Idea of Loving My Body Feels Impossible for Me. *Everyday Feminism*, 17 Sept. 2015, everydayfeminism.com/2015/09/im-a-fat-bulimic/.

Antiplatelet and Anticoagulant Drugs for Coronary Artery Disease.*DynaMed*, EBSCO Information Services, 26 Jan. 2018, www.dynamed.com/topics/dmp~AN~T114649/Antiplatelet-and-anticoagulant-drugs-for-coronary-artery-disease.

Antipolis, Sophia. Belly Fat Linked with Repeat Heart Attacks. *European Society of Cardiology*, 21 Jan. 2020, www.escardio.org/The-ESC/Press-Office/Press-releases/Belly-fat-linked-with-repeat-heart-attacks.

Appel, Lawrence J. Overweight, Obesity, and Weight Reduction in Hypertension.*UpToDate*, 24 Sept. 2018, www.uptodate.com/contents/overweight-obesity-and-weight-reduction-in-hypertension.

Aranceta, Javier, and Carmen Pérez-Rodrigo. Recommended Dietary Reference Intakes, Nutritional Goals and Dietary Guidelines for Fat and Fatty Acids: a Systematic Review. *British Journal of Nutrition*, vol. 107, no. S2, 2012, doi:10.1017/s0007114512001444.

Are Weight-Loss Drugs Worth Trying? - Harvard Health. *Harvard Health Publishing*, Harvard Medical School, 22 May 2018, www.health.harvard.edu/staying-healthy/are-weight-loss-drugs-worth-trying.

Arteaga, S. Sonia, et al. Childhood Obesity Research at the NIH: Efforts, Gaps, and Opportunities. *Translational Behavioral Medicine*, vol. 8, no. 6, 21 Nov. 2018, pp. 962–967, academic.oup.com/tbm/article/8/6/962/5134051, 10.1093/tbm/iby090.

Arthritis Foundation, arthritis.org/diseases/gout. Accessed 13 Mar. 2020.

Atapattu, Piyusha M. Obesity at Menopause: An Expanding Problem. *Journal of Patient Care*, vol. 01, no. 01, 2015, doi:10.4172/2573-4598.1000103.

Aubrey, Allison, and RhituChatterjee. Changing Your Diet Can Help Tamp Down Depression, Boost Mood. *National Public Radio*, 9 Oct. 2019, www.npr.org/sections/the-salt/2019/10/09/768665411/changing-your-diet-can-help-tamp-down-depression-boost-mood.

Avraham, Yosefa, and Sapir Nachum. Management of Obesity in Menopause: Lifestyle Modification, Medication, Bariatric Surgery and Personalized Treatment. *Current Topics in Menopause*, 2013, pp. 143–162., doi:10.2174/97816080545341130100 10.

Ayaz, Aylin, et al. How Does Food Addiction Influence Dietary Intake Profile? Plos One, vol. 13, no. 4, 2018, doi:10.1371/journal.pone.0195541.

Bacon, Linda, and Lucy Aphramor.*Body Respect: What Conventional Health Books Get Wrong, Leave Out, and Just Plain Fail to Understand about Weight.* Benbella, 2014.

Baker, Amanda, and Céline Blanchard. Men's Body Image: The Effects of an Unhealthy Body Image on Psychological, Behavioral, and Cognitive Health. *Weight Loss*, 5 Nov. 2018, doi:10.5772/intechopen.75187.

Baker, E.H., et al. A Pilot Study to Promote Walking among Obese and Overweight Individuals: Walking Buses for Adults. *Public Health*, vol. 129, no. 6, June 2015, pp. 822–824, 10.1016/j.puhe.2015.03.021.

Bales, Connie W, and Kathryn N Porter Starr. Obesity Interventions for Older Adults: Diet as a Determinant of Physical Function. *Advances in Nutrition*, vol. 9, no. 2, 1 Mar. 2018, pp. 151–159, 10.1093/advances/nmx016.

Bally, Michèle, et al. Risk of Acute Myocardial Infarction with NSAIDs in Real World Use: Bayesian Meta-Analysis of Individual Patient

Data. *BMJ*, 9 May 2017, p. j1909, doi: 10.1136/bmj.j1909.

Bandera, Elisa V, et al. Impact of Body Mass Index on Ovarian Cancer Survival Varies by Stage. *British Journal of Cancer*, vol. 117, no. 2, 6 June 2017, pp. 282–289., doi:10.1038/bjc.2017.162.

Bartelt, Alexander, and JoergHeeren.Adipose Tissue Browning and Metabolic Health.*Nature Reviews Endocrinology*, vol. 10, 2014, pp. 24-36, www.nature.com/nrendo/journal/v10/n1/full/nrendo.2013.204.html.

Batac, Joseph, et al. Abdominoplasty in the Obese Patient. *Plastic and Reconstructive Surgery*, vol. 143, no. 4, Apr. 2019, pp. 721e-726e, 10.1097/prs.0000000000005413.

Batch, Bryan C., et al. Outcome by Gender in the Veterans Health Administration Motivating Overweight/Obese Veterans Everywhere Weight Management Program.*Journal of Women's Health*, vol. 27, no. 1, Jan. 2018, pp. 32–39, 10.1089/jwh.2016.6212.

Batsis, John A. Obesity in the Older Adult: Special Issue. *Journal of Nutrition in Gerontology and Geriatrics*, vol. 38, no. 1, 2 Jan. 2019, pp. 1–5, 10.1080/21551197.2018.1564197.

Batsis, John A., and Alexandra B. Zagaria. Addressing Obesity in Aging Patients.*The Medical Clinics of North America*, vol. 102, no. 1, 1 Jan. 2018, pp. 65–85, www.ncbi.nlm.nih.gov/pmc/articles/PMC5724972/, 10.1016/j.mcna.2017.08.007.

Batuman, Vecihi. Diabetic Nephropathy.*Medscape*, 9 Oct. 2019, emedicine.medscape.com/article/238946-overview.

Beairsto, Rachael. AHA Recommends a Focus on Healthy Dietary Choices Over Cholesterol Cutoffs. *Endocrinology Advisor*, 16 Dec. 2019, www.endocrinologyadvisor.com/home/topics/cardiovascular-and-metabolic-disorders/american-heart-association-issues-science-advisory-on-dietary-cholesterol/.

Beckman, Joshua A., et al. Association of Human Immunodeficiency Virus Infection and Risk of Peripheral Artery Disease. *Circulation*, vol. 138, no. 3, 17 July 2018, pp. 255–265, 10.1161/circulationaha.117.032647.

Bell, Griffith A., et al. Intake of Long-Chain Omega-3 Fatty Acids From Diet and Supplements in Relation to Mortality. *American Journal of Epidemiology*, vol. 179, no. 6, 3 Feb. 2014, pp. 710–720., doi:10.1093/aje/kwt326.

Bencsath, Kalman, et al. Outcomes of Bariatric Surgery in Morbidly Obese Patients with Multiple Sclerosis. *Journal of Obesity*, vol. 2017, 2017, pp. 1–5, 10.1155/2017/1935204.

Bennie, Jason A., et al. Muscle Strengthening, Aerobic Exercise, and Obesity: A Pooled Analysis of 1.7 Million US Adults. *Obesity*, 11 Nov. 2019, www.onlinelibrary.wiley.com/doi/pdf/10.1002/oby.22673, 10.1002/oby.22673.

Bentley, R. Alexander, et al. Recent Origin and Evolution of Obesity-Income Correlation across the United States.*Palgrave Communications*, vol. 4, no. 1, 2018, doi:10.1057/s41599-018-0201-x.

Bentley, R. Alexander, et al. U.S. Obesity as Delayed Effect of Excess Sugar. *Economics & Human Biology*, vol. 36, 2020, p. 100818., doi:10.1016/j.ehb.2019.100818.

Benton, David, and Hayley A. Young. Reducing Calorie Intake May Not Help You Lose Body Weight. *Perspectives on Psychological Science*, vol. 12, no. 5, 28 June 2017, pp. 703–714., doi:10.1177/1745691617690878.

Berger, Nathan A. Obesity and Cancer Pathogenesis.*Annals of the New York Academy of Sciences*, vol. 1311, no. 1, 2014, pp. 57–76., doi:10.1111/nyas.12416.

Biobank Research Identifies Bipolar-Obesity Link. *Mayo Clinic*, Mayo Foundation for Medical Education and Research, 11 Nov. 2016, www.mayoclinic.org/medical-professionals/psychiatry-psychology/news/biobank-research-identifies-bipolar-obesity-link/mac-20429510.

Bjarnadottir, Adda. How GarciniaCambogia Can Help You Lose Weight and Belly Fat. *Healthline*, 6 Dec. 2018, www.healthline.com/nutrition/garcinia-cambogia-weight-loss.

Blair, Cindy K., et al. Obesity and Survival among a Cohort of Breast Cancer Patients Is Partially Mediated by Tumor Characteristics. *Npj Breast Cancer*, vol. 5, no. 1, 2 Oct. 2019, doi:10.1038/s41523-019-0128-4.

Bleich, Sara N., and Kelsey A. Vercammen. The Negative Impact of Sugar-Sweetened Beverages on Children's Health: an Update of the Literature. BMC Obesity, vol. 5, no. 1, 2018, doi:10.1186/s40608-017-0178-9.

Blesso, Christopher N., and Maria Luz Fernandez. Dietary Cholesterol, Serum Lipids, and Heart Disease: Are Eggs Working for or Against You? Nutrients, vol. 10, no. 4, 2018, p. 426., doi:10.3390/nu10040426.

Blokhin, Ilya O., and Steven R. Lentz.Mechanisms of Thrombosis in Obesity.*Current Opinion in Hematology*, vol. 20, no. 5, 2013, pp. 437–444., doi:10.1097/moh.0b013e3283634443.

BMI Classification.*Global Database on Body Mass Index.*World Health Organization. 27 July 2015.

Bode, B. W., et al. Patient-Reported Outcomes Following Treatment with the Human GLP-1 Analogue Liraglutide or Glimepiride in Monotherapy: Results from a Randomized Controlled Trial in Patients with Type 2 Diabetes. *Diabetes, Obesity and Metabolism*, vol. 12, no. 7, 7 Jan. 2010, pp. 604–612, 10.1111/j.1463-1326.2010.01196.x.

Body Mass Index (BMI).*Centers for Disease Control and Prevention.* 15 May 2015.

Bohannon, Nancy. Overview of the Gliptin Class (Dipeptidyl Peptidase-4 Inhibitors) in Clinical Practice.*Postgraduate Medicine*, vol. 121, no. 1, Jan. 2009, pp. 40–45, 10.3810/pgm.2009.01.1953.

Bohler, Henry Jr., et al. Adipose Tissue and Reproduction in Women.*Fertility and Sterility*, vol. 94, no. 3, Aug. 2010.

Bolster, Marcy. Gout.*American College of Rheumatology*, Mar. 2019, www.rheumatology.org/I-Am-A/Patient-Caregiver/Diseases-Conditions/Gout.

Bonanno, Lilla, et al. Assessment of Sleep and Obesity in Adults and Children. *Medicine*, vol. 98, no. 46, Nov. 2019, p. e17642, 10.1097/md.0000000000017642.

BondkePersson, A., et al. Therapeutic Arteriogenesis in Peripheral Arterial Disease: Combining Intervention and Passive Training. *Vasa*, vol. 40, no. 3, 1 May 2011, pp. 177–187, 10.1024/0301-1526/a000092.

Boston University School of Medicine.Evidence of Behavioral, Biological Similarities between Compulsive Overeating and Addiction.*ScienceDaily*, 17 Oct. 2019, www.sciencedaily.com/releases/2019/10/191017125240.htm.

Botros, Nader, et al. Obstructive Sleep Apnea as a Risk Factor for Type 2 Diabetes. *The American Journal of Medicine*, vol. 122, no. 12, Dec. 2009, pp. 1122–1127, www.ncbi.nlm.nih.gov/pmc/articles/PMC2799991/, 10.1016/j.amjmed.2009.04.026.

Bozzini, Sara, et al. Cardiovascular Characteristics of Chronic Fatigue Syndrome. *Biomedical Reports*, 28 Nov. 2017, doi:10.3892/br.2017.1024.

Bracci, Paige M. Obesity and Pancreatic Cancer: Overview of Epidemiologic Evidence and Biologic Mechanisms. *Molecular Carcinogenesis*, vol. 51, no. 1, 12 Jan. 2013, pp. 53–63., doi:10.1002/mc.20778.

Braithwaite, Irene, et al. Fast-Food Consumption and Body Mass Index in Children and Adolescents: an International Cross-Sectional Study. BMJ Open, vol. 4, no. 12, 2014, doi:10.1136/bmjopen-2014-005813.

Bramante, Carolyn T., et al. Treatment of Obesity in Patients With Diabetes. *Diabetes Spectrum*, vol. 30, no. 4, 2017, pp. 237–243., doi:10.2337/ds17-0030.

Bray, George A, et al. The Science of Obesity Management: An Endocrine Society Scientific Statement. *Endocrine Reviews*, vol. 39, no. 2, 6 Mar. 2018, pp. 79–132, academic.oup.com/edrv/article/39/2/79/4922247.

Bray, George A. Is Sugar Addictive? Diabetes, vol. 65, no. 7, 2016, pp. 1797–1799., doi:10.2337/dbi16-0022.

Bray, George A., and Barry M. Popkin. Dietary Sugar and Body Weight: Have We Reached a Crisis in the Epidemic of Obesity and Diabetes? *Diabetes Care*, vol. 37, no. 4, 20 Apr. 2014, pp. 950–956., doi:10.2337/dc13-2085.

Bray, George A., and Barry M. Popkin. Dietary Sugar and Body Weight: Have We Reached a Crisis in the Epidemic of Obesity and Diabetes? Diabetes Care, vol. 37, no. 4, 2014, pp. 950–956., doi:10.2337/dc13-2085.

Brazier, Yvette. What Causes Fatigue, and How Can I Treat It? *Medical News Today*, 15 Aug. 2017, www.medicalnewstoday.com/articles/248002.

Brogan, Kelly. The Role of the Microbiome in Mental Health: A Psychoneuroimmunologic Perspective. *Alternative and Complementary Therapies*, vol. 21, no. 2, 2015, pp. 61–67., doi:10.1089/act.2015.21204.

Brown, Harriet. *Body of Truth: How Science, History and Culture Drive Our Obsession with Weight—And What We Can Do about It.* De Capo, 2015.

Brownell, Kelly D., and B. Timothy Walsh.*Eating Disorders and Obesity a Comprehensive Handbook.* 3rd ed., The Guilford Press, 2017.

Buttitta, Flavio, et al. Usefulness of Carotid Intima-Media Thickness Measurement and Peripheral B-Mode Ultrasound Scan in the Clinical Screening of Patients with Coronary Artery Disease. *Angiology*, vol. 51, no. 4, Apr. 2000, pp. 269–279, 10.1177/000331970005100401.

Byrd, Angel S., et al. Racial Disparities in Obesity Treatment. *Current Obesity Reports*, vol. 7, no. 2, 31 July 2018, pp. 130–138., doi:10.1007/s13679-018-0301-3.

Cai, Xiaoling, et al. Baseline Body Mass Index and the Efficacy of Hypoglycemic Treatment in Type 2 Diabetes: A Meta-Analysis. *Plos One*, vol. 11, no. 12, 9 Dec. 2016, doi:10.1371/journal.pone.0166625.

Callaghan, Brian C., et al. Diabetes and Obesity Are the Main Metabolic Drivers of Peripheral Neuropathy. *Annals of Clinical and Translational Neurology*, vol. 5, no. 4, 14 Feb. 2018, pp. 397–405., doi:10.1002/acn3.531.

Campos, Marcelo. Ketogenic Diet: Is the Ultimate Low-Carb Diet Good for You? *Harvard Health Blog*, Harvard Medical School, 30 July 2019.

Canale, Maria Paola, et al. Obesity-Related Metabolic Syndrome: Mechanisms of Sympathetic Overactivity. *International Journal of Endocrinology*, vol. 2013, 2013, pp. 1–12., doi:10.1155/2013/865965.

Carbone, Salvatore, et al. Obesity and Heart Failure: Focus on the Obesity Paradox. *Mayo Clinic Proceedings*, vol. 92, no. 2, 2017, pp. 266–279., doi:10.1016/j.mayocp.2016.11.001.

Carbone, Salvatore, et al. Obesity Paradox in Cardiovascular Disease: Where Do We Stand? *Vascular Health and Risk Management*, vol. 15, 2019, pp. 89–100., doi:10.2147/vhrm.s168946.

Cardiac CT for Calcium Scoring.*Radiologyinfo.Org*, Radiological Society of North America, 28 Jan. 2020, www.radiologyinfo.org/en/info.cfm?pg=ct%5Fcalscoring.

Cardiac Medications. *American Heart Association*, 15 Jan. 2020, www.heart.org/en/health-topics/heart-attack/treatment-of-a-heart-attack/cardiac-medications.

Cardiac Procedures and Surgeries.*American Heart Association*, 31 Mar. 2017, www.heart.org/en/health-topics/heart-attack/treatment-of-a-heart-attack/cardiac-procedures-and-surgeries#.Wp2C22rwbIU.

Cardiac Procedures and Surgeries. *American Heart Association*, 31 Mar. 2017, www.heart.org/en/health-topics/heart-attack/treatment-of-a-heart-attack/cardiac-procedures-and-surgeries.

Cardiovascular Disease Major Risk Factors. *DynaMed*, EBSCO Information Systems, 12 June 2017, www.dynamed.com/condition/cardiovascular-disease-major-risk-factors.

Cardiovascular Disease Major Risk Factors. *DynaMed*, EBSCO Information Services, 20 Aug. 2018, www.dynamed.com/condition/cardiovascular-disease-major-risk-factors.

Cardiovascular Disease Possible Risk Factors. *DynaMed*, EBSCO Information Services, 26 Feb. 2018, www.dynamed.com/prevention/cardiovascular-disease-possible-risk-factors.

Cardiovascular Disease Possible Risk Factors. *DynaMed*, EBSCO Information Services, 28 Nov. 2018, www.dynamed.com/prevention/cardiovascular-disease-possible-risk-factors.

Cardiovascular Disease Prevention Overview. *DynaMed*, EBSCO Information Services, 22 Feb. 2018, www.dynamed.com/prevention/cardiovascular-disease-prevention-overview.

Carey, Mariko, et al. Prevalence of Comorbid Depression and Obesity in General Practice: a Cross-Sectional Survey. *British Journal of General Practice*, vol. 64, no. 620, 24 Mar. 2014, doi:10.3399/bjgp14x677482.

Carmel, Molly. *Breaking up with Sugar: a Plan to Divorce the Diets, Drop the Pounds, and Live Your Best Life.*Avery, 2019.

Carreau, Anne-Marie, et al. Late Reactive Hypoglycemia (RHG) as a Common Early Sign of

Glycemic Dysfunction in Obese Adolescent Girls.*Diabetes*, vol. 67, no. Supplement 1, 2018, doi:10.2337/db18-1361-p.

Carson-DeWitt, Rosalyn. Overweight in Adults. *Health Library*. EBSCO, 27 May 2014.

Carter, P., et al. Fruit and Vegetable Intake and Incidence of Type 2 Diabetes Mellitus: Systematic Review and Meta-Analysis. *BMJ*, vol. 341, no. aug18 4, 19 Aug. 2010, pp. c4229–c4229, www.bmj.com/content/341/bmj.c4229, 10.1136/bmj.c4229.

Carvalhana, Sofia, and Helena Cortez-Pinto. From Obesity to Fatty Liver/NASH: Two Parallel Epidemics. *World Gastroenterology Organisation*, July 2013, www.worldgastroenterology.org/publications/e-wgn/e-wgn-expert-point-of-view-articles-collection/from-obesity-to-fatty-liver-nash-two-parallel-epidemics.

Castillo, Michelle. Doctors Warn Obese Teens May Be at Higher Risk for Anorexia, Bulimia. *CBS News*, 9 Sept. 2013, www.cbsnews.com/news/doctors-warn-obese-teens-may-be-at-higher-risk-for-anorexia-bulimia/.

Catalán, V., et al. Adipose Tissue Immunity and Cancer.*Frontiers in Physiology*, Oct. 2013.

Cercato, C., and F. A. Fonseca.Cardiovascular Risk and Obesity.*Diabetology & Metabolic Syndrome*, vol. 11, no. 1, 28 Aug. 2019, doi:10.1186/s13098-019-0468-0.

Chang, Chi-Jen, et al. Evidence in Obese Children: Contribution of Hyperlipidemia, Obesity-Inflammation, and Insulin Sensitivity. *Plos One*, vol. 10, no. 5, 2015, doi:10.1371/journal.pone.0125935.

Chang, Sarah, and Kristin Koegel. Back to Basics: All About MyPlate Food Groups. *Journal of the Academy of Nutrition and Dietetics*, vol. 117, no. 9, 2017, pp. 1351–1353., doi:10.1016/j.jand.2017.06.376.

Chao, Anthony Tl, et al. Effect of Bariatric Surgery on Diabetic Nephropathy in Obese Type 2 Diabetes Patients in a Retrospective 2-Year Study: A Local Pilot. *Diabetes and Vascular Disease Research*, vol. 15, no. 2, 18 Nov. 2017, pp. 139–144., doi:10.1177/1479164117742315.

Chattu, Vijayk, et al. Nutritional Aspects of Depression in Adolescents - A Systematic Review. *International Journal of Preventive Medicine*, vol. 10, no. 1, 2019, p. 42., doi:10.4103/ijpvm.ijpvm_400_18.

Chen, Michael A. Coronary Heart Disease. *MedlinePlus*, U.S. National Library of Medicine, 13 Feb. 2018, medlineplus.gov/ency/article/007115.htm.

Chiu, Chih-Hui, et al. Benefits of Different Intensity of Aerobic Exercise in Modulating Body Composition among Obese Young Adults: A Pilot Randomized Controlled Trial. *Health and Quality of Life Outcomes*, vol. 15, no. 1, 24 Aug. 2017, www.ncbi.nlm.nih.gov/pmc/articles/PMC5571495/, 10.1186/s12955-017-0743-4.

Choquet, H., and Meyre, D. Genetics of Obesity: What Have We Learned? *Current Genomics*, vol. 12, no. 3, 2011, pp: 169–179.

Christian, James G. Clinic-Based Support to Help Overweight Patients With Type 2 Diabetes Increase Physical Activity and Lose Weight. *Archives of Internal Medicine*, vol. 168, no. 2, 28 Jan. 2008, p. 141, 10.1001/archinternmed.2007.13.

Clark, B. Ruth, et al. Obesity and Aerobic Fitness among Urban Public School Students in Elementary, Middle, and High School.*PLOS ONE*, vol. 10, no. 9, 17 Sept. 2015, p. e0138175, 10.1371/journal.pone.0138175.

Coelho, Marisa, et al. Biochemistry of Adipose Tissue: An Endocrine Organ. *Archives of Medical Science*, vol. 9, no. 2, 2013.

Colchicine.*DynaMed*, EBSCO Information Services, 6 Feb. 2017, www.dynamed.com/drug-monograph/colchicine.

Colesevelam.*DynaMed*, EBSCO Information Services, 6 Sept. 2016, www.dynamed.com/drug-monograph/colesevelam.

Collier, Jasmin. Being Overweight or Obese May Improve Stroke Survival. *Medical News Today*, 6 Mar. 2019, www.medicalnewstoday.com/articles/324628.

Cooper, Christopher B, et al. Sleep Deprivation and Obesity in Adults: A Brief Narrative Review. *BMJ Open Sport & Exercise Medicine*, vol. 4, no. 1, Oct. 2018, p. e000392, 10.1136/bmjsem-2018-000392.

Corbin, Karen D, et al. Obesity in Type 1 Diabetes: Pathophysiology, Clinical Impact, and

Mechanisms. *Endocrine Reviews*, vol. 39, no. 5, 27 July 2018, pp. 629–663., doi:10.1210/er.2017-00191.

Corliss, Julie. Eating Too Much Added Sugar Increases the Risk of Dying with Heart Disease. *Harvard Health Blog*, Harvard Medical School, 27 Aug. 2019, www.health.harvard. edu/blog/eating-too-much-added-sugar-increases-the-risk-of-dying-with-heart-disease-201402067021.

Coronary Artery Bypass Graft (CABG) Surgery. *DynaMed*, EBSCO Information Services, 28 Dec. 2017, www.dynamed.com/procedure/coronary-artery-bypass-graft-cabg-surgery.

Coronary Artery Bypass Graft (CABG) Surgery. *DynaMed*, EBSCO Information Services, 20 Feb. 2019, www.dynamed.com/procedure/coronary-artery-bypass-graft-cabg-surgery.

Coronary Artery Bypass Grafting.*National Heart, Lung, and Blood Institute*, U.S. Department of Health & Human Services, 18 Nov. 2014, www.nhlbi.nih.gov/health-topics/coronary-artery-bypass-grafting.

Coronary Artery Disease - Coronary Heart Disease. *American Heart Association*, 26 Apr. 2017, www.heart.org/en/health-topics/consumer-health-care/what-is-cardiovascular-disease/coronary-artery-disease#.Wp14QmrwbIV.

Coronary Artery Disease (CAD).*DynaMed*, EBSCO Information Services, 28 Feb. 2018, www.dynamed.com/topics/dmp~AN~T116156/Coronary-artery-disease-CAD.

Coronary Heart Disease.*National Heart, Lung, and Blood Institute*, U.S. Department of Health & Human Services, www.nhlbi.nih.gov/health-topics/coronary-heart-disease.Accessed 6 Mar. 2020.

Correia de FariaSantarém, G, et al. Correlation between Body Composition and Walking Capacity in Severe Obesity. *PLOS ONE*, vol. 10, no. 6, 22 June 2015, p. e0130268, 10.1371/journal.pone.0130268.

Corvera, Sylvia, and Olga Gealekman. Adipose Tissue Angiogenesis: Impact on Obesity and Type-2 Diabetes. *Molecular Basis of Disease*, vol. 1842, no. 3, Mar. 2014, www.science direct.com/science/article/pii/S0925443913002111.

Costanzo, Maria Rosa, et al. TransvenousNeuro-stimulation for Central Sleep Apnoea: A Randomised Controlled Trial. *The Lancet*, vol. 388, no. 10048, Sept. 2016, pp. 974–982, 10.1016/s0140-6736(16)30961-8.

Cox, Carla E. Role of Physical Activity for Weight Loss and Weight Maintenance.*Diabetes Spectrum*, vol. 30, no. 3, Aug. 2017, pp. 157–160, 10.2337/ds17-0013.

Cramer, Holger, et al.A Systematic Review of Yoga for Heart Disease.*European Journal of Preventive Cardiology*, vol. 22, no. 3, 3 Feb. 2014, pp. 284–295, 10.1177/2047487314523132.

Crandall, Jill P, et al. Alcohol Consumption and Diabetes Risk in the Diabetes Prevention Program.*The American Journal of Clinical Nutrition*, vol. 90, no. 3, 29 July 2009, pp. 595–601, 10.3945/ajcn.2008.27382.

C-Reactive Protein (CRP) and Other Biomarkers as Cardiac Risk Factors. *DynaMed*, EBSCO Information Services, 25 Feb. 2016, www.dynamed.com/evaluation/c-reactive-protein-crp-and-other-biomarkers-as-cardiac-risk-factors.

Creagan, Edward T. How to Manage Stress and Avoid Overeating When Stressed. *Mayo Clinic*, Mayo Foundation for Medical Education and Research, 20 July 2017, www.mayoclinic.org/healthy-lifestyle/stress-management/expert-answers/stress/faq-20058497.45

Csige, Imre, et al. The Impact of Obesity on the Cardiovascular System.*Journal of Diabetes Research*, vol. 2018, 4 Nov. 2018, pp. 1–12., doi:10.1155/2018/3407306.

Cunningham, Aimee. Ban on Artificial Trans Fats in NYC Restaurants Seems to Be Working. *Science News*, 8 Aug. 2019, www.sciencenews.org/article/ban-artificial-trans-fats-nyc-restaurants-appears-be-working.

Cusimano, Maria C, et al. Barriers to Care for Women with Low-Grade Endometrial Cancer and Morbid Obesity: a Qualitative Study. *BMJ Open*, vol. 9, no. 6, 2019, doi:10.1136/bmjopen-2018-026872.

Cvetkovi , N., et al. Exercise Training in Overweight and Obese Children: Recreational Football and High-Intensity Interval Training Provide Similar Benefits to Physical Fitness. *Scandinavian Journal of Medicine & Science in Sports*, vol. 28, 6 July 2018, pp. 18–32, onlinelibrary.wiley.com/doi/full/10.1111/sms.13241, 10.1111/sms.13241.

Dalvand, Sahar, et al. Assessing Factors Related to Waist Circumference and Obesity: Application of a Latent Variable Model. Journal of Environmental and Public Health, vol. 2015, 2015, pp. 1–9., doi:10.1155/2015/893198.

Dance Therapy and Obesity. *Clinical Trials*, U.S. National Library of Medicine, 16 Dec. 2014, clinicaltrials.gov/ct2/show/NCT01451892. Accessed 5 Mar. 2020.

Daniel, Sunil. Obesity and Heart Disease. *Obesity Action Coalition*, 2015, www.obesityaction.org/community/article-library/obesity-and-heart-disease/.

Daubenmier, Jennifer, et al. Mindfulness Intervention for Stress Eating to Reduce Cortisol and Abdominal Fat among Overweight and Obese Women: An Exploratory Randomized Controlled Study. *Journal of Obesity*, vol. 2011, 2011, pp. 1–13, www.ncbi.nlm.nih.gov/pmc/articles/PMC3184496/, 10.1155/2011/651936.

Davies, M J, et al. Effectiveness of the Diabetes Education and Self Management for Ongoing and Newly Diagnosed (DESMOND) Programme for People with Newly Diagnosed Type 2 Diabetes: Cluster Randomised Controlled Trial. *BMJ*, vol. 336, no. 7642, 14 Feb. 2008, pp. 491–495, 10.1136/bmj.39474.922025.be.

Davies, Nicola. Mental Illness and Obesity. *Psychiatry Advisor*, 17 Dec. 2018, www.psychiatryadvisor.com/home/conference-highlights/aaic-2015-coverage/mental-illness-and-obesity/.

Davies, Nicola. Mental Illness and Obesity. *Psychiatry Advisor*, 26 Feb. 2016, www.psychiatryadvisor.com/home/conference-highlights/aaic-2015-coverage/mental-illness-and-obesity/.

Davis, Caroline. From Passive Overeating to 'Food Addiction': A Spectrum of Compulsion and Severity. ISRN Obesity, 2013, pp. 1–20., doi:10.1155/2013/435027.

Davis, Kathleen. What to Know about Hyperlipidemia. *Medical News Today*, 15 July 2019, www.medicalnewstoday.com/articles/295385.

Davis, Kathleen. What's to Know about Body Dysmorphic Disorder. *Medical News Today*, 12 Mar.

2019, www.medicalnewstoday.com/articles/309254.

Dehghan, Mahshid, et al. Associations of Fats and Carbohydrate Intake with Cardiovascular Disease and Mortality in 18 Countries from Five Continents (PURE): a Prospective Cohort Study. *The Lancet*, vol. 390, no. 10107, 2017, pp. 2050–2062., doi:10.1016/s0140-6736(17)32252-3.

Diabetes Mellitus Type 2 in Adults. *DynaMed*, EBSCO Information Services, 29 Aug. 2016, www.dynamed.com/condition/diabetes-mellitus-type-2-in-adults.

Dietary Guidelines for Americans 2015–2020. *U.S. Department of Health and Human Services*, Office of Disease Prevention and Health Promotion, Dec. 2015, health.gov/our-work/food-nutrition/2015-2020-dietary-guidelines/guidelines/.

Dinicolantonio, James J, and James H O'Keefe. Effects of Dietary Fats on Blood Lipids: a Review of Direct Comparison Trials. *Open Heart*, vol. 5, no. 2, 2018, doi:10.1136/openhrt-2018-000871.

Does Metabolism Matter in Weight Loss? *Harvard Health Blog*, Harvard Medical School, July 2015, www.health.harvard.edu/diet-and-weight-loss/does-metabolism-matter-in-weight-loss.

Doheny, Kathleen. Osteoarthritis and Obesity: Anticipated Comorbidities with New Clues to Care. *EndocrineWeb*, 5 Feb. 2019, www.endocrineweb.com/professional/obesity/new-clues-obesity-osteoarthritis.

Donnelly, Joseph E., et al. Aerobic Exercise Alone Results in Clinically Significant Weight Loss for Men and Women: Midwest Exercise Trial 2. *Obesity*, vol. 21, no. 3, Mar. 2013, pp. E219–E228, 10.1002/oby.20145.

Drake, Matthew T. Hypothyroidism in Clinical Practice. *Mayo Clinic Proceedings*, vol. 93, no. 9, 2018, pp. 1169–1172., doi:10.1016/j.mayocp.2018.07.015.

DREAM (Diabetes REduction Assessment with ramipril and rosiglitazone Medication) Trial Investigators. Effect of Rosiglitazone on the Frequency of Diabetes in Patients with Impaired Glucose Tolerance or Impaired Fasting Glucose: A Randomised Controlled Trial. *The Lancet*, vol.

368, no. 9541, Sept. 2006, pp. 1096–1105, 10.1016/s0140-6736(06)69420-8.

Du, Xuan, et al. Abdominal Obesity and Gastro-esophageal Cancer Risk: Systematic Review and Meta-Analysis of Prospective Studies. *Bioscience Reports*, vol. 37, no. 3, 2017, doi:10.1042/bsr20160474.

Dubroff, Robert. A Reappraisal of the Lipid Hypothesis. *The American Journal of Medicine*, vol. 131, no. 9, 2018, pp. 993–997., doi:10.1016/j.amjmed.2018.04.027.

Dunne, Annette. Food and Mood: Evidence for Diet-Related Changes in Mental Health. *British Journal of Community Nursing*, vol. 17, no.Sup11, 2012, doi:10.12968/bjcn.2012.17.sup11.s20.

Dutheil, Frédéric, et al. Stress Management in Obesity during a Thermal Spa Residential Programme (ObesiStress): Protocol for a Randomised Controlled Trial Study. *BMJ Open*, vol. 9, no. 12, Dec. 2019, p. e027058, 10.1136/bmjopen-2018-027058.

DynaMed.Morbid Obesity.*DynaMed*. EBSCO, 9 May 2014.

DynaMed.Obesity in Children and Adolescents. *DynaMed*.EBSCO , 24 Mar. 2014.

Ebbing, Marta. Cancer Incidence and Mortality After Treatment With Folic Acid and Vitamin B$_{12}$. *JAMA*, vol. 302, no. 19, 18 Nov. 2009, p. 2119, 10.1001/jama.2009.1622.

Ecker, Brett L., et al. Impact of Obesity on Breast Cancer Recurrence and Minimal Residual Disease. *Breast Cancer Research*, vol. 21, no. 1, 13 Mar. 2019, doi:10.1186/s13058-018-1087-7.

Editorial Staff.Compulsive Overeating.*American Addiction Centers*, 3 Feb. 2020, americanaddictioncenters.org/compulsive-overeating.

Eenfeldt, Andreas. FDA Approves Bulimia Device as Treatment of Obesity. *Diet Doctor*, 15 June 2016, www.dietdoctor.com/fda-approves-bulimia-device-treatment-obesity.

Eibl, Guido, et al. Diabetes Mellitus and Obesity as Risk Factors for Pancreatic Cancer. *Journal of the Academy of Nutrition and Dietetics*, vol. 118, no. 4, 2018, pp. 555–567., doi:10.1016/j.jand.2017.07.005.

Ekelund, Ulf, et al. Does Physical Activity Attenuate, or Even Eliminate, the Detrimental Association of Sitting Time with Mortality? A Harmonised Meta-Analysis of Data from More than 1 Million Men and Women. *The Lancet*, vol. 388, no. 10051, Sept. 2016, pp. 1302–1310, www.thelancet.com/journals/lancet/article/PIIS0140-6736(16)30370-1/fulltext, 10.1016/s0140-6736(16)30370-1.

El-Menyar, Ayman, et al. Role of Overweight and Obesity in Occurrence and Outcomes of Venous Thromboembolism.*Journal of the American College of Surgeons*, vol. 223, no. 4, 2016, doi:10.1016/j.jamcollsurg.2016.08.167.

Emdin, Connor A., et al. Meta-Analysis of Anxiety as a Risk Factor for Cardiovascular Disease. *The American Journal of Cardiology*, vol. 118, no. 4, Aug. 2016, pp. 511–519, 10.1016/j.amjcard.2016.05.041.

Engin, Atilla. The Definition and Prevalence of Obesity and Metabolic Syndrome.*Obesity and Lipotoxicity Advances in Experimental Medicine and Biology*, 2017, pp. 1–17., doi:10.1007/978-3-319-48382-5_1.

European Association for the Study of Obesity. Analysis of New Studies Including 250,000 People Confirms Sugar-Sweetened Drinks Are Linked to Overweight and Obesity in Children and Adults. *ScienceDaily*, 23 Dec. 2017.

Evidence-Based Nutrition Principles and Recommendations for the Treatment and Prevention of Diabetes and Related Complications.*Diabetes Care*, vol. 25, no. Suppl1, 1 Jan. 2002, pp. S50–S60, doi: 10.2337/diacare.25.2007.s50.

Exenatide.*DynaMed*, EBSCO Information Services, 6 Sept. 2016, www.dynamed.com/drug-monograph/exenatide.

Farmer, Andrew, et al. Impact of Self Monitoring of Blood Glucose in the Management of Patients with Non-Insulin Treated Diabetes: Open Parallel Group Randomised Trial. *BMJ*, vol. 335, no. 7611, 25 June 2007, p. 132, 10.1136/bmj.39247.447431.be.

Febuxostat.*DynaMed*, EBSCO Information Services, 27 Sept. 2016, www.dynamed.com/drug-monograph/febuxostat.

Ferrario, Carrie R. Food Addiction and Obesity. Neuropsychopharmacology, vol. 42, no. 1, 2016, pp. 361–361., doi:10.1038/npp.2016.221.

Ferri, Fred F. Hypothyroidism. *Ferri's Clinical Advisor 2020: 5 Books in 1*, edited by Fred F. Ferri, Elsevier, 2020, pp. 769–770.

Finer, Nicholas.Weight Loss for Patients with Obesity and Heart Failure.*European Heart Journal*, vol. 40, no. 26, 10 June 2019, pp. 2139–2141., doi:10.1093/eurheartj/ehz406.

Fish and Omega-3 Fatty Acids. *American Heart Association*, 23 Mar. 2017, www.heart.org/en/healthy-living/healthy-eating/eat-smart/fats/fish-and-omega-3-fatty-acids.

Flegal, Katherine M., Brian K. Kit, Heather Orpana, and Barry I. Graubard. Association of All-Cause Mortality with Overweight and Obesity Using Standard Body Mass Index Categories: A Systematic Review and Meta-analysis. *The Journal of the American Medical Association*, vol. 309, no. 1, 2013, pp: 71–82.

Foong, Ke Wei, and Helen Bolton. Obesity and Ovarian Cancer Risk: A Systematic Review. *Post Reproductive Health*, vol. 23, no. 4, 18 July 2017, pp. 183–198., doi:10.1177/2053369117709225.

Forjuoh, Samuel N., et al. Determinants of Walking among Middle-Aged and Older Overweight and Obese Adults: Sociodemographic, Health, and Built Environmental Factors. *Journal of Obesity*, vol.2017,2017,pp.1–11,10.1155/2017/9565430.

Forkert, Elsie C. O., et al. Skipping Breakfast Is Associated with Adiposity Markers Especially When Sleep Time Is Adequate in Adolescents. *Scientific Reports*, vol. 9, no. 1, 23 Apr. 2019, doi:10.1038/s41598-019-42859-7.

Forouhi, Nita G, et al. Dietary Fat and Cardiometabolic Health: Evidence, Controversies, and Consensus for Guidance. *BMJ*, 13 June 2018, doi:10.1136/bmj.k2139.

Fox, Maggie. Cutting Processed Sugar for Just 9 Days May Improve Health. *Today*, NBC Universal, 4 Oct. 2016, www.today.com/health/cutting-processed-sugar-just-9-days-has-striking-effect-health-t52516.

Franceschelli, ennifer E.The Skinny on 'Fatty' Liver Disease.*Obesity Action Coalition*, 2013, www.obesityaction.org/community/article-library/the-skinny-on-fatty-liver-disease/.

Franco, Viviane Carvalho, et al. Obesity and Clozapine Use in Schizophrenia.*Obesity Research - Open Journal*, vol. 3, no. 2, 13 July 2016, pp. 24–29., doi:10.17140/oroj-3-124.

Friedman, Jeffrey M. Leptin and the Endocrine Control of Energy Balance.*Nature Metabolism*, vol. 1, no. 8, 2019, pp. 754–764., doi:10.1038/s42255-019-0095-y.

Fung, Teresa T., et al. Sweetened Beverage Consumption and Risk of Coronary Heart Disease in Women. *The American Journal of Clinical Nutrition*, vol. 89, no. 4, 1 Apr. 2009, pp. 1037–1042, www.ncbi.nlm.nih.gov/pubmed/19211821/, 10.3945/ajcn.2008.27140.

Galgani, Jose E., et al. Carbohydrate, Fat, and Protein Metabolism in Obesity.*Metabolic Syndrome*, 2016, pp. 327–346., doi:10.1007/978-3-319-11251-0_21.

Gander, Kashmira. This Revolutionary Weight-loss Aid Is Extremely Controversial. *The Independent*, Independent Digital News and Media, 15 Dec. 2016, www.independent.co.uk/lifestyle/health-and-families/health-news/medical-bulimia-aspireassist-weight-obesity-crisis-quick-fix-eating-disorders-diets-health-a7475161.html.

Garvin, Jane T., et al. Characteristics Influencing Weight Reduction Among Veterans in the MOVE!® Program. *Western Journal of Nursing Research*, vol. 37, no. 1, 18 May 2014, pp. 50–65, 10.1177/0193945914534323.

G sior-Perczak, Danuta, et al.The Impact of BMI on Clinical Progress, Response to Treatment, and Disease Course in Patients with Differentiated Thyroid Cancer.*Plos One*, vol. 13, no. 10, 1 Oct. 2018, doi:10.1371/journal.pone.0204668.

Geliebter, Allan, et al. Physiological and Psychological Changes Following Liposuction of Large Volumes of Fat in Overweight and Obese Women. *Journal of Diabetes and Obesity*, vol. 2, no. 4, 2015, pp. 1–7., doi:10.15436/2376-0494.15.032.

Geliebter, Allan. Physiological and Psychological Changes Following Liposuction of Large Volumes of Fat in Overweight and Obese Women. *Journal of Diabetes and Obesity*, vol. 2, no. 4, 2015, pp. 1–7, 10.15436/2376-0494.15.032.

Get the Facts: Sugar-Sweetened Beverages and Consumption. Centers for Disease Control and Prevention, 27 Feb. 2017, www.cdc.gov/nutrition/

data-statistics/sugar-sweetened-beverages-intake.html.

Getting the Most Out of Your Doctor Appointment. *FamilyDoctor.Org*, American Academy of Family Physicians, 19 Jan. 2018, familydoctor.org/tips-for-talking-to-your-doctor/.

Getting the Most Out of Your Doctor Appointment. *FamilyDoctor.Org*, American Academy of Family Physicians, 19 Jan. 2018, familydoctor.org/tips-for-talking-to-your-doctor/.

Gibson-Smith, Deborah, et al. The Relation between Obesity and Depressed Mood in a Multi-Ethnic Population.The HELIUS Study.*Social Psychiatry and Psychiatric Epidemiology*, vol. 53, no. 6, 11 Apr. 2018, pp. 629–638., doi:10.1007/s00127-018-1512-3.

Giuseppe, Rachele De, et al. Pediatric Obesity and Eating Disorders Symptoms: The Role of the Multidisciplinary Treatment. A Systematic Review.*Frontiers in Pediatrics*, vol. 7, 3 Apr. 2019, doi:10.3389/fped.2019.00123.

Gjuladin-Hellon, Teuta, et al. Effects of Carbohydrate-Restricted Diets on Low-Density Lipoprotein Cholesterol Levels in Overweight and Obese Adults: a Systematic Review and Meta-Analysis. Nutrition Reviews, vol. 77, no. 3, 2018, pp. 161–180., doi:10.1093/nutrit/nuy049.

Gohil, Anisha, and Tamara S. Hannon. Poor Sleep and Obesity: Concurrent Epidemics in Adolescent Youth. *Frontiers in Endocrinology*, vol. 9, 10 July 2018, 10.3389/fendo.2018.00364.

Golden, N. H., et al. Preventing Obesity and Eating Disorders in Adolescents.*PEDIATRICS*, vol. 138, no. 3, 22 Aug. 2016, pp. e20161649–e20161649, 10.1542/peds.2016-1649.

Goldman, Lee, and Dennis Ausiello, eds. *Cecil Medicine.*23d ed. Saunders, 2008.

Goroll, Allan H., and Albert G. Mulley, Jr., eds. *Primary Care Medicine: Office Evaluation and Management of the Adult Patient.*7th ed. Wolters, 2014.

Gout Management - Prevention of Recurrent Attacks.*DynaMed*, EBSCO Information Services, 4 Nov. 2016, www.dynamed.com/management/gout-management-prevention-of-recurrent-attacks.

Gout Management - Prevention of Recurrent Attacks.*DynaMed*, EBSCO Information Services,

4 Nov. 2016, www.dynamed.com/management/gout-management-prevention-of-recurrent-attacks.

Gout Management - Treatment of Acute Attack. *DynaMed*, EBSCO Information Services, 13 Oct. 2014, www.dynamed.com/management/gout-management-treatment-of-acute-attack.

Gout.*DynaMed*, EBSCO Information Services, 2 Sept. 2016, www.dynamed.com/condition/gout.

Greco, Marta, et al. Early Effects of a Hypocaloric, Mediterranean Diet on Laboratory Parameters in Obese Individuals.*Mediators of Inflammation*, 4 Mar. 2014, pp. 1–8., doi:10.1155/2014/750860.

Greenberg, Andrew S., and Martin S. Obin.Obesity and the Role of Adipose Tissue in Inflammation and Metabolism.*The American Journal of Clinical Nutrition*, vol. 83, no. 2, Feb. 2006.

Gregory, John W. Prevention of Obesity and Metabolic Syndrome in Children. *Frontiers in Endocrinology*, vol. 10, 1 Oct. 2019, doi:10.3389/fendo.2019.00669.

Gruzdeva, Olga, et al. Leptin Resistance: Underlying Mechanisms and Diagnosis. *Diabetes, Metabolic Syndrome and Obesity: Targets and Therapy*, vol. 12, 2019, pp. 191–198., doi:10.2147/dmso.s182406.

Gunta, Sujana S. Hypertension in Children with Obesity. *World Journal of Hypertension*, vol. 4, no. 2, 2014, p. 15., doi:10.5494/wjh.v4.i2.15.

Guo, Yan, et al. Overweight and Obesity in Young Adulthood and the Risk of Stroke: a Meta-Analysis. *Journal of Stroke and Cerebrovascular Diseases*, vol. 25, no. 12, 2016, pp. 2995–3004., doi:10.1016/j.jstrokecerebrovasdis.2016.08.018.

Gupta, Arjun, et al. Obesity and Mortality in Patients with Esophageal Cancer: A Systematic Review and Meta-Analysis. *Journal of Clinical Oncology*, vol. 34, no. 4_suppl, 2016, pp. 20–20., doi:10.1200/jco.2016.34.4_suppl.20.

Haas, Tara L., et al. Exercise Training and Peripheral Arterial Disease. Comprehensive *Physiology*, vol. 2, no. 4, Oct. 2012, www.ncbi.nlm.nih.gov/pmc/articles/PMC3767482/, 10.1002/cphy.c110065.

Habibzadeh, Nasim, and HassnDaneshmandi.The Effects of Exercise in Obese Women with Bulimia

Nervosa.*Asian Journal of Sports Medicine,* vol. 1, no. 4, 2010, doi:10.5812/asjsm.34829.

Hall, John E., et al. Obesity-Induced Hypertension. *Circulation Research,* vol. 116, no. 6, 13 Mar. 2015, pp. 991–1006., doi:10.1161/circresaha.116.305697.

Hayes, Jacqueline F., et al. Disordered Eating Attitudes and Behaviors in Youth with Overweight and Obesity: Implications for Treatment. *Current Obesity Reports,* vol. 7, no. 3, 1 Sept. 2018, pp. 235–246., doi:10.1007/s13679-018-0316-9.

Haywood, Cilla J, et al. Very Low Calorie Diets for Weight Loss in Obese Older Adults—A Randomized Trial.*The Journals of Gerontology: Series A,* vol. 73, no. 1, 20 Feb. 2017, pp. 59–65., doi:10.1093/gerona/glx012.

HDL (Good), LDL (Bad) Cholesterol and Triglycerides.*American Heart Association,* 30 Apr. 2017, www.heart.org/en/health-topics/cholesterol/hdl-good-ldl-bad-cholesterol-and-triglycerides.

Heart Attack Symptoms in Women. *American Heart Association,* 31 July 2015, www.heart.org/en/health-topics/heart-attack/warning-signs-of-a-heart-attack/heart-attack-symptoms-in-women.

Heart Attack Tools and Resources. *American Heart Association,* www.heart.org/en/health-topics/heart-attack/heart-attack-tools-and-resources.

Heart Attack.*National Heart Lung and Blood Institute,* U.S. Department of Health and Human Services, www.nhlbi.nih.gov/health-topics/heart-attack.

Heart-Health Screenings.*American Heart Association,* 22 Mar. 2019, www.heart.org/en/health-topics/consumer-healthcare/what-is-cardiovascular-disease/heart-health-screenings#.Wp2AzmrwbIU.

Heart-to-Heart: Talking to Your Doctor. *American Heart Association,* 26 Oct. 2015, www.heart.org/en/health-topics/consumer-healthcare/doctor-appointments-questions-to-ask-your-doctor/heart-to-heart-talking-to-your-doctor#.Wp2G-UmrwbIU.

Heerden, Ingrid van. Body Dysmorphic Disorder Can Lead to Obsessive Dieting. *Health24,* 19 Mar. 2015, www.health24.com/Diet-and-nutrition/Healthy-foods/Body-dysmorphic-disorder-can-lead-to-obsessive-dieting-20150319.

Heid, I. M., A. U. Jackson, J. C. Randall, et al. Meta-Analysis Identifies 13 New Loci Associated with Waist-Hip Ratio and Reveals Sexual Dimorphism in the Genetic Basis of Fat Distribution. *Nature America,* 10 Oct. 2010.

Henry, Zachary H., and Stephen H. Caldwell. Obesity and Hepatocellular Carcinoma: A Complex Relationship. *Gastroenterology,* vol. 149, no. 1, 2015, pp. 18–20., doi:10.1053/j.gastro.2015.05.024.

Hensrud, Donald. The Truth about Slow Metabolism.*Mayo Clinic,* Mayo Foundation for Medical Education and Research, 21 Feb. 2019, www.mayoclinic.org/healthy-lifestyle/weight-loss/expert-answers/slow-metabolism/faq-20058480.

Hilger-Kolb, Jennifer, et al. Associations between Dietary Factors and Obesity-Related Biomarkers in Healthy Children and Adolescents - a Systematic Review. *Nutrition Journal,* vol. 16, no. 1, Dec. 2017, 10.1186/s12937-017-0300-3.

Hills, Alexander J, et al. Peripheral Arterial Disease. *British Journal of Hospital Medicine,* vol. 70, no. 10, Oct. 2009, pp. 560–565, 10.12968/hmed.2009.70.10.44622.

Homocysteine and Cardiovascular Disease. *DynaMed,* EBSCO Information Services, 23 Aug. 2016, www.dynamed.com/evaluation/homocysteine-and-cardiovascular-disease.

Hopkins, Laura C., et al. Breakfast Consumption Frequency and Its Relationships to Overall Diet Quality, Using Healthy Eating Index 2010, and Body Mass Index among Adolescents in a Low-Income Urban Setting. *Ecology of Food and Nutrition,* vol. 56, no. 4, 12 Dec. 2017, pp. 297–311., doi:10.1080/03670244.2017.1327855.

Hosoi, Toru, and MargheritaMaffei. Editorial: Leptin Resistance in Metabolic Disorders: Possible Mechanisms and Treatments. *Frontiers in Endocrinology,* vol. 8, 2 Nov. 2017, doi:10.3389/fendo.2017.00300.

How Is Sleep Apnea Treated.*National Heart, Lung, and Blood Institute,* US Department of Health & Human Services, 10 Dec. 2018, www.nhlbi.nih.gov/health-topics/sleep-apnea.

Howard, Jacqueline. How Bulimics' Brains Are Different. *CNN,* Cable News Network, 24 July 2017, www.cnn.com/2017/07/18/health/bulimia-brain-stress-food-study/index.html.

Hozumi, Jun, et al. Relationship between Neuropathic Pain and Obesity. *Pain Research and Management*, vol. 2016, 2016, pp. 1–6., doi:10.1155/2016/2487924.

Hruby, Adela, and Frank B. Hu. The Epidemiology of Obesity: A Big Picture. *PharmacoEconomics*, vol. 33, no. 7, 4 Dec. 2014, pp. 673–689, www.ncbi.nlm.nih.gov/pmc/articles/PMC4859313/, 10.1007/s40273-014-0243-x.

Hudgel, David W., et al. The Role of Weight Management in the Treatment of Adult Obstructive Sleep Apnea.An Official American Thoracic Society Clinical Practice Guideline.*American Journal of Respiratory and Critical Care Medicine*, vol. 198, no. 6, 15 Sept. 2018, doi:10.1164/rccm.201807-1326st.

Hypertension Alternative Treatments. *DynaMed*, EBSCO Information Services, 17 Nov. 2017, www.dynamed.com/management/hypertension-alternative-treatments.

Hypertension Medication Selection and Management.*DynaMed*, EBSCO Information Services, 8 Feb. 2018, www.dynamed.com/management/hypertension-medication-selection-and-management.

Illegal Drugs and Heart Disease. *American Heart Association*, 3 May 2018, www.heart.org/HEARTORG/Conditions/More/MyHeartandStrokeNews/Cocaine-Marijuana-and-Other-Drugs-and-Heart-Disease_UCM_428537_Article.jsp#.XJuGvVVKgzx.

Insel, Paul M. *Discovering Nutrition.*4th ed. Jones & Bartlett Learning, 2013.

Insulin Basics.*American Diabetes Association*, 16 July 2015, www.diabetes.org/diabetes/medication-management/insulin-other-injectables/insulin-basics.

Insulin, Medicines, & Other Diabetes Treatments. *National Institute of Diabetes and Digestive and Kidney Diseases*, US Department of Health & Human Services, Dec. 2016, www.niddk.nih.gov/health-information/diabetes/overview/insulin-medicines-treatments?dkrd=hiscr0023.

Invokana.*DailyMed*, US National Library of Medicine, 4 Aug. 2016, dailymed.nlm.nih.gov/dailymed/search.cfm?labeltype=all&query=Invokana.

Isgin, K., et al. Breakfast Skipping Linked to the Risk of Obesity in School-Aged Children. *Journal of the Academy of Nutrition and Dietetics*, vol. 117, no. 9, 2017, doi:10.1016/j.jand.2017.06.352.

Jääskeläinen, Anne, et al. Stress-Related Eating, Obesity and Associated Behavioural Traits in Adolescents: A Prospective Population-Based Cohort Study. *BMC Public Health*, vol. 14, no. 1, 7 Apr. 2014, bmcpublichealth.biomedcentral.com/articles/10.1186/1471-2458-14-321, 10.1186/1471-2458-14-321.

Jang, Sun-Hwa, et al. Effects of Aerobic and Resistance Exercises on Circulating Apelin-12 and Apelin-36 Concentrations in Obese Middle-Aged Women: A Randomized Controlled Trial. *BMC Women's Health*, vol. 19, no. 1, 29 Jan. 2019, 10.1186/s12905-019-0722-5.

Jasmin, Luc. Hypothalamus.*MedlinePlus*, 2 Nov. 2012.

Jiang, Shu-Zhong, et al. Obesity and Hypertension. *Experimental and Therapeutic Medicine*, vol. 12, no. 4, 6 Sept. 2016, pp. 2395–2399., doi:10.3892/etm.2016.3667.

Joshi, Shivam, et al. The Ketogenic Diet for Obesity and Diabetes—Enthusiasm Outpaces Evidence. *JAMA Internal Medicine*, vol. 179, no. 9, 15 July 2019, p. 1163., doi:10.1001/jamainternmed.2019.2633.

Juo, Yen-Yi, et al. Obesity Is Associated with Early Onset of Gastrointestinal Cancers in California. *Journal of Obesity*, vol. 2018, 19 Sept. 2018, pp. 1–6., doi:10.1155/2018/7014073.

Jurado, Javier A., et al. Radiation-Induced Peripheral Artery Disease. *Catheterization and Cardiovascular Interventions*, vol. 72, no. 4, 1 Oct. 2008, pp. 563–568, 10.1002/ccd.21681.

Kakoschke, Naomi, et al. The Cognitive Drivers of Compulsive Eating Behavior.*Frontiers in Behavioral Neuroscience*, vol. 12, 2019, doi:10.3389/fnbeh.2018.00338.

Kang, Jenny H., and Quang A. Le.Effectiveness of Bariatric Surgical Procedures.*Medicine*, vol. 96, no. 46, Nov. 2017, p. e8632, journals.lww.com/md-journal/Fulltext/2017/11170/Effectiveness_of_bariatric_surgical_ procedures__A.48.aspx, 10.1097/md.0000000000008632.

Karczewski, Jacek, et al. Obesity and the Risk of Gastrointestinal Cancers.*Digestive Diseases and Sciences*, vol. 64, no. 10, 9 Apr. 2019, pp. 2740–2749., doi:10.1007/s10620-019-05603-9.

Karr, Samantha. Epidemiology and Management of Hyperlipidemia.*American Journal of Managed Care*, vol. 23, no. 9, 21 June 2017, pp. 139–148.

Kearns, Ann. Can Certain Foods Increase Thyroid Function in People with Hypothyroidism? *Mayo Clinic*, Mayo Foundation for Medical Education and Research, 4 Sept. 2019, www.mayoclinic.org/diseases-conditions/hypothyroidism/expert-answers/hypothyroidism-diet/faq-20058554.

Keller, Amélie, and Sophie Bucher Della Torre. Sugar-Sweetened Beverages and Obesity among Children and Adolescents: A Review of Systematic Literature Reviews. Childhood Obesity, vol. 11, no. 4, 2015, pp. 338–346., doi:10.1089/chi.2014.0117.

Kelly, Janis C. Obesity Doubles Gout Risk, Reduces Age of Onset. *Medscape*, 12 Aug. 2011, www.medscape.com/viewarticle/747967.

Khalid, MirzaUmair, et al. The Obesity Paradox in Heart Failure: Why Does It Clinically Matter? *American College of Cardiology*, 7 May 2015, www.acc.org/latest-in-cardiology/articles/2015/05/06/10/22/the-obesity-paradox-in-heart-failure.

Khalsa, Amrik Singh, et al. Attainment of '5-2-1-0' Obesity Recommendations in Preschool-Aged Children.*Preventive Medicine Reports*, vol. 8, Dec. 2017, pp. 79–87, 10.1016/j.pmedr.2017.08.003.

Khattab, Ahmed, and Mark A. Sperling. Obesity in Adolescents and Youth: The Case for and against Bariatric Surgery. *The Journal of Pediatrics*, vol. 207, Apr. 2019, pp. 18–22, 10.1016/j.jpeds.2018.11.058.

Khera, Rohan, et al. Association of Pharmacological Treatments for Obesity With Weight Loss and Adverse Events: A Systematic Review and Meta-Analysis. *JAMA*, vol. 315, no. 22, 2016, pp. 2424–34, www.ncbi.nlm.nih.gov/pubmed/27299618, 10.1001/jama.2016.7602.

Kim, Hee Soon, et al. What Are the Barriers at Home and School to Healthy Eating? *Journal of Nursing Research*, vol. 27, no. 5, Apr. 2019, p. 1, 10.1097/jnr.0000000000000321.

Kim, Seong Hwan, et al. Obesity and Cardiovascular Disease: Friend or Foe? *European Heart Journal*, vol. 37, no. 48, 18 Dec. 2015, pp. 3560–3568., doi:10.1093/eurheartj/ehv509.

King, Rhodri J, and Ramzi A Ajjan. Vascular Risk in Obesity: Facts, Misconceptions and the Unknown. *Diabetes and Vascular Disease Research*, vol. 14, no. 1, 14 Nov. 2016, pp. 2–13., doi:10.1177/1479164116675488.

Kirkpatrick, Carol F., et al. Review of Current Evidence and Clinical Recommendations on the Effects of Low-Carbohydrate and Very-Low-Carbohydrate (Including Ketogenic) Diets for the Management of Body Weight and Other Cardiometabolic Risk Factors: A Scientific Statement from the National Lipid Association Nutrition and Lifestyle Task Force. *Journal of Clinical Lipidology*, vol. 13, no. 5, 2019, doi:10.1016/j.jacl.2019.08.003.

Kitahara, Cari M, et al. Impact of Overweight and Obesity on U.S. Papillary Thyroid Cancer Incidence Trends (1995-2015). *JNCI: Journal of the National Cancer Institute*, 5 Dec. 2019, doi:10.1093/jnci/djz202.

Kizy, Scott, et al. Bariatric Surgery: A Perspective for Primary Care. *Diabetes Spectrum*, vol. 30, no. 4, Nov. 2017, pp. 265–276, 10.2337/ds17-0034.

Kloner, Robert A., and Bernard Chaitman.Angina and Its Management.*Journal of Cardiovascular Pharmacology and Therapeutics*, vol. 22, no. 3, 14 Dec. 2016, pp. 199–209.

Knight, Helen. A Metabolic Master Switch Underlying Human Obesity.*MIT News*, 19 Aug. 2015, news.mit.edu/2015/pathway-controls-metabolism-underlying-obesity-0819.

Koch, Sabine C., et al. Effects of Dance Movement Therapy and Dance on Health-Related Psychological Outcomes.A Meta-Analysis Update.*Frontiers in Psychology*, vol. 10, 20 Aug. 2019, 10.3389/fpsyg.2019.01806.

Kodama, Satoru. Cardiorespiratory Fitness as a Quantitative Predictor of All-Cause Mortality and Cardiovascular Events in Healthy Men and

Women. *JAMA*, vol. 301, no. 19, 20 May 2009, p. 2024, 10.1001/jama.2009.681.

Kohn, Jill Balla. What Do I Tell My Clients Who Want to Follow a Low Glycemic Index Diet? *Journal of the Academy of Nutrition and Dietetics*, vol. 117, no. 1, 2017, p. 164., doi:10.1016/j.jand.2016.10.019.

Koliaki, Chrysi, et al. Obesity and Cardiovascular Disease: Revisiting an Old Relationship. *Metabolism*, vol. 92, 2019, pp. 98–107., doi:10.1016/j.metabol.2018.10.011.

Kong, A. P. S., et al. Role of Low-Glycemic Index Diet in Management of Childhood Obesity. *Obesity Reviews*, vol. 12, no. 7, 2010, pp. 492–498., doi:10.1111/j.1467-789x.2010.00768.x.

Koolhaas, Chantal M, et al. Impact of Physical Activity on the Association of Overweight and Obesity with Cardiovascular Disease: The Rotterdam Study. *European Journal of Preventive Cardiology*, vol. 24, no. 9, 28 Feb. 2017, pp. 934–941, 10.1177/2047487317693952.

Korn, Leslie E. *Nutrition Essentials for Mental Health: a Complete Guide to the Food-Mood Connection.* W.W. Norton & Company, 2016.

Koski, Marja, and HannuNaukkarinen. The Relationship between Stress and Severe Obesity: A Case-Control Study. *Biomedicine Hub*, vol. 2, no. 1, 3 Mar. 2017, pp. 1–13., doi:10.1159/000458771.

Kossoff, Eric. Ketogenic Diet. *Epilepsy Foundation*, 25 Oct. 2017, www.epilepsy.com/learn/treating-seizures-and-epilepsy/dietary-therapies/ketogenic-diet.

Kotsis, Vasilios, et al. Mechanisms of Obesity-Induced Hypertension. *Hypertension Research*, vol. 33, no. 5, 2010, pp. 386–393., doi:10.1038/hr.2010.9.

Kreatsoulas, Catherine, et al. Interpreting Angina: Symptoms along a Gender Continuum. *Open Heart*, vol. 3, no. 1, 2016, doi:10.1136/openhrt-2015-000376.

Krishnan, Sridevi, et al. Zumba® Dance Improves Health in Overweight/Obese or Type 2 Diabetic Women. *American Journal of Health Behavior*, vol. 39, no. 1, 1 Jan. 2015, pp. 109–120, 10.5993/ajhb.39.1.12.

Krueger, Patrick M., and Eric N. Reither. Mind the Gap: Race/Ethnic and Socioeconomic Disparities in Obesity. *Current Diabetes Reports*, vol. 15, no. 11, 16 Nov. 2015, doi:10.1007/s11892-015-0666-6.

Kulkarni, Kunal, et al. Obesity and Osteoarthritis. *Maturitas*, vol. 89, 2016, pp. 22–28., doi:10.1016/j.maturitas.2016.04.006.

Kwon, Hyemi, et al. Weight Change Is Significantly Associated with Risk of Thyroid Cancer: A Nationwide Population-Based Cohort Study. *Scientific Reports*, vol. 9, no. 1, 7 Feb. 2019, doi:10.1038/s41598-018-38203-0.

LaChance, Laura R., and Drew Ramsey. Food, Mood, and Brain Health: Implications for the Modern Clinician. *Missouri Medicine*, vol. 112, no. 2, Mar. 2015, pp. 111–115.

Laclaustra, Martin, et al. LDL Cholesterol Rises With BMI Only in Lean Individuals: Cross-Sectional U.S. and Spanish Representative Data. Diabetes Care, vol. 41, no. 10, 2018, pp. 2195–2201., doi:10.2337/dc18-0372.

Lafrenière, Jacynthe, et al. The Effects of Food Labelling on Postexercise Energy Intake in Sedentary Women. *Journal of Obesity*, vol. 2017, 2017, pp. 1–10, 10.1155/2017/1048973.

Largest Ever Genome-Wide Study Strengthens Genetic Link to Obesity. *Broad Institute*, 11 Feb. 2015.

LaRosa, John C., et al. Comparison of 80 versus 10 Mg of Atorvastatin on Occurrence of Cardiovascular Events After the First Event (from the Treating to New Targets [TNT] Trial). *The American Journal of Cardiology*, vol. 105, no. 3, Feb. 2010, pp. 283–287, 10.1016/j.amjcard.2009.09.025.

Laskey, R. A., et al. Obesity-Related Endometrial Cancer: an Update on Survivorship Approaches to Reducing Cardiovascular Death. *BJOG: An International Journal of Obstetrics &Gynaecology*, vol. 123, no. 2, 29 Dec. 2015, pp. 293–298., doi:10.1111/1471-0528.13684.

Lau, Erica Y., et al. Maternal Weight Gain in Pregnancy and Risk of Obesity among Offspring: A Systematic Review. *Journal of Obesity*, vol. 2014, 2014, pp. 1–16, 10.1155/2014/524939.

Learmonth, Yvonne C., et al. Physical Education and Leisure-Time Sport Reduce Overweight and Obesity: A Number Needed to Treat Analysis.

International Journal of Obesity, vol. 43, no. 10, 8 Jan. 2019, pp. 2076–2084, 10.1038/s41366-018-0300-1.

Lee, Jennifer, et al. Visceral Fat Obesity Is Highly Associated with Primary Gout in a Metabolically Obese but Normal Weighted Population: a Case Control Study. *Arthritis Research & Therapy*, vol. 17, no. 1, 24 Mar. 2015, doi:10.1186/s13075-015-0593-6.

Lee, Kyuwan, et al. The Impact of Obesity on Breast Cancer Diagnosis and Treatment. *Current Oncology Reports*, vol. 21, no. 5, 27 Mar. 2019, doi:10.1007/s11912-019-0787-1.

Leitner, Deborah R., et al. Obesity and Type 2 Diabetes: Two Diseases with a Need for Combined Treatment Strategies - EASO Can Lead the Way. *Obesity Facts*, vol. 10, no. 5, 2017, pp. 483–492., doi:10.1159/000480525.

Leitzmann, Michael F., et al. Body Mass Index and Risk of Ovarian Cancer. *Cancer*, vol. 115, no. 4, 2009, pp. 812–822., doi:10.1002/cncr.24086.

Leng, Owain, and Salman Razvi. Hypothyroidism in the Older Population. *Thyroid Research*, vol. 12, no. 1, 8 Feb. 2019, doi:10.1186/s13044-019-0063-3.

Leptin. *Hormone Health Network*, Endocrine Society, Nov. 2018, www.hormone.org/your-health-and-hormones/glands-and-hormones-a-to-z/hormones/leptin.

Lerma-Cabrera, Jose Manuel, et al. Food Addiction as a New Piece of the Obesity Framework. Nutrition Journal, vol. 15, no. 1, 2015, doi:10.1186/s12937-016-0124-6.

Lerma-Cabrera, Jose Manuel, et al. Food Addiction as a New Piece of the Obesity Framework. Nutrition Journal, vol. 15, no. 1, 2015, doi:10.1186/s12937-016-0124-6.

Li, Tricia Y., et al. Regular Consumption of Nuts Is Associated with a Lower Risk of Cardiovascular Disease in Women with Type 2 Diabetes. *The Journal of Nutrition*, vol. 139, no. 7, 6 May 2009, pp. 1333–1338, 10.3945/jn.108.103622.

Lin, X.-J., et al. Body Mass Index and Risk of Gastric Cancer: A Meta-Analysis. *Japanese Journal of Clinical Oncology*, vol. 44, no. 9, 20 June 2014, pp. 783–791., doi:10.1093/jjco/hyu082.

Lindström, Jaana, et al. Sustained Reduction in the Incidence of Type 2 Diabetes by Lifestyle Intervention: Follow-up of the Finnish Diabetes Prevention Study. *The Lancet*, vol. 368, no. 9548, Nov. 2006, pp. 1673–1679, 10.1016/s0140-6736(06)69701-8.

Liraglutide. *DynaMed*, EBSCO Information Services, 27 Sept. 2016, www.dynamed.com/drug-monograph/liraglutide.

Littleberry, Merrill. Beyond the Looking Glass: An Honest View of Body Dysmorphic Disorder. *Obesity Action Coalition*, 2019, www.obesityaction. org/community/article-library/beyond-the-looking-glass-an-honest-view-of-body-dysmorphic-disorder/.

Liu, Ann G., et al. A Healthy Approach to Dietary Fats: Understanding the Science and Taking Action to Reduce Consumer Confusion. *Nutrition Journal*, vol. 16, no. 1, 30 Aug. 2017, doi:10.1186/s12937-017-0271-4.

Liu, Ann G., et al. A Healthy Approach to Dietary Fats: Understanding the Science and Taking Action to Reduce Consumer Confusion. *Nutrition Journal*, vol. 16, no. 1, 2017, doi:10.1186/s12937-017-0271-4.

Liu, Po-Hong, et al. Association of Obesity With Risk of Early-Onset Colorectal Cancer Among Women. *JAMA Oncology*, vol. 5, no. 1, 11 Oct. 2018, p. 37., doi:10.1001/jamaoncol.2018.4280.

Liu, Zhen, et al. The Association between Overweight, Obesity and Ovarian Cancer: a Meta-Analysis. *Japanese Journal of Clinical Oncology*, 21 Oct. 2015, doi:10.1093/jjco/hyv150.

Loimaala, Antti, et al. Effect of Long-Term Endurance and Strength Training on Metabolic Control and Arterial Elasticity in Patients With Type 2 Diabetes Mellitus. *The American Journal of Cardiology*, vol. 103, no. 7, Apr. 2009, pp. 972–977, 10.1016/j.amjcard.2008.12.026.

Loke, Y. K., et al. Long-Term Use of Thiazolidinediones and Fractures in Type 2 Diabetes: A Meta-Analysis. *Canadian Medical Association Journal*, vol. 180, no. 1, 6 Jan. 2009, pp. 32–39, 10.1503/cmaj.080486.

Long, Elizabeth, and Ian L.p.Beales.The Role of Obesity in Oesophageal Cancer Development. *Therapeutic Advances in Gastroenterology*, vol. 7, no.

6, 2014, pp. 247–268., doi:10.1177/1756283x14538689.

Look AHEAD Research Group. Effects of a Long-Term Lifestyle Modification Programme on Peripheral Neuropathy in Overweight or Obese Adults with Type 2 Diabetes: the Look AHEAD Study. *Diabetologia*, vol. 60, no. 6, 27 Mar. 2017, pp. 980–988., doi:10.1007/s00125-017-4253-z.

Lovejoy, Jessica. Body Image Issues Are Not Just For Women. *The Huffington Post*, 26 May 2014, www.huffingtonpost.com/jessica-lovejoy/body-image-issues-are-not-just-for-women_b_5034285.html.

Luca, Leonardo De, et al. Characteristics, Treatment and Quality of Life of Stable Coronary Artery Disease Patients with or without Angina: Insights from the START Study. *Plos One*, vol. 13, no. 7, 12 July 2018, doi:10.1371/journal.pone.0199770.

Luger, Maria, et al. Sugar-Sweetened Beverages and Weight Gain in Children and Adults: A Systematic Review from 2013 to 2015 and a Comparison with Previous Studies. *Obesity Facts*, vol. 10, no. 6, 2017, pp. 674–693., doi:10.1159/000484566.

Luz, Felipe Da, et al. Obesity with Comorbid Eating Disorders: Associated Health Risks and Treatment Approaches. *Nutrients*, vol. 10, no. 7, 27 June 2018, p. 829., doi:10.3390/nu10070829.

Luz, Felipe Da, et al. Obesity with Comorbid Eating Disorders: Associated Health Risks and Treatment Approaches. *Nutrients*, vol. 10, no. 7, 27 June 2018, p. 829., doi:10.3390/nu10070829.

Maciejewski, Matthew L., et al. Bariatric Surgery and Long-Term Durability of Weight Loss. *JAMA Surgery*, vol. 151, no. 11, 1 Nov. 2016, p. 1046, 10.1001/jamasurg.2016.2317.

Mahajan, Rajiv, et al. Complex Interaction of Obesity, Intentional Weight Loss and Heart Failure: a Systematic Review and Meta-Analysis. *Heart*, vol. 106, 17 Sept. 2019, pp. 58–68.

Maki, Kevin C, et al. Consumption of Diacylglycerol Oil as Part of a Reduced-Energy Diet Enhances Loss of Body Weight and Fat in Comparison with Consumption of a Triacylglycerol Control Oil. *The American Journal of Clinical Nutrition*, vol. 76, no. 6, 1 Dec. 2002, pp. 1230–1236, 10.1093/ajcn/76.6.1230.

Management of Stable Angina.*DynaMed*, EBSCO Information Services, 15 Nov. 2017, www.dynamed.com/management/management-of-stable-angina.

Mandal, Ananya.Obesity and Deep Vein Thrombosis (DVT).*News-Medical.Net*, 14 June 2019, www.news-medical.net/health/Obesity-and-deep-vein-thrombosis-(DVT).aspx.

Mangge, Harald, et al. Weight Gain During Treatment of Bipolar Disorder (BD)—Facts and Therapeutic Options. *Frontiers in Nutrition*, vol. 6, 11 June 2019, doi:10.3389/fnut.2019.00076.

Mannan, Munim, et al. Prospective Associations between Depression and Obesity for Adolescent Males and Females- A Systematic Review and Meta-Analysis of Longitudinal Studies.*Plos One*, vol 11, no. 6, 10 June 2016, doi:10.1371/journal.pone.0157240.

Mantovani, Alessandro, et al. Nonalcoholic Fatty Liver Disease and Risk of Incident Type 2 Diabetes: A Meta-Analysis. *Diabetes Care*, vol. 41, no. 2, 22 Jan. 2018, pp. 372–382, 10.2337/dc17-1902.

Marcello, M. A., et al. Obesity and Thyroid Cancer. *Endocrine Related Cancer*, vol. 21, no. 5, 16 Oct. 2014, doi:10.1530/erc-14-0070.

Maric-Bilkan, Christine. Obesity and Diabetic Kidney Disease.*Medical Clinics of North America*, vol. 97, no. 1, 2013, pp. 59–74., doi:10.1016/j.mcna.2012.10.010.

Martí-Carvajal, Arturo J, et al. Homocysteine-Lowering Interventions for Preventing Cardiovascular Events. *Cochrane Database of Systematic Reviews*, vol. 8, 17 Aug. 2017, 10.1002/14651858.cd006612.pub5.

Martinez-Useros, Javier, and Jesus Garcia-Foncillas. Obesity and Colorectal Cancer: Molecular Features of Adipose Tissue. *Journal of Translational Medicine*, vol. 14, no. 1, 22 Jan. 2016, doi:10.1186/s12967-016-0772-5.

Masab, Muhammad. How Does Obesity Affect the Risk for Esophageal Adenocarcinoma? *Medscape*, 5 Aug. 2019, www.medscape.com/answers/277930-38122/how-does-obesity-affect-the-risk-for-esophageal-adenocarcinoma.

Masheb, Robin, and Marney A. White.Bulimia Nervosa in Overweight and Normal-Weight Women. *Comprehensive Psychiatry*, vol. 53, no. 2, 2012, pp.

181–186., doi:10.1016/j.comp-psych.2011.03.005.

Mayer, Emeran A. *The Mind-Gut Connection: How the Hidden Conversation within Our Bodies Impacts Our Mood, Our Choices, and Our Overall Health.* HarperWave, 2018.

Mayo Clinic Staff. Metabolic Syndrome. *Mayo Clinic,* Mayo Foundation for Medical Education and Research, 14 Mar. 2019, www.mayoclinic.org/diseases-conditions/metabolic-syndrome/symptoms-causes/syc-20351916?page=0&citems=10.

Mazur, Erin E., et al., editors. Diet and Cancer. *Lutz's Nutrition and Diet Therapy,* 7th ed., F.A. Davis, 2018, pp. 375–388.

Mcaninch, Elizabeth A., and Antonio C. Bianco. The History and Future of Treatment of Hypothyroidism. *Annals of Internal Medicine,* vol. 164, no. 1, 5 Jan. 2016, p. 50., doi:10.7326/m15-1799.

McCaslin, James E, et al. Cryoplasty for Peripheral Arterial Disease. *Cochrane Database of Systematic Reviews,* 11 Aug. 2013, 10.1002/14651858.cd005507.pub3.

McConville, Sharon. Body Dysmorphia and Its Link to Eating Disorders: How Do They Relate? *Eating Disorder Hope,* 10 June 2019, www.eatingdisorderhope.com/information/body-image/body-dysmorphia.

Mcfarlane, Samy I, et al. Obstructive Sleep Apnea and Obesity: Implications for Public Health. *Sleep Medicine and Disorders: International Journal,* vol. 1, no. 4, 12 Dec. 2017, doi:10.15406/smdij.2017.01.00019.

McGuire, Jane. Binge Eating Disorder & Body Dysmorphic Disorder Connection. *Eating Disorder Hope,* 12 Oct. 2017, www.eatingdisorderhope.com/blog/bed-bdd-connection.

McGuire, Jane. Teens, Eating Disorders, and Obesity. *Eating Disorder Hope,* 25 Apr. 2018, www.eatingdisorderhope.com/blog/teens-eating-disorders-obesity.

McIntosh, James. How Do Race and Ethnicity Influence Childhood Obesity? *Medical News Today,* 23 Apr. 2013, www.medicalnewstoday.com/articles/292913.

McKenna, Rebecca A, et al. Food Addiction Support: Website Content Analysis. *JMIR Cardio,* vol.

2, no. 1, 24 Apr. 2018, p. e10, 10.2196/cardio.8718.

McQuillan, Susan. How Your Culture Affects Your Weight. *Psychology Today,* 12 May 2016, www.psychologytoday.com/us/blog/cravings/201605/how-your-culture-affects-your-weight.

Measuring Physical Activity Intensity. *Centers for Disease Control and Prevention,* 29 Jan. 2020, www.cdc.gov/physicalactivity/basics/measuring/index.html.

Menayang, Adi. New Report Supports Chromium Picolinate's Weight Management Benefits. *NutraIngredients-USA,* 2 Jan. 2019, www.nutraingredients-usa.com/Article/2019/01/02/New-report-supports-chromium-picolinate-s-weight-management-benefits.

Mendizábal, Brenda, and Elaine M. Urbina. Subclinical Atherosclerosis in Youth: Relation to Obesity, Insulin Resistance, and Polycystic Ovary Syndrome. *The Journal of Pediatrics,* vol. 190, 2017, pp. 14–20., doi:10.1016/j.jpeds.2017.06.043.

Meynier, Anne, and Claude Genot. Molecular and Structural Organization of Lipids in Foods: Their Fate during Digestion and Impact in Nutrition. *Ocl,* vol. 24, no. 2, 2017, doi:10.1051/ocl/2017006.

Minges, Karl E., et al. Overweight and Obesity in Youth With Type 1 Diabetes. *Annual Review of Nursing Research,* vol. 31, no. 1, 2013, pp. 47–69., doi:10.1891/0739-6686.31.47.

Mitchell, Andrew B., et al. Obesity Increases Risk of Ischemic Stroke in Young Adults. *Stroke,* vol. 46, no. 6, 2015, pp. 1690–1692., doi:10.1161/strokeaha.115.008940.

Mohan, Viswanathan, and Joshi Shilpa. Ketogenic Diets: Boon or Bane? *Indian Journal of Medical Research,* vol. 148, no. 3, 2018, p. 251., doi:10.4103/ijmr.ijmr_1666_18.

Moholdt, Trine, et al. Sustained Physical Activity, Not Weight Loss, Associated With Improved Survival in Coronary Heart Disease. *Journal of the American College of Cardiology,* vol. 71, no. 10, 2018, pp. 1094–1101., doi:10.1016/j.jacc.2018.01.011.

Molnar, Miklos Z, et al. Association of Incident Obstructive Sleep Apnoea with Outcomes in a Large Cohort of US Veterans. *Thorax,* vol. 70, no.

9, 2 June 2015, pp. 888–895, 10.1136/thoraxjnl-2015-206970.

Moore, Catherine F., et al. Neuropharmacology of Compulsive Eating. *Philosophical Transactions of the Royal Society B: Biological Sciences*, vol. 373, no. 1742, 29 Jan. 2018, p. 20170024., doi:10.1098/rstb.2017.0024.

Moore, Catherine F., et al. Neuroscience of Compulsive Eating Behavior. *Frontiers in Neuroscience*, vol. 11, 24 Aug. 2017, doi:10.3389/fnins.2017.00469.

Moreno, Megan. Early Infant Feeding and Obesity Risk.*JAMA Pediatrics*, vol. 168, no. 11, 1 Nov. 2014, p. 1084, 10.1001/jamapediatrics.2013.3379.

Mottalib, Adham, et al. Weight Management in Patients with Type 1 Diabetes and Obesity. *Current Diabetes Reports*, vol. 17, no. 10, 23 Aug. 2017, doi:10.1007/s11892-017-0918-8.

Mulik, Kranti, and Lindsey Haynes-Maslow. The Affordability of MyPlate: An Analysis of SNAP Benefits and the Actual Cost of Eating According to the Dietary Guidelines. *Journal of Nutrition Education and Behavior*, vol. 49, no. 8, 2017, doi:10.1016/j.jneb.2017.06.005.

Mulugeta, Anwar, et al. Obesity and Depressive Symptoms in Mid-Life: a Population-Based Cohort Study. *BMC Psychiatry*, vol. 18, no. 1, 17 Sept. 2018, doi:10.1186/s12888-018-1877-6.

Muscogiuri, Giovanna, et al. The Management of Very Low-Calorie Ketogenic Diet in Obesity Outpatient Clinic: a Practical Guide. *Journal of Translational Medicine*, vol. 17, no. 1, 29 Oct. 2019, doi:10.1186/s12967-019-2104-z.

Myers, Amy. *The Thyroid Connection: Why You Feel Tired, Brain-Fogged, and Overweight – and How to Get Your Life Back.* Little, Brown and Company, 2016.

Nagle, C M, et al. Obesity and Survival among Women with Ovarian Cancer: Results from the Ovarian Cancer Association Consortium. *British Journal of Cancer*, vol. 113, no. 5, 7 July 2015, pp. 817–826., doi:10.1038/bjc.2015.245.

Nall, Rachel. Unstable Angina.*Healthline*, 30 May 2017, www.healthline.com/health/unstable-angina.

Nascimento, E. R., et al. Sexual Dysfunction and Cardiovascular Diseases: A Systematic Review of Prevalence. *Clinics*, vol. 68, no. 11, 1 Nov. 2013, pp. 1462–1468, 10.6061/clinics/2013(11)13.

National Institute of Arthritis and Musculoskeletal and Skin Diseases, National Institutes of Health, 12 Apr. 2017, www.niams.nih.gov/health-topics/gout.

Nemiary, Deina, et al. The Relationship Between Obesity and Depression Among Adolescents. *Psychiatric Annals*, vol. 42, no. 8, 1 Aug. 2012, pp. 305–308., doi:10.3928/00485713-20120806-09.

Neumark-Sztainer, Dianne. Higher Weight Status and Restrictive Eating Disorders: An Overlooked Concern. *Journal of Adolescent Health*, vol. 56, no. 1, 2015, pp. 1–2., doi:10.1016/j.jadohealth.2014.10.261.

Newman, Tim. Does Depression Cause Obesity or Does Obesity Cause Depression? *Medical News Today*, 13 Nov. 2018, www.medicalnewstoday.com/articles/323668.

Newton, Suzy, et al. Socio-Economic Status over the Life Course and Obesity: Systematic Review and Meta-Analysis. *Plos One*, vol. 12, no. 5, 16 May 2017, doi:10.1371/journal.pone.0177151.

Ngo, Nealie Tan. What Historical Ideals of Women's Shapes Teach Us About Women's Self-Perception and Body Decisions Today. *AMA Journal of Ethics*, vol. 21, no. 10, 1 Oct. 2019, doi:10.1001/amajethics.2019.879.

Nguyen, Ngan. Don't Fixate on Fifteen: Healthy Lifestyle Choices for College Freshmen. *University of Michigan School of Public Health*, 9 Sept. 2019, sph.umich.edu/pursuit/2019posts/freshman-fifteen.html.

Nielsen, Sabrina, et al. Weight Loss for Overweight and Obese Individuals with Gout: a Systematic Review of Longitudinal Observational Studies. *Annals of the Rheumatic Diseases*, vol. 76, 2017, pp. 1870–1882., doi:10.1136/annrheumdis-2017-eular.2651.

Nissen, Steven E., and Kathy Wolski.Effect of Rosiglitazone on the Risk of Myocardial Infarction and Death from Cardiovascular Causes.*New England Journal of Medicine*, vol. 356, no. 24, 14 June 2007, pp. 2457–2471, 10.1056/nejmoa072761.

Nordqvist, Joseph. How Much Sugar Is in Your Food and Drink? *Medical News Today*, 7 July 2013, www.medicalnewstoday.com/articles/262978.php.

Norris, T, et al. Obesity in Adolescents with Chronic Fatigue Syndrome: an Observational Study. *Archives of Disease in Childhood*, vol. 102, no. 1, 21 Sept. 2016, pp. 35–39., doi:10.1136/archdischild-2016-311293.

Norwood, Diane Voyatzis. Diabetes Insipidus. *Health Library*, 15 Mar. 2013.

Nutrition Overview. *American Diabetes Association*, 2019, www.diabetes.org/nutrition.

NYU School of Medicine. How Far Schoolkids Live from Junk Food Sources Tied to Obesity. ScienceDaily, 29 Oct. 2019, www.sciencedaily.com/releases/2019/10/191029080737.htm.

O'Connor, Anahad. The Keto Diet Is Popular, but Is It Good for You? *The New York Times*, 20 Aug. 2019, www.nytimes.com/2019/08/20/well/eat/the-keto-diet-is-popular-but-is-it-good-for-you.html.

Obesity & Heart Disease. *Cleveland Clinic*, 2 Jan. 2019, my.clevelandclinic.org/health/articles/17308-obesity–heart-disease.

Obesity Independently Drives NASH and Hepatocellular Carcinoma. *Cancer Discovery*, vol. 8, no. 12, 2018, doi:10.1158/2159-8290.cd-rw2018-190.

Obstructive Sleep Apnea (OSA) in Adults. *DynaMed*, EBSCO Information Services, 5 Oct. 2016, www.dynamed.com/condition/obstructive-sleep-apnea-osa-in-adults.

Øen, Gudbjørg, et al. Adolescents' Perspectives on Everyday Life with Obesity: A Qualitative Study. *International Journal of Qualitative Studies on Health and Well-Being*, vol. 13, no. 1, Jan. 2018, p. 1479581, 10.1080/17482631.2018.1479581.

Oesch, Lisa, et al. Obesity Paradox in Stroke – Myth or Reality? A Systematic Review. *Plos One*, vol. 12, no. 3, 14 Mar. 2017, doi:10.1371/journal.pone.0171334.

Office of Dietary Supplements. Chromium. *National Institutes of Health*, U.S. Department of Health and Human Services, 27 Feb. 2020, ods.od.nih.gov/factsheets/Chromium-HealthProfessional/.

Ogilvie, Rachel P., and Sanjay R. Patel. The Epidemiology of Sleep and Obesity. *Sleep Health*, vol. 3, no. 5, 1 Oct. 2017, pp. 383–388, www.sciencedirect.com/science/article/abs/pii/S2352721817301481?via%3Dihub, 10.1016/j.sleh.2017.07.013.

Ohio State University Center for Clinical and Translational Science. Childhood Obesity Influenced by How Kids Are Fed, Not Just What They Eat. *ScienceDaily*, 13 May 2015, www.sciencedaily.com/releases/2015/05/150513093358.htm.

Onakpoya, Igho, et al. Pyruvate Supplementation for Weight Loss: A Systematic Review and Meta-Analysis of Randomized Clinical Trials. *Critical Reviews in Food Science and Nutrition*, vol. 54, no. 1, 4 Nov. 2013, pp. 17–23, 10.1080/10408398.2011.565890.

Onstad, Michaela A., et al. Addressing the Role of Obesity in Endometrial Cancer Risk, Prevention, and Treatment. *Journal of Clinical Oncology*, vol. 34, no. 35, 2016, pp. 4225–4230., doi:10.1200/jco.2016.69.4638.

Ordway, Denise-Marie. The Freshman 15: Does College Cause Students to Gain Weight? *Journalist's Resource*, 7 Feb. 2017, journalistsresource.org/studies/society/public-health/freshman-15-college-student-weight-gain/.

Oussaada, Sabrina M., et al. The Pathogenesis of Obesity. *Metabolism*, vol. 92, 2019, pp. 26–36., doi:10.1016/j.metabol.2018.12.012.

Owen, James P. *Just Move! A New Approach to Fitness after Fifty*. National Geographic, 2017.

Pajk, Barbara. Obesity among Patients with Schizophrenia: When We Fix One Problem and Create Another. *Clinical and Experimental Psychology*, vol. 2, no. 3, 2016, doi:10.4172/2471-2701.1000135.

Pallazola, Vincent A., et al. A Clinician's Guide to Healthy Eating for Cardiovascular Disease Prevention. *Mayo Clinic Proceedings: Innovations, Quality & Outcomes*, vol. 3, no. 3, 2019, pp. 251–267., doi:10.1016/j.mayocpiqo.2019.05.001.

Pandita, Aaakash, et al. Childhood Obesity: Prevention Is Better than Cure. *Diabetes, Metabolic Syndrome and Obesity: Targets and Therapy*, vol. 9, Mar. 2016, p. 83, www.ncbi.nlm.nih.gov/pmc/articles/PMC4801195/, 10.2147/dmso.s90783.

Park, Chan Seok, et al. Relation Between C-Reactive Protein, Homocysteine Levels, Fibrinogen, and Lipoprotein Levels and Leukocyte and Platelet Counts, and 10-Year Risk for Cardiovascular Disease Among Healthy Adults in the USA. *The American Journal of Cardiology*, vol. 105, no. 9, May 2010, pp. 1284–1288, 10.1016/j.amjcard.2009.12.045.

Parziale, Andrea, and GorikOoms. The Global Fight against Trans-Fat: the Potential Role of International Trade and Law. *Globalization and Health*, vol. 15, no. 1, 11 July 2019, doi:10.1186/s12992-019-0488-4.

Pediatric Sleep-Disordered Breathing.*ENT Health*, American Academy of Otolaryngology–Head and Neck Surgery Foundation, Dec. 2018, www.enthealth.org/conditions/pediatric-sleep-disordered-breathing/.Accessed 16 Mar. 2020.

Pegloticase.*DynaMed*, EBSCO Information Services, 6 Feb. 2017, www.dynamed.com/drug-monograph/pegloticase.

Percutaneous Coronary Intervention (PCI) Procedure.*DynaMed*, EBSCO Information Services, 26 July 2017, www.dynamed.com/procedure/percutaneous-coronary-intervention-pci-procedure.

Percutaneous Coronary Intervention (PCI) Procedure. *DynaMed*, EBSCO Information Services, 18 Jan. 2019, www.dynamed.com/procedure/percutaneous-coronary-intervention-pci-procedure.

Pereira, ElisângelaVitoriano, et al. Effect of Glycemic Index on Obesity Control. *Archives of Endocrinology and Metabolism*, vol. 59, no. 3, 2015, pp. 245–251., doi:10.1590/2359-3997000000045.

Peripheral Artery Disease (PAD) of Lower Extremities.*DynaMed*, EBSCO Information Services, 23 Aug. 2018, www.dynamed.com/condition/peripheral-artery-disease-pad-of-lower-extremities.

Peripheral Artery Disease (PAD) of Lower Extremities.*DynaMed*, EBSCO Information Services, 23 Aug. 2018,

Peripheral Artery Disease (PAD) of Lower Extremities.*DynaMed*, EBSCO Information Services, 23 Aug. 2018, www.dynamed.com/condition/peripheral-artery-disease-pad-of-lower-extremities.

Peripheral Artery Disease.*National Heart, Lung, and Blood Institute*, US Department of Health & Human Services, 23 Jan. 2019, www.nhlbi.nih.gov/health/health-topics/topics/pad.

Petersen, Ruth, et al. Racial and Ethnic Disparities in Adult Obesity in the United States: CDC's Tracking to Inform State and Local Action. *Preventing Chronic Disease*, vol. 16, 11 Apr. 2019, doi:10.5888/pcd16.180579.

Phung, O. J., et al. Oral Anti-Diabetic Drugs for the Prevention of Type 2 Diabetes.*Diabetic Medicine*, vol. 28, no. 8, 13 July 2011, pp. 948–964, 10.1111/j.1464-5491.2011.03303.x.

Picon-Ruiz, Manuel, et al. Obesity and Adverse Breast Cancer Risk and Outcome: Mechanistic Insights and Strategies for Intervention. *CA: A Cancer Journal for Clinicians*, vol. 67, no. 5, 1 Aug. 2017, pp. 378–397., doi:10.3322/caac.21405.

Poli, Vanessa FadanelliSchoenardie, et al. The Excessive Caloric Intake and Micronutrient Deficiencies Related to Obesity after a Long-Term Interdisciplinary Therapy. *Nutrition*, vol. 38, 2017, pp. 113–119., doi:10.1016/j.nut.2017.01.012.

Polyzos, Stergios A., et al. Obesity and Nonalcoholic Fatty Liver Disease: From Pathophysiology to Therapeutics. *Metabolism*, vol. 92, 2019, pp. 82–97., doi:10.1016/j.metabol.2018.11.014.

Position Statement: Surgical Management of Obstructive Sleep Apnea. *American Academy of Otolaryngology-Head and Neck Surgery*, 20 Mar. 2014, www.entnet.org/content/surgical-management-obstructive-sleep-apnea.

Pothuraju, Ramesh, et al. Pancreatic Cancer Associated with Obesity and Diabetes: an Alternative Approach for Its Targeting. *Journal of Experimental & Clinical Cancer Research*, vol. 37, no. 1, 2018, doi:10.1186/s13046-018-0963-4.

Poti, Jennifer M, et al. The Association of Fast Food Consumption with Poor Dietary Outcomes and Obesity among Children: Is It the Fast Food or the Remainder of the Diet? The American Journal of Clinical Nutrition, vol. 99, no. 1, 2013, pp. 162–171., doi:10.3945/ajcn.113.071928.

Prediabetes.*American Diabetes Association*, 2019, www.diabetes.org/diabetes-risk/prediabetes.

Prediabetes.*DynaMed*, EBSCO Information Services, 16 Nov. 2018, www.dynamed.com/condition/prediabetes.

Preparing for Medical Visits.*American Heart Association*, 8 Jan. 2018, www.heart.org/en/health-topics/cardiac-rehab/communicating-with-professionals/preparing-for-medical-visits#.Wp2Ga2rwbIU.

Preparing for Medical Visits. *American Heart Association*, 31 Jan. 2018, www.heart.org/en/health-topics/cardiac-rehab/communicating-with-professionals/preparing-for-medical-visits.

Prevention and Treatment of PAD.*American Heart Association*, 31 Oct. 2016, www.heart.org/en/health-topics/peripheral-artery-disease/prevention-and-treatment-of-pad.

Probenecid.*DynaMed*, EBSCO Information Services, 6 Feb. 2017, www.dynamed.com/drug-monograph/probenecid.

Prushinski, G., et al. 'The Freshman Fifteen:' Prevalence and Predictors of Weight Gain Among College Freshmen Students. *Journal of the Academy of Nutrition and Dietetics*, vol. 117, no. 9, 2017, doi:10.1016/j.jand.2017.06.336.

Qi, Lu. Personalized Nutrition and Obesity.*Annals of Medicine*, vol. 46, no. 5, 10 Apr. 2014, pp. 247–252, www.ncbi.nlm.nih.gov/pmc/articles/PMC5330214/, 10.3109/07853890.2014.891802.

Quarta, Carmelo, et al. Renaissance of Leptin for Obesity Therapy. *Diabetologia*, vol. 59, no. 5, 16 Mar. 2016, pp. 920–927., doi:10.1007/s00125-016-3906-7.

Rapaport, Lisa. More Evidence Linking Stress to Obesity.*Reuters*, 30 Mar. 2017, www.reuters.com/article/us-health-stress-cortisol-obesity/more-evidence-linking-stress-to-obesity-idUSKBN17130P.

Rapaport, Lisa. Obesity, Drinking and Unhealthy Diet Add to Gout Risk. *Reuters*, 20 Sept. 2019, www.reuters.com/article/us-health-gout-prevention/obesity-drinking-and-unhealthy-diet-add-to-gout-risk-idUSKBN1W52AA.

Rathi, SunanadaSurendra, et al. Development and Validation of Integrated Yoga Module for Obesity in Adolescents.*International Journal of Yoga*, vol. 11, no. 3, 2018, p. 231, 10.4103/ijoy.ijoy_38_17.

Ratziu, Vlad, and GiulioMarchesini.When the Journey from Obesity to Cirrhosis Takes an Early Start.*Journal of Hepatology*, vol. 65, no. 2, 2016, pp. 249–251.

Redif, Zibe. Overeaters Anonymous Saved My Life — But Here's Why I Quit. *Healthline*, 30 July 2019, www.healthline.com/health/mental-health/leaving-overeaters-anonymous#1.

Reichel, Chloe. Journalist's Resource. *Journalist's Resource*, 4 Apr. 2018, journalistsresource.org/studies/environment/food-agriculture/food-labels-junk-nafta-obesity/.

Renehan, A. G., et al. Obesity and Endometrial Cancer: Unanswered Epidemiological Questions. *BJOG: An International Journal of Obstetrics &Gynaecology*, vol. 123, no. 2, 2015, pp. 175–178., doi:10.1111/1471-0528.13731.

Rennert, Nancy J. Hypothalamus. *MedlinePlus*, 11 Dec. 2011.

Revascularization for Coronary Artery Disease (CAD).*DynaMed*, EBSCO Information Services, 1 Feb. 2018, www.dynamed.com/management/revascularization-for-coronary-artery-disease-cad.

Riaz, Haris, et al. Association Between Obesity and Cardiovascular Outcomes. *JAMA Network Open*, vol. 1, no. 7, 2018, doi:10.1001/jamanetworkopen.2018.3788.

Ricci, Natalie L., and Melanie Jay. Fast and Furious: Rapid Weight Loss Via a Very Low Calorie Diet May Lead to Better Long-Term Outcomes Than a Gradual Weight Loss Program. *Journal of Clinical Outcomes Management*, vol. 22, no. 8, Aug. 2015, pp. 346–350.

Richard-Davis, Gloria A. Obesity and Menopause: A Growing Concern. *The North American Menopause Society*, 14 Dec. 2016, www.menopause.org/for-women/menopause-take-time-to-think-about-it/consumers/2016/12/14/obesity-and-menopause-a-growing-concern.

Richardson, Laura A., et al. Effect of an Exercise and Weight Control Curriculum: Views of Obesity among Exercise Science Students. *Advances in Physiology Education*, vol. 39, no. 2, June 2015, pp. 43–48, 10.1152/advan.00154.2014.

Ridker, Paul M., et al. Comparison of C-Reactive Protein and Low-Density Lipoprotein

Cholesterol Levels in the Prediction of First Cardiovascular Events. *New England Journal of Medicine*, vol. 347, no. 20, 14 Nov. 2002, pp. 1557–1565, 10.1056/nejmoa021993.

Roberto, C A, and N Khandpur.Improving the Design of Nutrition Labels to Promote Healthier Food Choices and Reasonable Portion Sizes. *International Journal of Obesity*, vol. 38, no.S1, July 2014, pp. S25–S33, 10.1038/ijo.2014.86.

Robinson, S. M. Infant Nutrition and Lifelong Health: Current Perspectives and Future Challenges. *Journal of Developmental Origins of Health and Disease*, vol. 6, no. 5, 19 June 2015, pp. 384–389, 10.1017/s2040174415001257.

Rodríguez-Martín, Boris C., and BelénGallego-Arjiz. Overeaters Anonymous: A Mutual-Help Fellowship for Food Addiction Recovery. *Frontiers in Psychology*, vol. 9, 20 Aug. 2018, 10.3389/fpsyg.2018.01491.

Roever, Leonardo S., et al. Abdominal Obesity and Association With Atherosclerosis Risk Factors. *Medicine*, vol. 95, no. 11, 2016, doi:10.1097/md.0000000000001357.

Rogers, Tony B. MOVE! Weight Management Program Home.*MOVE!*, U.S. Department of Veterans Affairs, 2020, www.move.va.gov/.

Rooke, Thom W., et al. 2011 ACCF/AHA Focused Update of the Guideline for the Management of Patients With Peripheral Artery Disease (Updating the 2005 Guideline). *Journal of the American College of Cardiology*, vol. 58, no. 19, Nov. 2011, pp. 2020–2045, 10.1016/j.jacc.2011.08.023.

Rosenbloom, Christine, and Bob Murray.*Food and Fitness after 50: Eat Well, Move Well, Be Well*. Academy of Nutrition and Dietetics, 2018.

Ross, A. Catharine, et al., eds. *Dietary Reference Intakes for Calcium and Vitamin D*. National Academies Press, 2011.

Ross, A., et al. A Different Weight Loss Experience: A Qualitative Study Exploring the Behavioral, Physical, and Psychosocial Changes Associated with Yoga That Promote Weight Loss. *Evidence-Based Complementary and Alternative Medicine*, vol. 2016, 2016, pp. 1–11, www.ncbi.nlm.nih.gov/pmc/articles/PMC4995338/, 10.1155/2016/2914745.

Rouhani, Mohammad Hossein, et al. The Effect of Low Glycemic Index Diet on Body Weight Status and Blood Pressure in Overweight Adolescent Girls: a Randomized Clinical Trial. *Nutrition Research and Practice*, vol. 7, no. 5, 2013, p. 385., doi:10.4162/nrp.2013.7.5.385.

Rshikesan, P. B. Yoga Practice for Reducing the Male Obesity and Weight Related Psychological Difficulties-A Randomized Controlled Trial. *Journal of Clinical and Diagnostic Research*, vol. 10, no. 11, 2016, 10.7860/jcdr/2016/22720.8940.

Ruanpeng, D., et al. Sugar and Artificially Sweetened Beverages Linked to Obesity: a Systematic Review and Meta-Analysis. *QJM: An International Journal of Medicine*, vol. 110, no. 8, 11 Apr. 2017, pp. 513–520., doi:10.1093/qjmed/hcx068.

Rubin, Rita. Postmenopausal Women With a 'Normal' BMI Might Be Overweight or Even Obese. *JAMA*, vol. 319, no. 12, 27 Mar. 2018, p. 1185., doi:10.1001/jama.2018.0423.

Rumsey, Alissa. Should You Add MCT Oil to Your Diet? *US News & World Report*, 2019, health.usnews.com/health-news/blogs/eat-run/articles/should-you-add-mct-oil-to-your-diet.

Runenko, Svetlana D., et al. Efficiency of Dance Therapy for Weight Loss and Improvement of the Psychological and Physiological State in Overweight or Obese Young Women.*Journal of Physical Education and Sport*, vol. 18, no. 2, June 2018.

Russell-Mayhew, Shelly, et al. How Does Overeaters Anonymous Help Its Members? A Qualitative Analysis.*European Eating Disorders Review*, vol. 18, no. 1, Jan. 2010, pp. 33–42, 10.1002/erv.966.

Sackner-Bernstein, Jonathan, et al. Dietary Intervention for Overweight and Obese Adults: Comparison of Low-Carbohydrate and Low-Fat Diets. A Meta-Analysis.*Plos One*, vol. 10, no. 10, 20 Oct. 2015, doi:10.1371/journal.pone.0139817.

Said, Mohamed Ahmed, et al. Multidisciplinary Approach to Obesity: Aerobic or Resistance Physical Exercise? *Journal of Exercise Science & Fitness*, vol. 16, no. 3, Dec. 2018, pp. 118–123, 10.1016/j.jesf.2018.11.001.

Saitta, Carlo, et al. Obesity and Liver Cancer.*Annals of Hepatology*, vol. 18, no. 6, 2019, pp. 810–815.

Salas-Salvado, J., et al. Reduction in the Incidence of Type 2 Diabetes With the Mediterranean Diet: Results of the PREDIMED-Reus Nutrition Intervention Randomized Trial. *Diabetes Care,* vol. 34, no. 1, 7 Oct. 2010, pp. 14–19, 10.2337/dc10-1288.

Sandoiu, Ana. Cardiovascular Disease: Dietary Cholesterol May Not Raise Risk. *Medical News Today,* 20 Dec. 2019, www.medicalnewstoday.com/articles/327329.

Sarwar, Raiya, et al. Obesity and Nonalcoholic Fatty Liver Disease: Current Perspectives. *Diabetes, Metabolic Syndrome and Obesity: Targets and Therapy,* vol. 11, 2018, pp. 533–542., doi:10.2147/dmso.s146339.

Sattler, Elisabeth LilianPia. Weight Management in Overweight and Obese Breast Cancer Survivors. *Advances in Obesity, Weight Management & Control,* vol. 7, no. 3, 2017, doi:10.15406/aowmc.2017.07.00200.

Schlenker, Eleanor D. Williams' Essentials of Nutrition and Diet Therapy. *Williams' Essentials of Nutrition and Diet Therapy,* edited by Eleanor D. Schlenker and Joyce Gilbert, 12th ed., Elsevier, 2018, pp. 55–67.

Schwartz, Allan. Obesity, An Addiction? *MentalHelp. net,* American Addiction Centers, 2019, www.mentalhelp.net/blogs/obesity-an-addiction/.

Schwingshackl, Lukas, et al. Effects of Low Glycaemic Index/Low Glycaemic Load vs. High Glycaemic Index/ High Glycaemic Load Diets on Overweight/Obesity and Associated Risk Factors in Children and Adolescents: a Systematic Review and Meta-Analysis. *Nutrition Journal,* vol. 14, no. 1, 25 Aug. 2015, doi:10.1186/s12937-015-0077-1.

Scott, Karen A., et al. Effects of Chronic Social Stress on Obesity. *Current Obesity Reports,* vol. 1, no. 1, 11 Jan. 2012, pp. 16–25, www.ncbi.nlm.nih.gov/pmc/articles/PMC3428710/, 10.1007/s13679-011-0006-3.

Scripps Research Institute. Little-Known Protein Appears to Play Important Role in Obesity and Metabolic Disease. *ScienceDaily,* 20 Nov. 2019.

Secondhand Smoke (SHS) Facts. *Centers for Disease Control and Prevention,* 17 Jan. 2018, www.cdc. gov/tobacco/data_statistics/fact_sheets/secondhand_smoke/general_facts/index.htm.

Selhub, Eva. Nutritional Psychiatry: Your Brain on Food. *Harvard Health Blog,* Harvard Medical School, 5 Apr. 2018, www.health.harvard.edu/blog/nutritional-psychiatry-your-brain-on-food-201511168626.

Severe Obesity Revealed as a Stand-Alone High-Risk Factor for Heart Failure. *Johns Hopkins Medicine,* 22 Aug. 2016, www.hopkinsmedicine.org/news/media/releases/severe_obesity_revealed_as_a_stand_alone_high_risk_factor_for_heart_failure.

Shattat, Ghassan F. A Review Article on Hyperlipidemia: Types, Treatments and New Drug Targets. *Biomedical and Pharmacology Journal,* vol. 7, no. 2, 2014, pp. 399–409., doi:10.13005/bpj/504.

Shen, Hsiu-Nien, et al. Risk of Diabetes Mellitus after First-Attack Acute Pancreatitis: A National Population-Based Study. *American Journal of Gastroenterology,* vol. 110, no. 12, Dec. 2015, pp. 1698–1706, 10.1038/ajg.2015.356.

Shiroma, Paulo R, et al. Antidepressant Effect of the VA Weight Management Program (MOVE) Among Veterans With Severe Obesity. *Military Medicine,* 20 Feb. 2020, 10.1093/milmed/usz475.

Sievert, Katherine, et al. Effect of Breakfast on Weight and Energy Intake: Systematic Review and Meta-Analysis of Randomised Controlled Trials. *BMJ,* 30 Jan. 2019, p. 142., doi:10.1136/bmj.l42.

Sitagliptin. *DynaMed,* EBSCO Information Services, 27 Sept. 2016, www.dynamed.com/drug-monograph/sitagliptin.

Sleep Apnea Information Page. *National Institute of Neurological Disorders and Stroke,* National Institutes of Health, 27 Mar. 2019, www.ninds.nih.gov/Disorders/All-Disorders/Sleep-Apnea-Information-Page.

Sleep Apnea Information. *American Sleep Apnea Association,* 5 Apr. 2019, www.sleepapnea.org/learn/sleep-apnea/.

Sleep Apnea. *National Heart, Lung, and Blood Institute,* US Department of Health & Human Services, 10 Dec. 2018, www.nhlbi.nih.gov/health-topics/sleep-apnea.

Smith-Jackson, Terisue, and Justine J. Reel. Freshmen Women and the 'Freshman 15': Perspectives on Prevalence and Causes of College Weight Gain. *Journal of American College Health*, vol. 60, no. 1, 2012, pp. 14–20., doi:10.1080/074 48481.2011.555931.

Snoring, Sleeping Disorders, and Sleep Apnea.*ENT Health*, American Academy of Otolaryngology–Head and Neck Surgery Foundation, Aug. 2018, www.enthealth.org/conditions/snoring-sleeping-disorders-and-sleep-apnea/.

Soliman, Ghada. Dietary Cholesterol and the Lack of Evidence in Cardiovascular Disease. Nutrients, vol. 10, no. 6, 2018, p. 780., doi:10.3390/nu10060780.

Soltani, Ghodratollah, et al. Obesity, Diabetes and the Risk of Colorectal Adenoma and Cancer. *BMC Endocrine Disorders*, vol. 19, no. 1, 29 Oct. 2019, doi:10.1186/s12902-019-0444-6.

Son, Sungmin, et al. Effects of a Walking Exercise Program for Obese Individuals with Intellectual Disability Staying in a Residential Care Facility. *Journal of Physical Therapy Science*, vol. 28, no. 3, 2016, pp. 788–793, 10.1589/jpts.28.788.

Sontheimer, Daniel L. Peripheral Vascular Disease: Diagnosis and Treatment. *American Family Physician*, vol. 73, no. 11, 1 June 2006, pp. 1971–1976.

Souza, Russell J De, et al. Intake of Saturated and Trans Unsaturated Fatty Acids and Risk of All Cause Mortality, Cardiovascular Disease, and Type 2 Diabetes: Systematic Review and Meta-Analysis of Observational Studies. *BMJ*, 11 Aug. 2015, doi:10.1136/bmj.h3978.

Sponholtz, Todd R., et al. Body Size, Metabolic Factors, and Risk of Endometrial Cancer in Black Women.*American Journal of Epidemiology*, vol. 183, no. 4, 2016, pp. 259–268., doi:10.1093/aje/kwv186.

Standards of Medical Care in Diabetes–2010.*Diabetes Care*, vol. 33, no.Suppl 1, Jan. 2010, pp. S11–S61, 10.2337/dc10-s011.

Standards of Medical Care in Diabetes—2018.*Diabetes Care*, vol. 41, no.Suppl 1, Jan. 2018, pp. S1–S172.

Stang, Jamie, and Laurel G. Huffman. Position of the Academy of Nutrition and Dietetics: Obesity, Reproduction, and Pregnancy Outcomes. *Journal of the Academy of Nutrition and Dietetics*, vol. 116, no. 4, Apr. 2016, pp. 677–691, 10.1016/j.jand.2016.01.008.

Stanhope, Kimber L. Sugar Consumption, Metabolic Disease and Obesity: The State of the Controversy. *Critical Reviews in Clinical Laboratory Sciences*, vol. 53, no. 1, 17 Sept. 2015, pp. 52–67., doi:10.3109/10408363.2015.1084990.

Start Simple with MyPlate. *ChooseMyPlate*, U.S. Department of Agriculture, 2020, www.choosemyplate.gov/eathealthy/start-simple-myplate.

Statins for Primary and Secondary Prevention of Cardiovascular Disease.*DynaMed*, EBSCO Information Services, 22 Feb. 2018, dynamed.com/prevention/statins-for-primary-and-secondary-prevention-of-cardiovascular-disease.

Statins. *DynaMed*, EBSCO Information Services, 5 Apr. 2018, www.dynamed.com/drug-review/statins.

Statistics About Diabetes. *American Diabetes Association*, 22 Mar. 2018, www.diabetes.org/resources/statistics/statistics-about-diabetes.

Steinke, Elaine E., et al. Sexual Counselling for Individuals with Cardiovascular Disease and Their Partners. *European Heart Journal*, vol. 34, no. 41, 29 July 2013, pp. 3217–3235, 10.1093/eurheartj/eht270.

ST-Elevation Myocardial Infarction (STEMI). *DynaMed*, EBSCO Information Services, 10 July 2018, www.dynamed.com/condition/st-elevation-myocardial-infarction-stemi.

Stiles, Laura. Prediabetes, Obesity May Impact Risk of Polyneuropathy. *Neurology Advisor*, 15 Feb. 2020, www.neurologyadvisor.com/topics/neuropathy/prediabetes-obesity-may-impact-risk-of-polyneuropathy/.

Stoll, Walt, and Jan DeCourtney.*Recapture Your Health*. Sunrise Health Coach, 2006.

Stone, Trevor W., et al. Obesity and Cancer: Existing and New Hypotheses for a Causal Connection. *EBioMedicine*, vol. 30, 2018, pp. 14–28., doi:10.1016/j.ebiom.2018.02.022.

Strassler, Douglas. Greater Cognitive Decline in Individuals at Risk for Bipolar Disorder With Obesity. *Psychiatry Advisor*, 17 Dec. 2018, www.psychiatryadvisor.com/home/topics/mood-disorders/bipolar-disorder/

greater-cognitive-decline-in-individuals-at-risk-for-bipolar-disorder-with-obesity/.

Strassnig, Martin, et al. Obesity Rates Higher in Schizophrenia, Bipolar Disorder. *Bipolar Disorders*, vol. 19, no. 5, 29 Aug. 2017, pp. 336–343., doi:10.1111/bdi.12505.

Sugary Drinks.The Nutrition Source, Harvard School of Public Health, 16 Oct. 2019, www.hsph.harvard.edu/nutritionsource/healthy-drinks/sugary-drinks/.

Sun, Beicheng, and Michael Karin.Obesity, Inflammation, and Liver Cancer.*Journal of Hepatology*, vol. 56, no. 3, 2012, pp. 704–713., doi:10.1016/j.jhep.2011.09.020.

Sun, Li, et al. Body Mass Index and Prognosis of Breast Cancer. *Medicine*, vol. 97, no. 26, 2018, doi:10.1097/md.0000000000011220.

Sundbøll, Jens, et al. Changes in Childhood Body Mass Index and Risk of Venous Thromboembolism in Adulthood.*Journal of the American Heart Association*, vol. 8, no. 6, 19 Mar. 2019, doi:10.1161/jaha.118.011407.

Swaab, Dick F. *Human Hypothalamus: Basic and Clinical Aspects, Part 2: Handbook of Clinical Neurology.* Elsevier, 2003.

Sweis, Ranya N. Acute Myocardial Infarction (MI). *Merck Manuals Professional Edition*, Merck Manuals, 2018, www.merckmanuals.com/professional/cardiovascular-disorders/coronary-artery-disease/acute-myocardial-infarction-mi.

Symon, B, et al. Does the Early Introduction of Solids Promote Obesity? *Singapore Medical Journal*, vol. 58, no. 11, Nov. 2017, pp. 626–631, 10.11622/smedj.2017024.

Symptoms and Diagnosis of PAD.*American Heart Association*, 31 Oct. 2016, www.heart.org/en/health-topics/peripheral-artery-disease/symptoms-and-diagnosis-of-pad.

Talking to Your Doctor.*National Institutes of Health*, 8 May 2015, www.nih.gov/institutes-nih/nih-office-director/office-communications-public-liaison/clear-communication/talking-your-doctor. Accessed 10 Dec. 2018.

Talking to Your Doctor.*National Institutes of Health*, U.S. Department of Health & Human Services, 8 May 2015, www.nih.gov/institutes-nih/

nih-office-director/office-communications-public-liaison/clear-communication/talking-your-doctor.

Tapsell, Linda C, et al. Foods, Nutrients, and Dietary Patterns: Interconnections and Implications for Dietary Guidelines. *Advances in Nutrition*, vol. 7, no. 3, 1 May 2016, pp. 445–454., doi:10.3945/an.115.011718.

Tawonsawatruk, T., et al. Adipose Derived Pericytes Rescue Fractures from a Failure of Healing—Non-union. *Scientific Reports*, vol. 6, 21 Mar. 2016.

Telles, Shirley, et al. Twelve Weeks of Yoga or Nutritional Advice for Centrally Obese Adult Females. *Frontiers in Endocrinology*, vol. 9, 17 Aug. 2018, 10.3389/fendo.2018.00466.

Thavendiranathan, Paaladinesh, et al. Primary Prevention of Cardiovascular Diseases With Statin Therapy. *Archives of Internal Medicine*, vol. 166, no. 21, 27 Nov. 2006, p. 2307, 10.1001/archinte.166.21.2307.

The Geisel School of Medicine at Dartmouth. Fast Food Intake Leads to Weight Gain in Preschoolers. ScienceDaily, 14 Feb. 2020, www.sciencedaily.com/releases/2020/02/200214134723.htm.

The Sweet Danger of Sugar.Harvard Health Publishing, Harvard Medical School, 6 Nov. 2015, www.health.harvard.edu/heart-health/the-sweet-danger-of-sugar.

The Use of Garcinia Extract (Hydroxycitric Acid) as a Weight Loss Supplement: A Systematic Review and Meta-Analysis of Randomised Clinical Trials. *Journal of Obesity*, vol. 2011, 2011, pp. 1–9, www.hindawi.com/journals/jobe/2011/509038/, 10.1155/2011/509038.

Thijssen, E., et al. Obesity and Osteoarthritis, More than Just Wear and Tear: Pivotal Roles for Inflamed Adipose Tissue and Dyslipidaemia in Obesity-Induced Osteoarthritis. *Rheumatology*, vol. 54, no. 4, 11 Dec. 2014, pp. 588–600., doi:10.1093/rheumatology/keu464.

Thompson, Amy E. Hypoglycemia. *Jama*, vol. 313, no. 12, 24 Mar. 2015, p. 1284., doi:10.1001/jama.2015.0876.

Three Ways Obesity Contributes to Heart Disease. *Penn Medicine*, 25 Mar. 2019, www.pennmedicine.org/updates/blogs/

metabolic-and-bariatric-surgery-blog/2019/march/obesity-and-heart-disease.

Tips for Parents–Ideas to Help Children Maintain a Healthy Weight. *Centers for Disease Control and Prevention*, 18 July 2018, www.cdc.gov/healthy-weight/children/index.html.

Todd, Alwyn, et al. Overweight and Obese Adolescent Girls: The Importance of Promoting Sensible Eating and Activity Behaviors from the Start of the Adolescent Period. *International Journal of Environmental Research and Public Health*, vol. 12, no. 2, 17 Feb. 2015, pp. 2306–2329, www.ncbi.nlm.nih.gov/pmc/articles/PMC4344727/, 10.3390/ijerph120202306.

Todd, Jennifer N., et al. Genetic Evidence for a Causal Role of Obesity in Diabetic Kidney Disease. *Diabetes*, vol. 64, no. 12, 25 Dec. 2015, pp. 4298–4246., doi:10.2337/db15-0254.

Torre, Sophie Bucher Della, et al. Sugar-Sweetened Beverages and Obesity Risk in Children and Adolescents: A Systematic Analysis on How Methodological Quality May Influence Conclusions. Journal of the Academy of Nutrition and Dietetics, vol. 116, no. 4, 2016, pp. 638–659., doi:10.1016/j.jand.2015.05.020.

Towner, Elizabeth K., et al. Treating Obesity in Preschoolers. *Pediatric Clinics of North America*, vol. 63, no. 3, June 2016, pp. 481–510, 10.1016/j.pcl.2016.02.005.

Traina, Andrea N., and Michael P. Kane. Primer on Pramlintide, an Amylin Analog. *The Diabetes Educator*, vol. 37, no. 3, 6 Apr. 2011, pp. 426–431, 10.1177/0145721711403011.

Tran, Bach Xuan, et al. Global Evolution of Obesity Research in Children and Youths: Setting Priorities for Interventions and Policies. *Obesity Facts*, vol. 12, no. 2, 2019, pp. 137–149, 10.1159/000497121.

Treatment for Tobacco Use. *DynaMed*, EBSCO Information Services, 17 Oct. 2018, www.dynamed.com/management/treatment-for-tobacco-use-19.

Tsai, Tsung-Cheng, et al. Body Mass Index–Mortality Relationship in Severe Hypoglycemic Patients With Type 2 Diabetes. *The American Journal of the Medical Sciences*, vol. 349, no. 3, 2015, pp. 192–198., doi:10.1097/maj.0000000000000382.

Tully, Agnes, et al. Interventions for the Management of Obesity in People with Bipolar Disorder. *Cochrane Database of Systematic Reviews*, 12 Apr. 2018, doi:10.1002/14651858.cd013006.

Turner, Robert W., et al. Reported Sports Participation, Race, Sex, Ethnicity, and Obesity in US Adolescents From NHANES Physical Activity (PAQ_D). *Global Pediatric Health*, vol. 2, 6 Apr. 2015, p. 2333794X1557794, www.ncbi.nlm.nih.gov/pmc/articles/PMC4784630/, 10.1177/2333794x15577944.

Type 2 Diabetes. *American Diabetes Association*, www.diabetes.org/diabetes/type-2?loc=DropDownDB-type2.

Types of Diabetes. *National Institute of Diabetes and Digestive and Kidney Diseases*, US Department of Health & Human Services, 11 Nov. 2019, www.niddk.nih.gov/health-information/diabetes/overview/what-is-diabetes#types.

Tzoulaki, I., et al. Risk of Cardiovascular Disease and All Cause Mortality among Patients with Type 2 Diabetes Prescribed Oral Antidiabetes Drugs: Retrospective Cohort Study Using UK General Practice Research Database. *BMJ*, vol. 339, no. dec03 1, 3 Dec. 2009, pp. b4731–b4731, 10.1136/bmj.b4731.

U.S. Department of Health and Human Services and U.S. Department of Agriculture. *2015 – 2020 Dietary Guidelines for Americans.* 8th ed. USDA and HHS, 2015. https://health.gov/our-work/food-and-nutrition/2015-2020-dietary-guidelines/.

U.S. Department of Health and Human Services. *Physical Activity Guidelines for Americans.* 2nd ed. US Department of Health and Human Services, 2018.

Ueland, Venke, et al. Living with Obesity — Existential Experiences. *International Journal of Qualitative Studies on Health and Well-Being*, vol. 14, no. 1, 1 Aug. 2019, p. 1651171., doi:10.1080/17482631.2019.1651171.

Understand Your Risk for PAD. *American Heart Association*, 31 Oct. 2016, www.heart.org/en/health-topics/peripheral-artery-disease/understand-your-risk-for-pad.

Understand Your Risks to Prevent a Heart Attack. *American Heart Association*, 30 June 2016, www.heart.org/en/health-topics/heart-attack/understand-your-risks-to-prevent-a-heart-attack.

University of Cambridge.Children Who Walk to School Less Likely to Be Overweight or Obese. *ScienceDaily*, 21 May 2019, www.sciencedaily.com/releases/2019/05/190521101344.htm.

University of South Australia.'Strongest Evidence Yet' That Being Obese Causes Depression.*ScienceDaily*, 12 Nov. 2018, www.sciencedaily.com/releases/2018/11/181112095951.htm.

University of Texas Health Science Center at Houston.Negative Body Image, Not Depression, Increases Adolescent Obesity Risk.*ScienceDaily*, 9 Nov. 2015, www.sciencedaily.com/releases/2015/11/151109083418.htm.

Uranga, RominaMaría, and Jeffrey Neil Keller. The Complex Interactions Between Obesity, Metabolism and the Brain. *Frontiers in Neuroscience*, vol. 13, 24 May 2019, doi:10.3389/fnins.2019.00513.

Vadeboncoeur, Claudia, et al. A Meta-Analysis of Weight Gain in First Year University Students: Is Freshman 15 a Myth? *BMC Obesity*, vol. 2, no. 1, 28 May 2015, doi:10.1186/s40608-015-0051-7.

Valk, Eline S. Van Der, et al. Stress and Obesity: Are There More Susceptible Individuals? *Current Obesity Reports*, vol. 7, no. 2, 16 Apr. 2018, pp. 193–203., doi:10.1007/s13679-018-0306-y.

Van Gaal, Luc, and EvelineDirinck.Pharmacological Approaches in the Treatment and Maintenance of Weight Loss.*Diabetes Care*, vol. 39, no. Supplement 2, 19 July 2016, pp. S260–S267, 10.2337/dcs15-3016.

Ventricular Assist Devices (VADs). *Texas Heart Institute*, www.texasheart.org/heart-health/heart-information-center/topics/ventricular-assist-devices/.

Ventriglio, Antonio, et al. Metabolic Issues in Patients Affected by Schizophrenia: Clinical Characteristics and Medical Management. *Frontiers in Neuroscience*, vol. 9, 3 Sept. 2015, doi:10.3389/fnins.2015.00297.

Vincent, Heather K. Advising the Obese Patient on Starting a Running Program. *Current Sports Medicine Reports*, vol. 14, no. 4, 2015, p. 278, 10.1249/jsr.0000000000000171.

Viola, Gaia Claudia Viviana, et al. Are Food Labels Effective as a Means of Health Prevention? *Journal of Public Health Research*, vol. 5, no. 3, 21 Dec. 2016, www.ncbi.nlm.nih.gov/pmc/articles/PMC5206777/, 10.4081/jphr.2016.768.

Volger, Sheri, et al. Early Childhood Obesity Prevention Efforts through a Life Course Health Development Perspective: A Scoping Review. *PLOS ONE*, vol. 13, no. 12, 28 Dec. 2018, p. e0209787, www.ncbi.nlm.nih.gov/pmc/articles/PMC6310279/, 10.1371/journal.pone.0209787.

Walking: Trim Your Waistline, Improve Your Health. Mayo Clinic.Mayo Foundation for Medical Education and Research. 18 Apr. 2013, http://www.mayoclinic.org/healthy-lifestyle/fitness/in-depth/walking/art-20046261

Wanders, Anne, et al. Trans Fat Intake and Its Dietary Sources in General Populations Worldwide: A Systematic Review.*Nutrients*, vol. 9, no. 8, 5 Aug. 2017, p. 840, doi:10.3390/nu9080840.

Wang, Liang, et al. Ethnic Differences in Risk Factors for Obesity among Adults in California, the United States. *Journal of Obesity*, vol. 2017, 2017, pp. 1–10., doi:10.1155/2017/2427483.

Wang, Shiming, and XianyiBao. Hyperlipidemia, Blood Lipid Level, and the Risk of Glaucoma: A Meta-Analysis. *Investigative Opthalmology& Visual Science*, vol. 60, no. 4, 21 Mar. 2019, p. 1028., doi:10.1167/iovs.18-25845.

Warning Signs of a Heart Attack. *American Heart Association*, 30 June 2016, www.heart.org/en/health-topics/heart-attack/warning-signs-of-a-heart-attack.

Watson, Stephanie. Weight Loss, Breathing Devices Still Best for Treating Obstructive Sleep Apnea. *Harvard Health Publishing*, Harvard Medical School, 18 Mar. 2019, www.health.harvard.edu/blog/weight-loss-breathing-devices-still-best-for-treating-obstructive-sleep-apnea-201310026713.

Wee, Yong, et al. Medical Management of Chronic Stable Angina. *Australian Prescriber*, vol. 38, no. 4, 1 Aug. 2015, pp. 131–136., doi:10.18773/austprescr.2015.042.

Weinberger, Natascha-Alexandra, et al. Body Dissatisfaction in Individuals with Obesity Compared to Normal-Weight Individuals: A Systematic Review and Meta-Analysis. *Obesity Facts*, vol. 9, no. 6, 2016, pp. 424–441., doi:10.1159/000454837.

Wen, Li Ming, et al. The Effect of Early Life Factors and Early Interventions on Childhood Overweight and Obesity 2016. *Journal of Obesity*, vol. 2017, 2017, pp. 1–3, 10.1155/2017/3642818.

Westcott, Wayne L., and Thomas R. Baechle. *Strength Training Past Fifty*. 2nd ed. Human Kinetics, 2015.

Westwater, Margaret L., et al. Sugar Addiction: the State of the Science. European Journal of Nutrition, vol. 55, no. S2, 2016, pp. 55–69., doi:10.1007/s00394-016-1229-6.

What Are Purines and How Are They Related to Food and Health? *World's Healthiest Foods*, The George Mateljan Foundation, www.whfoods. org/genpage.php?tname=george&dbid-51.

What Are the Signs and Symptoms of Sleep Apnea. *National Heart, Lung, and Blood Institute*, US Department of Health & Human Services, 10 Dec. 2018, www.nhlbi.nih.gov/health-topics/sleep-apnea.

What Is MyPlate. *Choose MyPlate*, US Department of Agriculture, 7 Jan. 2016, www.choosemyplate.gov/.

What Is Peripheral Artery Disease. *National Heart, Lung, and Blood Institute*, US Department of Health & Human Services, 23 Aug. 2018, www. nhlbi.nih.gov/health/health-topics/topics/pad.

What Is Peripheral Artery Disease? *National Heart, Lung, and Blood Institute*, US Department of Health & Human Services, 23 Jan. 2019, www. nhlbi.nih.gov/health-topics/peripheral-artery-disease.

Whiteman, Honor. Chronic Stress May Raise Obesity Risk. *Medical News Today*, 27 Feb. 2017, www.medicalnewstoday.com/articles/316074.

Whitlock, Kevin, et al. The Association between Obesity and Colorectal Cancer. *Gastroenterology Research and Practice*, 2012, pp. 1–6., doi:10.1155/2012/768247.

Who Is at Risk for Sleep Apnea. *National Heart, Lung, and Blood Institute*, US Department of Health & Human Services, 10 Dec. 2018, www. nhlbi.nih.gov/health-topics/sleep-apnea.

Why Stress Causes People to Overeat. *Harvard Health Blog*, Harvard Medical School, 18 July 2018, www.health.harvard.edu/staying-healthy/why-stress-causes-people-to-overeat.

Wiklund, Petri. The Role of Physical Activity and Exercise in Obesity and Weight Management: Time for Critical Appraisal. *Journal of Sport and Health Science*, vol. 5, no. 2, June 2016, pp. 151–154, www.sciencedirect.com/science/article/pii/S2095254616300060.

Wiklund, Petri. The Role of Physical Activity and Exercise in Obesity and Weight Management: Time for Critical Appraisal. *Journal of Sport and Health Science*, vol. 5, no. 2, June 2016, pp. 151–154, www.sciencedirect.com/science/article/pii/S2095254616300060, 10.1016/j.jshs.2016.04.001.

Winter, Yaroslav, et al. Obesity and Abdominal Fat Markers in Patients with a History of Stroke and Transient Ischemic Attacks. *Journal of Stroke and Cerebrovascular Diseases*, vol. 25, no. 5, 2016, pp. 1141–1147., doi:10.1016/j.jstrokecerebrovasdis.2015.12.026.

Wiss, David A., et al. Sugar Addiction: From Evolution to Revolution. Frontiers in Psychiatry, vol. 9, 2018, doi:10.3389/fpsyt.2018.00545.

Wittgrove, Alan. Dear Doctor, Why Doesn't Liposuction Cure Obesity? *Obesity Action Coalition*, 2014, www.obesityaction.org/community/article-library/dear-doctor-why-doesnt-liposuction-cure-obesity/.

Wolfe, Bruce M., et al. Treatment of Obesity. *Circulation Research*, vol. 118, no. 11, 27 May 2016, pp. 1844–1855, 10.1161/circresaha.116.307591.

Wolfram, Taylor. Body Image and Young Women. *EatRight*, Academy of Nutrition and Dietetics, 31 May 2019, www.eatright.org/health/diseases-and-conditions/eating-disorders/body-image-and-young-women.

Wolters Kluwer Health. No Increase in Complications with 'tummy Tuck' in Obese Patients. *ScienceDaily*, 22 Apr. 2019, www.sciencedaily.com/releases/2019/04/190422151038.htm.

Wooton, Angela Kaye, and Lynne M. Melchior. Obesity and Type 2 Diabetes in Our Youth: A Recipe for Cardiovascular Disease. *The Journal for Nurse Practitioners*, vol. 13, no. 3, 2017, pp. 222–227., doi:10.1016/j.nurpra.2016.08.035.

Wyne, Kathleen l.The Lesser-Known Consequences of Obesity.*EmPower*, 2014, pp. 7–9.

Xenaki, Niovi, et al. Impact of a Stress Management Program on Weight Loss, Mental Health and Lifestyle in Adults with Obesity: A Randomized Controlled Trial. *Journal of Molecular Biochemistry*, vol. 7, no. 2, 3 Oct. 2018, pp. 78–84.

Xenaki, Niovi, et al. Impact of a Stress Management Program on Weight Loss, Mental Health and Lifestyle in Adults with Obesity: a Randomized Controlled Trial. *Journal of Molecular Biochemistry*, vol. 7, no. 2, 3 Oct. 2018, pp. 78–84.

Xu, Furong, et al. A Community-Based Nutrition and Physical Activity Intervention for Children Who Are Overweight or Obese and Their Caregivers.*Journal of Obesity*, vol. 2017, 2017, pp. 1–9, www.ncbi.nlm.nih.gov/pmc/articles/PMC5651117/, 10.1155/2017/2746595.

Yale University. Biology of Leptin, the Hunger Hormone, Revealed. *ScienceDaily*, 18 June 2019, www.sciencedaily.com/releases/2019/06/190618113120.htm.

Yale University. School-Based Nutritional Programs Reduce Student Obesity. *ScienceDaily*, 17 Dec. 2018, www.sciencedaily.com/releases/2018/12/181217101814.htm.

Yang, Genyan, et al. The Effects of Obesity on Venous Thromboembolism: A Review. *Open Journal of Preventive Medicine*, vol. 02, no. 04, 2012, pp. 499–509., doi:10.4236/ojpm.2012.24069.

Yanovski, Susan Z., and Jack A. Yanovski.Long-Term Drug Treatment for Obesity.*JAMA*, vol. 311, no. 1, 1 Jan. 2014, p. 74, 10.1001/jama.2013.281361.

Yetley, Elizabeth A, et al. Options for Basing Dietary Reference Intakes (DRIs) on Chronic Disease Endpoints: Report from a Joint US-/Canadian-Sponsored Working Group. *The American Journal of Clinical Nutrition*, vol. 105, no. 1, 7 Dec. 2016, doi:10.3945/ajcn.116.139097.

Your Weight History May Predict Your Heart Failure Risk. *Johns Hopkins Medicine*, 12 Dec. 2018, www.hopkinsmedicine.org/news/newsroom/news-releases/your-weight-history-may-predict-your-heart-failure-risk.

Zalewska, Magdalena, and El bietaMaciorkowska. Selected Nutritional Habits of Teenagers Associated with Overweight and Obesity. *PeerJ*, vol. 5, 22 Sept. 2017, p. e3681, 10.7717/peerj.3681.

Zebrack, James S, et al. C-Reactive Protein and Angiographic Coronary Artery Disease: Independent and Additive Predictors of Risk in Subjects with Angina. *Journal of the American College of Cardiology*, vol. 39, no. 4, Feb. 2002, pp. 632–637, 10.1016/s0735-1097(01)01804-6.

Zhao, Sitong, et al. Association of Obesity with the Clinicopathological Features of Thyroid Cancer in a Large, Operative Population. *Medicine*, vol. 98, no. 50, 2019, doi:10.1097/md.0000000000018213.   145

Zhao, Zhuoxian, et al. The Potential Association between Obesity and Bipolar Disorder: A Meta-Analysis. *Journal of Affective Disorders*, vol. 202, 2016, pp. 120–123., doi:10.1016/j.jad.2016.05.059.

Zhou, Lin, et al. The Impact of Changes in Dietary Knowledge on Adult Overweight and Obesity in China.*PLOS ONE*, vol. 12, no. 6, 23 June 2017, p. e0179551, 10.1371/journal.pone.0179551.

■ Journals

Advances in Nutrition
Editor: Katherine Tucker
Publisher: American Society for nutrition
ISSN: 2161-8313 (print)
2156-5376 (web)
https://academic.oup.com/advances
advances@nutrition.org

American Journal of Cardiology
Editor: William C. Roberts
Publisher: Elsevier
ISSN: 0002-9149 (print)
1879-1913 (web)
https://www.ajconline.org/
Jill.Rutherford2@bswhealth.org

American Journal of Respiratory and Critical Care Medicine
Editor: Jadwiga A. Wedzicha
Publisher: American Thoracic Society
ISSN: 1073-449X (print)
1535-4970 (web)
https://www.atsjournals.org/journal/ajrccm

Arteriosclerosis, Thrombosis, and Vascular Biology
Editor: Alan Daugherty
Publisher: Lippencott
ISSN: 1079-5642 (print)
1524-4636 (web)
https://www.ahajournals.org/journal/atvb
atvb@atvb.org

Childhood Obesity
Editor: Tom Baranowski
Publisher: Mary Ann Liebert, Inc.
ISSN: 2153-2168 (print)
2153-2176 (web)
https://home.liebertpub.com/publications/childhood-obesity/384/overview

Circulation
Editor: Joseph A. Hill
Publisher: Lippincott Williams & Wilkins
ISSN: 0009-7322 (print)
1524-4539 (web)
https://www.ahajournals.org/journal/circ
circ@circulationjournal.org

Diabetes
Editor: Martin G. Myers, Jr.
Publisher: American Diabetes Association

ISSN: 0012-1797 (print)
1939-372X (web)
https://diabetes.diabetesjournals.org/

Diabetes, Obesity and Metabolism
Editor: R. Donnelly, A. Garber
Publisher: Wiley-Blackwell
ISSN: 1462-8902 (print)
1463-1326 (web)
https://dom-pubs.onlinelibrary.wiley.com/journal/14631326
Susan.Lane@nottingham.ac.uk

Heart
Editor: Catherine Otto
Publisher: BMJ Group
ISSN: 1355-6037 (print)
1468-201X (web)
https://heart.bmj.com/
info.heart@bmj.com

International Journal of Behavioral Nutrition and Physical Activity
Editor: Hidde van der Ploeg
Publisher: BioMed Central
ISSN: 1479-5868
https://ijbnpa.biomedcentral.com/
info@biomedcentral.com

International Journal of Obesity
Editor: R. L. Atkinson, I. Macdonald
Publisher: Nature Publishing Group
ISSN: 0307-0565 (print)
1476-5497 (web)
https://www.nature.com/ijo/

International Journal of Sport Nutrition and Exercise Metabolism
Editor: Ronald J. Maughan
Publisher: Human Kinetics Publishers
ISSN: 1526-484X (print)
1543-2742 (web)
https://journals.humankinetics.com/view/journals/ijsnem/ijsnem-overview.xml

Journal of Clinical Endocrinology and Metabolism
Editor: R. Paul Robertson
Publisher: The Endocrine Society
ISSN: 0021-972X (print)
1945-7197 (web)
https://academic.oup.com/jcem
publications@endocrine.org

Journal of Hypertension
Editor: Alberto Zanchetti
Publisher: Lippincott Williams & Wilkins
ISSN: 0263-6352 (print)
1473-5598 (web)
https://journals.lww.com/jhypertension/pages/default.aspx
info@jhypertens.com

Journal of Nutrition
Editor: Teresa A. Davis
Publisher: American Society for Nutrition
ISSN: 0022-3166 (print)
1541-6100 (web)
https://academic.oup.com/jn
jnutr@bcm.edu

Journal of the American College of Cardiology
Editor: Valentin Fuster
Publisher: Elsevier on behalf of the American College of Cardiology
ISSN: 0735-1097 (print)
1558-3597 (web)
http://www.onlinejacc.org/
jacc@acc.org

Journal of the American Heart Association
Editor: Barry London
Publisher: John Wiley & Sons on behalf of the American Heart Association
ISSN: 2047-9980
https://www.ahajournals.org/journal/jaha
jaha@journalaha.org

Nutrition and Cancer
Editor: Leonard A. Cohen
Publisher: Routledge
ISSN: 0163-5581 (print)
1532-7914 (web)
https://www.tandfonline.com/toc/hnuc20/current

Obesity
Editor: Eric Ravussin
Publisher: Wiley-Blackwell on behalf of The Obesity Society
ISSN: 1930-7381 (print)
1930-739X (web)
https://onlinelibrary.wiley.com/journal/1930739x
editorial@obesity.org

Obesity Reviews
Editor: David York
Publisher: Wiley-Blackwell
ISSN: 1467-7881 (print)
1467-789X (web)
https://onlinelibrary.wiley.com/journal/1467789x
obr@worldobesity.org

Obesity Surgery
Editor: Scott Shikora
Publisher: Springer Science+Business Media
ISSN: 0960-8923 (print)
1708-0428 (web)
https://www.springer.com/journal/11695
victoria.ferrara@springer.com

Surgery for Obesity and Related Diseases
Editor: Harvey Sugerman, Raul J. Rosenthal
Publisher: Elsevier
ISSN: 1550-7289 (print)
1878-7533 (web)
https://www.soard.org/
Obesity@Stellarmed.com

The American Journal of Clinical Nutrition
Editor: Dennis M. Bier
Publisher: American Society for Nutrition
ISSN: 0002-9165 (print)
1938-3207 (web)
https://academic.oup.com/ajcn
ajcnsubmit@nutrition.org

Glossary

abdominal aortic aneurysms (AAA): a dilation of the aorta in the abdominal cavity.

acid pump inhibitors: a group of drugs that block the stomach cells' mechanism for producing hydrochloric acid.

adenohypophysis: another name for the anterior lobe of the pituitary gland.

adipose tissue: tissue that stores fat; occurs in humans beneath the skin, usually in the abdomen or in the buttocks.

adrenal: an endocrine gland located above each kidney; the inner part of each gland secretes epinephrine (adrenaline) and the outer part secretes hormones that help regulate blood pressure, blood sugar levels, and metabolism.

adventitia: the outer most collagen layer of the aortic vessel.

agglutination: a clumping of blood cells caused by antibodies joining with antigens on the cell surfaces.

albuminuria: the appearance of abnormal levels of protein into the urine.

alcohol: an organic compound containing a hydroxyl (-OH) group attached to a carbon atom.

allergen: any substance that causes an overreaction of the immune system; also called an antigen.

allergic reaction: the presence of adverse symptoms that are part of the body's overreaction to an antigen.

amaurosis fugax: temporary blindness in one eye.

amenorrhea: the absence of menstruation.

amyloidosis: the deposition of immunoglobulin fibrils in various tissues, including the kidneys.

anabolic: a part of metabolism that consists of biochemical reactions that synthesize molecules.

anaphylaxis: a severe allergic reaction involving the circulatory and respiratory systems; often fatal without immediate treatment.

angina: pain in the chest caused by insufficient blood flow to the heart muscle.

angiography: radiological modality to visualize the arteries in the body; involves the placement of a catheter in an artery and the injection of dye.

antianxiety medication: a medication that acts in the brain to decrease negative reactions to stress and anxiety and to decrease avoidance behavior.

antibody: a protein made by B lymphocytes that is found in blood; a specific antibody binds with a specific antigen.

anticoagulant: a substance that hinders the clotting of blood.

antidepressant: a medication that acts in the brain to decrease a sad or depressed mood and other behaviors associated with depression.

antigen: a substance that is capable of causing an immune response if it is foreign to the body that it enters; antigens may be free or located on cell surfaces.

antisera: the fluid portion of blood that contains specific antibodies.

aorta: largest artery in the body carrying freshly oxygenated blood to the peripheral vascular system.

apnea: lack of airflow for more than ten seconds.

atherosclerosis: fat deposition and pathologic changes in the arterial surface and walls of major blood vessels of the body.

atria: the chambers in the right and left top portions of the heart that receive blood from the veins and pump it to the ventricles.

autonomic nervous system: a branch of the nervous system that controls bodily functions that are not consciously directed.

B lymphocyte: a blood and lymphatic cell that plays a role in the secretion of antibodies.

basal metabolic rate (BMR): the standardized measure of metabolism in warm-blooded organisms.

beta cells: the insulin-producing cells located at the core of the islets of Langerhans in the pancreas; the alpha, or glucagon-producing, cells form an outer coat.

beta-agonists: chemicals that attach to the beta-receptors on cells; often used in inhalers, they cause the bronchioles to dilate, or open.

biphasic reaction: delayed allergic reaction to an allergen, between one to four hours after the initial reaction.

bipolar disorders: mood disorders characterized by symptoms of mania and symptoms of depression.

blood type: a blood classification group based on the presence or absence of certain antigens on red blood cells.

Bouchard's nodes: osteophytes or bony spurs that develop as a result of destruction of joint cartilage in proximal interphalangeal joints.

bronchioles: small air tubes leading to the air sacs of the lungs; the functional units of the airway that are involved in asthma.

calcification: the deposit of lime salts in organic tissue, leading to the buildup of calcium in the arterial wall.

calorie: a measurement of heat, particularly in measuring the value of foods for producing energy and heat in an organism.

carboxylic acid: an organic compound that contains the carboxyl ($-CO_2H$) group.

cardiac arrhythmia: a disturbance in the heartbeat.

cardiomyopathy: disease of the heart muscle.

cardiovascular: of, relating to, or involving the heart and blood vessels.

cartilage: a smooth material covering the ends of bone joints that cushions the bone, allowing the joint to move easily.

catabolism: the complete breaking down of molecules by an organism for the purpose of obtaining chemical building blocks.

cerebrovascular: of, or involving, the brain and the blood vessels supplying it.

cholesterol: a lipid substance that is a component of cell membranes and the surface of circulating lipoproteins.

cholesteryl ester: cholesterol linked to a fatty acid; it is stored in lipid droplets in the cytoplasm of cells and circulates in the core of lipoproteins.

cirrhosis: chronic degenerative liver disease in which normal cells are replaced by fibrous tissue and normal liver function is disrupted.

cognitive behavior psychotherapy: talk therapy consisting of cognitive interaction between a patient and a mental health professional.

colitis: inflammation of the large intestine (colon), which usually is associated with bloody diarrhea and fever.

collagen: a fibrous protein substance in connective tissue, bone, tendons, and cartilage.

computed tomography (CT): a scan that uses x-rays to visualize cross-sections of the body.

congestive heart failure: the stage of heart failure that occurs when a backup of pressure results in accumulation of fluid in the veins and tissues.

coronary arteries: blood vessels surrounding the heart that provide nourishment and oxygen to heart tissue.

crepitus: the scraping or grinding sound heard or felt when bone rubs over bone in joint spaces.

cretinism: a severe hypothyroidism in which infants are born with insufficiently developed thyroid tissue.

cross-linking: a chemical reaction, triggered by the binding of glucose to tissue proteins, that results in the attachment of one protein to another and the loss of elasticity in aging tissues.

cyclothymia: a mood disorder characterized by fewer and less intense symptoms of elevated mood and depressed mood than bipolar disorders.

degenerative: marked by progression to a state below what is considered normal or desirable.

diabetes mellitus type 2: peripheral resistance to insulin and increases in serum glucose and insulin concentrations, with damage to arteries in various organs.

diabetes mellitus: an endocrine disease that results from the production of insufficient quantities of the hormone insulin or an inability to properly response to physiological levels of insulin.

dialysis: the use of artificial membranes to remove metabolites from the blood when the kidneys fail; the peritoneum can also be used (peritoneal dialysis).

diarrhea: loose or watery stools, usually a decrease in consistency or increase in frequency from an individual baseline.

diastolic blood pressure: the pressure of the blood within the artery while the heart is at rest.

distal interphalangeal joints: the distal joints of the fingers.

distal: away from the point of origin.

diuretic: a drug that stimulates the kidneys to eliminate more salt and water from the body.

docospantaenoic acid (DHA): an omega-3 fatty acid with 22 carbons and six carbon-carbon double bonds.

dyslipidemia: abnormal blood lipid levels, especially characterized by high serum triglycerides and very lowdensity lipoproteins (VLDLs) and depressed serum high-density lipoprotein (HDL) cholesterol.

dysmorphic: abnormal in shape or appearance.

dysthymia: a mood disorder characterized by symptoms similar to depression that are fewer in number but last for a much longer period of time.

edema: the accumulation of fluid around the cells in tissue.

eicosapentaenoic acid(EPA): an omega-3 fatty acid with 20 carbons and five carbon-carbon double bonds.

ejection fraction: the ratio of the stroke volume to the residual volume, expressed as a percentage.

electroconvulsive therapy (ECT): the use of electric shocks to induce seizure in depressed patients as a form of treatment.

embolus: a small piece of atherosclerotic plaque, thrombus, or other debris that breaks off and lodges in a blood vessel.

endarterectomy: a surgical technique in which an atherosclerotic plaque is excised.

endocrine system: a series of ductless glands that deliver hormones to target cells directly through the bloodstream.

enzyme: a complex protein produced by living cells that catalyzes certain biochemical reactions at body temperature.

epinephrine: a hormone that acts as a vasoconstrictor and cardiac stimulant.

Epi-Pen: a device that administers a prescribed dose of injectable epinephrine.

essential fatty acid: a fatty acid that cannot be synthesized by humans.

essential nutrients: molecules that an organism needs for survival but cannot manufacture itself.

ester: the relatively non-water-soluble compound formed when an alcohol reacts with a carboxylic acid.

exocrine gland: a gland that releases its secretions via ducts to external surfaces.

extracellular fluid: the internal environment of the human body that surrounds the cells; the fluid contains ions, gases, and the nutrients needed by cells for proper functioning and is constantly circulated throughout the body by the blood and into tissues by diffusion.

false aneurysms: a weakening and dilation of an arterial vessel caused by trauma.

fast: to abstain from food.

fasting hypoglycemia: hypoglycemia that occurs when no food is available from the intestinal tract; usually caused by failure of the neural, hormonal, and/or enzymatic mechanisms that convert stored fuels (primarily glycogen) into glucose.

fatty acid: an organic compound that is composed of a long hydrocarbon chain with a carboxyl group at one end.

fibrillation: wild beating of the heart, which may occur when the regular rate of the heartbeat is interrupted.

fibrin: a fibrous insoluble protein formed from fibrinogen by the action of thrombin, especially in the clotting of blood.

fibrinogen: a protein produced in the liver that is present in blood plasma and is converted to fibrin during the clotting of blood.

filtration rate: the amount of fluid passing per minute from blood across the glomerular capillaries to form glomerular fluid.

food allergy action plan: a care plan outlining lifesaving strategies when experiencing a food allergy reaction.

fusiform aneurysm: dilation of the circumference of the arterial vessel.

glomeruli: structures consisting mainly of capillary blood vessels contained in a capsule, across whose walls water and solutes pass (filter) to form glomerular fluid.

glomerulonephritis: inflammation of glomeruli.

glucagon: a pancreatic hormone that signals an elevated concentration of glucose in the circulation.

gluconeogenesis: the synthesis of molecules of glucose from smaller carbohydrates and amino acids.

glucose: a simple sugar, readily converted to metabolic energy by most cells of the body and essential for the welfare of brain cells.

glucosuria: a condition in which the concentration of blood glucose exceeds the ability of the kidney to reabsorb it; as a result, glucose spills into the urine, taking with it body water and electrolytes.

glycerol: a three-carbon alcohol that has one hydroxyl compound on each carbon atom.

glycogen: a storage form of carbohydrate, composed of many molecules of glucose linked together; is found in many tissues of the body and serves as a major source of circulating glucose.

glycogenolysis: the cleavage of glycogen into its constituent molecules of glucose.

glycosuria: the presence of glucose in the urine.

gonads: ovaries in girls and testes in boys.

gout: a disease in which uric acid, a waste product that normally passes out of the body in urine, collects in the joints and the kidneys.

Graves' disease: a common type of hyperthyroidism in which the thyroid gland produces an oversupply of hormone.

great arteries and veins: large vessels channeling blood into and out of the heart, including the aorta (to the body), the pulmonary artery (to the lungs), the vena cava (from the body), and the pulmonary veins (from the lungs).

heart failure: a condition in which the heart cannot pump enough blood to meet the body's needs.

hematuria: the presence of red blood cells or red blood cell casts in the urine.

hemorrhagic: weakened blood vessel ruptures, as a result of aneurysm or arteriovenous malformation.

Herberden's nodes: osteophytes or bony spurs that develop as a result of destruction of joint cartilage in distal interphalangeal joints.

histamine II blockers: the general term used to describe various drugs that block the hormonal stimulation of histamine, one inducer of stomach acid.

Hodgkin's disease: a malignant disorder of lymphoid tissue, generally first appearing in cervical lymph nodes, which is characterized by the presence of the Reed-Sternberg cell.

homeostasis: the maintenance of a constant internal environment; the systems of the body work together to maintain a constant temperature, pH, oxygen availability, water content, ion concentrations, and so on.

homeostasis: the process by which a constant internal environment is maintained.

hormones: chemicals produced by glands such as the thyroid, pituitary, or adrenals that stimulate bodily changes or growth and that regulate body functions.

hydrocarbon: an organic compound composed of only hydrogen and carbon atoms that does not dissolve in water (water-insoluble).

hydrophilic: "water-loving" or "water-attracting"; a term given to molecules or regions of molecules that interact favorably with water.

hydrophobic: "water-hating" or "water-repelling"; a term given to molecules or regions of molecules that do not interact favorably with water.

hyperglycemia: excessive levels of glucose in the circulating blood.

hyperinsulinemia: an abnormally high serum insulin concentration.

hypertension: abnormally high blood pressure, especially high arterial blood pressure; also the systemic condition accompanying high blood pressure.

hypertrophic left ventricle: enlargement of the muscle tissue of the heart's main pumping chamber.

hypoglycemic unawareness: the occurrence of hypoglycemia without the warning symptoms of trembling, palpitations, hunger, or anxiety.

hypoglycemic unresponsiveness: inadequate recovery of the circulating glucose concentration after an episode of hypoglycemia.

hypopnea: a decrease in airflow greater than 50 percent.

hypothalamic hamartomas: tumors in the hypothalamic region of the brain, which are usually benign.

hypothalamus: the region of the brain that stimulates glands to secrete hormones.

hypothyroidism: a condition in which the thyroid gland produces an insufficient supply of hormone.

idiopathic: having an unidentified cause.

immunoglobulin antibody: a protein activated during allergic reactions by the immune system.

incubation period: the time between first exposure to an organism and onset of symptoms.

infarct: tissue death resulting from lack of blood flow.

inflammatory: irritation that causes swelling, heat, and discomfort.

inotropic agent: a drug that improves the ability of the heart muscle to contract.

insulin resistance: a lack of insulin action; a reduction in the effectiveness of insulin to lower blood glucose concentrations; characteristic of type 2 diabetes.

insulin: a pancreatic hormone that signals a reduced concentration of glucose in the circulation.

insulin-dependent diabetes mellitus (IDDM): type 1 diabetes, a state of absolute insulin deficiency in which the body does not produce sufficient insulin to move glucose into the cells.

insulitis: the selective destruction of the insulin-producing beta cells in type 1 diabetes.

intima: the innermost layer of endothelial cells in the aortic vessel.

ischemia: lack of blood in a particular tissue.

Islets of Langerhans: small islands of endocrine tissue scattered throughout the pancreas.

joints: the junctions at the ends of bones that allow for movement.

ketoacidosis: high levels of ketones in the blood that result from a lack of circulating insulin.

laxative: an agent that promotes evacuation of the bowel.

leukotriene: fatty acid-derived compounds that mediate inflammation and cause constriction of the bronchioles.

lipids: substances that are poorly soluble in water; in animal tissues, the principal lipids are triglycerides (fat), phospholipids, cholesterol, and cholesteryl esters.

lipoproteins: lipid aggregates that transport fat and cholesteryl esters in the circulation; associated apolipoproteins determine how rapidly they are taken up by the liver or other tissues.

lymphoma staging: a classification of lymphomas based upon the stage of the disease; used in the determination of treatment.

major depressive disorder: a pattern of major depressive episodes that form an identified psychiatric disorder.

manic episode: a syndrome of symptoms characterized by elevated, expansive, or irritable mood; required for the diagnosis of some mood disorders.

mast cells: cells in connective tissue capable of releasing chemicals that cause allergic reactions.

media: the middle layer of the aortic vessel made up of thick elastic tissue.

murmur: a sound made by the heart other than the normal two-step beat; murmurs are caused by the turbulent movement of blood and may indicate a heart defect.

myocardium: the muscle tissue that forms the walls of the heart, varying in thickness in the upper and lower regions.

negative feedback: a common physiological process by which the product of a process feeds back to inhibit further stimulation (or reverse) the process.

negative feedback: a homeostatic control system designed to respond to a stress by returning body conditions to normal physiologic levels.

nephrotic syndrome: a condition involving edema, the retention of water and of sodium and chloride ions, urinary protein losses greater than 3 grams per day, and hypoalbuminemia.

nervous system: the system in the body, including the brain, that receives and interprets stimuli and transmits impulses to other organs; the brain is the center of thinking and behavior.

neuroglycopenia: abnormal function of the brain, caused by an inadequate supply of glucose from the circulation.

neurohypophysis: another name for the posterior lobe of the pituitary gland.

neuropathy: nerve dysfunction resulting in numbness or weakness.

neurotransmitter: a chemical in the brain that sends a signal from one brain cell to another.

nodes: areas of electrochemical transmission within the heart that regulate the heartbeat.

non-Hodgkin's lymphoma: any malignant lympho-pro-liferative disorder other than Hodgkin's disease.

non-insulin-dependent diabetes mellitus (NIDDM): type 2 diabetes, which is the state of a relative insulin deficiency; although insulin is released, its target cells do not adequately respond to it by taking up blood glucose.

nonsteroidal anti-inflammatory drugs (NSAIDs): compounds that inhibit the synthesis of prostaglandins and thromboxanes.

nonulcerous dyspepsia: a condition that exhibits many of the symptoms of peptic ulcers but does not involve actual lesions in the linings of the stomach or intestines.

obese: having a body mass index (BMI), calculated as weight in kilograms divided by height in meters squared, that is greater than 30.

omega-3(ω-3 or n-3) fatty acid: an unsaturated fatty acidwith a carbon-carbon double bond, three carbons from the methyl end of the hydrocarbonchain.

optimal length: the length of a heart muscle cell at which stimulation can elicit the maximum possible force development.

osteopenia: reduced bone mass.

osteoporosis: demineralization of the bone.

overweight: having a BMI that is between 25 and 29.9.

oxygenation: the process of getting oxygen into the bloodstream.

pancreas: a gland located in the abdomen that secretes cocktails for enzymes for digestion and hormones that control blood sugar levels.

parathyroid: one of four small endocrine glands physically close to the thyroid that control the calcium balance of the body.

pepsin: the first component of gastric juice to be discovered, in the 1830s; the term "peptic ulcer" derives from the name of this digestive fluid.

peripheral vascular: of, relating to, involving, or forming the vasculature in the periphery (the external boundary or surface of a body); usually referring to circulation not involving cardiovascular, cerebrovascular, or major organ systems.

peripheralnerves: Nerves outside the brain and spinal cord.

pH: a measure of the acidity or alkalinity of a solution; equal to the negative logarithm of the hydrogen ion concentration (as measured in moles per liter).

pharmacotherapy: the treatment of disease with medication.

pituitary: the endocrine gland responsible for the functioning of the thyroid, along with many other central control activities.

plaque: a compound made up of fat, cholesterol, calcium, and other substances found in the blood. It can stick to the walls of arteries, partially or totally blocking blood flow.

platelet: a minute disk of vertebrate blood that assists in blood clotting.

prostacyclin: a fatty acid-derived compound that inhibit platelet aggregation and blood clotting and act as vasodilators.

prostaglandin: a fatty acid-derived compound that inhibit platelet aggregation and blood clotting, act as vasodilators, mediate inflammation and increase the perception of pain.

proteinuria: the presence of proteins, including globulins, in the urine; usually considered a sign of changes in the glomerular structures.

proximal interphalangeal joints: the proximal joints in the fingers.

proximal: toward the point of origin.

psychopharmacology: the drug treatment of psychiatric disorders.

psychosurgery: the surgical removal or destruction of part of the brain of depressed patients as a form of treatment.

psychotherapy: the "talk" therapies that target the emotional, social, and other contributors to and consequences of depression.

puberty: secondary sexual development that involves the maturation of the reproductive system and is typified by significant physical growth.

RAST: the most accurate blood test available to diagnose allergies.

reactive hypoglycemia: hypoglycemia that occurs within a few hours after ingestion of a meal.

Reed-Sternberg cell: a large atypical macrophage with multiple nuclei; found in patients with Hodgkin's disease.

renal blood flow: the amount of whole blood entering the renal arteries per minute; a fraction of water and solutes is removed to form urine.

renal failure: severe kidney insufficiency requiring the use of dialysis or transplantation to return and maintain composition of body fluids at or near normal values.

renal insufficiency: the inability of the kidneys to maintain a normal internal environment of the body and its fluids.

residual volume: the blood volume left in the heart chamber at the end of a heartbeat.

revascularization: procedures to reestablish the circulation to a diseased portion of the body.

saccular aneurysm: arterial wall dilation confined to one area causing a ballooning effect.

saponification: a reaction in which a strong basic solution splits a molecule into a carboxylic acid unit and an alcohol unit.

satiety: the state of feeling full or fed and free from hunger.

saturated fatty acid: a fatty acid with no carbon-carbon double bonds.

scientific method: a method of scientific investigation of a problem through observation, the formation of a hypothesis (a possible explanation to a problem), experimentation, and the reevaluation of data.

seasonal affective disorder (SAD):a mood disorder associated with the winter season, when the amount of daylight hours is reduced.

selective serotonin reuptake inhibitor (SSRI): a class of antidepressant medications effective in the treatment of anxiety disorders.

septum: a membrane that serves as a wall of separation; in the heart, the interatrial septum divides the two atria and the interventricular septum divides the two ventricles.

serotonin: the neurotransmitter associated with pain perception, sleep, impulsivity, and aggression; implicated in disorders associated with anxiety, depression, and migraines.

serum: the fluid part of blood without red blood cells and clotting factors.

side effect: a secondary and usually adverse effect (as of a drug); also known as an adverse effect or reaction.

sinoatrial node: the section of the right atrium that determines the appropriate rate of the heartbeat.

somatoform disorder: a mental disorder whose symptoms focus on the physical body.

sphygmomanometer: a device that uses a column of mercury to measure blood pressure force; pressure is measured in millimeters of mercury

standard metabolic rate (SMR): the standardized measure of metabolism in cold-blooded organisms.

steatohepatitis: an increased fat content in the liver independent of alcohol consumption.

sterols: a class of chemically related lipids; cholesterol is the principal sterol in vertebrates, but in plants its functions are served by related substances.

storage compounds: areas in the body that store nutrients not immediately required by an organism.

streptococci: bacteria responsible for the development of some cases of acute glomerulonephritis, but without infection of the kidneys.

stroke volume: the blood volume leaving either the right or the left side of the heart with each beat; each side usually ejects the same volume per beat.

sugar: crystalline carbohydrate obtained from plants used to sweeten food and drink.

sugarcane: stout tropical grass from which sugar is extracted.

syncope: fainting, passing out, temporary loss of consciousness.

synovial fluid: fluid contained in the synovium of joint margins that reduces friction during movement of the joints.

synovium: fluid-filled sacs in joint margins.

systolic blood pressure: the pressure of the blood within the artery while the heart is contracting.

T lymphocyte: a blood and lymphatic cell that functions in cell-mediated immunity, which involves the direct attack of diseased tissues; subclasses of T cells aid B lymphocytes in the production of antibodies.

thoracic aortic aneurysms (TAA): a dilation of the aorta in the thoracic cavity.

thrombin: an enzyme that facilitates the clotting of blood by catalyzing a conversion of fibrinogen to fibrin.

thrombosis: the aggregation of platelets and other blood cells to form a clot.

thromboxane: a fatty acid-derived compound that are vasodilators and promote platelet aggregation and blood clotting.

thyroiditis: Inflammation of the thyroid gland.

thyroxine: the chief hormone of the thyroid gland, an iodine-containing derivative of the amino acid tyrosine.

trans fatty acid: a fatty acid with at least one carbon-carbon double bond where the hydrogens attached to the carbons that participate in the double bond are on opposite sides of the double bond.

transfusion: the injection of whole blood or its parts into the bloodstream.

transient ischemic attacks(TIAs): commonly known as mini strokes; associated neurological deficits last less than twenty-four hours and usually only minutes.

transmission: the mode of acquiring a disease.

trigger: the substance or event that sets off an asthma attack; triggers may be allergens or some other type of stimulus.

true aneurysms: dilation of an arterial vessel caused by a congenital or acquired problem.

tubules: hollow structures conducting glomerular fluid to the collecting ducts and the renal pelvis; they produce composition and volume changes of glomerular fluid passing through them and may reabsorb some of the protein that crosses the glomerular capillaries.

ultrasound: a method of diagnostic imaging using high-frequency sound.

unsaturated fatty acid: a fatty acid with at least one carbon-carbon double bond.

vasodilator: a drug that relaxes blood vessels.

ventricles: heart chambers that pump blood out of the heart, the left to the body and the right to the lungs.

ventricles: the chambers in the right and left bottom portions of the heart that receive blood from the atria and pump it to the arteries.

watersoluble: a compound that dissolves in water. Water-soluble vitamins are not stored in the body the way fat-soluble vitamins are, so the body needs a regular supply of water-soluble vitamins.

Zollinger-Ellison syndrome: a rare condition in which secretions of acid are so sudden and excessive that normal gastric defenses cannot prevent the immediate ulceration of stomach membranes.

α-*linolenic* acid (ALA): an essential fatty acid from which EPA and DHA are synthesized.

γ-*linolenic acid (GLA)*: an essential fatty acid from which other fatty acids are synthesized.

Organizations

Academy of Nutrition and Dietetics
120 South Riverside Plaza
Suite 2190
Chicago, Illinois 60606-6995
1-800-877-1600
https://www.eatright.org/

Alliance for a Healthier Generation
2525 SW 1st Ave
Suite 120
Portland, OR 97201
1-888-543-4584
https://www.healthiergeneration.org/

America Walks
PO Box 70742
Bethesda, MD 20813
1-503-610-6619
https://americawalks.org/

American Academy of Family Physicians:
11400 Tomahawk Creek Parkway
Leawood, KS 66211-2680
1-800-274-2237
https://familydoctor.org/

American Academy of Otolaryngology—Head and Neck Surgery
1650 Diagonal Road
Alexandria, VA 22314
703-836-4444
http://www.entnet.org

American Association of Bariatric Counselors
110 Chestnut Ridge Road, Suite 137,
Montvale, NJ 07645
1-866-284-3682
https://www.aabc-certification.org/

American Board of Obesity Medicine
2696 S. Colorado Blvd.
Suite #340
Denver, CO 80222
1-303-770-9100
https://www.abom.org/

American Cancer Society
250 Williams Street NW
Atlanta, GA 30303
1-800-227-2345
https://www.cancer.org/

American Diabetes Association
2451 Crystal Drive
Suite 900
Alexandria, VA 22202
1-800-342-2383
http://www.diabetes.org

American Heart Association
7272 Greenville Avenue
Dallas, TX 75231
1-800-AHA-USA-1
http://www.heart.org

American Nutrition Association
211 West Chicago Avenue
Suite 217
Hinsdale, IL 60521
https://theana.org/

American Obesity Treatment Association
117 Anderson Court
Suite 1
Dothan, AL 36303
1-334-403-4057
https://www.americanobesity.org/

American Sleep Apnea Association
641 S Street NW
3rd Floor
Washington, DC 20001-5196
1-888-293-3650
https://www.sleepapnea.org

American Society for Metabolic and Bariatric Surgery
14407 SW 2nd Place
Suite F-3
Newberry, FL, 32669
1-352-331-4900
https://asmbs.org/

American Society for Nutrition
9211 Corporate Blvd., Suite 300
Rockville, Maryland, 20850, USA
1-240-428-3650
https://nutrition.org/

Arthritis Foundation
1355 Peachtree Street NE, Suite 600
Atlanta, GA 30309
800-283-7800
https://www.arthritis.org

Center for Health & Health Care in Schools
2175 K Street NW
Suite 200
Washington, DC 20037
1-202-994-4895
http://healthinschools.org/#sthash.zXT9Vmok.dpbs

Centers for Disease Control
1600 Clifton Rd.
Atlanta, GA 30333
1-800-CDC-INFO
http://www.cdc.gov

ChooseMyPlate
1320 Braddock Place
Alexandria, VA 22314
https://www.choosemyplate.gov/

Food Addicts in Recovery Anonymous
400 W. Cummings Park
Suite 1700
Woburn, MA 01801
1-781-932-6300
https://www.foodaddicts.org/

Food Policy Action
1436 U Street NW
Suite 200
Washington, DC 20009
https://foodpolicyaction.org/

Foot Health Facts—American College of Foot and Ankle Surgeons
8725 West Higgins Road, Suite 555
Chicago, IL 60631
800-421-2237
https://www.foothealthfacts.org

The Heart Foundation
31822 Village Center Road
Suite 208
Westlake Village, CA 91361
1-818-865-1100
https://theheartfoundation.org/

Heart and Stroke Foundation of Canada
110-1525 Carling Avenue
Ottawa, ON K1Z 8R9
1-888-473-4636
http://www.heartandstroke.ca

Joslin Diabetes Center
One Joslin Place
Boston, MA 02215
1-617-309-2400
http://www.joslin.harvard.edu

LEAD for Rare Obesity
222 Berkeley Street
Suite 1200
Boston, MA 02116
1-833-818-3222
https://www.leadforrareobesity.com/

National Association to Advance Fat Acceptance
P.O. Box 61586
Las Vegas, NV 89160
1-916-558-6880
https://www.naafaonline.com/dev2

National Coalition for Promoting Physical Activity
1150 Connecticut Ave, NW
Suite 300
Washington, DC 20036
http://www.ncppa.org/

National Collaborative on Childhood Obesity Research
https://www.nccor.org/

National Heart, Lung, and Blood Institute
Building 31
31 Center Drive
Bethesda, MD 20892
301-592-8573
https://www.nhlbi.nih.gov

National Institute of Diabetes and Digestive and Kidney Diseases
9000 Rockville Pike
Bethesda, MD 20892
301-496-3583
https://www.niddk.nih.gov

National Institute on Aging
Building 31, Room 5C27
31 Center Drive, MSC 2292
Bethesda, MD 20892
1-800-222-2225
https://www.nia.nih.gov/

National Sleep Foundation
https://sleepfoundation.org

Nutrition Obesity Research Centers
https://norccentral.org/

The Obesity Action Coalition
4511 North Himes Avenue
Suite 250
Tampa, FL 33614
1-800-717-3117
https://www.obesityaction.org/

Obesity Canada
2-126 Li Ka Shing Centre for Health Research Innovation
University of Alberta Edmonton, AB T6G2E1
1-780-492-8361
https://obesitycanada.ca/

Obesity Care Advocacy Network
https://obesitycareadvocacynetwork.com/

Obesity Medicine Association
101 University Blvd., Ste 330
Denver, CO 80206
1-303-770-2526
https://obesitymedicine.org/

The Obesity Society
1110 Bonifant Street, Suite 500
Silver Spring, MD 20910
1-301-563-6526
https://www.obesity.org/

Overeaters Anonymous
6075 Zenith Court NE
PO Box 44727
Rio Rancho, NM 87174-4727
1-505-891-2664
https://oa.org/

Partnership for a Healthier America
1203 19th Street NW
3rd Floor
Washington, DC 20036
1-202-842-9001
https://www.ahealthieramerica.org/

President's Council on Sports, Fitness & Nutrition
1101 Wootton Parkway
Suite 420
Rockville, MD 20852
1-240-276-9567
https://www.hhs.gov/fitness/index.html

Rudd Center for Food Policy & Obesity
University of Connecticut
One Constitution Plaza
Suite 600
Hartford, CT 06103
http://uconnruddcenter.org/

School Nutrition Association
2900 S. Quincy Street
Suite 700
Arlington, VA 22206
1-703-824-3000
https://schoolnutrition.org/

Society of Interventional Radiology
3975 Fair Ridge Drive
Suite 400 North
Fairfax, VA 22033
703-691-1805
https://www.sirweb.org

**Strategies to Overcome and Prevent (STOP)
Obesity Alliance**
950 New Hampshire Avenue, NW
3rd Floor
Washington, DC 20052
1-202-994-4308
https://stop.publichealth.gwu.edu/

US Department of Agriculture
1400 Independence Ave., S.W.
Washington, DC 20250
1-202-720-2791
https://www.usda.gov/

Vascular Cures
274 Redwood Shores Parkway
Suite 717
Redwood City, CA 94065
650-368-6022
http://vascularcures.org

World Obesity Federation
Unit 406, 107-111 Fleet Street
London, EC4A 2AB
United Kingdom
+44 20 7936 9987
https://www.worldobesity.org/

INDEXES

Category Index

Subject Index

U

unsaturated fat, 6, 8-9, 11, 19-21, 26, 33-35, 52, 59, 62, 67, 85

uterine cancer, 91

uvulopalatopharyngoplasty, 136, 265

V

valine, 37

vasodilator, 104, 108-110, 114-115, 224

vertical banded gastroplasty, 151-152

very low calorie diet (VLCD), 171

very-low-density lipoprotein (VLDL), 28

Veterans Health Administration (VHA), 178

vitamin A, 93, 145, 194

vitamin C, 35, 59, 96, 156, 205

vitamin D, 6, 33, 67, 128, 135, 138, 156, 185, 187, 190, 192, 196, 198-200

vitamin E, 95, 156

vitamin K, 6, 19

volume of oxygen, 158, 163

W

warfarin, 56, 68, 225, 246, 256